PERIOPERATIVE AND SUPPORTIVE CARE IN GYNECOLOGIC ONCOLOGY

PERIOPERATIVE AND SUPPORTIVE CARE IN GYNECOLOGIC ONCOLOGY:
Evidence-Based Management

Edited by

STEVEN A. VASILEV, M.D., M.B.A.
Clinical Professor
Division of Gynecologic Oncology
University of Southern California School of Medicine

Director of Gynecologic Oncology
Los Angeles Tertiary Referral Center
Southern California Permanente Medical Group

President and Medical Director
Global Health Systems, Inc.
EBM Practice Collaborative

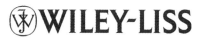

WILEY-LISS

A JOHN WILEY & SONS, INC., PUBLICATION
New York • Chichester • Weinheim • Brisbane • Singapore • Toronto

Library of Congress Cataloging-in-Publication Data:
Evidence-based perioperative and critical care gynecology : guidelines
 for clinical decision-making / edited by Steven A. Vasilev,
     p. cm.
  Includes bibliographical references and index.
  ISBN 0-471-24788-X (alk. paper)
  1. Generative organs, Female—Surgery. 2. Evidence-based
medicine. 3. Clinical medicine—Decision making. I. Vasilev,
Steven A.
  [DNLM: 1. Genital Neoplasms, Female—surgery. 2. CriticalCare—
methods. 3. Evidence-Based Medicine. 4. Gynecology—methods.
5. Perioperative Care—methods. WP 145 E93 1999]
  RG104.E94   1999
  618.1′45—dc21
  DNLM/DLC
  for Library of Congress   99-28929

Printed in the United States of America.

10 9 8 7 6 5 4 3 2 1

This work is dedicated to the living bookends of my life—enablers of projects such as this. For my mother, Katharina, a lifelong source of support and encouragement; and my two sons, Alex and Andrei, sources of emotional inspiration and vibrant reflections of a youthful zeal for learning.

CONTENTS

FOREWORD

This original scientific volume provides the reader with a comprehensive analysis of how to best provide preoperative, perioperative and postoperative care to women receiving treatment for gynecologic malignancies. The authors have utilized the principles of evidence based medicine to provide a foundation for the decisions regarding care. Therefore, the chapters in this volume are based mainly upon the results of scientific studies instead of personal experience. The first two chapters provide the reader with an excellent summary of the techniques used to provide management decisions which are based upon scientific evidence and how to quantify the strength of the recommendations according to the quality of the studies being analyzed. With this foundation, after reading the subsequent chapters, the clinician will be able to learn and understand the optimal principles and techniques to utilize when managing the patient with a gynecologic malignancy. Each chapter is written by individuals with expertise in their subject area in a manner that is easily understood by the reader. This volume is mainly intended to be read by clinicians caring for patients with gynecologic oncologic problems. Nevertheless the content is also of value to individuals performing any type of major gynecologic surgical procedure. All residents in obstetrics and gynecology would also benefit from reading this volume as many of the chapters provide current comprehensive knowledge of general surgical principles as well as those involving preoperative, perioperative and postoperative care of women undergoing laparotomy or laparoscopy to treat problems involving the reproductive organs.

DANIEL R. MISHELL JR., M.D.

*The Lyle G. McNeile Professor and
Chairman, Department of
Obstetrics and Gynecology
University of Southern California
School of Medicine*

CONTRIBUTORS

DENISE ABERLE, M.D., Professor, Department of Radiological Sciences, UCLA School of Medicine, 10833 Le Conte Avenue, Los Angeles, CA

ROBERT BURGER, M.D., Assistant Professor, Division of Gynecologic Oncology, UCI School of Medicine, 101 The City Drive, Orange, CA

ROY D. CANE, M.B., B.Ch., F.C.C.M., Professor of Anesthesiology, Director of Critical Care Services, University of South Florida School of Medicine, Tampa, FL

JOAN MICHELLE CHRISTIE, M.D., Assistant Professor, Department of Anesthesiology, University of South Florida School of Medicine, Tampa, FL

ANDREW DEUTSCH, M.D., M.B.A., Tower Radiology Inc., Los Angeles, CA

LASZLO Z. GALFFY, M.D. Pasadena Rehabilitation Institute, Pasadena, CA

MARK GENESEN, M.D., Gynecologic Oncology Associates, Riverside, CA

STEFAN HEINZE, M.D., Department of Radiological Sciences, UCLA School of Medicine, 10833 Le Conte Ave., Los Angeles, CA

DOROTHY N. KAMMERER-DOAK, M.D., Assistant Professor, Department of Ob/Gyn, University of New Mexico, Albuquerque, NM

PAUL P. KOONINGS, M.D., Director of Gynecologic Oncology, Kaiser Permanente, San Diego, CA

LEO LAGASSE, M.D., F.A.C.S., F.A.C.O.G., Cedars-Sinai Comprehensive Cancer Center, Professor of Gynecology, UCLA School of Medicine, Los Angeles, CA

PAUL LIN, M.D., Director, Department of Gynecologic Oncology, Division of Surgery, City of Hope National Medical Center, 1500 E. Duarte Rd., Duarte, CA

KATHRYN F. MCGONIGLE, M.D., F.A.C.S., F.A.C.O.G., Assistant Professor,

UCLA School of Medicine, Division of Gynecologic Oncology, 10833 Le Conte Avenue, Los Angeles, CA

JUDITH MCKAY, Ph.D., Clinical Psychologist, 294 Surrey Pl., Bonita, CA

BRADLEY J. MONK, M.D., Assistant Professor, Division of Gynecologic Oncology, UCI Medical Center, 101 The City Drive, Orange, CA

C. PAUL MORROW, M.D., F.A.C.S., F.A.C.O.G., Director of Gynecologic Oncology, University of Southern California School of Medicine, Los Angeles, CA

LEE S. ROSEN, M.D., Division of Hematology/Oncology, UCLA School of Medicine, Los Angeles, CA

JOHN B. SCHLAERTH, M.D., Women's Cancer Center, 2750 E. Washington Blvd., Suite 210, Pasadena, CA

SUBIR ROY, M.D., Professor of Obstetrics and Gynecology, University of Southern California School of Medicine, Women's Hospital, 1240 N. Mission Road, Los Angeles, CA

GARY SCHILLER, M.D., F.A.C.P., Associate Professor, Division of Hematology/ Oncology, UCLA School of Medicine, Los Angeles, CA

HOWARD SILBERMAN, M.D., F.A.C.S., Professor of Surgery, University of Southern California School of Medicine, Los Angeles, CA

HARRIET SMITH, M.D., Director of Gynecologic Oncology, University of New Mexico School of Medicine, Albuquerque, NM

CLAYTON A. VARGA, M.D., M.H.S.M., Pasadena Rehabilitation Institute, Pasadena, CA

STEVEN A. VASILEV, M.D., M.B.A., F.A.C.O.G., F.A.C.S., Director of Gynecologic Oncology, L. A. Tertiary Referral Center, Southern California Permanente Medical Group, Inc., Los Angeles, CA; Clinical Professor of Obstetrics and Gynecology, USC School of Medicine, Los Angeles, CA; President, Global Health Systems, Inc., EBM Practice Collaborative

PART I

GENERAL PRINCIPLES

CHAPTER 1

INTRODUCTION

STEVEN A. VASILEV, M.D., M.B.A.

Learning without thinking is useless. Thinking without learning is dangerous.
—Confucius

TOWARD EVIDENCE-BASED MEDICAL PRACTICE

The very roots of Osler's apprentice-based medical education and practice, to which we still largely adhere, are being severed. Lest this be interpreted as a call to arms, Osler noted that his 1918 textbook of medicine was based on "personal experience correlated with the general experience of others."[1a] This is a far cry from practice based on randomized clinical trials, or even scientific evidence from observational studies.

Health care is indeed undergoing a "frame-breaking" shift fueled by the steadily advancing moniker of managed care. In vehement opposition, many physicians argue that managed health care has nothing managed about it, and that it has no impact on reducing true total costs. In a recent survey by J. D. Power and Associates, encompassing 32,000 physicians in 22 markets, 9 out of 10 described themselves as being "anti–managed care."[1b] The study results indicated that physicians wanted to practice with minimum interference and maximum independence. Fully 42% of surveyed physicians felt that costs should *never* be considered in clinical decisions, and half stated that profiling regarding utilization "makes them angry." Nonetheless, radical changes will continue to take place in health care delivery. So far they have been initiated externally and are often based on business and cost considerations. Many changes have been out of the individual physician's control, or even understanding. As a result, health care is rapidly evolving from a cottage to a mainstream industry and the physician has largely been out of this evolutionary loop. Are physicians partly

Perioperative and Supportive Care in Gynecologic Oncology: Evidence-Based Management,
Edited by Steven A. Vasilev.
ISBN 0-471-24788-X   Copyright © 2000 by Wiley-Liss, Inc.

responsible for this loss of control? If so, why? Is it possible that maximum physician independence, revered above all else and at all costs, is undermining the ability for physicians to regain control of health care delivery? If physician independence means preserving unexplained practice variance, which is currently out of control, perhaps physicians *are* their own worst enemy.

What is unexplained practice variance and how is it managed? W. Edwards Deming, a statistician and management leader who taught quality as a system to the Japanese, spoke of variance management as being at the very core of quality improvement.[2] Of course, as opposed to manufacturing, zero tolerance for variance and defects is not often possible in medicine. The focus must instead be on narrowing the range between upper and lower limits of a process. To this end, when a procedure or diagnostic test falls within a reasonable range of indications and evidence, the system process is in control. When procedures fall well outside this range, or if the range is exceedingly wide, the system process is out of control. Such is the case with health care, both on a micro- and macroscale.

For decades, many studies have documented overuse of specific medical services, sometimes solely based on geographic location (e.g., certain cities have higher coronary bypass surgery rates with no increased epidemiologic risk factors to explain this). Essentially, these practice patterns are "unexplained" by reasonable common causes or indications. In other words, reasonable variation in practice patterns is exceeded too often. One study specifically noted that 10% to 27% of hysterectomies among women enrolled in seven health plans were performed for totally inappropriate reasons.[3] Multiple studies performed by the RAND Corporation and others document similar findings and illuminate a quality problem in that patients are being subjected to risk of adverse consequences without documented benefit.[4] It is worth repeating that the goal is not to achieve zero variance but merely to reduce practice variance to levels supported by existing evidence of benefit.

It has also been argued that the wrong primary questions are being asked in this evolution and the wrong goals set. For example, a central high-profile question today asks, "How can we reduce costs?" Instead, should we perhaps be asking, "How can we improve the quality of care, minimizing unjustifiable and unexplainable practice variance?" Is it possible that costs could be effectively reduced as a by-product of this alternative and more palatable primary question? If the correct goals were set, could there be an alignment of effort toward true physician-driven optimally managed care?

Is practice variance reduction and quality improvement via evidence-based guidelines just another medical management fad being forced upon physicians? After all, there is a veritable alphabet soup proliferation of managed care and business-based buzzwords, reflecting the driving forces in the evolution of health care delivery, usually not in concert with medical terminology. There are also over 1,500 practice guidelines in print and countless critical pathways. Most organizations seemingly have generated a set, but what has been the practical impact? Can these guidelines help? How can they help? Are guidelines the same as critical pathways? Are these pathways just a "nursing thing"? How can we expect externally applied forces, embodied by practice guidelines forged by "expert" consensus panels, to be truly incorporated into better practice patterns at the local level? Certainly, unless the very best concepts in guideline development and evidence-based practice are actually implemented, there is no net effect on patient care and cost efficiencies. Thus far, in fact, there has been no net impact. Perhaps the wrong approach is being taken as well as the wrong questions asked. Perhaps the best solutions will come from individual physicians self-adjusting practice patterns based on evidence and outcomes rather than from externally imposed guidelines.

Is there a paradigm among all of the confusion that is good? Is there a means by which the positive thrust toward value-added (outcomes/cost) care, as opposed to cheapest care, can be directed by physicians? One answer might be to practice the best medicine possible. Obviously this is not a new concept. However, as we generate more and more data and publish them in a forest of journals, the ability to keep up gives way to information overload. Additionally, not all data have the same strength and the quality varies; thus, the *data* may not translate into practical *information*. Along these lines, the randomized controlled clinical trial has been a gold standard and usually carries more weight than a case report/series or a consensus panel report. However, despite the estimated 250,000 or so randomized clinical trials that have confirmed the relative efficacy of many treatments, there is still a paucity of such studies to guide certain medical practice decisions. Without actually reading every single journal, often in specialties that do not normally cross our desk, it is simply impossible for the average clinician to keep up with what is proven and what is not, and with what strength of evidence.

Ideally, to optimally obtain and use information, physicians would need electronic databases with continually updated, properly analyzed and processed data. Most, if not all, practicing physicians do not have these resources readily available or are not facile in searching current literature.[5] Problem-based electronic database searches, with tools such as MEDLINE to answer specific questions, are still infrequently used and may be incomplete since full article text is often not immediately available. In practice, the tendency is to evaluate problems based only on personal and often antiquated experience, or to refer to respected authorities.[5] Commonly we refer to readily available resources such as textbooks to answer specific questions. The challenge inherent to this approach is in maintaining a full and up-to-date library, which is usually impossible.

Printed media such as this book may be criticized as being immediately outdated as of the print date, which is a potentially valid criticism. Much of what is summarized in this textbook is in fact not new, and in some areas quite dated but axiomatic. Nevertheless, it represents the best evidence known to the contributors to date. As long as the reader is aware of this limitation, by the 80/20 rule, 80% of evidence is relatively static and 20% represents new findings. In most cases, it is really the former scenario that is the bigger problem in practice variance minimization. In many instances, the main point is the *lack* of data to support efficacy of generally accepted common interventions. Of greater concern, despite strong data to support one point or another in patient care improvement, many physicians continue to practice status quo simply because "that is the way we have always done it." In some cases, the available evidence is rapidly evolving and in other areas solid evidence in existence for years or even decades has not been incorporated into general practice.

Are we discussing "cookbook medicine" here? Not at all. Medicine is both an art and science, and will continue to be as long as we treat human beings and not machines or biomechanical hybrids. However, we now have the operational tools to make it as much a science as possible to support the art in delivering compassionate and effective care. Some of these tools are introduced in this text, and the best evidence as of this printing for perioperative and supportive care issues is presented. Selective chapters contain more axiomatic material than others. We have attempted to highlight controversial areas. However, this book is a *synopsis* of evidence regarding general principles of perioperative care. As such, it is not intended to be comprehensive and the reader is referred to the excellent references within each chapter or to other works.

PERIOPERATIVE AND CRITICAL CARE ECONOMICS

Currently, an estimated 1% of the U.S. gross national product (GNP) is consumed by intensive care. A significant portion is taken up by oncologic and perioperative care, which extends onto the ward and outpatient settings. Those caring for gynecologic oncology and complicated gynecology patients directly influence all medical outcomes and 80% of the cost outcomes in the immediate perioperative and long-term-care periods.

At the societal decision-making level, we must ultimately balance the focus on *maximum* acute care with *optimal* care of an aging population. While some chronic and catastrophic diseases, such as cancer, often cannot be cured, patients still need relief from symptoms and minimization of disease-related complications and dysfunction. All of these issues touch upon supply and demand realities and opportunity costs. Maximizing efficiencies and minimizing unexplained practice variance will go a long way toward conservation of scarce resources and improved outcomes, and will contribute to overall cost reduction in health care delivery services.

If a classic economic marginal analysis approach is adopted toward mortality, morbidity, level and extent of intensive care, complications and avoidance thereof, the incremental impact of each decision on quality and costs can be determined. Key questions might be as follows: During preoperative evaluation, prevention of complications is key to decreased morbidity and length of stay. How much more, or perhaps less, is required as a diagnostic input to achieve a given superior-quality output? During perioperative care, what incremental opportunities exist for prevention with appropriate surveillance and management that are based on good evidence? In selecting new technologies, or even older technologies, what is the appropriate incremental use of such resources and what are their limitations toward optimizing outcomes?

The primary surgeon must be intimately involved in perioperative planning and delivery of care. A skill base is required for interpretation of data that influence critical perioperative care decisions. The surgeon must also know when to call for consultants to optimize care delivery. The physician must know how to treat the basics, recognize the more difficult problems early, and know how to care for the patient until consultants are available while initiating the most appropriate cost-effective diagnostic or therapeutic interventions.

OPERATIONAL TOOLS OVERVIEW

This textbook strives to present the best available evidence for decision making in perioperative and supportive care in the gynecologic oncology patient. It also introduces some operational mindsets and tools. Questions that are addressed include:

- What is evidence-based medicine? How can you find all the available data? What if there are no good data? How do you evaluate which evidence is best for the given situation?
- What evidence exists for minimizing unexplained variance and optimizing practice patterns?
- Are there any formal decision analysis methodologies that can help?
- Can these principles translate into practice guidelines that can actually be implemented and contribute to improvement?
- Is this just cookbook medicine, or is it a guide toward evolution of best practices specific to each physician's and patient's environment?

This textbook primarily addresses gynecologic oncology care but can readily apply to complicated gynecologic perioperative care. Key issues are associated with a level-of-evidence score within the text, or in algorithm form. Some chapters also contain more axiomatic information than others, and as such they are not always subject to grading. In other subject areas, the lack of extensive underlying evidence is striking. Chapter 2 addresses information gathering and interpretation tools. The subsequent clinical chapters present the contributing author's best efforts to gather and synthesize up-to-date information addresssing best approaches to common, as well as uncommon, problems in perioperative, supportive, and critical care. Some authors found data gathering and grading more second nature than others, and some biases remain. These areas should be apparent and interpreted to mean that the subject area is heavily influenced by descriptive studies and expert opinion. Editing cannot always alleviate this bias and may confuse the reader if expert opinion meaning is altered.

In summary, this book is an imperfect but focused and genuine effort to present the best available information to help decrease practice variance toward predictable, improved clinical outcomes. As presented, it is anticipated to be a kernel work in progress, constantly improved through revision, and a guide for reader-directed updating and local adaptation.

REFERENCES

1a. Osler W. *The Principles and Practice of Medicine*, 8th ed. New York: Appleton and Co., 1918.

1b. MEDSTAT Quality Catalyst Program. The MEDSTAT Group and J. D. Power and Associates. Sept 15, 1998. Ann Arbor, Mich.

2. Walton M. *The Deming Management Method*, 1st ed. New York: The Putnam Publishing Group, 1986.

3. Bernstein SJ. The appropriateness of hysterectomy: a comparison of care in seven health plans. *JAMA* 1993;269:2398–2402.

4. Chassin MR. Assessing strategies for quality improvement. *Health Affairs* 1997;16:151–161.

5. Olatunbosun OA, Edouard L, Pierson RA. Physician's attitudes toward evidence based obstetric practice: a questionnaire survey. *Br Med J* 1998;316:365–366.

CHAPTER 2

EVIDENCE-BASED MEDICINE AND DECISION SUPPORT

STEVEN A. VASILEV, M.D., M.B.A.

WHAT IS EVIDENCE-BASED MEDICINE?

Bertrand Russell noted, "The extent to which beliefs are based on evidence is very much less than believers suppose."[1a] It is easy to see how this statement may be directly applicable to medical practice.

Under the protective blanket of the "art" of medical practice, decision making has often been based on anecdotal experience and incomplete utilization of the best available objective data. Physicians tend to practice based more on what their attendings taught them rather than continually researching existing evidence.[1b,2] It then becomes a matter of unchanging practice to make decisions based mostly on personal experience and intuition. In effect, all physicians may be doing what they perceive to be their best, but that is not enough. The data suggest that many decisions are made contrary to available evidence and 51% of decisions are based on no evidence.[2,3] Therefore, it is essential that the medical educational process be carefully scrutinized to see if it requires transformation to optimize decision making and reproducible quality outcomes.[4–6] Unexplained practice variance is a significant problem, contributing to runaway costs and a wide range of outcomes.[6–13] W. Edwards Deming, a leader in cross-industry quality issues, stated that all of his work at the core was based on controlling variance via statistical process control (SPC).[14]

What is unexplained or assignable clinical practice variance? In any industry, to maintain quality of outcomes, operations and process must be continually inspected and tested to minimize defects. In health care, just as in other industries, there will be variability in outcomes. The goal in health care services might not be *zero defects* as proposed in some manufacturing scenarios but

Perioperative and Supportive Care in Gynecologic Oncology: Evidence-Based Management,
Edited by Steven A. Vasilev.
ISBN 0-471-24788-X   Copyright © 2000 by Wiley-Liss, Inc.

rather minimization of variability in outcomes such that the result as a whole is of acceptable quality. The question then becomes, "Is the outcome variability following a given intervention due to chance (random) variation or assignable (nonrandom) unexplained variation?" Chance variation is that which is built into a system, such as the range of normal hemoglobins in the physiologic system of a patient. Assignable variation occurs if some portion of the system is out of control and is amenable to intervention. One of the biggest challenges is to determine if a process or activity is out of control, requiring adjustment, or not.

During the 1920s and 1930s, while at Bell Telephone Laboratories, Walter Shewhart developed *statistical control charts* to help determine when assignable variation has occurred. A repetitive operation, such as caring for a set of patients with a particular problem, will seldom, if ever, produce exactly the same result. However, the outcome variability surrounding a mean value and standard deviation will often produce a normal distribution for the population. As in any other statistical scenario, periodically examining the entire population of interest for variation in the mean is not feasible. Instead, sampling is performed along with selection of an *upper control limit (UCL)* and a *lower control limit (LCL)*. If the sample mean exceeds control limits, typically set at ±3 standard deviations in most industries, the possibility that the variation is due to chance is <0.3%. Taken one step further, it is even possible to *predict* assignable variation prior to loss of system control. Also, in some cases, assignable variation can represent improvement in process rather than loss of control, and should also be investigated.

This brief discussion is meant to introduce the idea that unexplained clinical practice variance should be sought, the reasons should be identified, and a process improvement should be implemented. It could be on an individual practice, organizational, or even societal level. Details regarding statistical process control are beyond the scope of this textbook, and the interested reader is referred elsewhere.[15] The key point is that tools are available to assess how unexplained variance can influence outcomes and point to areas requiring attention and correction.

Unexplained variance due to assignable variation has the potential to be significantly influenced by evidence-based medical practice. How scientific can the base for the art of medicine get? It is estimated that less than 10% of clinical practice is based on randomized clinical trial (RCT) data.[3,16,17] While this may be a criticism of evidence-based medicine (EBM), it reflects a core misunderstanding of EBM intent.[18,19] In fact, the other 90% of clinical practice should still be based on the best available level of evidence, or at least the understanding that a particular practice pattern or intervention is not well grounded in evidence of any kind.[16,20] This understanding alerts clinicians that their convictions may be on shaky ground and that further evaluation may be required to minimize practice variance. What is more disturbing is that the 10% of clinical practice that *is* well grounded in solid RCT data is often not incorporated into standard patient care, and unexplained variance is seen in this group of interventions as well. Lag time between publication of compelling data and incorporation can exceed 10 years.[21]

Is evidence-based medicine a new managed care concept? On the contrary, the concept of EBM dates back more than a century.[22,23] Recently, largely due to managed care pressures, it has enjoyed a resurgence of interest among divergent groups: clinicians wishing to regain control of medical practice, payors wishing to limit variance and lower costs, health care purchasers wishing for quality initiatives for better value, and the public wishing to understand the best approach.[24] Numerous centers and Internet Web sites for evidence-based practice have been established in a variety of disciplines. For example, the Cochrane Collaboration, an international multicenter venture (www.cochrane.co.uk), reviews, synthesizes, and distributes data on health care practices on an ongoing basis.[25,26] A number of EBM journals have also been introduced. Additionally, recommendations for improvement in reporting clinical trials have been proposed.[27,28]

This resurgence of interest in EBM has certainly faced significant criticism.[29–32] Some have interpreted it to be a fad, a pure cost-cutting device; others label it "cookbook" medicine, which at its core is an antithesis to the "art" of medicine. Much of this criticism and negative reaction is based on misunderstanding of terminology and philosophy. It may also be negatively associated with the current backlash against managed care. However, lost among this controversy is the EBM philosophic thrust toward improvement in the quality of medical practice. Although some believe that quality de facto requires higher costs, the converse is likely to be true in most cases. There is no question that technology transfer will continue to affect health care costs. However, the correct application of new and emerging technology and limitation of poor management decisions will serve as a counterbalance. In the optimal scenario, overall quality improvement will decrease costs.[33,34] Additionally, convergence of information technology and computer-assisted decision analysis and support will likely accelerate and contribute to quality improvement and cost control.[35] Thus, it may be axiomatic that true improvements in quality and efficiency will control costs. As long as quality is better defined and becomes the lead issue, and costs are well described and assigned, a relationship between the two will become easier to evaluate and implement process improvement. Currently, neither is the case. Quality is not clearly defined and costs are usually imprecisely assigned.[36]

Thus, evidence-based medicine may be poised to utilize the boom in information technology and improve quality through unexplained variance reduction, but it is certainly in a state of evolution. Various interpretations and local adaptations are apparent and will continue while health care is in a state of reorganization. Thus, it may be helpful and illuminating to review what EBM can do and what it cannot do.

At its core, evidence-based medicine may be viewed as a process. This process combines systematically obtaining the best available refined data (i.e., information) on a defined topic with the clinical expertise of the clinician. The resulting knowledge base then is applied to patient care.[4,37] While this process may seem like good old-fashioned medical care, data gathering is the first significant challenge. In today's environment of data overload, physicians are challenged to keep up with the myriad of peer-reviewed journal articles, as well as the adequacy of each study and the strength of evidence presented. A new paradigm and skill set is required, including efficient access to published studies and systematic application of evidence strength analysis.[38]

The second challenge is to continually and systematically incorporate the best evidence into clinical practice. The application of clinical expertise and judgment, heretofore known as the "art" of medicine, is an integral part of compassionate health care delivery and cannot be summarily replaced by data-driven guidelines. Physicians must continue to combine research-based evidence with accumulated clinical expertise.[39–41] The physician is a knowledge worker and the goal should be development of a learning system within the individual a la modification of (Peter Senge's) *learning organization*, which is based on continually improving systems.[42,43] In a patient-centered environment, hard objective data may point toward one intervention, but based on clinical experience and patient input, the best outcomes may be realized by taking a different path for a given clinical situation. Optimally both data and expertise should be available, interventions applied, and outcomes assessed.

A common misperception is that EBM is equivalent to "cookbook" medicine. Pat prescriptions for any imaginable condition without regard for individual patient requirements or the physician's clinical expertise would fit that definition. However, EBM mandates *integration* of clinical experience with a commitment to using the best available data as a guide to continued improvement and incremental narrowing of practice variance patterns. Evidence-based medicine cannot and does not have cost reduction as its primary goal. Rather, more effective utilization of diagnostic and treatment resources has the by-product of possible cost reduction. This does not always occur and depends on how costs are defined and to whom they are assigned.

Evidence-based medicine does not rest entirely on external research findings with the randomized clinical trial as the gold standard. While it is true that well-designed and interpreted prospective studies should have a strong influence on shaping practice patterns, they are not the only factor. Neither is the compilation of this material via meta-analyses. The process goal is to define the best available external evidence that addresses specific clinical questions. The type of evidence depends on the clinical question at hand. Some questions require a randomized clinical trial, whereas others require a cohort study, and still others may merely require an observation of clear and undisputed efficacy of a given intervention.

Traditional continuing medical education (CME) has failed to keep physicians abreast of new developments, to the extent that these innovations are not readily integrated into practice.[44–46] Worse, the half-life of medical education is getting ever shorter. Without the best current evidence, practice patterns can become dangerous and costly in both an economic and morbidity sense.

EBM can help maintain the balance between the data-driven guidelines and the patient-centered "art" of medical practice.[47]

EBM is a philosophic approach to medical practice and education. It is not outcome research, but it can help delineate where evidence is lacking as a basis for future studies. It does so by distinguishing the type and strength of evidence that exists for a particular question and facilitating the gathering and grading of such evidence. As more supporting evidence becomes available, the validation of evidence-based medicine as a philosophy and generally accepted practice infrastructure appears to be warranted.[48,49]

According to Sackett, there are five key steps to incorporating evidence-based practice into daily medical care. First, the clinical problem must be framed into answerable questions. Second, the best available data that will help answer the question must be quickly and efficiently tracked down. Third, the evidence must be critically appraised for validity and usefulness as information. Fourth, the appraisal results must be incorporated into daily practice. Fifth, the results of this change in practice patterns must be evaluated for outcomes and other feedback regarding the new practice pattern.[50]

EXTERNAL DATA GATHERING AND RELEVANCE INTERPRETATION TOOLS

As the information age explodes, the total amount of readily available knowledge far exceeds the clinical experience of a single physician or consensus group of experts. Additionally, due to the electronic superhighway and multiple electronic storage media, it is no longer necessary to read through masses of journals and memorize key references in order to stay current.[51,52]

The following represents a synopsis of helpful sources and strategies for electronically searching the medical literature. For a slightly dated but more comprehensive discussion, refer to Sackett's *Evidence Based Medicine: How to Practice and Teach EBM*.[50] Helpful online tips are also offered at the sites listed in Table 2.1. In general, evidence must be current and credible, applicable to the practitioner's patient population, and clinically relevant above and beyond an acceptable *p* value.

TABLE 2.1. Online Primary Literature Search Sites

Grateful Med/Pub med	http://www.ncbi.nih.gov/PubMed/
	http://igm.nlm.nih.gov/
Silver Platter	http://www.silverplatter.com/
Paper Chase	http://www.Paperchase.com/
Healthgate	http://www.healthgate.com
Institute for Scientific Information	http://www.isinet.com
Physicians Online	http://www.po.com

Electronic searches have practically become synonymous with MEDLINE searches. As described below, MEDLINE is the largest and most well known database. However, other sources may be better for focused topic searches. For example, recent research topics and cutting edge information may be best found in Current Contents. On the other hand, for a general review on a particular topic, possibly with CME credit attached to help fulfill licensing requirements, Medscape or other online journal databases should be consulted (Table 2.2). Online structured reviews and guidelines provide an evidence based synthesis of available literature on a growing number of topics (Table 2.3). The overview provided in this chapter is pragmatically structured around available and useful web sites as of this printing rather than the more artificial constructs of database vs. search engine and like classifications.

MEDLINE

The most widely available tool to clinicians, which is often available directly to the public, is the searchable MEDLINE database through the National Library of Medicine. In addition to online Internet searching availability, CD-ROM versions are provided by many medical libraries. Unfortunately, not all peer-reviewed articles are referenced and some are misclassified.

Most electronic search engines that access this online portion of the National Library of Medicine (NLM) retrieve references by either text words or medical subject headings (MeSH). Searches can be initiated for specific article titles, authors, general subjects, or specific clinical questions.

The most popular and easy-to-use search engines are Grateful Med/PubMed, Paperchase, and OVID via Universities. Availability is usually free through services such as Physicians Online (http://www.po.com), the NLM (http://ncbi.nlm.nih.gov/PubMed; http://igm.nlm.nih.gov/), and Healthgate (http://www.healthgate.com/Healthgate/MEDLINE/search.shtml). Abstracts are available for 67% of the references, comprising over 3,600 journals indexed from 1966 on.

Search strategies can significantly influence the quantity and quality of data found.[53] First, the MEDLINE database articles recovered should reflect the available literature for the appropriate time period.[54] Second, *all* evidence for a given topic should be considered, from case series or consensus opinions to randomized double-blind prospective studies. Third, all evidence must describe the specific patient population or clinical problem in reasonable detail, which centers on entry of the appropriate key words and MeSH headings. Since the early 1990s, the MeSH vocabulary has expanded to include specific search string toggles for type of study (e.g., controlled trial vs. cohort) and publication (e.g., meta-analysis).[55]

Although the validity of studies should be individually appraised, by including these methodology toggles in their search, users of the MEDLINE and other online NLM databases can search by type of studies available. The Health Information Research Unit (HIRU) of McMaster University (http://hiru.hirunet.mcmaster.ca/ebm/) has suggested strategies for optimal retrieval of relevant citations by methodology-based MEDLINE searching.[53] For example, in order to maximize the retrieval of relevant citations, the search strategy (included with other key words or MeSH headings) EXPLODE SENSITIVITY and SPECIFICITY OR PREDICTIVE VALUE (TEXTWORD) can be used. If a personally performed search does not provide appropriate information, librarian consultation should be sought.

Current Contents

A more robust and up-to-date index of approximately 6,000 journals is available through the Institute for Scientific Information (http://www.isinet.com). However, it may not be beginner-level user friendly, optimally requiring very specific search requests. A free interactive trial is offered.

EMBASE

EMBASE, an international database of approximately 3,500 journals, indexed from 1988 on, is available through Silver Platter (http://www.silverplatter.com/) and other vendors for a subscription fee. Search structure is similar to MEDLINE, and information is available by multiple specialties, including pharmaceutical utilization research, in CD-ROM and Internet access format.

Online Journals

A very brief list of available full text journals pertaining to perioperative care is listed in Table 2.2. Most come with an online search engine; many are free and indexed back to 1995 or earlier.

TABLE 2.2. Full Electronic Text Journals

Medscape (multiple e-journals)	http://medscape.com
Anesthesia and Intensive Care	http://www.aaic.net.au/home.html
Anesthesiology	http://www.anesthesiology.org/index.html
Annals of Internal Medicine	http://www.acponline.org/
Chest	http://journals.chestnet.org/chest/
Journal of the American Medical Association	http://www.ama-assn.org/public/journals/jama/ jamahome.htm
New England Journal of Medicine	http://www.nejm.org/
British Medical Journal	http://www.bmj.com/index.html
Canadian Medical Association Journal	http://www.cma.ca/journals/cmaj/
American Journal of Managed Care	http://www.ajmc.com/

Textbooks

Textbooks have the distinct advantage of presenting synthesized information that is quickly accessible. The disadvantages are that some information may be outdated before publication or the required textbook(s) may not be at hand. However, if EBM philosophy is applied and explicit links to evidence are identified, textbooks are still a valuable resource. In particular, there is relative stability of supporting data for 80% of clinical interventions. The other 20% is subject to periodic change, although this ratio may change depending on the subject. Thus, a textbook synthesis of EBM information can facilitate incorporation into clinical practice those interventions that are clearly well grounded and can facilitate removal from clinical practice those interventions that are clearly without basis. In order to capture a current compendium regarding clinical problems and interventions, rapidly updated CD-ROM or online textbooks offer a distinct advantage.

Meta-analysis

A meta-analysis is a secondary systematic review of published primary data, optimally including randomized controlled trials. Often smaller studies are grouped together in order to apply statistical analysis tools to an increased pooled sample size.[56] While meta-analysis has gained widespread acceptance, the utility of this method has been questioned.[57,58] Additionally, the results are limited by the quality of the primary data publications. Therefore, the review must include a description of how the primary data sources were identified, and must provide enough information for the reader to be able to assess the possibility of selection and analysis distortion due to various biases. Continuous compilation of clinical trial results and analysis of the results have been suggested and are provided on multiple subject areas by the Cochrane Collaboration.[59] Although not meta-analysis per se, the ACP Journal Club provides online abstracted reviews of primary literature.

EBM Guidelines and Structured Reviews

Evidence-based guidelines represent an attempt to distill the best available evidence via a structured process for a particular clinical question.[60] Many, if not most, published guidelines (approximately 1,500) do not employ such a rigorous process and should be interpreted accordingly.[61] Also, guidelines written by external sources do not enjoy widespread implementation. However, with these caveats in mind, the Society of Critical Care Medicine operates a good online guidelines site pertaining to issues on perioperative and critical care. Additional resources are listed in Table 2.3, including the *Health Services Technology Assessment Text (HSTAT)*, which provides *National Institutes of Health (NIH) Consensus Statements* and *AHCPR Evidence Based Guidelines*, representing the two extremes of guideline development process.

TABLE 2.3. Online Structured Reviews and Guidelines

Society of Critical Care Medicine	http://www.sccm.org/accm/guidelines/guide_home_set.html
Evidence Based Medicine	http://www.acponline.org/journals/ebm
ACP Journal Club	http://www.acponline.org/journals/acpjc
Turning Practice into Research (TRIP)	http://www.gwent.nhs.gov.uk/trip/test-search.html
Health Services Technology Assessment Text (HSTAT)	http://text.nlm.nih.gov/
Cochrane Collaborative database	http://www.cochrane.co.uk

Grading the Data

Once a representative data set of published references is obtained, it must be systematically reviewed to determine the quality of data presented. The key question is, "Which *data* set translates into the best *information* available for the specific question at hand?" *Best* may be defined as relevant and with the least methodological flaws. These flaws differ depending on the type of study design (see below). Extensive discussion regarding clinical research design is well beyond the scope of this textbook. Interested readers may refer to the many excellent textbooks and reviews.[62-66] A particularly comprehensive review series of articles, entitled "User's Guide to the Medical Literature," published by the Evidence-Based Medicine Working Group from McMaster University,[67-80] is highly recommended.

The studies must then be evaluated for strength of evidence and categorized by EBM level. This textbook uses guidelines proposed by the U.S. Preventive Services Task Force.[81] Although this system was proposed for evaluation of clinical preventive services, it is generally applicable to other interventions. These EBM levels may be noted in the text or in the decision algorithm or both, depending on the chapter and material (e.g., Level I; 3 and Level II-3; 6). When available, the number of "best" studies/reports used to support the evidence is noted after a semicolon.

Level I: Evidence obtained from at least one properly designed randomized controlled trial.

Level II-1: Evidence obtained from well-designed controlled trials without randomization.

Level II-2: Evidence obtained from well-designed cohort or case-controlled analytic studies, preferably from more than one center or research group.

Level II-3: Evidence obtained from multiple time series with or without the intervention. Dramatic results in uncontrolled experiments could also be regarded as this type of evidence.

Level III: Opinions of respected authorities, based on clinical experience, descriptive studies, or reports of expert committees.

An alternative grading system is based on the Canadian Task Force on the periodic health examination, is more detailed, and is presented here for completeness of discussion. It is not used in this textbook, but the similarities are readily apparent.

Level I: Evidence obtained from meta-analysis of multiple, well-designed, controlled studies or from high-power, randomized, controlled clinical trials.

Level II: Evidence obtained from at least one well-designed experimental study or low-power, randomized, controlled clinical trial.

Level III: Evidence obtained from at least one well-designed quasi-experimental study, such as nonrandomized, controlled single-group, pre-post, cohort, time, or matched case-controlled series.

Level IV: Evidence from well-designed nonexperimental studies, such as comparative and correlational descriptive and case studies.

Level V: Evidence from case reports and clinical examples.

A letter grade may then be assigned, based on the overall strength of evidence. The grades below are based on the Canadian system. Modifications of this grading system have also been used for the U.S. Public Health Service (USPHS) system. Most have been specific for the preventive services or screening question at hand. Nonetheless, a general appreciation for the use of levels of evidence as they translate into grades can be achieved by reviewing the following information. In this textbook, letter grades are not assigned, leaving readers to make their own assessment based on EBM level of evidence.

Grade A: There is evidence of Level I or consistent findings from multiple studies of Levels II, III, or IV.

Grade B: There is evidence of Levels II, III, or IV and findings are generally consistent.

Grade C: There is evidence of Levels II, III, or IV, but findings are inconsistent.

Grade D: There is little or no systematic empirical evidence.

WHAT IS THE "BEST" EVIDENCE?

The "best" level of evidence is generally considered to be the randomized clinical trial (RCT). This study design provides very useful information with the least bias vulnerability, but it is not the appropriate answer to all questions. Many interventions or other clinical questions have not and will not ever be investigated at that level, or the clinical question being asked may not be appropriate for evaluation in a randomized controlled fashion. Examples are abundant and include low-prevalence conditions, treatment or diagnostic decisions of low impact, low-morbidity conditions, and highly complicated, very high-cost low-volume interventions. For example, the Pap smear was never evaluated by RCT. However, enough observational epidemiologic evidence exists such that its role in reducing the incidence of invasive cervical cancer is not generally questioned. Similarly, certain other questions require answers not from RCTs but from observational cohort and case-controlled studies, outcomes data within a local practice setting, questionnaire or interview-based data, problem-modeling data, and other formats.

Intuitively, it is important to consider what type of information an RCT provides. Usually the RCT compares two or more treatments, which are felt to differ relatively minimally in efficacy, in order to determine which is the better intervention. The true effectiveness of an RCT treatment arm is often inversely proportional to the number of RCTs it has been a part of. Thus, if a significant advance occurs, such as the introduction of the Pap smear or of antibiotics/penicillin, an RCT is not mandated to demonstrate efficacy.

EBM grading schemes place high value on RCTs, but this should not overshadow the fact that some questions are better answered by alternative study designs. Total homage to and reverence for the RCT p value is not realistic. Instead, asking the appropriate question usually determines the appropriate study design or data source and is a philosophic underpinning of EBM practice.

Evaluating Prospective Randomized Controlled Trials (EBM Level I)

Clinical trials are intervention based by definition, with the subjects prospectively assigned to experimental and control arms. The subjects in both arms should be similar in all or most characteristics, allowing outcomes of a given intervention to be accurately assessed between the arms. Although blinded studies are more difficult to design and implement, unblinded studies overestimate benefit by up to 17%.

Major advantages of this study design include (1) bias elimination by random assignment of intervention; (2) blinding of the investigators as well as the participants whenever possible, further reducing bias; and (3) the facilitation of statistical probability analysis in determining strength of the cause-effect relationship.

Study design flaws to watch for may include (1) invalid methods of randomization, (2) subjects not matched by key variables, (3) sample size too small to detect potentially important differences, and (4) compliance problems or loss to follow-up rate affecting the outcome analysis.

Evaluating Controlled Prospective Nonrandomized Studies (EBM Level II-1)

Level II-1 studies are also interventional in nature. However, the study and control groups are not prospectively and randomly assigned, introducing biases.

When using historical or otherwise unmatched control groups, the reported effects of the intervention being studied are often exaggerated.[82,83]

Study design flaws may include those listed under the Level I category. The main detraction from the highest reliability rating is the nonrandom assignment between the study and control groups, which could unevenly distribute known and unknown variables and factors sufficiently to sway the outcome analysis and interpretation.

Evaluating Observational Studies (EBM Levels II-2, II-3, and III)

These studies represent the bulk of evidence available for the majority of diagnostic and treatment interventions. They include both prospective and retrospective study designs.

Level II-2

Case-Controlled Studies   The design of these studies is generally retrospective. First, the research question is identified and explicitly framed. Then the objective is to identify subjects with and without a disease or condition. A sample population is identified as well as a matched sample population without the condition but with similar demographics. The background of each group is then reviewed in order to find out why the cases developed a given condition and the controls did not. The odds that a given intervention or exposure produced the condition in the case group is compared with the control group (Table 2.4). As such the output of the study is the *odds ratio*, which approximates the *relative risk* rather well if the prevalence of a condition is not excessively high.

Advantages are that the study can be rapidly performed and is useful when studying rare conditions. Major study flaws include (1) unknown factors that inadvertently influence the development of a condition are not taken into consideration; (2) selection bias preferentially includes or excludes subjects in either the case or control group; and (3) differential recall bias may affect the ability of either group to remember, admit to, or include certain key exposures under investigation.

Cohort Studies   Cohort studies can be either prospective or retrospective. In each case, a group of subjects is followed through time, usually made up of exposed and unexposed subjects to a given risk factor or intervention. In a *prospective* cohort study, these risk-factor exposures have been identified, and the incidence of outcomes such as a finding or disease state in both groups is recorded as it occurs. In a *retrospective* cohort study, the risk-factor exposure as well as the outcome has already occurred in a well-delineated cohort assembled for another purpose. Most often the control group is internal, since comparisons are made between subjects within the single cohort. The outcome is reported as a *relative risk*.

Major study flaws include (1) this method is an expensive and inefficient

TABLE 2.4. Ratios

Group	Outcome Event		Total
	Yes	No	
Control	a	b	a + b
Experimental (or case)	c	d	c + d

Number needed to treat (NNT)
$$= \frac{1}{(a/a+b) - (c/c+d)} = \frac{1}{ARR}$$

(in order to achieve a benefit or harm/risk)

Relative risk reduction (RRR)
$$= \frac{[(a/a+b) - (c/c+d)]}{a/a+b} = \frac{\text{untreated} - \text{treated}}{\text{untreated}}$$

(cohort studies)

Absolute risk reduction (ARR) $= (a/a+b) - (c/c+d) = \text{untreated} - \text{treated}$
(cohort studies)

Odds ratio
$$= \frac{\text{odds of outcome in case group}}{\text{odds of outcome in control group}} = \frac{c/d}{a/b}$$

(case-controlled studies)

way to study rare diseases or states; (2) confounding variables may exist that obscure the cause-effect relationship between risk factor and outcome; (3) outcome assessment between groups can be biased; and (4) criteria for risk-factor exposure may not be accurate.

Level II-3   The following studies fall between classic observational studies (case controlled and cohort) and pure descriptive accounts.

Uncontrolled Experiments   Uncontrolled observations of intervention or exposure results that show dramatic outcomes may point to a valid question requiring hypothesis testing. However, since no exact information is provided about exposure and no control groups exist, other methods must be employed to test the hypothesis for a cause-effect relationship. Other factors may have caused the outcome rather than the intervention or exposure being considered.

Cross-Sectional Studies   These observational studies collect data at a single point in time, comparing presence or absence of an exposure or intervention with a given outcome. It is difficult or impossible to assess a temporal relationship, although serial cross-sectional surveys can evaluate general changes over time. This design is hypothesis generating rather than testing and generates prevalence or relative prevalence.

Level III   The least persuasive studies, which offer almost no insight into an exposure-outcome relationship, include (1) pure descriptive studies, (2) case series and reports, and (3) expert opinion or consensus panel reports. Consensus conferences that use EBM strategies provide recommendations based on structured review of available evidence. In this setting, the strength of recommendations is much higher than that coming from a simple round-table discussion or expert opinion. In communicating the EBM review results, standards may be set based on Level I data, guidelines may be introduced based on Level II data, and options may be suggested based on Level III data.[84]

STATISTICS ISSUES: DESIGN, POWER, SAMPLE SIZE, AND CLINICAL UTILITY

A review of basic statistics, even briefly, is well beyond the scope of this textbook. A brief and very readable synopsis of statistics for the nonstatistician is provided within an excellent review series published recently in the *British Medical Journal*.[85,86]

Without delving into the specifics of statistical analysis tools, several key issues can be addressed in assessing the quality of published research. Common errors in study design and reporting involve (1) inadequate sample size, (2) inadequate power, (3) inadequate follow-up, and (4) statistically significant but clinically irrelevant results.

Sample size should be large enough to provide a high probability of detecting *clinically* relevant effects of a given intervention, if they exist. This is accomplished via published nomograms or computer programs, and is determined by the desired power of the study—that is, what sample size is required to find a true clinical difference between the groups at a moderate, high, or very high probability.[66] Too often a power of 80% to 90% is not achieved and the given study is prone to a Type II (β) error, meaning the intervention is reported as having no effect when in fact it did have an effect. Type I (α) errors are less common, defined as reporting a significant difference when in fact no true difference exists.

A study may not be conducted for a sufficiently long period of time or may be hampered by subjects who are lost to follow-up. This results in incomplete detection of late effects and bias within the group not followed to the established endpoint. The latter bias is often in favor of the intervention. Thus, it is standard to analyze results based on intention to treat rather than actual treatment provided.[87] Additionally, the statistical handling of outliers should be specifically addressed in the study methods section.

Regarding significance, the p value for an intervention may be statistically significant, but the difference fails to approach clinical relevance. Depending on secondary issues such as various assigned costs, the proposed intervention may not be appropriate to recommend. Conversely, a p value that is not significant means there is no difference or the sample size is too small to demonstrate a difference. Unfortunately, a nonsignificant p value does not distinguish between these results. Since the p value is not a measure of association and is an arbitrary construct based on a cutoff-point "yes-no" dichotomy, many have questioned its value. Instead, *confidence intervals* (*CI*) provide a better assessment of evidence strength and definitiveness of the study at hand.[88] A 95% confidence interval implies high probability that the value given is included within the specified range. The larger the clinical trial, the narrower the confidence interval, increasing the likelihood that the result is definitive. If the confidence interval overlaps zero difference (e.g., 95% CI = −2.0 to 10) between groups under study, the strength of inference is far weaker than a situation with no overlap. Despite the advantages, CI reporting is still not prevalent in the medical literature.

Finally, the ideal clinical interpretation of treatment or diagnostic efficacy includes the likelihood that an effect will be realized if a given intervention is applied. These statements of likelihood are embodied in (1) the number needed to treat (NNT), (2) the relative and absolute risk reduction (RRR and ARR) in cohort studies, and (3) the odds ratio (OR) in case-controlled studies. These inter-related calculations allow comparison of practical clinical applicability between available interventions—that is, if a given treatment or test is proposed for a patient, what is the probability that the intervention will be effective (Table 2.4).

The relative significance of the odds ratio (case control) or relative risk (cohort or RCT) in determining strength of evidence depends upon the clinical scenario. The more the effect carries clinically important consequences, the lower the number which may be considered significant. Also, since a case control study has greater potential for bias than a cohort study or RCT, a significant odds ratio should exceed 3 or 4. In comparison, a relative risk for a cohort study or RCT may be considered significant at a level of 1 to 2.

However, statements about risk reduction do not always help in making decisions about when to offer a treatment to a particular patient. Thinking about clinical problems using the NNT construct provides the clinician with an idea of how applicable a risk reduction is to a given population or even a particular patient. The NNT is calculated by taking the inverse of the ARR (Table 2.4). It tells us how many patients need to be treated with the intervention in question to achieve one additional benefit (i.e. marginal benefit). For example, assume the risk of outcome (O) for new treatment (y) is 40%, and the risk for the same outcome (O) is 65% for control treatment (x). The ARR is: $x - y = 25\%$. Since NNT is the inverse of this number we arrive at $1/0.25 = 4$. In other words, four patients would need to receive treatment y in order to achieve the outcome (O). As the ARR increases, fewer patients need to be treated to achieve the desired outcome. Ideally the NNT calculation should be bounded by a 95% CI in order to appreciate the precision of the number. The broader the CI, the less convincing the argument is for an intervention or for a statement regarding harm.

Unfortunately, methodology of NNT reporting is not uniform in the literature and several caveats are critical. First, the NNT can only be calculated from an ARR not a RRR or an OR. The ARR allows the NNT to assess the clinical magnitude of the outcome or treatment effect. The RRR does not discriminate between a 70% reduction of an outcome from 90% to 20% vs. 0.00090% to 0.00020%. In the former situation the NNT is $1/70 = 1.4$ (i.e. less than 2 patients need to be treated), and in the latter it is $1/.00070 = 1429$ (i.e. more than 1400 patients need to be treated). In case control studies, OR may be converted to NNT if the particular population patient expected even rate (PEER) is known by the following formula, in which RRR × PEER = ARR[50]:

$$NNT = \frac{1 - [PEER \times (1 - OR)]}{(1 - PEER) \times PEER \times (1 - OR)}$$

Rapid calculation of these values, and those related to the following discussion regarding diagnostic tests, is made possible via free or low cost software for personal digital assistants (PDA) such as the hand held Palm PILOT (http://i.am/healthypalmpilot/).

The NNT outcome event noted in Table 2.4 can be favorable (benefit) or unfavorable (risk or harm), sometimes denoted as NNH or number needed to harm. It may be desirable to know how many patients would require treatment to yield that one additional (marginal) benefit, harm, or both. Thus, an additional modification to the NNT formula, which addresses both the marginal benefit and the marginal harm or risk of a given intervention, yields:

$$NNT = \frac{1}{(benefit_1 - benefit_2) + (risk_1 - risk_2)}$$

Alternatively, the NNT can be compared to the NNH in order to define the relative benefit associated with providing a treatment. Decision thresholds for the absolute NNT or NNH will depend upon the clinical situation, and the physician's and patient's risk aversion profile. For example, if the adverse outcome is significant or severe enough in terms of harm (i.e. morbidity, mortality or costs), it may be prudent to increase the threshold for an acceptable NNH before considering the treatment (e.g. NNH = 100 rather than NNH = 5). Of course, all of this depends upon the available alternatives. In-depth consideration of multiple parameters involving risks, benefits and costs requires formal decision analysis, which is introduced later in this chapter.

DIAGNOSTIC TEST ANALYSIS

Evaluation of diagnostic tests is based on the outcome possibilities of true positive and negative results versus false positive and negative results. These give rise to the following familiar formulas:

Sensitivity = true positive/(true positive + false negative) = true positive rate

Specificity = true negative/(true negative + false positive) = true negative rate

Most tests have a range which overlaps a diseased vs. non-diseased state.

Thus, both sensitivity and specificity are influenced by the choice of a test's normal vs. abnormal cutoff point within this overlapping range of values. Ideally, the cutoff is set to minimize both false positive and false negative results. The exact point may be influenced by the medical or economic consequences of an excess in sensitivity or specificity. For example, would too high of a sensitivity lead to excess additional testing, resulting in higher cost and possible morbidity. Assuming an appropriate cutoff point, a negative test result of a highly sensitive test effectively rules out a condition. Conversely, a positive result of a highly specific condition rules in a diagnosis.

Prevalence of a disease state is approximated by the *prior probability* or estimated likelihood that the patient has the disease prior to performing the test, and has a major impact on the usefulness or predictive value of a test.

$$\text{Positive predictive value} = \frac{\text{patients with positive test and disease}}{\text{all patients with positive test}}$$

$$\text{Negative predictive value} = \frac{\text{patients with negative test and no disease}}{\text{all patients with negative test}}$$

With high prevalence conditions, the positive predictive value of a test is high and the negative predictive value low. The converse holds true for low prevalence conditions. However, better tests have good positive predictive value even if prevalence is low.

With respect to assessment of diagnostic testing modalities, the marginal role of each test is to increase diagnostic certainty. How much more information does that one additional test provide and at what value cutoff point? None of our testing tools are 100% accurate, so the information obtained from a given test can best be assessed by receiver operating characteristic (ROC) curves. The ROC curve plots sensitivity versus the false positive rate. The inverse relationship between sensitivity and specificity becomes obvious in evaluating an ROC curve, with the perfect test having an area under the curve (AUC) of 1.0, representing sensitivity = 1 and specificity = 1. Thus, the most ideal attainable test value approaches the upper left-hand corner of the curve (Fig. 2.1).

A poor test has a curve of 45° at a diagonal left to right, with an equal loss of specificity for each marginal gain in sensitivity. For most tests, there is a steep ascending portion of the curve that represents excellent gains in sensitivity with minimal loss in specificity. The best cutoff value for a test is the point at which the curve turns and flattens out, representing greater losses of specificity for minimal marginal improvement in sensitivity. In Figure 2.1, a test value around 60 would be ideal. An attractive feature of ROC curves in diagnostic test selection is that the curves can be compared to determine which test gets closest to the upper left-hand corner and has the largest AUC (i.e., the "best" test). A clinically useful way to approach test result analysis is to look at that point/value beyond which the condition or disorder in question becomes highly

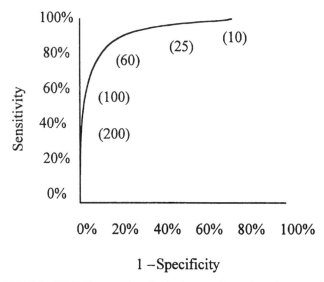

FIGURE 2.1. ROC Curve. Hypothetical test values given in parentheses.

probable or improbable. This approach moves beyond Gaussian distributions and standard deviations or cutoff points. It minimizes use of redundant testing modalities by introducing an incremental or marginal analysis mind set. In other words, how much more certain am I going to be of the diagnosis after a given test? Does additional testing beyond this result improve my diagnostic yield by 1% or 20%?

The first task is to estimate, calculate or use established/published pre-test odds that a condition exists. For example, a new 5 × 6 cm adnexal mass in a 60 yo patient, with smooth, cystic and mobile characteristics, may represent a 50% chance of malignancy. The 50% odds may have been published in a significant series of adnexal masses or may be calculated if supporting information is provided in the form of a 2 × 2 table, such as Table 2.4.

$$\text{Prevalence} = (a + c)/(a + b + c + d) = \text{outcome present/all patients in sample population}$$
$$\text{Pre-test odds} = \text{prevalence}/(1 - \text{prevalence})$$

Can this level of diagnostic certainty be improved such that pre-operative planning is optimized? A pelvic ultrasound is quite commonly ordered in these situations. As an illustrative example, a pelvic ultrasound may have a sensitivity of 90% and a specificity of 70% for predicting malignancy findings at surgery. A derivative of these numbers is the likelihood ratio (LR) for a positive or negative test:

$$LR+ = sensitivity/(1 - specificity)$$
$$LR- = (1 - sensitivity)/specificity$$

Basically, 30% of patients (100%–70%) with ultrasound characteristics suggestive of malignancy do not turn out to have ovarian cancer. So the LR+ = 90/30% = 3. Therefore, the pre-test odds of malignancy were 50%, or 1 : 1 by convention. The post test odds are a product of the LR and the pre-test odds. In this case, post test odds = 3 × 1 : 1 = 3 : 1. The post test probability that the condition exists is 3/3 + 1 = 75%. The probability of malignancy is now 75%, making this a test which added significant marginal value. Conversely, in order to rule out a cancer, the likelihood ratio of a negative test result (i.e. an ultrasound not suggestive of ovarian cancer) can be calculated in a similar fashion as follows:

$LR- = 10/70\% = 0.14$

Post-test odds = $1 \times 0.14 = 0.14$

Post-test probability that ovarian cancer exists = $0.14/1.14 = 12\%$

The same logic can be applied to determine if CA125, other tumor markers, computerized tomography, or magnetic resonance imaging would provide significant incremental value. Several tests may be equal in incremental value as the primary test, but involve cost considerations. These economic analysis issues are addressed later in this chapter, and the testing sequence may be best determined via formal multi-factorial decision analysis.

Diagnostic test results may report multilevel likelihood ratios from a very positive result, through a range of neutral or indeterminate results, to a highly negative result. The pulmonary ventilation-perfusion (V-Q) scan is an example of reporting the probability of pulmonary embolism in this fashion. The V-Q scan results must be correlated with the clinical picture (i.e. pre-test odds) in order to make an optimal treatment decision. In general, a highly positive LR (i.e. >10) with pre-test probability of >33% will generate post-test probabilities in excess of 83%. On the other hand, with a highly negative LR (i.e. <0.1), pre-test probability of <33% translates into a post-test probability of <5%. In the indeterminate LR range, a series of clinical decision sequelae is possible, but depending on the pre-test odds, additional testing may be required. Ideally, for any test, the range of LR and pre-test probabilities must be correlated in order to determine the post-test probability, the marginal clinical impact and need for further testing. Not doing so, instead relying on the high sensitivity or specificity of a seemingly good test at a given cutoff, may lead to a sub-optimal decision. This is because the precise value obtained within the test's range may represent an indeterminate LR approaching 1, reflecting a zero marginal benefit for the test. In other words, the pre-test probability equals the post-test probability at best. For an in-depth discussion of diagnostic test analysis, interested readers are referred to other works.[66,89]

DECISION ANALYSIS PRIMER

Lack of a formal manner by which to approach multifactorial risk decisions is akin to attempting preparation of an annual income tax statement in your head. Some clinical decisions are straight forward, or at least seem to be. However, when multiple diagnostic tests and findings are entertained, a free-form decision will fail to take all issues into weighed consideration.

Decision analysis rests upon the concept of *expected value*. Using computer-assisted modeling, such as DATA^{TM} from TreeAge Software Inc.[90] (Williamstown, MA), all uncertainties are put into perspective and analyzed using Markov (recursive) processes.[91] A Markov model is a recursively defined system with a finite number of states. It is used to model changes to an individual or population over time. An influence diagram is usually initially constructed, defining all factors that affect the decision and how they are related. Then a decision tree is created that includes the following tenets:

1. Time flows from left to right and events are placed in proper sequence.
2. All clinically important final outcomes must be represented.
3. Nodes are designated as a decision, an uncertainty, or an outcome.
4. Branches emanating from a decision node represent all available options.
5. Branches emanating from a chance node represent all possible clinically important outcomes.
6. Probabilities of events are assigned at each chance node and payoffs are assigned at each terminal outcome node.

Figure 2.2 represents a very rudimentary tree in which colorectal cancer screening tests are ordered in several possible combinations. Probabilities, based on best available evidence via EBM approach, are assigned to each chance node. The tree can then be "rolled back" by the computer program in order to determine which path is the most likely to provide the best desired outcome, and at what expected value (i.e., the outcome value that can be expected on average). The utility outcome or payoff measure may be defined as optimal detection, minimal morbidity, optimal cost structure, quality of life, and so on. For any decision or chance node branch, a sensitivity analysis may be performed and a tornado diagram created, graphically displaying which decision and chance points have the greatest relative uncertainty effects on the final outcome. Each variable undergoing analysis is represented by a horizontal bar, summarizing the range of possible model outcomes generated by varying the related variable. A wide bar indicates that the associated variable has a large potential effect on the expected value of the model. The graph is called a tornado diagram because the horizontal bars are arranged in order. The widest bar, representing the most critical uncertainty, is displayed at the top. The result is a funnel shaped visual aid displaying a sensitivity analysis comparing key variable impact on the model.

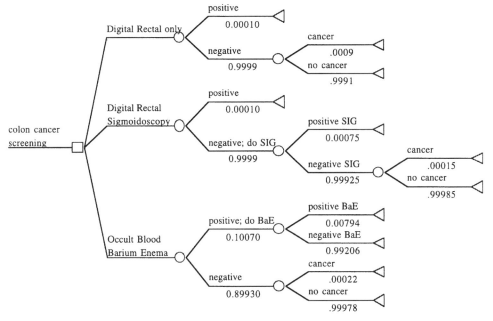

FIGURE 2.2. Basic decision analysis tree.

Validity of decision analysis must be iteratively reviewed during model construction as well as at the time of analysis. The following key questions should be kept in mind:

1. Was the appropriate decision model used?
2. Were all appropriate strategies included and in a clinically appropriate sequence?
3. Were all clinically relevant outcomes considered?
4. Was an explicit and appropriate process used to collect and transform the available evidence into the probabilities used within the tree?
5. Were appropriate utilities assigned to the possible outcomes?
6. Were the appropriate sensitivity analyses conducted?

The last item is particularly important since the quality of input equals the quality of output. If the entire result is overly dependent on a chance or decision data point that is not very precise or not well substantiated, the definitiveness of the result is in question.

Serious limitations of decision analysis include (1) availability and quality of data in formulation of chance node probabilities is questionable, (2) complex medical decisions may be overly simplified, and (3) assignment of utilities to the outcomes can be very subjective. Although decision analysis is a very complex subject, information technology and user-friendly, inexpensive computer programs are leveling the playing field. Several very useful references can provide enough background such that basic decision analysis can be readily incorporated into relatively complex clinical decision making.[21,89,92–96]

ECONOMIC ANALYSIS PRIMER

An economic analysis concentrates on choices and trade-offs in resource allocation, possibly including established diagnostic testing, treatment intervention, or application of emerging technologies. The ultimate economic outcome of interest is usually cost in relation to some utilization or outcome parameter. This is the first problem. Costs are exceedingly difficult to correctly define and assign.[97,98] Furthermore, the perspective (e.g., payor vs. provider vs. patient vs. society) of the analysis determines the types of costs considered. Table 2.5 lists types of costs generally considered in various analyses and their definitions. The list is by no means exhaustive. For example, if a study on cost-effectiveness is conducted over a long period of time, issues such as short-term versus long-term costs arise. These two time frames have a different intrinsic distribution of fixed and variable direct costs. Additionally, the economic cost accrued today is not the same as that over a period of time due to inflation and cost of money provided (i.e., interest or hurdle rates), at which point discounting methods, need to be employed.[99,100] If the study period exceeds 1 year, a discount rate to adjust for present value should be applied, with published estimates ranging from 3% to 7%.[101]

Due to difficulties in measuring the subjective costs of pain, suffering, morbidity/mortality, and some opportunity costs, most analyses concentrate on the direct costs of providing a medical service. However, this policy can skew the true clinical meaning and validity of a given study.

The population type also influences the cost issue. For example, older gynecologic cancer patients are often Medicare beneficiaries. Therefore, many economic analyses from the payor perspective have been based on cost estimates from Medicare data. These are based on diagnosis-related groups (DRG) and are paid by Medicare in a fixed amount per hospitalization. It follows that any additional costs incurred by the provider would not be considered in an analysis based on Medicare DRG cost data, even though they will clearly affect the provider's profit/loss. In general, indirect reference-based measures of cost, such as *cost-to-charge ratios*, can be very misleading due to charge fluctuations and an inconsistent relationship between true costs for rendering a service and a charge.[102] For this reason, economic analysis validity is enhanced greatly when a direct measurement of cost, such as activity-based costing/management, is used.[103]

It should be apparent that even the seemingly simple task of accurately defining and assigning a cost structure is foreboding. However, once it is performed, the next equally challenging step is assigning a value to a given health benefit from an intervention or test. If there is an objective medical measurement such as blood pressure readings, it must be accurately defined and used. In the

TABLE 2.5. Cost Definitions

Cost	A sacrifice of resources, regardless of whether it is accounted for as an asset or expense (not equal to expense per se)
Expense	A cost charged against a revenue in a given accounting period (not equal to cost per se)
Direct medical cost	Costs of medical services provided
Direct nonmedical cost	Costs of additional related services such as transportation, transfer of materials
Indirect cost	Costs indirectly impacting patient care such as administration, housekeeping, engineering
Direct variable cost	Costs that change in direct proportion with changes in volume of service provided
Direct fixed cost	Costs that do not change as volume changes within a relevant range of activity
Semifixed/step cost	Costs that increase in steps with volume or outcome, such as academic salary adjustments
Total cost	Variable costs + fixed costs
Average cost	Total cost divided by the total quantity of output
Marginal cost	Addition to total cost that results from one additional unit of output or benefit
Opportunity cost	A foregone benefit that could have been realized from the best foregone alternative use of a resource: time, money, health benefit, etc.
Intangible cost	Costs of pain and suffering
Morbidity cost	Costs of economic loss due to work missed
Mortality cost	Costs of economic productivity loss due to death

absence of objective measurements, or as a supplement, quality-adjusted life years (QALY) provide a very common metric for differentiating interventions that require a patient's subjective preferences for a specific outcome.[104–106] An alternative is the health years equivalent (HYE), which incorporates the likelihood of deterioration or improvement in condition over time.[107] These metrics have been determined by patient utility preferences as well as community-defined preferences, with no consensus as to which one is better.[104,108] Unfortunately, there is no good way to assess QALYs and HYEs per intervention when a patient has multiple disabling conditions. Both methods have their critics, but a better alternative is elusive.

Economic analysis studies are often mislabeled. Several different types exist and depend on the goal of the study. First and foremost, prior to any economic analysis, well-documented evidence-based data regarding pure clinical effectiveness should be sought. Once clinical effectiveness is established, the goal of economic assessment is defined and questions are formulated, yielding the appropriate study design as summarized in Table 2.6.

TABLE 2.6. Economic Analyses[a]

Question	Outcome Units	Study Design
Which of several similar interventions that yield similar outcomes should be chosen?	Equal medical outcomes	Cost-minimization analysis (CMA)
Which of several interventions that yield clinically different outcomes should be chosen?	Medical units e.g., mmHg pressure	Cost-effectiveness analysis (CEA)
Which of several similar interventions that affect quality of life or patient preferences should be chosen?	Quality-adjusted life years (QALY) or health years equivalent (HYE)	Cost-utility analysis (CUA)
Which of several different interventions with differing outcomes, also expressed in terms of cost, should be chosen?	Monetary	Cost-benefit analysis (CBA)

[a]Cost units for *all* study designs are in monetary terms (e.g., dollars).

Cost-Minimization Analysis

The simplest analysis determines which is the least costly of clinically equivalent interventions. An example might be comparison of equivalent same-generation, same–side effects, same–coverage spectrum antibiotics from several vendors.

Cost-Effectiveness Analysis

When comparing several interventions with different clinical outcomes, the effectiveness of the intervention is compared using clinical effect on the same medical units (e.g., medication A and medication B effect on mmHg reduction in blood pressure). If the outcome units differ, some common denominator must be sought, such as survival.

Once a cost and clinical effect for the study interventions are determined, a cost-effectiveness ratio (C/E) is reported.[106,109–111] Although most often an *average* total cost is used in reporting cost-effectiveness, the optimal assessment should be based on *marginal* cost versus marginal benefit. In other words, how much more cost is associated with one more unit of benefit or with the next most effective option?[89,112]

An additional requirement of appropriate reporting of C/E studies is presentation of alternative scenario–based sensitivity analyses. This factor indicates the stability or definitiveness of the reported findings.[110]

Cost-Utility Analysis

When utility or preference is the outcome, reported as QALY or HYE, the analysis becomes a specific type of cost-effectiveness assessment. It determines the clinical outcome benefits gained in terms of a *time trade-off* of preference for raw life years gained versus the quality of life in those years. The alternative is a *standard gamble* technique, which asks the patient to rate the utility of a sure outcome (e.g., chronic pain) versus a gamble on a possible alternative outcome with an intervention (e.g., motor nerve damage with surgical intervention).

Cost-Benefit Analysis

This method of analysis is less frequently used because of the difficulty of assigning a monetary amount to an outcome, such as a QALY gained or medical complication avoided. The intervention cost and benefit are both expressed in monetary terms, such that the interventions can be compared for best value for dollars spent in health care delivery.

Finally, a decision analysis tree can be structured rather than a pure spreadsheet cost model. This analysis offers greater versatility by visually representing the decision and chance issues (nodes) and can calculate effectiveness, cost-effectiveness, dollars per QALY for a given intervention, and so forth.

TOWARD EFFECTIVE GUIDELINE DEVELOPMENT AND IMPLEMENTATION

Guidelines merely point toward a path of decreasing clinical practice variance. They are *not* standards. This difference is critical. A *standard* may be proposed when the outcomes of intervention are known at EBM Level I and there is unanimous agreement that exceptions are rare. *Guidelines* are recommended when the outcomes are mixed, the evidence is generally EBM Level II, and there is agreement that exceptions are fairly common. Lastly, *options* may be advanced when the outcomes are unknown or the evidence is generally based on Level III data. The latter may be regarded as pure opinion, although the options are still based on expert review and are still "guides" in principle when compared to free-form intervention decision making.

Currently there are more than 1,500 published guidelines, which in general have failed to reduce clinical practice variance.[113] The most often cited reason is that the guidelines have been externally generated, thus failing to achieve significant local approval. Furthermore, most guidelines are developed without a defined systematic EBM process, instead being generated via consensus approach, which is wide open to bias.[60] Even when the development process is defined, the written guidelines often fail to note which recommendations are based on high-level evidence and which are opinions.[114] In addition, guidelines will not have an impact unless the outcomes are measurable such that pro-

TABLE 2.7. Guideline Attributes for Development or Assessment

Can provide guidance toward decreasing assignable practice variance
Are systematically developed, evidence based, and current
Are clearly defined and optimally categorized by strength of evidence
• Standards
• Guidelines
• Options
Provide flexibility at guideline and option levels, with exceptions noted
The guidelines are implementable
The outcomes are measurable

cess improvement can be initiated via guideline modification—that is, guideline implementation should be a dynamic rather than a static process.

Is there a mechanism by which guidelines can be meaningfully generated and implemented? First, it must be decided which practice patterns have significant reducible, assignable practice variance. Second, the attributes of good guidelines and their purpose must be understood (Table 2.7). Third, it must be decided if appropriate guidelines already exist for the problem at hand or if new guidelines are required. Fourth, guidelines must be designed, generated, or modified. Fifth, guidelines must be implemented.[77,115]

Since guideline development is a time- and resource-intensive process, a more efficient approach at the local practitioner level may be existing guideline assessment and/or modification. First, it is important to determine who developed the guidelines and whether the guidelines fit the population at hand. Second, the methodology of guideline development should be determined. The underlying evidence for the guidelines must be substantiated as described in this chapter and explicitly noted. This process may require an updated search of primary literature in order to ensure that the recommendations are current. Third, the established measurable outcomes should coincide with the goals for guideline requirement. For example, if a set of guidelines is developed to improve quality or manage variance, it may not fulfill needs for a cost-containment or optimal utilization program. Fourth, the guidelines should close the gap between the current clinical practice outcomes and the outcomes desired. Fifth, the guidelines should be implemented in a cost-efficient and practical fashion. If the effort and use of resources required to implement the guidelines exceed the anticipated benefits, the implementation should be reconsidered.

Implementation is generally regarded as the most difficult phase of the guideline development or incorporation process. Even before development or appropriateness assessment of existing guidelines, the organizational dynamics must be considered. Often, the organization must be prepared for implementation, obtaining buy-in for the process from top to bottom. Additionally, understanding physician behavior modification is a separate skill set that must be sought and developed by the organization.

Table 2.8 represents the relative effectiveness of development, dissemination,

TABLE 2.8. Guideline Strategies

Development Strategy	Dissemination Strategy	Implementation Strategy
Internal	Specific education	Patient-specific reminder at time of visit
Intermediate	Continuing medical education (CME)	Patient-specific feedback
External, local	Mailing targeted groups	General feedback
External, national	Journal publications	General reminder

and implementation strategies.[116] If a set of guidelines fails within an organization, the question should not be, "what is wrong with the practitioners," but rather, "what is wrong with the guidelines and the implementation process?" The guideline process is dynamic and even relative successes should be viewed as works in progress. As new information becomes available, modifications are required.

BEST PRACTICES LOOP MODEL

Synthesizing all of the information-gathering, evidence-grading, and analysis tools yields a useful framework toward continually improved best practices. Elements of the cross-industry plan-do-check/study-act (PDCA/PDSA) improvement-cycle loop are employed.[43] The resulting continuous-loop feedback model (Fig. 2.3) promotes the collection, interpretation, and integration into practice of valid, important, and relevant patient-reported, clinician-observed, and research-based evidence. The best available evidence, moderated by specific clinical circumstances and judgment, is integrated into evolving practice patterns. The outcomes are continually assessed, which modify the loop along with any newly available and relevant external evidence.

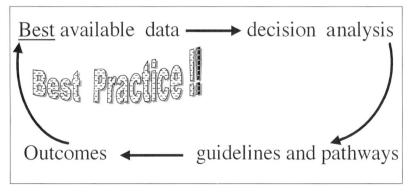

FIGURE 2.3. Evidence-based continuous-loop feedback model.

REFERENCES

1a. Russell B. Sceptical Essays. New York, NY. W. W. Norton and Company, Inc. 1928.

1b. Covell DG, Uman GC, Manning PR. Information needs in office practice: Are they being met? *Ann Intern Med* 1985;103:596–599.

2. Olatunbosun OA, Edouard L, Pierson RA. Physician's attitudes toward evidence based obstetric practice: a questionnaire survey. *Br Med J* 1998;316:365–366.

3. Field MJ, Lohr KN. *Guidelines for Clinical Practice. Institute of Medicine.* Washington, DC: National Academy Press, 1992, p. 34.

4. Bordley DR, Fagan M, Theige D. Evidence-based medicine: a powerful educational tool for clerkship education. *Am J Med* 1997;102:427–432.

5. Chassin MR, Galvin RW. The urgent need to improve healthcare quality. *JAMA* 1998;280:1000–1005.

6. Chassin MR, Brook RH, Park RE, Keesey J, Fink A, Kosecoff J, et al. Variations in the use of medical and surgical services by the Medicare population. *N Eng J Med* 1986;314:285–290.

7. Hampton JR. Evidence based medicine, practice variations and clinical freedom. *J Eval Clin Practice* 1997;3:123–131.

8. Marwick C. Proponents gather to discuss practicing evidence based medicine. *JAMA* 1997;278;531–532.

9. Weinstein MW. Checking medicine's vital signs. *New York Times Magazine*, April 19, 1998, pp. 36–37.

10. Wennberg DE. Variations in the delivery of health care: the stakes are high. *Ann Intern Med* 1998;128:866–868.

11. Wennberg J. Dealing with medical practice variations: a proposal for action. *Health Aff Millwood* 1984;3(2):6–32.

12. Eddy DM. *Clinical Decision Making: From Theory to Practice: A Collection of Essays from JAMA.* Boston: Jones and Bartlett Publishers, 1996, p. 5.

13. Stafford RS, Singer DE. National patterns of warfarin use in atrial fibrillation. *Arch Intern Med* 1996;156:2537–2541.

14. Walton, M. *The Deming Management Method.* New York: Putnam Publishing Co., 1986.

15. Shafer SM, Meredith JR. Quality control. In Shafer SM, Meredith JR (Eds), *Operations Management.* New York. John Wiley and Sons, 1998, pp. 741–747.

16. Naylor CD. Grey zones of clinical practice: some limits to evidence based medicine. *Lancet* 1995;345:840–842.

17. Rodarte JR. Evidence based surgery. *Mayo Clin Proc* 1998;73:603.

18. Smith R. Where is the wisdom: the poverty of medical evidence. *Br Med J* 1991;303:798–799.

19. Woolf SH. Practice guidelines, a new reality in medicine: II. Methods of developing guidelines. *Arch Intern Med* 1992;152:946–952.

20. Sackett DL, Rosenberg WMC, Gray JAM, et al. Evidence-based medicine: what it is and what it isn't. *Br Med J* 1996;312:71–72.

21. Deedwania PC. Underutilization of evidence based therapy in heart failure. An

opportunity to deal a winning hand with an ace up your sleeve. *Arch Intern Med* 1997;157;2409–2412.

22. Kaska SC, Weinstein JN. Historical perspective. Ernest Amory Codman, 1869–1940. A pioneer of evidence based medicine: the end result idea. *Spine* 1998;23:629–633.

23. Rangachari PK. Evidence based medicine: Old French wine with a new Canadian label? *J Royal Soc Med* 1997;90:280–284.

24. Auplish S. Using clinical audit to promote evidence based medicine and clinical effectiveness: an overview of one health authority's experience. *J Eval Clin Prac* 1997;3:77–82.

25. Bero L, Rennie D. The Cochrane Collaboration: Preparing, maintaining and disseminating systematic reviews of the effects of health care. *JAMA* 1995;274:1935–1938.

26. Jadad AR, Haynes RB. The Cochrane Collaboration: advances and challenges in improving evidence based decision making. *Med Decision Making* 1998;18:2–9.

27. Freemantle N, Mason JM, Haines A, Eccles MP. CONSORT: an important step toward evidence based health care. Consolidated standards of reporting trials. *Ann Intern Med* 1997;126:81–83.

28. Rosenberg W, Donald A. Evidence based medicine: an approach to clinical problem solving. *Br Med J* 1995;310:1122–1126.

29. Feinstein AR, Horwitz RI. Problems in the "evidence" of "evidence based medicine." *Am J Med* 1997;103:529–535.

30. Kernick DP. Lies, damned lies, and evidence based medicine. *Lancet* 1998;351:1824.

31. Horwitz RI. The dark side of evidence based medicine. *Clev Clin J Med* 1996;63:320–323.

32. Shahar E. A Popperian perspective of the term "evidence based medicine." *J Eval Clin Prac* 1997;3:109–116.

33. Baird MA. Physician-patient-family trust: the bridge to reach evidence based medicine. *Fam Med* 1996;28:682–683.

34. Ellrodt G, Cook DJ, Lee J, Cho M, Hunt D, Weingarten S. Evidence based disease management. *JAMA* 1997;278:1687–1692.

35. Cohen JJ. Higher quality at lower cost: maybe there is a way. *Acad Med* 1998;73:414–419.

36. Carpenter CE, Bender DA, Nash DB, Cornman JM. Must we choose between quality and costs? *Quality in Healthcare* 1996;5:223–229.

37. Evidence Based Medicine Working Group. Evidence-based medicine: a new approach to teaching the practice of medicine. *JAMA* 1992;268:2420–2425.

38. Rafuse J. Evidence based medicine means MDs must develop new skills, attitudes, CMA conference told. *CMAJ* 1994;150:1479–1481.

39. Cook D. Evidence based critical care medicine: a potential tool for change. *New Horizons* 1998;6:20–25.

40. Cook DJ, Sibbald WJ, Vincent JL, Cerra FB. Evidence based critical care medicine: What is it and what can it do for us? Evidence based medicine in critical care group. *Crit Care Med* 1996;24:334–337.

41. Vanderbroucke JP. Observational research and evidence based medicine: What should we teach young physicians? *J Clin Epidemiol* 1998;51:467–472.

42. Senge PM. *The Fifth Discipline: The Art and Practice of the Learning Organization.* New York: Bantam Doubleday Dell Publishing Group Inc., 1990.

43. Berwick DM. Developing and testing changes in the delivery of care. *Ann Intern Med* 1998;128:833–838.

44. Davis D. *The Physician as a Learner.* Chicago: AMA Press, 1994.

45. Davis DA, Thomson MA, Oxman AD, et al. Changing physician performance. A systematic review of the effect of continuing medical education strategies. *JAMA* 1995;274:700–705.

46. Davis DA, Thomson MA, Oxman AD, et al. Evidence for the effectiveness of CME: a review of 50 randomized controlled trials. *JAMA* 1992;268:1111–1117.

47. Green ML, Ellis PJ. Impact of an evidence based medicine curriculum based on adult learning theory. *J Gen Intern Med* 1997;12:742–750.

48. Bennett RJ, Sackett DL, Haynes RB, Neufeld VR. A controlled clinical trial of teaching critical appraisal of clinical literature to medical students. *JAMA* 1987;257:2451–2454.

49. Shin JH, Haynes RB, Johnston ME. Effect of problem based, self directed undergraduate education on life-long learning. *Can Med Assoc J* 1993;148:969–976.

50. Sackett DL. *Evidence Based Medicine: How to Practice and Teach EBM.* London: Churchill Livingstone, 1998.

51. Hersh W. Evidence based medicine and the Internet. *ACP J Club* 1996;125:A14–A16.

52. Kiley R. Evidence based medicine on the Internet. *J Royal Soc Med* 1998;91:74–75.

53. Haynes RB, et al. Developing optimal search strategies for detecting clinically sound studies in MEDLINE. *J Am Med Informatics Assoc* 1994;1:447–458.

54. MacPherson DW. Evidence based medicine. CMAJ 1995;152:201–204.

55. Nwosu CR, Khan KS, Chien PFW. A two term MEDLINE search strategy for identifying randomized trials in obstetrics and gynecology. *Obstet Gynecol* 1998;91:618–622.

56. Thacker SB, Peterson HB, Stroup DF. Meta-analysis for the obstetrician gynecologist. *Am J Obstet Gynecol* 1996;174:1403–1407.

57. Ohlsson A. Systematic reviews—theory and practice. *Scan J Clin Lab Invest* 1994;54(219):25–32.

58. Lelorier J, Gregoire G, Benhaddad A, Lapierre J, Derderian F. Discrepancies between meta-analyses and subsequent large randomized controlled trials. *N Engl J Med* 1997;337:536–542.

59. Lau J, Antman EM, Jimeniez-Silva J, et al. Cumulative meta-analysis of therapeutic trials for myocardial infarction. *N Engl J Med* 1992;327:248–254.

60. Heffner JE. Does evidence based medicine help the development of clinical practice guidelines? *Chest* 1998;113:172S–178S.

61. Berg AO. Clinical practice guidelines: believe only some of what you read. *Family Pract Manage* 1996;3(4):58–70.

62. Begg C, Cho M, Eastwood S, et al. Improving the quality of reporting of randomized controlled trials: the CONSORT statement. *JAMA* 1996;276:637–639.

63. Chalmers TC, Smith H, Blackburn B, et al. A method for assessing the quality of a randomized controlled trial. *Control Clin Trials* 1981;2:31–49.

64. Chalmers I, Dickerson K, Chalmers TC. Getting to grips with Archie Cochrane's agenda. *Br Med J* 1992;304:786–788.

65. Ingelfinger JA, Mosteller F, Thibodeau LA, et al. Reading a report of a clinical trial. In *Biostatistics in Clinical Medicine*, 3rd ed. New York: McGraw Hill, 1994, pp. 259–279.

66. Hulley SB, Cummings SR. *Designing Clinical Research.* Baltimore: Williams and Wilkins, 1988.

67. Oxman AD, Sackett DL, Guyatt GH. User'sguide to the medical literature. I. How to get started. *JAMA* 1993;270:2093–2095.

68. Guyatt GH, Sackett DL, Cook DJ. Evidence-Based Medicine Working Group: User's guide to the medical literature. II. How to use an article about therapy or prevention. A. Are the results of the study valid? *JAMA* 1993;270(21):2598–2601.

69. Guyatt GH, Sackett DL, Cook DJ. User's guide to the medical literature. II. How to use an article about therapy or prevention. B. What were the results and will they help me in caring for my patients? *JAMA* 1994;271:59–63.

70. Jaeschke R, Gyatt GH, Sackett DL. User'sguide to the medical literature. III. How to use an article about a diagnostic test. A. Are the results of the study valid? *JAMA* 1994;271:389–391.

71. Jaeschke R, Gyatt GH, Sackett DL. User's guide to the medical literature. III. How to use an article about a diagnostic test. B. What are the results and will they help me in caring for my patients? *JAMA* 1994;271:703–707.

72. Levine M, Walter S, Lee H, Haines T, Holbrokk A, Moyer V. User's guide to the medical literature. IV. How to use an article about harm. *JAMA* 1994;271:1615–1619.

73. Laupacis A, Wells G, Richardson S, Tugwell P. User's guide to the medical literature. V. How to use an article about prognosis. *JAMA* 1994;272:234–237.

74. Oxman AD, Cook DJ, Guyatt GH. User's guide to the medical literature. VI. How to use an overview. *JAMA* 1994;272:1367–1371.

75. Richardson WS, Detsky AS. User's guide to the medical literature. VII. How to use a clinical decision analysis. A. Are the results of the study valid? *JAMA* 1995;273:1292–1295.

76. Hayward RSA, Wilson M, Tunis SR, Bass EB, Guyatt G. User's guide to the medical literature. VIII. How to use clinical practice guidelines. A. Are the recommendations valid? *JAMA* 1995;274:570–574.

77. Wilson M, Hayward RSA, Tunis S, Bass EB, Guyatt G. User's guide to the medical literature. VIII. How to use clinical practice guidelines. B. What are the recommendations and will they help you in caring for your patients? *JAMA* 1995;274:1630–1632.

78. Guyatt GH, Sackett DL, Sinclair JC, Hayward R, Cook DJ, Cook RJ. User's guide to the medical literature. IX. A method for grading health care recommendations. *JAMA* 274:1800–1804.

79. Naylor CD, Guyatt GH. User's guide to the medical literature. X. How to use an article reporting variations in the outcomes of health services. JAMA 1996;275:554–558.

80. Naylor CD, Guyatt GH. User's guide to the medical literature. XI. How to use an article about clinical utilization review. *JAMA* 1996;275:1435–1439.

81a. U.S. Preventive Health Services Task Force. *Guide to Clinical Preventive Services*, 2nd ed. Baltimore: Williams and Wilkins, 1995.

81b. Schultz KF, Chalmers I, Hayes RJ, et al. Dimensions of methodological quality with estimates of treatment effects in controlled trials. *JAMA* 1995;273:412–415.

82. Colditz GA, Miller JN, Mosteller F. How study design affects outcomes in comparisons of therapy. I. *Med Stat Med* 1989;8:441–454.

83. Miller JN, Colditz GA, Mosteller F. How study design affects outcomes in comparisons of therapy. II. *Surg Stat Med* 1989;8:455–466.

84. Bullock DR, Chestnut R, Clifton G, et al. Guidelines for the management of severe head injury. *Eur J Emerg Med* 1996;3:109–127.

85. Greenhalgh T. Statistics for the non-statistician I. *Br Med J* 1997;315:364–366.

86. Greenhalgh T. Statistics for the non-statistician. II: "Significant" relations and their pitfalls. *Br Med J* 1997;315:422–425.

87. Stewart LA, Parmar MKB. Bias in the analysis and reporting of controlled trials. *Int J Health Tech Assess* 1996;12:264–275.

88. Guyatt G, Jaenschke R, Heddle N, Cook D, Shannon H, Walter S. Basic statistics for clinicians. I. Hypothesis testing. *Can Med Assoc J* 1995;152:27–32.

89. Sox HC Jr, Blatt MA, Higgins MC, Marton KI. *Medical Decision Making*. Newton, MA: Butterworth-Heinemann, 1988, pp. 103–145.

90. DATA^{TM} Decision Analysis program from TreeAge Software. Williamstown, MA; tel 413/458-0104; http://www.treeage.com.

91. Sonnenberg FA, Beck JR. Markov models in decision making: a practical guide. *Med Decision Making* 1993;13:322–328.

92. Detsky AS, Naglie G, Krahn MD, Naimark D, Redelmeier DA. Primer on medical decision analysis: Part 1. Getting started. *Med Decision Making* 1997;17:123–125.

93. Detsky AS, Naglie G, Krahn MD, Redelmeier DA, Naimark D. Primer of medical decision analysis: Part 2. Building a tree. *Med Decision Making* 1997;17:126–135.

94. Naglie G, Murray D, Krahn MD, Naimark D, Redelmeier DA, Detsky AS. Primer on medical decision analysis. Part 3. Estimating probabilities and utilities. *Med Decision Making* 1997;17:136–141.

95. Krahn MD, Naglie G, Naimark D, Redelmeier DA, Detsky AS. Primer on medical decision analysis. Part 4. Analyzing the model and interpreting the results. *Med Decision Making* 1997;17:142–151.

96. Naimark D, Krahn MD, Naglie G, Redelmeier DA, Detsky AS. Primer on medical decision analysis. Part 5. Working with Markov processes. *Med Decision Making* 1997;17:152–159.

97. Schuette HL, Tucker TC, Brown ML. The costs of cancer care in the United States: implications for action. *Oncology* 1995;9(11):19–22.

98. Doubilet PM, Weinstein MC, McNeil BJ. Use and abuse of the term "cost-effective" in medicine. *N Engl J Med* 1986;314:253–256.

99. Keeler EB, Cretin S. Discounting of lifesaving and other monetary benefits. *Manage Sci* 1983;29:300–306.

100. Samuelson WF, Marks SG. *Time Valve of Money in Managerial Economics*, 2nd

ed. Orlando: The Dryden Press/Harcourt Brace College Publishers, 1995, pp. 700–715.

101. Gold MR, Siegel JE, Russell LB. *Cost-Effectiveness in Health and Medicine.* New York: Oxford University Press, 1996.

102. Finkler SA. The distinction between cost and charges. *Ann Intern Med* 1982;96:102–109.

103. Maher M. *Cost Accounting. Creating Value for Management,* 5th ed. McGraw-Hill, 1997, pp. 231–185.

104. Boyle MH, Torrance GW, Sinclair JC, Horwood SP. Economic evaluation of neonatal intensive care very-low-birth-weight infants. *N Engl J Med* 1983;308:1330–1337.

105. Oldridge N, Furlong W, Feeny D. Economic evaluation of cardiac rehabilitation soon after myocardial infarction. *Am J Cardiol* 1993;72:154–161.

106. Russell LB, Gold MR, Siegel JE, Daniels N, Weinstein MC. Panel on cost-effectiveness in health and medicine: the role of cost-effectiveness analysis in health and medicine. *JAMA* 1996;276(14):1172–1177.

107. Mehrez A, Gafni A. Quality adjusted life years, utility theory and health year equivalents. *Med Decision Making* 1989;9:142–149.

108. Nease RF Jr, Kneeland T, O'Connor GT. The Ischemic Heart Disease Patient Outcomes Research Team: variation in patient utilities for outcomes of the management of chronic stable angina: implications for clinical practice guidelines. *JAMA* 1995;273:1185–1190.

109. Weinstein MC, Siegel JE, Gold MR, Kamlet MS, Russell LB. Panel on Cost-Effectiveness in Health and Medicine: recommendations on cost-effectiveness in health and medicine. *JAMA* 1996;275(15):1253–1258.

110. Siegel JE, Weinstein MC, Russell LB, Gold MR. Panel on Cost-Effectiveness in Health and Medicine: recommendations for reporting cost-effectiveness analysis. *JAMA* 1996;276(16):1339–1341.

111. Smith WJ, Blackmore CC. Economic analysis in obstetrics and gynecology. *Obstet Gynecol* 1998;91(3):472–478.

112. Weinstein MC. Principles of cost effective resource allocation in health care organizations. *Int J Technol Assess Health Care* 1990;6:93–103.

113. Kosecoff J, Kanouse DE, Rogers WH, McCloskey L, Winslow CM, Brook RH. Effects of the National Institutes of Health Consensus Development Program on physician practice. *JAMA* 1987;258(19):2708.

114. Winn RJ, Botnick WZ, Brown NH. The NCCN Guideline Program 1998. *Oncology* 1998;12:30–34.

115. Hutchinson A. The philosophy of clinical practice guidelines: purposes, problems, practicality and implementation. *J Qual Clin Pract* 1998;18:63–73.

116. Grimshaw JM, Russell IT. Effects of clinical guidelines on medical practice: a systematic review of rigorous evaluations. *Lancet* 1993;342:1317–1322.

CHAPTER 3

VASCULAR ACCESS AND OTHER INVASIVE PROCEDURES

PAUL KOONINGS, M.D.

Venous access is an important technique in the care and management of gynecological patients. There are two major types of venous access available: peripheral and central.[1] Peripheral venous access is the preferred method unless there is a contraindication to its use. In general, the closer venous access is toward the heart, the greater the frequency and severity of complications.

SHORT-TERM CENTRAL VENOUS CATHETERIZATION

Central venous catheterization has emerged as an integral part of the management of gynecological oncology patients.[2] As many house officers and patients can attest, multiple venipunctures and the prolonged administration of intravenous agents leads to venous irritation. The resultant phlebitis produces a gradual sclerosis with subsequent destruction of these peripheral veins.[3] Hyperosmolar solutions, chemotherapeutic agents, and other irritating intravenous agents are particularly destructive. This absence of adequate peripheral veins may not only delay the administration of chemotherapeutic agents but can result in a higher complication rate secondary to the extravasation of these particularly toxic drugs.

Central venous catheterization has been used in many of these situations to circumvent problems, allowing for reliable venous catheterization, albeit placement and maintenance is not without risk. Indications for central venous catheterization include the absence of peripheral veins, prolonged intravenous therapy, parenteral hyperalimentation, hemodynamic monitoring, and the administration of intensive chemotherapy. Short-term (less than 30 days) catheterization is pri-

Perioperative and Supportive Care in Gynecologic Oncology: Evidence-Based Management,
Edited by Steven A. Vasilev.
ISBN 0-471-24788-X   Copyright © 2000 by Wiley-Liss, Inc.

marily used in the perioperative or immediate postoperative period. The usual indications for short-term central venous catheterization include infusion of large amounts of intravenous solutions including blood products, the need to monitor central venous pressure, or placement of a Swan–Ganz catheter. Short-term parenteral hyperalimentation may also be given through these devices.

There are two primary approaches to central venous catheterization used in the gynecological patient: internal jugular and subclavian. Familiarity with each method is recommended; however, most institutions utilize either the internal jugular or subclavian vein exclusively.[3,4] Needless to say, it is of great importance to understand the anatomy involving each approach. It is precisely because of anatomy that the right side is preferred for each technique. On the left side, the dome of the lung and pleura are elevated while the thoracic duct empties nearby, exposing these structures to possible trauma. Moreover, there is a more direct route to the right atrium when using the right internal jugular approach. This approach should be exclusively used on ventilator patients requiring a central venous line, since a lung puncture can result in a tension pneumothorax.

General Preparation of the Patient

Once the decision for central venous access has been made, informed consent should be obtained from the patient or guardian. Informed consent, including risks, benefits, and alternatives, should be addressed, as well as questions from the patient or guardian.

Following informed consent, an area of 5–10 cm surrounding the proposed introduction site is prepared with an antiseptic solution. Hirsute sites should be depilated with electric clippers. Insertion discomfort should be dealt with aggressively. Intravenous medication (e.g., morphine sulfate and midazolam [Versed]) along with a generous amount of local anesthetic will usually suffice. After the local anesthetic is drawn up in a syringe, it is injected slowly, subcutaneously, using a 25 gauge or smaller needle along the proposed needle tract.

Once the area has been adequately prepped and anesthetized, the clinician should use sterile gloves. If the procedure is nonemergent, the use of sterile drapes, gown, cap, and mask is recommended.

The clinician should be familiar with the prepackaged kits available. A spare kit should be available during insertion in case the original becomes unusable.

Internal Jugular Vein Approach

Anatomy The internal jugular vein extends from the base of the skull adjacent to the carotid artery entering the chest to join the subclavian vein behind the clavicle. It is initially lateral to the carotid artery and moves anterior to the internal carotid artery at the level of C6. It lies posterior to the sternocleidomastoid muscle.

Procedure   The patient undergoes general preparation and is placed in Trendelenburg position (15–30°). The patient's head is turned contralateral to the insertion site, approximately 45°. The anatomical landmarks are identified, including the apex of the triangle formed by the sternocleidomastoid muscle and the base of the trapezius near the clavicle. If the ipsilateral carotid artery can be palpated, it is gently retracted medially. The needle is inserted at the apex of the triangle at a 20–30° angle to the frontal plane, aiming just lateral to the ipsilateral nipple. It is advanced with continuous gentle negative pressure. The jugular vein is usually entered within 3 cm; if the needle catheter is inserted beyond 5 cm, the risk of pneumothorax or arterial puncture increases. Once the vein has been identified and blood may be easily aspirated, the modified Seldinger technique is used to insert the selected catheter. A J-shaped guidewire is gently passed through the needle. This wire must never be forced as vessel rupture could result. Moreover, the wire should never be retracted with the needle in place as this may result in wire shearing. If the guidewire is advanced too far, it may cause premature ventricular beats. In these circumstances, it should be retracted so that the ectopic beats abate. The wire should be constantly held through these maneuvers. The needle is removed and replaced with the vein dilator and catheter. Occasionally the skin puncture site needs to be enlarged sharply. Once the catheter is in place, the dilator and guidewire are removed. Flow of blood is then confirmed and the catheter is connected to the appropriate intravenous solution. The catheter is then anchored to the skin and covered with a gauze dressing. A mandatory end-expiration chest X ray is checked for proper catheter placement and the presence of a pneumothorax.[5–7] Figure 3.1 shows the ideal location of a central venous catheter.

Subclavian Vein Approach

Anatomy   The subclavian vein, a continuation of the axillary vein, arches gently across the first rib in front of the anterior scalene muscle and inferior to the clavicle. Its course approximates that of the deeper subclavian artery, which can be palpated posterior to the clavicular head of the sternocleidomastoid muscle. The thoracic duct enters at the junction of the left subclavian and internal jugular veins.[9–11]

Procedure   The patient is prepared and positioned similar to that for internal jugular intravenous catheterization except that a small pillow is placed between the scapula to elevate the clavicular heads. The puncture site should be located lateral to the midpoint of the clavicle, approximately 1–2 cm below it. Once inserted, the needle should be parallel to the frontal plane just below the clavicle. It is unnecessary to "walk" the needle under the clavicle as this causes extreme pain and discomfort. The index finger may be placed gently in the suprasternal notch to indicate the target area. Mild constant aspiration is applied during needle advancement. Once the free flow of blood is achieved, the needle is advanced 5 mm farther to confirm intraluminal placement. The needle bevel

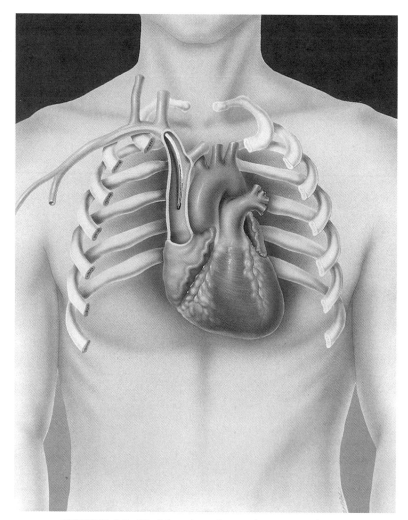

FIGURE 3.1. Ideal location of central venous catheter.

is then oriented toward the heart. A guidewire is threaded through the needle while the patient valsalvas to prevent an air embolus. The needle is replaced with a vein dilator followed by the catheter. It is extremely important not to let go of the guidewire during this procedure. Once the catheter is placed, the guidewire is removed. Blood flow is confirmed and the catheter is connected to the appropriate intravenous solution. The catheter is then anchored and covered. Position and the absence of a pneumothorax are confirmed by a postprocedure end-expiration chest X ray. The catheter tip should be in the superior vena cava above the pericardial reflection (1–2 cm; see Fig. 3.1 for ideal location).

Complications

Complications of central venous catheterization occur during insertion or continued catheter presence. Insertion complications include the inability to cannulize the vein, cardiac arrhythmias, pneumothorax, arterial puncture, and air embolization. It appears that a failed initial insertion is the biggest predictor of complication. Insertion complications can be avoided with increasing experience and meticulous attention to details. It is the responsibility of the surgeon to not only be able to diagnose these complications but to treat them in a timely manner.

Inability to Identify or Cannulize the Central Vein Rarely, the physician is unable to identify and aspirate the central vein after several attempts. In these incidences, the anatomy should be reviewed to make sure that landmarks are correctly identified. The patient's position is checked to make sure that she is in steep Trendelenburg position with her head turned toward the opposite side. If the patient has a peripheral venous catheter, hydration is useful. If these exercises are unsuccessful, there are two further approaches the physician may use. The first approach is to utilize ultrasound to identify the intended central vein.[12,13] A 5 to 7.5 megahertz transducer may identify the vein and allow easier targeting. Failing this, an internal jugular anterior, middle or posterior approach may be used.[14] This should be performed on the ipsilateral side if the subclavian vein catheterization was attempted to obviate the risk of bilateral pneumothorax or paratracheal hematoma.

Cardiac Arrhythmia Occasionally, premature ventricular beats are encountered during catheter placement. These ectopic beats are primarily due to ventricular irritation from the guidewire. Withdrawing the guidewire will usually halt these beats. Rarely are antiarrhythmia agents required.

Pneumothorax The risk of pneumothorax appears inversely related to the experience of the physician.[15] It has been estimated that experienced physicians have one-half the complication rate of inexperienced physicians. Therefore, a physician experienced in central line placement should be present during the actual procedure. The risk of pneumothorax is also related to the approach used. The subclavian approach appears to have a higher preponderance of pneumothorax compared to the internal jugular approach.[16] As previously mentioned, left-sided placements have a higher pneumothorax rate. Chest X ray is the gold standard for diagnosing a pneumothorax. An end-expiration film enhances the diagnosis of pneumothorax. After central venous catheterization has been attempted or completed, it is prudent to obtain a chest X ray. Clinically the patient may complain of sudden onset of chest pain with radiation to the neck as well as shortness of breath. Physical findings occasionally reveal absent breath sounds with tactile fremitus. The treatment for pneumothorax is discussed under "Chest Tube Placement."

Hematoma   The risk of massive hematoma following central venous placement is low.[17] A thorough understanding of the anatomy combined with experience and good technique will reduce this complication. Any history of a bleeding disorder should be evaluated with the appropriate coagulation studies before this procedure is undertaken.

Occasionally, internal jugular venous cannulization can result in an inadvertent carotid artery puncture. Palpation and medial retraction of the carotid artery is helpful. If the carotid artery is inadvertently punctured, direct pressure is usually adequate to control bleeding. Subclavian site bleeding is more difficult to control since direct pressure of the involved vessel is difficult. An expanding hematoma may result in respiratory embarrassment secondary to a paratracheal hematoma. Thoracic surgery consultation should be considered to assist in the management of this complication.

Air Embolism   The deadliest, rarest, and most preventable complication associated with central venous placement is air embolism. Air embolism occurs when there is a break in the circuit, allowing atmospheric pressure to push air into the circulation. A fatal dose of air (100 ml) can be delivered in less than 1 second. The primary opportunities for this devastating condition occur during insertion or removal of the catheter and during line breaks when the intravenous components are changed. Careless technique or equipment failure allows air to enter the venous circulation, which is then pumped into the right ventricular, thereby interrupting blood flow. The patient may complain of chest pain with shortness of breath as well as anxiety. Clinical findings reveal hypotension tachycardia and cog-wheel cardiac murmur.

Air embolism can be prevented during vein cannulation by placing the vein in a dependent position while the patient exhales. Once air embolism is diagnosed or suspected, the patient should be placed in the left lateral Trendelenburg position and given 100% oxygen immediately. The source of the air leak should be located and closed off. A thoracic surgery consult should be considered as well as direct percutaneous suction of the heart.

Complications Related to Catheter Presence   Infection, thrombosis, and positional obstruction are the most common problems associated with catheter presence.[18] The physician who places these catheters needs to know how to recognize and treat these challenges to patient well-being.

Infection   It is estimated that anywhere from 5% to 25% of venous catheters become infected.[19-24] The incidence of infection is directly time related and becomes more common after 72 hours. Diagnosis is made by physical examination, primarily from the catheter site as well as the patient's temperature. Blood and catheter cultures are obtained to confirm the diagnosis. A basic line sepsis algorithm is shown in Figure 3.2, and the topic discussed further in Chapter 11. There appear to be several maneuvers available that decrease the infection rate. Subclavian vein catheters have a lower infection rate than internal jugular

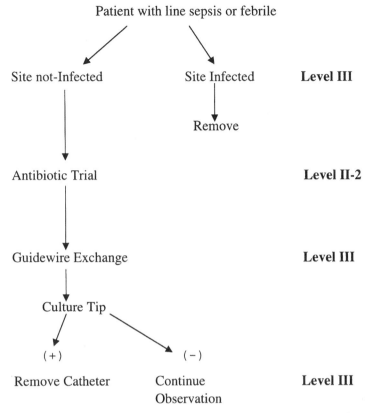

FIGURE 3.2. Suggested management of central venous line sepsis.

venous catheterization. This is believed secondary to the difficulty in keeping the neck area sterile. Therefore, the subclavian approach should be considered, especially in neutropenic patients.

Several studies have examined whether changing the catheter site, changing the catheter over a guidewire, or use of the same site until removal is clinically indicated is of benefit in decreasing the infection rate.[25–28] Studies have not revealed any differences between these aforementioned techniques. An arbitrary rule dictating catheter change every 3 to 7 days appears to be of little, if any, benefit. Therefore, the catheter should be left in place unless there are clinical signs of infection. After the initial enthusiasm for semipermeable dressings for central vein catheterization, recent studies have revealed no advantage over the plain gauze dressing. They may in fact lead to increased infection rate. It is therefore recommended that the catheter exit site be covered with an antibiotic ointment if desired and then covered with a plain gauze dressing. Another issue is whether single-, double-, or triple-lumen catheters have a higher infection rate (Fig. 3.3). In general, the multilumen catheters require more connections,

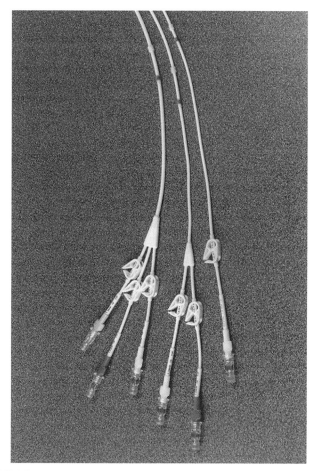

FIGURE 3.3. Examples of one-, two-, and three-channel Hickman catheters.

thereby permitting more opportunities for technique breakdown and bacterial contamination. Therefore, as in other situations, the right catheter for the right job should be selected.

Thrombosis Secondary to Catheter Presence The incidence of catheter-related thrombosis is related to the length of time that the catheter is left in place.[29] Significant thrombosis is unusual in catheters left in place for 2 weeks or less. The signatures of central venous thrombosis are edema, erythema, and pain in either upper extremity. Duplex ultrasound will diagnose venous obstruction while radiographic dye infusion through the catheter will characterize the thrombus. Other clinical clues to the presence of thrombosis include the inability to aspirate and inject through the catheter. Once the diagnosis of catheter-related thrombosis is made, treatment is indicated (Figure 3.4). The patient is

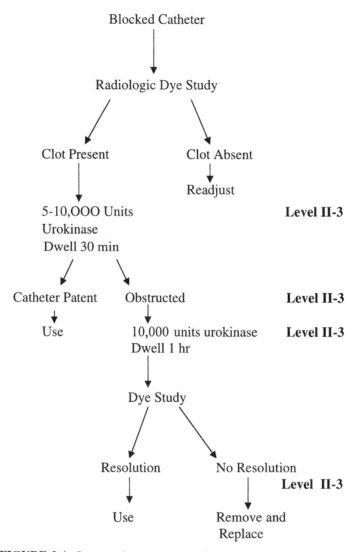

FIGURE 3.4. Suggested management of central venous line blockage.

heparinized with catheter removal until asymptomatic and then placed on warfarin (Coumadin) for approximately 3 months.[30] If continued catheter use is warranted in the face of thrombosis, urokinase or streptokinase infusion may resolve the thrombosis; however, a bleeding diathesis may be significant. Ultimately, if the catheter is not removed, the thrombosis will recur.

Positional Obstruction. Positional obstruction can occur with subclavian catheters.[31] It is related to the medial location of the catheter. This allows the catheter to be pinched off between the clavicle and the first rib. This obstruction is usually intermittent and is relieved when the shoulder is elevated. If not corrected, this condition may result in catheter fracture with subsequent embolus. This complication can be avoided by using an alternate access site once positional obstruction is recognized. To prevent this complication, the venous puncture should be made lateral to the midclavicular line so that the catheter will be inside the lumen of the subclavian vein and therefore protected as it passes over the first rib.

LONG-TERM CENTRAL VENOUS CATHETERIZATION

Over the past two decades, long-term venous catheterization devices have emerged as the benchmark for reliable venous access in patients requiring lengthy intravenous therapy. The decision of whether to place a long-term central venous catheterization device in the patient is dependent on many factors. These factors include the patient's current condition, the availability of effective therapy, and the patient's life expectancy. Patients with malignancy requiring chemotherapy, administration of blood products, and parenteral nutrition have an improved quality of life with these devices. They may also be used for blood draws. It is estimated that approximately 400,000 long-term intravenous catheters are implanted yearly in the United States alone.[1]

Once the decision to place the long-term central venous catheter has been made, a device needs to be selected. Currently, there are two major catheter systems used: those with and without a reservoir. A Mediport is an example of the reservoir type. The reservoir system is completely buried underneath the epidermis. The advantages of this system include minimal maintenance, freedom from dressings and activity restrictions, better cosmesis, and minimal maintenance when compared to the nonreservoir system. A special needle (Huber) that displaces rather than punctures the diaphragm is used to access the reservoir. The major disadvantage of the reservoir type is the increased time (approximately 15 minutes) required to place the reservoir and technical skill. Also, in larger patients transcutaneous access may become a challenge, especially if the port shifts in position. However, its advantages easily outweigh its disadvantages, leading it to become the device of choice. Examples of the nonreservoir type include a Broviac or Hickman catheter. The nonreservoir system usually requires frequent flushing and dressing changes. Moreover, it traverses the epidermis, constantly reminding the patient of her disease, and limits physical activities including swimming and showering.

Procedure

Informed consent should be obtained. The site of the reservoir or exit site of the nonreservoir system should be identified. It is best to do this while the patient wears her brassiere so that the device can be located in such a manner that it will not interfere with or irritate the patient. The reservoir/exit site should not be so far lateral that the patient rubs the device when moving her arm from the device. In patients with large breasts, the port should be located medially so that it can be easily palpated for access. The internal jugular or subclavian vein is located and accessed as previously mentioned, leaving the J-wire in situ with a clamp to prevent migration. The proposed reservoir/exit site is infiltrated with bupivacaine (Marcaine) and an incision is made. If a reservoir port is going to be used, the incision should be approximately 4 to 5 cm long. A 21 gauge spinal needle is then used to infiltrate Marcaine along the proposed catheter track. An introducer/dilator is introduced from the exit of the J-wire to the proposed reservoir/exit site of the catheter. The catheter is attached to the dilator and tunneled in the subcutaneous tissue to where the J-wire is located. The Dacron cuff is placed well within the tunnel. If a reservoir is used, a small crevice is made for it to prevent migration. The reservoir must be anchored to the chest fascia using nonabsorbable monofilament sutures. The catheter is then placed on the chest along its proposed course through the vascular system. It is tailored to a length usually 1 or 2 cm below the sternal notch, approximating the location of the superior vena cava. A peel-away catheter introducer is then inserted along the J-wire into the venous system. The J-wire is removed and the catheter is threaded while the patient valsalvas. The peel-away introducer is retracted, peeled, and removed. Catheter placement is then confirmed using fluoroscopy. The catheter tip should be in the superior vena cava 1 to 2 cm from the right atrium. The incision sites are then closed using either Steri-Strips or subcuticular stitches. The reservoir or catheter can be accessed following a chest X ray to confirm position and to rule out pneumothorax. This should only be done with a Huber needle in the case of the reservoir.

Complications

For practical purposes, recognition, prevention and management of long term catheter complications is similar to that described under short term catheterization.

PULMONARY ARTERY CATHETERIZATION

The Swan–Ganz catheter was first developed and described over a quarter-century ago.[32] Although indications for its use are myriad, its benefits may be elusive.[33] The common theme of most published series is use of the Swan–Ganz in a judicious manner.[33–35] Like most tools in medicine, if not totally familiar with its use, consultation should be obtained. The Swan–Ganz catheter can be inserted via any vein used for central venous catheterization.

Procedure

Informed consent should be obtained from the patient. The equipment should be checked to make sure that all the necessary parts are present for insertion and use and are in working order. Technical difficulties with the equipment are frustrating and easily avoided by examining the equipment prior to use. It is mandatory to examine the catheter balloon for leakage, size, and shape by injecting it with 1.5 ml of air prior to insertion. The expiration date on the catheter should also be checked. Do not inject fluid into the balloon port. All ports must be flushed and checked for patency. The internal jugular vein or subclavian vein is accessed with the J-wire as previously mentioned. The skin incision is then enlarged and a vessel dilator with an introducer stealth is advanced along the J-wire into the vein. Do not let go of the J-wire. The J-wire and dilator are then removed and replaced by the pulmonary artery catheter. The pulmonary artery catheter is gently threaded through the introducer. The tip will approximate the right atrium when it is 10 to 15 cm from the entrance of either the internal jugular or subclavian vein. The balloon is then inflated to 1.5 ml. It is advanced smoothly and rapidly using continuous electrocardiographic and pressure monitoring. The catheter will transverse the tricuspid valve, enter and exit the right ventricle at approximately 35 to 40 cm, traverse the pulmonary artery, and ultimately wedge at approximately 60 cm. Proper position is identified using the characteristic pressure changes. Congestive heart failure may require fluoroscopic assistance.

Balloon deflation should reveal a pulmonary artery pressure pattern. If the catheter continues to reveal a wedge pressure, it should be retracted slowly. Once a correct positioning has been confirmed, using the pressure tracing, a postprocedure chest X ray must be obtained. The catheter can be secured and covered in the usual fashion.

Complications of the Swan-Ganz Catheter

Complications associated with cannulizing the appropriate central vein are similar to those previously described for short-term venous catheterization. Placement of the Swan–Ganz catheter itself is associated with its own unique complications. Arrhythmias associated with Swan–Ganz insertion placement are common.[36] The majority of arrhythmias encountered during placement can be avoided by inflating the catheter balloon. Although antiarrhythmic drugs are rarely needed, they should be readily available. It is incumbent upon the physician to be able to diagnose and manage arrhythmias. They are primarily of ventricular origin secondary to cardiac muscle irritation. Arrhythmias are more common when the patient has underlying cardiac disease and a previous history of them.

Thrombosis is occasionally encountered. Its management is similar to that described for short-term central venous catheterization. Increased thrombosis rates are associated with left-sided central catheterization and prolonged duration of catheterization. Whether low-dose heparin or Coumadin is of benefit in this setting is unknown. Infections complicating Swan–Ganz presence may also occur. The discussion under short-term central venous catheterization is applicable in this situation. Sterile technique is mandatory to help reduce this problem. Unfortunately, even with sterile technique, prolonged catheterization will result in infection, which should be treated on an individual basis and may involve removal of the catheter and use of antibiotics. Pulmonary infarction is fortunately rare when the catheter is routinely inspected to ensure proper location. The pressure pattern is key in this situation. Prolonged wedging will result in pulmonary infarction. It is mandatory that the monitors be regularly checked to rule out persistent wedging.

Balloon malfunction is another complication of Swan–Ganz catheters. Balloon rupture occurs primarily with repeated inflations or excessive inflation volumes. The average balloon capacity is less than 1.5 ml and should not be exceeded. If balloon rupture is encountered, the decision should be made on whether pulmonary artery diastolic pressures are sufficient in lieu of wedge pressures before replacement is contemplated. Less common complications include pulmonary artery rupture, which occasionally occurs in patients who have pulmonary hypertension. It is associated with balloon inflation and excess catheter looping. Therefore, only inflate the balloon for short periods of time with the right volume and avoid catheter redundancy.

Complete heart block is an unusual complication associated with preexisting left-bundle-branch block. Pacemaker insertion is the treatment of choice in this situation. Cardiac tissue injury usually occurs when the balloon is not deflated and the catheter is roughly withdrawn. The catheter may disrupt the cordia in this circumstance. Balloon deflating before catheter withdrawal will avoid this devastating complication. Catheter knotting, a rare but serious complication, is associated with patients with congestive heart failure with large hearts.[37] When this situation is encountered, it is prudent to place the Swan–Ganz catheter with fluoroscopic guidance. If a knot is encountered, it can involve one of the tricuspid cordia. Occasionally, it can be loosened with gentle traction. If this procedure is unsuccessful, atriotomy is necessary to release the catheter. Force should never be used, as it may rupture the cordia, resulting in massive heart failure with death.

PLEURAL CAVITY PROCEDURES

Thoracentesis

Thoracentesis is the most common invasive pulmonary procedure performed by gynecologists. There are two major types of thoracentesis: diagnostic and therapeutic.[38] Diagnostic thoracentesis is performed when the pleural effusion is of unknown etiology. Once fluid is obtained, it is evaluated for lactic dehydrogenase (LDH), protein, infection, and malignant cells. This evaluation allows for differentiation between transudate and exudate. Transudates are usually related to cardiac, liver, or renal dysfunction. Once the responsible organ dysfunction has been corrected, the effusion will correct. An exudative pleural effusion requires a thorough investigation to determine its origin. The vast majority of exudative pleural effusions encountered in gynecology are associated with ovarian malignancy. These effusions are usually associated with ascites. Occasionally, benign ovarian disease can cause a pleural effusion. Meig described the classic syndrome of ovarian fibroma, ascites, and pleural effusion. It is important for the physician to determine whether the pleural effusion is malignant, as this will have an impact on the patient's treatment and survival.

A therapeutic thoracentesis is primarily performed to relieve the symptoms of dyspnea. It may be combined with a diagnostic thoracentesis, if not previously performed, by sending the aspirated fluid for the appropriate laboratory evaluation. A patient who undergoes a therapeutic thoracentesis will accumulate pleural fluid in 3 to 7 days if the underlying disorder is not corrected. Multiple therapeutic thoracentesis can be performed for continued relief of symptoms. Persistent, recurrent pleural effusions should be treated with a chest tube as described in the pleurodesis section.

Procedure A chest X ray including a lateral decubitus film should be obtained. Classic findings include a hemithorax opacification, which follows the effect of gravity, ruling out loculations. If the fluid layers to less than 1 cm, ultrasound guidance should be used.[39] If the patient has an abnormal bleeding history or is receiving anticoagulant therapy, coagulation studies should be ordered and acted upon in a judicious manner. Informed consent should be obtained. The patient is placed in a comfortable sitting position with arms supported at shoulder height and the head resting on the pillow. If the patient leans too far forward, the fluid accumulates beyond the reach of the needle. The needle entrance should be placed one to two rib spaces below where the percussion note becomes dull, but not below the ninth rib. It should be inserted superior to the inferior rib to prevent damage to the neurovascular bundle. Numerous thoracentesis kits are available. The physician should be familiar with them and have an extra one on hand. The proposed thoracentesis site is cleansed with antiseptic solution and draped appropriately. A skin wheal is created using Marcaine with a 25 gauge needle. This is followed by injection along the proposed needle tract. The thoracentesis needle is then slowly introduced while gently aspirating. Once fluid is withdrawn, stabilize the needle, have the patient exhale, and advance the plastic catheter into the pleural space. Aspiration is performed with a three-way stopcock and vacuum bottles. Aspirated fluid is processed in the appropriate manner. Once the fluid has been aspirated, the needle should be withdrawn quickly and a bandage applied. A postthoracentesis expiratory chest X ray should be obtained to rule out pneumothorax.

Complications Pneumothorax is the most common complication following thoracentesis.[40,41] Approximately 10% of patients undergoing thoracentesis will develop a pneumothorax. Optimally, only one-fifth of these patients will ulti-mately require a chest tube. A common cause of pneumothorax during tho-racentesis is faulty technique, which is usually due to a break in the system, allowing atmospheric pressure to enter into the pleural space. Lung laceration secondary to needle trauma is a rare cause of pneumothorax. Other complica-tions encountered during thoracentesis include cough and vasovagal reaction. These are both felt to be secondary to pleural irritation. Removal of the needle will usually result in resolution of the cough. A vasovagal reaction may require the administration of atropine in rare instances. Infrequently, laceration to the abdominal organs may occur, which is a result of improper needle placement. A dry tap may be corrected using ultrasound guidance.

Chest Tube Placement

Chest tubes have been used since the dawn of medicine and were described in the time of Hippocrates.[42] Pneumothorax represents one of the most com-mon causes for chest tube insertion in gynecology. Central-line placement and mechanical ventilation barotrauma are the usual causes of pneumothorax. Clas-sical teaching recommended chest tube insertion for all pneumothoraces. Recent studies have indicated that a pneumothorax does not automatically require a chest tube insertion.[43] Asymptomatic nonventilated patients with an iatrogenic pneumothorax of less than 25% can be safely observed in most cases. Approx-imately 1.5% of the initial volume of the pneumothorax will be absorbed every 24 hours. Therefore, it will take approximately 3 weeks for the pneumothorax to resolve. Chest X ray should be repeated in 4 to 6 hours to confirm that the pneumothorax is not enlarging and in 1 to 2 days to document absorption.

The patient with a symptomatic pneumothorax or one larger than 25% may undergo an aspiration thoracentesis. If unsuccessful, or if chest tube placement is indicated, the tube is left in place for a minimum of 24 hours following lung expansion with air seal and then removed. All patients on mechanical ventilators developing pneumothoraxes should undergo chest tube placement. The rationale for this decision is that tension pneumothorax can develop rapidly with positive pressure ventilation.

Another indication for chest tube placement is symptomatic recurrent pleural effusion from ovarian cancer. Tube placement is used as a precursor to pleu-rodesis. Once the chest tube is inserted and the lung is reexpanded for a mini-mum of 24 hours, pleurodesis may be attempted. The two most common areas for chest tube insertion are the third intercostal space in the midclavicular line or the fifth intercostal space in the midaxillary line. The midaxillary, although initially uncomfortable to the patient, has better cosmesis. It is important for the physician not to place the tube posterior to the midaxillary line as this will result in the patient not being able to lay comfortably on her back.

Procedure   The patient should be given the rationale for placement of the chest tube and informed consent should be obtained. The proposed location for chest tube placement should be identified and the area fully anesthetized with Marcaine as previously mentioned. The pleura should be generously anesthetized where the tube will penetrate. A 3 cm incision can be made parallel to the interspace above the superior edge of the inferior rib. The incision should be taken down to the muscle without cutting it. A hemostat may then be used to dissect the intercostal muscle to the parietal pleural. The chest tube is grasped with the hemostat and pushed through the parietal pleura into the pleural space. The chest tube should be anchored and covered with sterile petroleum gauze to ensure an airtight seal. The tube is then connected to a pleuravac unit or comparable unit. A postprocedure chest X ray is obtained to confirm placement. The decision to remove the chest tube is made once the pneumothorax or drainage from the pleural effusion has resolved with complete lung expansion for a minimum of 24 hours. The tube is quickly removed while the patient valsalvas and the wound site is covered with petroleum gauze.

Complications   The major complication of chest tube insertion and placement is patient discomfort. Adequate anesthesia during insertion and placement will easily rectify this problem. If local anesthesia is not effective, an intravenous combination of midazolam and morphine sulphate are effective. Ectopic chest tube location is unusual. Once recognized, this situation should be corrected by removal and correct insertion. Infectious complications can occur and should be treated with antibiotics and timely removal of the chest tube. Occasionally, subcutaneous emphysema may develop when the catheter holes are not all in the pleural space. Careful placement may avoid this problem.

Pleurodesis

Pleurodesis is used primarily for recurrent pneumothoraces and malignant pleural effusions. Chest tube placement is first accomplished, and once the lung has reexpanded for a minimum of 24 hours, pleurodesis considered. Classically, tetracycline has been the pleural irritant used.[44,45] Recently, it has been removed from the market. The agents that are now commonly used in lieu of tetracycline are bleomycin or a talc slurry.

Procedure   The lung has to be completely reexpanded before an attempt is made to perform pleurodesis. If the lung has not reexpanded, pleurodesis is futile and a pleurectomy is indicated. Once the lung has reexpanded, lidocaine 3–4 mg per kg is infused into the pleural space through the chest tube. The tube is then clamped and for the next 10 minutes the patient is repositioned so that the entire parietal pleura is anesthetized. The patient is given intravenous sedation as well. Bleomycin 60 units is then infused into the pleural space. The chest tube is clamped for 2 hours and the patient is repositioned frequently to ensure that this sclerotic agent contacts all pleural surfaces, resulting in pleural space obliteration. Once the tube is released, it is attached to negative pressure

20 cm of H_2O for a minimum of 24 hours. Once the pleural drainage is less that 150 cc per day, the chest tube can be removed.

Complications   The major complication of pleurodesis is pain. Intrapleural lidocaine is effective in most cases. Occasionally, intravenous Versed with morphine sulfate is required. Failure rates are increased if the lung is not expanded or if there is a pleural effusion. Adequate chest expansion with drainage prior to pleurodesis is the key to success of this procedure. The reported failure rate for both bleomycin and talc slurry is approximately 10% to 20%. Other adverse effects associated with bleomycin infusion are fever, nausea, alopecia, and skin rash. Fever can be controlled with antipyretic agents.

ABDOMINAL CAVITY PROCEDURES

Paracentesis

A contraindication for this procedure is paramount. An undiagnosed abdominal pelvic mass is not an indication for paracentesis. Paracentesis in this picture can change a potentially curable localized neoplasm into an incurable metastatic disease. The extenuating circumstances that justify an exception to this tenet are indeed rare.

The most common gynecologic indication for this procedure is the relief of postoperative ascites, which causes respiratory embarrassment.[46] This is particularly justified if the patient has not yet received chemotherapy. Once chemotherapy is initiated, the ascites will usually resolve. Patients with end-stage malignancy not responding to treatment who develop symptomatic ascites can be temporarily relieved with paracentesis. Unfortunately, the ascites will reaccumulate, requiring multiple taps. Prudent use of this technique is required in order to balance immediate patient relief with future procedures. Recently, considerable discussion with regard to the amount of fluid removed has appeared in the literature.[47–49] While the majority of this work has been done on patients with liver disease, it does appear applicable to ovarian cancer patients. Recent studies have shown that removal of large amounts of fluid (greater than 5 L) are not detrimental to the patient's health. Whether the intravenous infusion of albumin should be done currently is debatable. Each case should be managed on an individual basis.

Procedure   The patient should be informed of the need for paracentesis and informed consent should be obtained. Ultrasound examination of the abdomen will reveal the deepest fluid pocket and any loculations should be noted. The area through which the needle is to be introduced should be cleansed and a sterile towel should be placed around the site. Prepackaged kits are available and an extra kit should be available. Local anesthesia should be infused into the skin and along the proposed needle track using a small gauge needle. A Z-track method should be used to prevent postprocedure leakage. A 14 to 16 gauge 3 inch needle with a flexible catheter should be introduced with ultrasound guidance. The fluid is then removed either manually using a syringe or with the use of vacuum bottles. After the fluid has been removed, the needle can be removed and a Band-Aid applied. Initially, the patient should have intravenous access available during this procedure.

Complications The major complication is infection. It can be prevented using sterile technique. If infection is encountered, it can be treated in the appropriate method after cultures have been obtained. Bowel injury can be avoided by ultrasound guidance. If the bowel is struck by the needle, the needle can be inserted at a different angle to avoid the bowel. Another complication is continued leakage of intraperitoneal fluid, which may be reduced by the Z-track technique.

Intraperitoneal Catheterization

With the cure for ovarian cancer still elusive, different methods of chemotherapy administration have been sought. Among these methods, intraperitoneal chemotherapy is currently being evaluated in patients with ovarian cancer in an attempt to improve survival.[50,51] Although initial enthusiasm for this approach has recently waned, studies continue searching for a meaningful role for this treatment. Theoretically, intraperitoneal chemotherapy administration offers the advantage of increased dose concentration to intraperitoneal tumor compared to systemic administration. There are three major types of catheters available for intraperitoneal chemotherapy: Tenckoff, Groshong, and Mediport. These catheters are similar in appearance to catheters used for long-term central venous catheterization therapy. If intraperitoneal chemotherapy is only to be given once, as in the administration of P32, a Tenckoff-type catheter is recommended. These catheters have no subcutaneous port. Alternatively, a Jackson Pratt drain can be utilized for this function. The rationale for the decision to use either a catheter or a port-type system is similar to that as discussed in "Long-term Venous Catheterization" section.

Procedure The rationale for placement of the intrabdominal catheter is given to the patient and informed consent is obtained. Local anesthesia is injected at the exit site and along the catheter's tract at the level of the umbilicus, lateral to the intrabdominal rectus abdominus muscle. The catheter is placed into the abdomen through a small incision. A subcutaneous tunnel is then made on the ipsilateral side to the lower quadrant. The Decron cuff is placed in subcutaneous tissue 2 cm from the exit site. Implanted subcutaneous ports are placed on the ipsilateral side along the lower rib cage on the midclavicular line. The port is then anchored to the chest wall fascia and closed in the subcuticular manner and Steri-Strips are placed.

Complications   Most abdominal access complications are similar to those encountered with central venous access devices. However, bowel perforation is encountered in approximately 3% of patients. Etiology is believed to be catheter erosion. Peritonitis is reported 5% to 10% of the time and usually mandates catheter removal.

Subcutaneous infections are unusual. However, if associated with a tunnel infection, removal appears indicated. A decision on whether to place an intraperitoneal catheter with large-bowel surgery has been discussed by several authors.[50,51] Although there is no definite evidence that catheter placement with large-bowel surgery will increase the risk of peritonitis, it appears prudent to delay placement.

Long-term complications include infusion and aspiration difficulties. A fibrous sheath coating the catheter is usually responsible. If intraluminal wire placement is unsuccessful in dislodging the obstruction, laparoscopy may be helpful; otherwise, catheter replacement is required.

REFERENCES

1. Groeger J, Lucas A, et al. Venous access in the cancer patient. *Prin Pract Oncol* 1991;5(3):2–14.

2. Gleeson N, Fiorica J, et al. Externalized Groshong catheters and Hickman ports for central venous access in gynecologic oncology patients. *Gynecol Oncol* 1993;51:372–376.

3. Koonings P, Given F. Long term experience with a totally implanted catheter system in gynecologic oncologic patients. *J Am Coll Surgeons* 1994;178:164–166.

4. Brothers T, Von Moll L, et al. Experience with subcutaneous infusion ports in three hundred patients. *Surg Gynecol Obstet* 1988;166:295–301.

5. Civetta J, Gable J, et al. Internal-jugular-vein puncture with a margin of safety. *Anesthesiology* 1972;36:622–625.

6. Vaughan RW, Weygandt GR. Reliable percutaneous central venous pressure measurement. *Anesthesia and Analgesia, Curr Res* 1973;52:709–712.

7. Prince SR, Sullivan RL, et al. Percutaneous catheterization of the internal jugular vein in infants and children. *Anesthesiology* 1976;44:170–174.

8. Seldinger SI. Catheter replacement of needle in percutaneous arteriography: new technique. *Acta Radiol* 1962;39:368.

9. Wilson JN, Grow JB, et al. Central venous pressure in optimal blood volume maintenance. *Archiv Surg* 1962;85:563.

10. Tofield J. A safer technique of percutaneous catheterization of the subclavian vein. *Surg, Gynecol Obstet* 1969;128:1069.

11. Mogil R, Delaurentis D, et al. The infraclavicular venipuncture. *Archiv Surg* 1967;95:320.

12. Sherer D, Abulafia O, et al. Ultrasonographically guided subclavian vein catheterization in critical care obstetrics and gynecologic oncology. *Am J Obstet Gynecol* 1993;169:1246–1248.

13. Mansfield P, Hohn D, et al. Complications and failures of subclavian-vein catheterization. *New Engl J Med* 1994;331:1735–1738.

14. Vyskocil J, Kruse, J, et al. Alternative techniques for gaining venous access. *J Crit Illness* 1993;8(3):435–442.

15. Laffer U, Durig H, et al. Vascular access problems and implantable devices. *Rec Results Cancer Res* 1991;121:189–197.

16. Nelson B, Mayer A, et al. Experience with the intravenous totally implanted port in patients with gynecologic malignancies. *Gynecol Oncol* 1994;53:98–102.

17. Eastridge B, Lefor A, et al. Complications of indwelling venous access devices in cancer patients. *J Clin Oncol* 1995;13(1):233–238.

18. Richardson D, Bruso P. Vascular access devices. *J Intravenous Nursing* 1993;16(1):44–49.

19. Keung Y, Watkins K, et al. Comparative study of infectious complications of different types of chronic central venous access devices. *Cancer* 1994;73(11):2832–2837.

20. Johnson A, Oppenheim B. Vascular catheter-related sepsis: diagnosis and prevention. *J Hosp Infection* 1992;20:67–78.

21. Garrison RN, Wilson MA. Intravenous and central catheter injections. *S Clin N America* 1994;74(3):557–570.

22. Schwartz C, Henrickson K, et al. Prevention of bacteremia attributed to luminal colonization of tunneled central venous catheters with vancomycin-susceptible organisms. *J Clin Oncol* 1990;8(9):1591–1597.

23. Lecciones J, Lee J, et al. Vascular catheter-associated fungemia in patients with cancer: analysis of 155 episodes. *Clin Infect Dis* 1992;14:875–883.

24. Mueller B, Skelton J, et al. A prospective randomized trial comparing the infectious and noninfectious complications of an externalized catheter versus a subcutaneously implanted device in cancer patients. *J Clin Oncol* 1992;10:1943–1948.

25. Cobb D, High K, et al. A controlled trial of scheduled replacement of central venous and pulmonary catheters. *New Engl J Med* 1992;327:1062–1068.

26. Eyer S, Brummit C, et al. Catheter-related sepsis: prospective, randomized study of three methods of long-term catheter maintenance. *Crit Care Med* 1990;18:1073–1079.

27. Gregory J, Schiller W. Subclavian catheter changes every third day in high risk patients. *Am J Surg* 1985;51:534–536.

28. Carlisle E, Blake P, et al. Septicemia in long-term jugular hemodialysis catheters: eradicating infection by changing the catheter over a guidewire. *Int J Artificial Organs* 1991;14(3):150–153.

29. Lokich J, Becker B. Subclavian vein thrombosis in patients treated with infusion chemotherapy for advance malignancy. *Cancer* 1983;52:1586–1589.

30. Bern M, Lokich J, et al. Very low doses of warfarin can prevent thrombosis in central venous catheters. *Ann Int Med* 1990;112:423–428.

31. Aitken D, Minton J, et al. The "pinch off sign": a warning of impending problems with permanent subclavian catheters. *Am J Surg* 1984;148:633–636.

32. Swan H, Ganz W, Forrester J, et al. Catheterization of the heart in man with use of a flow-directed balloon-tipped catheter. *N Engl J Med* 1970;283:447–451.

33. Shoemaker W. Use and abuse of the balloon tip pulmonary artery (Swan–Ganz)

catheter: Are patients getting their money's worth? *Crit Care Med* 1990;18(11): 1294–1296.

34. Berlauk J, Abrams J, et al. Preoperative optimization of cardiovascular hemodynamics improves outcome in peripheral vascular surgery. *Ann Surg* 1991;214(3):289–299.

35. Rosen M, Berger D, et al. Practice guidelines for pulmonary artery catheterization. *Anesthesiology* 1993;78:380–394.

36. Bennett D, Boldt J, et al. Expert panel: the use of the pulmonary artery catheter. *Intensive Care Med* 1991;17:I–VIII.

37. Tremblay N, Taillefer J, et al. Successful non-surgical extraction of a knotted pulmonary artery catheter trapped in the right ventricle. *Can J Anaesthesiol* 1992;39(3):293–295.

38. Grogan D, Irwin R, et al. Complications associated with thoracentesis. *Arch Intern Med* 1990;150:873–877.

39. Kohan J, Poe R, et al. Value of chest ultrasonography versus decubitus roentgenography for thoracentesis. *Am Rev Respir Dis* 1986;133:1124–1126.

40. Grogan D, Irwin R, et al. Complications associated with thoracentesis. *Arch Intern Med* 1990;150:873–877.

41. Collins T, Sahn S. Thoracentesis: clinical value, complications, technical problems, and patient experience. *Chest* 1987;91(6):817–822.

42. Silver M, Bone R. Techniques for chest tube insertion and pleurodesis. *J Crit Illn* 1993;8:631–637.

43. Light R. Iatrogenic pneumothorax. In *Pleural Diseases*, 2nd ed. Philadelphia: Lea & Febinger, 1990, pp. 251–253.

44. Lynch T. Management of malignant pleural effusions. *Chest* 1993;103(4):385S–389S.

45. Keller S. Current and future therapy for malignant pleural effusion. *Chest* 1993;103(1):63S–67S.

46. Lifshitz S, Buchsbaum H. The effect of paracentesis on serum proteins. *Gynecol Oncol* 1976;4:347–353.

47. Berkowitz K, Butensky M, et al. Pulmonary function changes after large volume paracentesis. *Am J Gastroenterol* 1993;88(6):905–907.

48. Panos M, Moore K, et al. Single, total paracentesis for tense ascites: sequential hemodynamic changes and right atrial size. *Hepatology* 1990;11(4):662–667.

49. Reynolds T. Renaissance of paracentesis in the treatment of ascites. *Adv Intern Med* 1990;35:365–374.

50. Pfeifle C, Howell S, et al. Totally implantable system for peritoneal access. *J Clin Oncol* 1984;2(11):1277–1280.

51. Naumann R, Alvarez R, et al. The Groshong catheter as an intraperitoneal access device in the treatment of ovarian cancer patients. *Gynecol Oncol* 1993;50(3):291–293.

52. Weiner, ES. Catheter sepsis: The central venous line Achilles' heel. *Semin Pediatr Surg* 1995;4(4):297–314.

53. Bagnall-Reeb H, Ruccione K: Practical application of an algorithm for the thrombolytic treatment of occluded vascular access devices. *J Ped Oncol Nurs* 1993;10(2):79–82.

CHAPTER 4

IMAGING OF THE ABDOMEN, PELVIS, SPINE, AND CENTRAL NERVOUS SYSTEM

ANDREW DEUTSCH, M.D., M.B.A., AND RACHAEL E. GORDON, M.D.

Diagnostic imaging is frequently utilized to help in the evaluation of patients with gynecological malignancies. Its role is magnified in the setting of acute illness and suspected complications in the perioperative period. The patient's condition may reflect a direct manifestation of her malignancy or could be related to an unassociated concurrent process. This chapter attempts to provide a practical diagnostic approach to the acutely ill patient with a gynecologic malignancy. The organization is in several broad categories: abdominal/pelvic, central nervous system, and spine. Emphasis is placed on the diagnostic approach to problem solving: what tests should be utilized for what clinical concern. Emphasis, where appropriate, is placed on the significance and implications of specific imaging findings as a practical guide to the practicing clinician.

The objective of this text is to provide clinicians with the evidence available to assist them in making the best possible decision. Traditionally, evidenced-based medicine (EBM) has been associated with randomized clinical trials and meta-analysis which may be appropriate in certain settings, particularly in the evaluation of different therapeutic options, but it is not necessarily a prerequisite in the evaluation of many diagnostic tests. To determine the accuracy of a diagnostic test, it is not necessary to perform a randomized trial but rather to identify and study the proper cross-sectional group of patients considered on clinical grounds to harbor the relevant disorder. This procedure is reflected in the radiology literature cited throughout this chapter.

The focus of diagnostic radiologists is on the relative accuracy of different examinations in establishing a specific diagnosis and the relative value of different diagnostic criteria to be employed in the interpretation of the studies.

Perioperative and Supportive Care in Gynecologic Oncology: Evidence-Based Management,
Edited by Steven A. Vasilev.
ISBN 0-471-24788-X   Copyright © 2000 by Wiley-Liss, Inc.

As such, the emphasis is on sensitivity and specificity and positive and negative predictive values of different examinations. This practice is utilized to help establish the relative value of one examination compared to another. The bulk of the diagnostic imaging literature is case study in nature. While studies are increasingly prospective, they are rarely randomized and controlled. As such, overwhelmingly, the studies cited in this chapter are Level II-3, although all subtypes of the level are included as are works of Levels I and III.

THE ABDOMEN AND PELVIS

The Plain Abdominal Radiograph

The time-honored imaging approach to the patient presenting with acute abdominal signs and symptoms has been the plain-film abdominal series. The examination is widely available, is of relatively low cost, and can provide quite critical and specific information in many cases. Given the surgical orientation of most of the likely readers of this chapter, particular emphasis is placed on plain radiographic findings, since many readers will be directly involved in the interpretation of these studies. The principal application of the plain X ray is in the assessment of the intestinal gas pattern. Plain radiographs may provide information on the presence or absence of intestinal obstruction. They are also the first imaging test most commonly utilized to assess for the presence of gas in other than an intraluminal location (e.g., free in the peritoneal cavity or within the bowel wall).

Based on the findings of the plain radiographic series, the diagnostic evaluation may be complete or may lead to the use of additional imaging examinations such as ultrasonography or computed tomography. An approach based on the plain radiographic findings is advanced in this section and the significance of plain radiographic findings is considered in detail. In subsequent sections of this chapter, specific consideration is given to the assessment of distinct clinical concerns (e.g., bowel obstruction, renal disease, abscess) and the most appropriate imaging techniques to be employed in their further assessment beyond that which can be accomplished with the plain film examination.

Bowel Gas Pattern   As is well appreciated, intestinal gas either representing swallowed air or gas liberated by bacterial fermentation is normally present throughout the lumen of the gastrointestinal tract. As a consequence, gas is normally depicted in the stomach, frequently throughout the colon, and typically selectively throughout the small bowel. The radiological approach to the acute abdomen has emphasized the need for images in at least two projections, typically one supine and the second upright or left lateral decubitus. A chest radiograph, if properly centered and thus including a view of the diaphragm, may also be extremely valuable in the assessment of the acute abdomen, but is typically difficult to obtain in the upright projection in significantly ill patients.

On upright and decubitus projection, air fluid levels are commonly normally depicted in the fundus of the stomach, within the first portion of the duodenum, and in the colon. Air fluid levels depicted in the small bowel other than in the first portion of the duodenum are considered abnormal. The presence of bowel distention is also well evaluated on conventional radiographs. Disproportionate distention of bowel is abnormal. Conventional abdominal radiographs have traditionally been most commonly utilized as the first imaging procedure in patients with suspected obstruction.

Plain radiographs have the advantages of relative simplicity, universal access, and relatively low cost. Plain radiographic analysis may provide sufficient diagnostic information for clinical purposes in approximately 60% of cases (Level III).[2] Bowel obstruction is manifest on plain radiographs by demonstration of bowel dilatation and the presence of air fluid levels. Mechanical obstruction of bowel is differentiated from paralytic ileus by the disproportionate distention of bowel in mechanical obstruction. Diffuse and symmetric dilatation is more suggestive of ileus (Fig. 4.1). In up to 20% of patients, however, there may be no evidence of obstruction on plain radiographs (Level III).[1]

When plain radiographic analysis is not confirmatory and the clinical picture remains uncertain, further imaging diagnosis is typically entertained. This can be accomplished with positive contrast studies (e.g., barium evaluation of small and large bowel) as well as more recently with computerized tomography (CT), which is further considered in a section devoted to imaging of suspected bowel obstruction.

Extraluminal Gas   Gas located in any other than an intraluminal location (e.g., within the bowel wall, free within the peritoneal cavity) should be regarded as abnormal. An important role of diagnostic imaging in the acutely ill patient with abdominal symptoms is the detection of such extraluminal gas. Conventional radiographs of the abdomen have been the mainstay of diagnosis for the detection of extraluminal gas and represent a widely available and relatively inexpensive means for detection. Plain films, however, are not the most sensitive examination for the detection of collections of gas residing outside the lumen of the gastrointestinal tract and increasingly CT has become a valuable adjunct in this evaluation.

Pneumoperitoneum   As the cause of free air may range from the innocuous to the life-threatening, its presence must be interpreted within the appropriate clinical setting. The most common cause of free intraperitoneal air is recent abdominal surgery. Following surgery, air is gradually reabsorbed over the course of 3 to 7 days but may be detected for up to 2 to 4 weeks if a large amount was present initially.[1,2] A prolonged postoperative pneumoperitoneum is more commonly seen in thin rather than obese patients (Level III).[1] The degree of free air postoperatively should progressively decrease and as such an increase in the amount of free air several days after surgery should be considered abnormal and likely reflective of a complication.

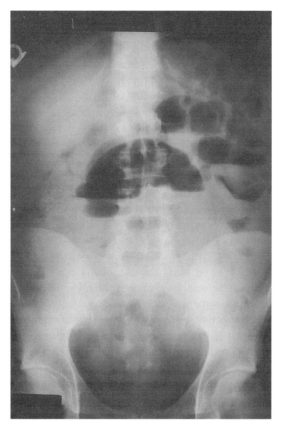

FIGURE 4.1. Small bowel obstruction. Upright radiograph of the abdomen reveals multiple air-fluid levels within moderately dilated small-bowel loops. There is a paucity of gas within nondistended large bowel. The findings are highly characteristic of small-bowel obstruction.

Spontaneous pneumoperitoneum is most commonly caused by the perforation of a hollow viscus, with the major cause representing a perforated duodenal or gastric ulcer (70% of cases). Other common causes include colon perforation secondary to obstruction, gross adynamic ileus, infection, infarction, and ulcerated neoplasm. In two common conditions associated with perforation and abdominal distress, namely appendicitis and diverticulitis, free air is uncommonly depicted (Level III).[1] Although the demonstration of free intraperitoneal air is most commonly associated with a ruptured viscus, a wide variety of benign causes have been reported, and thus the finding of a pneumoperitoneum must be closely correlated with the patient's overall clinical findings to avoid unnecessary exploration. Benign causes of pneumoperitoneum include (1) bowel overdistention with intact mucosa (gastric dilatation), (2) pneumatosis cystoides intestinalis (rupture of serosal cyst), and (3) chronic obstructive pulmonary disease (COPD), (4) pneumothorax, (5) recent tracheal intubation, and (6) head and neck surgery (Level III).[1]

Upright chest and left lateral decubitus radiographs of the abdomen have been considered the time-honored projections for the diagnosis of free air (Fig. 4.2). Miller and Nelson have shown that as little as 1 to 2 ml of free air can be detected (Level II-3).[3] This requires, however, proper technique including the need for the patient to be upright or in a decubitus position for up to 10 to 20 minutes, which is rarely accomplished in clinical practice with busy departments and patients too ill to tolerate the positioning for prolonged periods of time. Free air can also be appreciated on supine radiographs, although it is frequently subtle and a wide number of diagnostic signs have been described for its detection (e.g., Rigler's sign, falciform ligament sign). The right upper quadrant is most common and frequently the only place that free air can be depicted on supine-only radiographs; this region and the associated signs of free air must be carefully scrutinized and applied. Supine-only radiographs allow depiction of free intraperitoneal air in approximately 60% of cases Level III.[4]

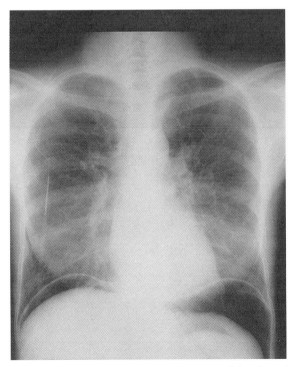

FIGURE 4.2. Free intraperitoneal air. Upright radiograph of the chest demonstrates gas beneath both hemidiaphragms (arrows). The findings are classic for free intraperitoneal air. Ideally the examination, when performed to assess for free intraperitoneal air, should be centered at the level of the hemidiaphragm.

CT is an extremely sensitive method for the depiction of free intraperitoneal air. In a study comparing CT with upright chest radiographs in patients following diagnostic peritoneal lavage for trauma, CT demonstrated free air in 100% of patients whereas chest radiography demonstrated free air in only 27% of patients with air collections less than 13 ml in diameter.[5] On CT scans, free air is often best depicted in the midabdomen and over the peritoneal surface of the liver (Level III).[1] Numerous tiny collections of free air trapped within the various peritoneal recesses may be depicted exclusively by CT.

Bowel-Wall Gas   Gas within the bowel wall may be associated with a wide variety of conditions and can occur in any portion of the gastrointestinal tract (Fig. 4.3). In infants, the finding most often is indicative of necrotizing enterocolitis. In adults, the detection of linear gas in the bowel wall suggests bowel infarction (Level III).[1] In recent years, however, there has been increasing

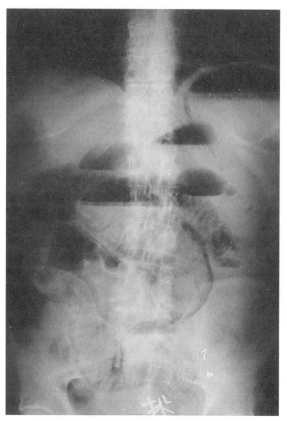

FIGURE 4.3. Ischemic bowel. Upright radiograph demonstrates air-fluid levels in proximal small bowel (arrows). In the midabdomen a dilated loop is present with linear gas within the bowel wall (arrow).

recognition of benign forms of intestinal-wall gas. It may be seen in patients with pulmonary as well as gastrointestinal obstructive disease including patients recently status postbowel surgery (particularly jejunoileal bypass or placement of feeding jejunostomy).

Pneumatosis has also been reported in patients with progressive systemic sclerosis (in which it represents a grave prognostic sign), Crohn's disease, peptic ulcer, and following traumatic gastrointestinal endoscopy (Level III).[1] A variety of medications including steroids and chemotherapeutic agents also have been associated with mural gas. An uncommon benign entity, pneumatosis cystoides intestinalis, usually seen in adults and affecting the left colon, is characterized by the presence of multiple thin-walled gas-filled cysts in the subserosa or submucosa that do not communicate with the lumen (Level III).[1]

In the secondary form of pneumatosis, the gas collections are most commonly linear and parallel the lumen, in contrast to the appearance of pneumatosis cystoides intestinalis, in which the gas appears as round or ovoid lucencies. Plain-film radiography has most commonly been utilized to identify bowel-wall gas, but more recently CT has been shown to be more sensitive and specific with regard to the detection of mural gas as well as associated surrounding abnormalities (Level II-3).[6] Bubbles of gas trapped in stool, in a chain of sigmoid diverticula, or within the mostly fluid-filled small bowel, where it is arrayed in a line underneath the valvulae conniventes, can mimic the appearance of pneumatosis (Level III).[1]

Portal Venous Gas   Gas within the portal venous system is usually an ominous finding indicating bowel infarction. Other reported causes include (1) diverticulitis, (2) acute gastric or intestinal dilatation, (3) inflammatory bowel diseases following barium enema or colonoscopy, and (4) hepatic transplant recipients (in the absence of bowel disease or transplant rejection) (Level III).[1] Despite these other causes, the radiographic depiction of portal venous gas should be considered a potentially ominous sign until demonstrated otherwise. In differentiating portal venous gas from gas located in the biliary tree, the central positioning of the latter collection compared with the peripheral branching pattern of portal venous gas is most helpful. This pattern can be recognized on both plain radiographs and CT. More recently, Doppler sonography has been used to detect gas in the portal vein, which is appreciated as a branching pattern of high-amplitude echoes (Level II-3).[7]

Air in the Biliary Tree   The most common cause of air in the biliary system is surgical creation of a biliary-enteric fistula (Level III).[1] Other reported causes include (1) erosion of a gallstone in the bowel, (2) peptic ulcer penetration of the common bile duct, and (3) traumatic or neoplastic fistulization between the gallbladder or bile duct and the gastrointestinal tract. Cholangitis with gas-forming organism is a reported but rarely seen cause. Air in the biliary tree is well demonstrated radiographically and usually is confined to the major ducts and virtually never extends to the periphery of the liver, which is an important diagnostic feature, allowing differentiating from gas seen in the portal venous system (Level III).[1] Air in the gallbladder wall, in contrast to the lumen, is seen exclusively in emphysematous cholecystitis (see separate discussion of biliary disease).

Abscess　Plain radiography can be utilized to depict gas in abscess cavities with a reported success rate of 70% to 80% (Level III).[8] Gas in abscess cavities can appear as multiple bubbles aggregated in an ill-defined area or as single large lucency filling the abscess cavity. The depiction of collections of gas bubbles outside the normal location of the small or large bowel should be considered suspicious for abscess unless proven otherwise. On occasion, gas can form in necrotic tumors, especially after chemotherapy, radiation therapy, or vascular embolization. It may be related to ischemic complications or to the effect of chemotherapeutic agents on the mucosal integrity and bacterial overgrowth or fermentation. Gas trapped within a retained surgical sponge or a bioabsorbable hemostatic agent such as oxidized cellulose (Surgicel) placed at the bleeding site can be seen as a focal collection of gas that could mimic an abscess.

The remainder of this section on the abdomen and pelvis centers on discussions of specific conditions and clinical concerns that may be encountered in the perioperative patient with a gynecological malignancy and may necessitate more sophisticated imaging beyond that which can be accomplished utilizing plain-film radiography.

Gallbladder and Biliary Tract: Emphasis on Acute Disease

The acutely ill patient with a gynecological malignancy can present with right upper-quadrant pain reflective of biliary disease. Indeed, 10% to 15% of adults have gallstones, and more than 600,000 cholecystectomies are performed in the United States each year. Imaging assessment of the patient with pain of suspected biliary origin involves establishing the presence of gallstones, diagnosing acute cholecystitis and its complications, and assessing the biliary ducts for dilatation and evidence of obstruction related to stone disease or neoplasm.

Cholelithiasis　Ultrasonography is the most commonly employed examination for the detection of gallstones and has largely supplanted oral cholecystography for this purpose, particularly in the acutely ill patient. Following pain radiographs, which can detect 15% of all gallstones, ultrasound is the initial examination of choice. An accuracy for the detection of gallstones exceeding 96% has been reported since the earliest series on the subject (Level II-3).[9] In addition, valuable information on the gallbladder wall, pericholecystic abnormalities, and adjacent structures including the biliary system, liver, kidney, and pancreas can be readily obtained.

Gallstones are diagnosed by ultrasound upon the demonstration of an intraluminal echogenic focus that demonstrates both acoustic shadowing and gravity dependence (Fig. 4.4). A common sonographic finding related to cholelithiasis

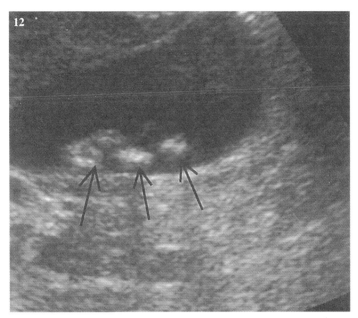

FIGURE 4.4. Cholelithiasis. Single image from a real-time ultrasound examination of the gallbladder reveals multiple dependent high-echogenicity foci with posterior acoustic shadowing (arrows). The findings are classic for multiple gallstones. The gallbladder wall is normal in thickness and there is no pericholecystic fluid.

is that of biliary sludge, which is manifest as echogenic foci that do not demonstrate acoustic shadowing and is believed to represent lithogenic bile. Sludge is generally attributed to biliary stasis and has several known etiologies including intravenous hyperalimentation, prolonged fasting, and biliary outlet obstruction. Although sludge is significantly questioned as a cause of acute cholecystitis, it has been incriminated as a cause of pancreatitis.

Cholecystitis   The major sonographic features of acute cholecystitis include cholelithiasis, maximal pain over the gallbladder at the time of sonographic examination, and gallbladder-wall edema. The combination of the sonographic depiction of a Murphy sign (elicited by compression of the gallbladder) and the presence of gallstones has a 92% positive predictive value for acute cholecystitis (Level II-3).[10] Considerable controversy surrounds the utility of the depiction of gallbladder-wall edema in the diagnosis of acute cholecystitis, as it may also be seen in a variety of other conditions, including chronic cholecystitis, hepatitis, hypoproteinemia, and physiologic contraction (gallbladder ultrasound is ideally performed following at least an 8 hour fast). It has been recently suggested that color-flow Doppler ultrasound may improve the recognition of acute cholecystits when increased arterial flow is seen (Level II-3).[9,11]

Direct radionuclide imaging of the biliary system and gallbladder may be

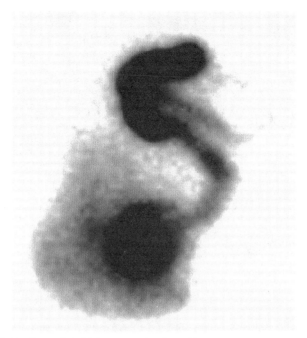

FIGURE 4.5. Radionuclide biliary examination. Single static image obtained 40 minutes following the intravenous administration of the isotope. There is visualization of the gallbladder, extrahepatic biliary system, and isotope within the small bowel. Such findings would strongly exclude acute cholecystitis.

accomplished utilizing technetium 99m-labeled derivatives of hepato-iminodiacetic acid (HIDA, DISIA) that are directly excreted into the biliary system and can demonstrate patency of the cystic duct with a high degree of accuracy (Level II-3).[12] Following the administration of the radioisotope, its concentration within the liver can be detected within 5 to 10 minutes, and usually by 40 to 60 minutes there is visualization of the gallbladder, biliary system, and the presence of detectable activity within the proximal small bowel (Fig. 4.5). Nonvisualization of the gallbladder after 1 hour is usually indicative of cystic duct obstruction. Delayed visualization of the gallbladder beyond 1 hour after common bile duct and small-bowel visualization does not necessarily rule out the possibility of acute cholecystitis, although such a finding would be unusual. More commonly, delayed visualization of the gallbladder is associated with chronic cholecystits (Level II-3).[9,12]

Cholecystitis in the absence of gallstones occurs in approximately 5% of cases and may be more commonly encountered in children (Level II-3).[13] It is certainly a consideration in postoperative patients, who have been reported to have a higher incidence than the general population (Level II-3).[9] The signs and symptoms may be identical to acute cholecystitis secondary to stone disease. Given the lack of stones, the diagnosis may be difficult. Ultrasound has a reported accuracy of 60% to 70% (Level II-3).[13] The diagnostic criterion in the absence of stones has centered on the thickness of the gallbladder wall, a finding that has proven increasingly less specific.

While radionuclide imaging has been suggested as a more useful procedure for the diagnosis of acalculous cholecystitis since it is not dependent on the direct visualization of gallstones, its reported accuracy is in a similar range to that of diagnostic ultrasound (Level II-3).[13] Although it has been shown to be highly sensitive (90%), gallbladder distention and stasis result in a high number of false positive examinations, lowering the overall accuracy of scintigraphy (Level II-3).[14] The morbidity and mortality of acute acalculous cholecystitis is higher than that associated with stone disease. This may well be accounted for by the difficulty in establishing an early diagnosis.

Five to ten percent of cases of acute cholecystitis may be complicated by perforation, which is associated with a morality of 20% to 24% (Level II-3).[15] Patients may initially feel transient improvement as the bile leak decompresses the gallbladder. Once bile peritonitis develops, however, the patient is seen to rapidly deteriorate. Ultrasound may be of use in demonstrating pericholecystic fluid collections and abscesses elsewhere in the peritoneal cavity. Radionuclide techniques can be used to demonstrate extravasation of isotopes, which may outline Morison's pouch.

Emphysematous cholecystitis is a rare condition that clinically presents with sudden and rapidly progressive right upper-quadrant pain accompanied by fever and leukocytosis. Diagnosis and treatment must be expeditiously accomplished, as the mortality rate is significantly higher than for acute calculus cholecystitis. On plain radiographs, the critical finding is that of gas contained within the gallbladder wall, typically seen as bubbles and streaks. Mottled gas can be seen around the gallbladder fossa. This condition is to be distinguished from the commonly benign finding of pneumobilia (representing gas within the gallbladder lumen), which is frequently encountered in less symptomatic patients and is most frequently seen secondary to a prior diverting surgical procedure upon the biliary tract.

Biliary Tract Obstructive Disease   Patients with gynecologic malignancies may also present with clinical signs and symptoms suggested of obstruction of the biliary tract. As with the assessment of the gallbladder, ultrasound is frequently the initially employed examination technique, and the demonstration of both intrahepatic and extrahepatic biliary distention is readily accomplished. It is determined whether the distention is on an obstructive or nonobstructive basis, and if obstructive, the etiology for the obstruction frequently requires additional diagnostic measures. Computed tomography can be utilized for this purpose and is quite sensitive to the detection of intrahepatic biliary dilatation; the common bile duct can be directly visualized, as well as the peripancreatic region. In the absence of a mass in the region of the pancreatic head or direct demonstration of a gallstone in the common bile duct, the precise etiology for the presumed obstruction may elude diagnosis by CT.

In this setting, visualization of the biliary system by means of direct contrast opacification is frequently employed. It is most commonly accomplished utilizing either endoscopic retrograde cholangiography or transhepatic cholangiography. Both techniques can precisely demonstrate both intraluminal and extraluminal causes of biliary obstruction (Level II-3).[14] The most common cause of intraluminal obstruction is stone disease. Hemorrhage into the biliary system can result in a variety of appearances, ranging from an isolated filling defect to a total cast of the lumen. The most common causes include trauma, instrumentation, tumor, and vascular abnormalities. Filling defects may be seen also on the basis of benign polypoid lesions, which are typically rare, as well as on the basis of parasites, which are becoming more common.

Extrinsic narrowing of the biliary system may be seen secondary to a wide variety of etiologies including postinflammatory, postsurgical, ampullary, and periampullary processes, adjacent malignant lesions, and primary cholangiocarcinoma (Level II-3).[14] Chronic pancreatitis is one of the most frequent causes of common bile duct obstruction. Other causes of stricture resulting from inflammation/fibrosis include trauma secondary to stone passage as well as ischemic and inflammatory damage that can occur as a result of hepatic artery chemotherapy infusion.

Sclerosing pancreatitis, a progressive inflammatory process involving all or parts of the bile duct system, is commonly associated with a number of systemic conditions, the most common of which is ulcerative colitis (Level II-3).[9] The condition is characterized by diffuse or localized regions of narrowing and relative dilatation involving both the intra- and extrahepatic portions of the biliary system. The resulting changes in the biliary system can be indistinguishable from those associated with secondary or ascending cholangitis. These latter patients are usually critically ill, with a biliary system filled with pus at the peak of the infection. While the treatment of the septic process is primary, definitive treatment consists of relieving the distal obstructive process. More recently, nonbacterial forms of ascending cholangitis have been described in patients with human immunodeficiency virus (HIV) disease, with a radiological picture quite similar to sclerosing cholangitis. This is commonly on the basis of biliary Cryptosporidium in the HIV population (Level II-3).[16]

Metastatic spread in the porta hepatis or the peripancreatic or periduodenal region can also, on occasion, cause sufficient compression to cause bile duct narrowing and obstruction. Of the gynecological malignancies, breast cancer is the most commonly reported cause (Level II-3).[9] Other principal causes of extrinsic obstruction include tumors arising in adjacent organs (liver, pancreas) as well as primary cholangiocarcinoma.

Pancreatic Disease

Pancreatic disease, most commonly related to acute pancreatitis, may be encountered in the perioperative patient with a gynecological malignancy.

Cross-sectional imaging techniques have revolutionized pancreatic imaging by allowing direct visualization of the pancreas. Percutaneous drainage of pancreatic or peripancreatic fluid collections and aspiration or biopsy of pancreatic masses are also widely performed using ultrasound guidance or CT.

Although an advantage of ultrasound over CT is that of lower cost, visualization of the pancreas is often poor or incomplete secondary to patient body habitus or overlying bowel gas. Optimized imaging of the pancreas using CT requires the administration of oral contrast material to opacify the stomach, duodenum, and proximal small bowel and frequently the intravenous administration of iodinated contrast material for vascular and parenchymal opacification. With the recent advent of helical CT techniques, the study can be expeditiously accomplished, even in the most critically ill patients.

Pancreatitis   The common abnormality of the pancreas that is likely to be encountered in the perioperative patient with a gynecological malignancy is pancreatitis. Acute pancreatitis may cause either focal or diffuse enlargement of the pancreas. Abdominal plain films are often nonspecific but may demonstrate a generalized or focal ileus (sentinel loop and/or colon cutoff sign). Chest radiographic findings include basilar atelectasis, pleural fluid, and diaphragmatic elevation. On a conventional gastrointestinal contrast examination, acute pancreatitis may cause widening of the duodenal sweep, thickening and/or effacement of duodenal folds, and anterior displacement of the stomach.

Ultrasound of acute pancreatitis typically demonstrates diffuse or focal pancreatic enlargement, hypoechoic parenchyma, and poorly defined contour, Ultrasound in these patients, however, is often limited by overlying bowel gas related to intestinal ileus. CT should be considered the imaging method of choice for the assessment of acute pancreatitis and its complications (Level II-3).[13] In addition to demonstrating pancreatic enlargement and poor definition of the pancreatic parenchyma, CT may reveal inflammatory infiltration of peripancreatic fat and fascial planes. With acute pancreatitis, the pancreatic parenchyma usually demonstrates decreased attenuation secondary to edema or necrosis, but on contrast-enhanced examinations the pancreas may appear diffusely hyperdense because of hyperemia (Fig. 4.6). In acute hemorrhagic pancreatitis, a severe form of pancreatitis characterized by parenchymal hemorrhage, inflammation, and destruction, focal areas of increased attenuation are frequently seen on nonenhanced examinations.

Although usually a diffuse process, acute pancreatitis may cause focal enlargement of the pancreas. The localized pancreatic mass may appear solid, cystic, or inhomogeneous on CT and hyperechoic, normal, or hypoechoic on ultrasound. Pancreatic phlegmon represents diffuse pancreatic enlargement and peripancreatic inflammation secondary to acute pancreatitis. It appears inhomogeneous on ultrasound and CT, and may resolve completely or worsen, contributing to fluid collections, necrosis, or abscess formation. Acute fluid collections occur secondary to release of pancreatic secretions from disrupted pancreatic ductules. Although these collections may be confined to the pancreas,

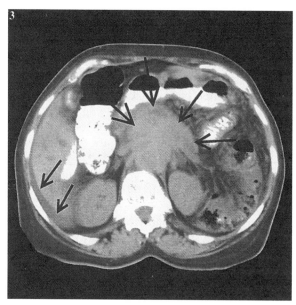

FIGURE 4.6. Pancreatic inflammatory disease. Axial CT section through the midabdomen reveals a poorly defined mass involving the head and body of the pancreas (arrows). There are streaky linear bands of high attenuation infiltrating the peripancreatic fat. They are highly characteristic for inflammatory processes. A small degree of free fluid is seen surrounding the tip of the liver.

they frequently extend throughout the retroperitoneum. Acute pancreatic fluid collections, in contrast to pseudocysts, lack a fibrous capsule.

Gastrointestinal Tract: Specific Conditions

Colitis   While colitis may occur on an infectious or noninfectious basis, the most commonly encountered form in patients with gynecological malignancies is radiation colitis as a complication of radiation therapy for carcinoma of the cervix (Level 11-3).[13] Barium enema examinations remain the primary imaging method for diagnosis, although CT has been applied to the evaluation of inflammatory bowel disease (Level 11-3).[13] On barium studies the findings are nonspecific and mostly consist of edema and erythema. With more severe involvement, the colon tends to lose its haustral pattern and become somewhat tubular. Frequently there is widening of the presacral space. Ulceration may be present in both the acute and chronic phase.

Pseudomembranous colitis, also referred to as antibiotic-associated colitis, results from the overgrowth of *Clostridium difficile*, which produces a toxin that causes mucosal inflammation, necrosis, and formation of pseduomembranes. In the appropriate clinical setting, endoscopic examination of the rectosigmoid is usually diagnostic and radiographic evaluation is often not performed. Plain radiographs demonstrate bowel dilatation, haustral fold thickening, and thumb printing.[17]

Diverticulitis Diverticulitis represents one of the two principal complications of diverticulosis, the other being lower gastrointestinal hemorrhage. The condition occurs as a result of occlusion of a diverticulum by stool, contributing to peridiverticular inflammatory changes associated with microperforations. This process can progress to frank pericolic abscess formation.

Until relatively recently, the contrast enema examination was the principal radiographic means utilized for the diagnosis. Although this procedure allows assessment of mucosal detail and the detection of sinus tracts, it is unable to adequately stage the extent of inflammation, because the pathologic process is pericolonic in location and thus extramucosal. If extravasation of contrast from a ruptured diverticulum is not seen, the presence of intramural or pericolonic involvement can only be indirectly inferred by the presence of mass effect. Additionally, the barium examination may be contraindicated if there is concern for possible perforation. In this setting, water-soluble contrast may be employed, but it allows for lower sensitivity in the detection of mucosal detail and sinus tracts. Therefore, CT in many centers has emerged as the initial imaging test of choice.

Compared to the barium enema examination, several studies have now demonstrated higher diagnostic sensitivity utilizing CT. In a study comparing CT and barium enema examination, Cho and colleagues found CT to demonstrate a higher sensitivity for the diagnosis of diverticulitis than barium enema (93% compared with 80%), as well as a specificity for the diagnosis of 100% (Level II-3).[18] The diagnostic criteria utilizing the contrast enema include the presence of diverticula, spasm or narrowing or the lumen, and mass effect. Many of these findings are associated with a more advanced stage of disease. A major advantage of CT is its ability to directly visualize the bowel wall. Mild degrees of bowel-wall thickening, as well as associated early changes in the adjacent pericolonic fat, allow for an earlier-stage CT diagnosis.

CT is less invasive and more readily tolerated by patients than is the contrast enema. It is better able to delineate the presence and extent of the associated pericolic inflammatory process and is more robust in the detection of extracolonic disease (Level II-3).[19] A major impact of CT has been its ability to consistently identify patients with pericolic abscesses. CT is also a useful aid for planning percutaneous or surgical drainage of pericolic abscesses. Of the diagnostic pitfalls, the most commonly reported is related to excessive thickening of the colonic wall. While in most cases wall thickening in diverticulitis does not exceed 4 to 5 mm, in some cases wall thickening up to 3 cm may be encountered (Level II-3).[19] In these cases, distinction from colon carcinoma may be difficult and sigmoidoscoy may be required for a diagnosis.

Appendicitis The traditional radiographic approach to the diagnosis of acute appendicitis has been the contrast enema examination, performed with either water-soluble contrast or more commonly barium enema examination. Complete filling of the appendix on a barium enema examination occurs in approximately 60% of cases and essentially excludes the diagnosis of appendicitis (Level II-3).[19] With the use of a postevacuation film, additional demonstration of the appendix is achieved in approximately 20% of cases. Incomplete filling of the appendix on barium examination, however, does not exclude appendicitis. Most commonly, on barium examinations of patients with acute appendicitis, spasm at the cecal tip and mass effect from an adjacent abscess are demonstrable.

More recently, both ultrasound and CT have been quite successfully in the diagnosis of appendicitis (Level II-3).[19] The ultrasound technique employs graduated compression of the right lower quadrant during a real-time ultrasound examination. Direct demonstration of an enlarged and noncompressible appendix 7 mm or greater in anteroposterior diameter is the primary criterion for the diagnosis of acute appendicitis (Level II-3).[20] An appendix measuring 6 mm in anteroposterior diameter is probably normal and these patients can likely be followed conservatively. The presence of an appendicolith is always considered to represent a positive study no matter what the diameter of the appendix. Most studies demonstrate sensitivity greater than 85% and specificity greater than 90% (Level II-3).[19]

The CT examination has been accomplished utilizing a variety of techniques including the use of oral water-soluble contrast material, retrograde administration of diluted water-soluble contrast, as well as techniques that have required no administration of contrast. The CT examination is well performed in obese patients in whom the ultrasound examination can prove to be more difficult. CT is also excellent for delineation of the full extent of periappendiceal abscess formation and can serve as a guide to percutaneous drainage procedures (Fig. 4.7).

Bowel Obstruction Obstruction of the bowel is a common condition and one in which the diagnosis is most typically suspected based on the patient's clinical presentation. Eighty percent of all intestinal obstructions are caused by adhesion (50%), hernias (15%), or neoplasms (15%) and approximately 35% of all cases are caused by multiple etiologies (Level II-3).[21] Diagnostic imaging procedures must address whether obstruction is present, and if so, the level of the obstruction and the likely cause.

Conventional abdominal radiographs have traditionally been utilized as the first imaging procedure in patients with suspected obstruction. Plain radiographs have the advantages of relative simplicity, universal access, and relatively low cost. At least two projections, typically one performed with the patient supine and a second with the patient upright or in a left lateral decubitus position, are required for comprehensive diagnosis (e.g., detection of air-fluid levels, free intraperitoneal air). Plain radiographic analysis may provide sufficient diagnostic information for clinical purposes in approximately 60% of cases (Level II-3).[22] In up to 20% of patients, however, there may be no evidence of obstruction on plain radiographs (Level II-3).[21]

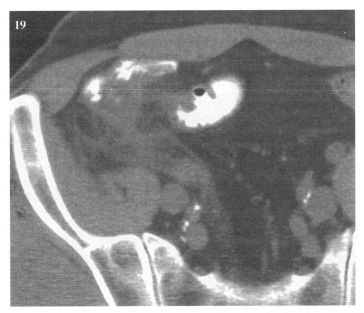

FIGURE 4.7. Appendicitis. Axial section from a CT examination demonstrating contrast within the distal small bowel and right colon. There is a poorly defined increased attenuation mass representing the dilated appendix and periappendiceal inflammatory process (arrows).

When plain radiographic analysis is not confirmatory and the clinical picture remains uncertain, further imaging diagnosis is typically entertained. Traditionally, intraluminal contrast radiography has been performed in this setting. Such examinations can be performed with both barium sulfate and water-soluble agents. Barium sulfate is contraindicated if bowel perforation is suspected, and the presence of barium is frequently objected to by surgeons contemplating the need for emergent surgery following the diagnostic procedures. Dilutional effects typically limit the effectiveness of water-soluble agents in the small bowel, although these agents are generally effectively utilized in retrograde examination of the colon. Oral barium studies are relatively rapid in early obstruction when exaggerated peristalsis is present. As motor activity decreases in later stages of obstruction, transit time increases and results not only in prolonged examination times but in compromised studies secondary to increasing dilution effects.

Enteroclysis examinations of the small bowel have been increasingly advocated for assessment of small-bowel disease and studies have demonstrated an overall accuracy of 85% in the diagnosis of small-bowel obstruction (Fig. 4.8). This technique, however, is contraindicated in patients with complete obstructions and in those suspected of strangulation (Level II-3).[22] The large amounts of barium required may also delay cross-sectional imaging examinations for

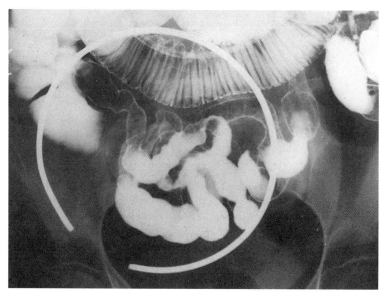

FIGURE 4.8. Enteroclysis study of the small bowel. There is a marked disparity in size of proximal and more distal small-bowel loops. The study is able to precisely delineate the area of transition in this patient with recurrent partial small-bowel obstructions.

assessment of extraintestinal disease and may pose difficulty for the surgeon contemplating immediate intervention.

There has been increasing interest and experience in the use of CT for assessment of patients with suspected bowel obstruction. CT has been shown to be useful in revealing the site, level, and cause of obstruction and in displaying signs of threatened bowel viability (Level II-3).[22,23] CT can be performed with or without the use of intraluminal contrast. In many cases of obstruction, there is sufficient fluid within the obstructed bowel to allow accurate visualization of obstructed loops and prediction of the level of obstruction. If contrast material is utilized, either a diluted solution of barium sulfate (1.2%) or 2% iodinated water-soluble contrast medium is employed. Either contrast agent is sufficiently dilute to obviate the concerns with regard to intraluminal contrast that traditionally have been raised with the use of full-strength barium. With the new generation of helical (spiral) CT scanners, the complete examination can be performed literally within minutes and can be tolerated by even the most severely ill patients. Intravenous contrast material is highly desirable for assessment of the presence of strangulation.

The CT diagnosis of bowel obstruction is based on the demonstration of discrepancy in caliber of the bowel loops (Fig. 4.9). In the majority of patients, this discrepancy is quite marked, making the determination of bowel obstruction relatively straightforward. Many studies have attested to the value of approaching the interpretation of CT for bowel obstruction in a retrograde fashion begin-

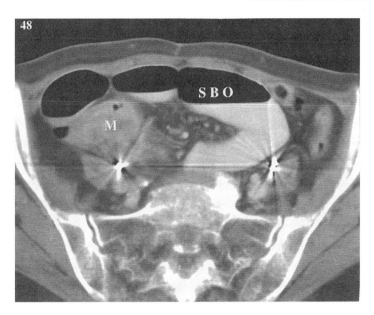

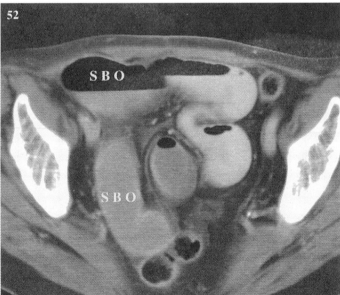

FIGURE 4.9. Small-bowel obstruction secondary to recurrent tumor. (A) On an axial scan section through the distal abdomen, several dilated loops of small bowel are seen proximal to a mass (M) of recurrent tumor. Artifact is introduced related to surgical clips. (B) On a more distal CT section through the midpelvis, multiple dilated loops of small bowel are seen. While these loops are seen in the pelvis, they are located proximal to the level of obstruction.

ning at the rectum and working toward the cecum. In cases of small-bowel obstruction, the transverse colon will typically be compressed against the anterior abdominal wall by the tensely distended small-bowel loops. With regard to assessment of the small bowel, a common mistake is to assume that loops on more caudal images are ileal loops and loops on more proximal images are jejunal loops. In actuality, as the bowel dilates, the loops align themselves along the small-bowel mesentery, and as a consequence, jejunal loops may appear in the pelvis and ileal loops in the right upper quadrant. The retrograde evaluation technique is valuable in avoiding this type of diagnostic error.

Modern scanners also allow the images to be paged through in a serial or simulated "cine" mode that can also be extremely helpful for viewing and correctly interpreting the multiple images obtained. A prospective series evaluating the utility of CT in the diagnosis of bowel obstruction has demonstrated a sensitivity of 94%, a specificity of 96%, and an overall accuracy of 95% (Level II-3).[24]

After the presence of obstruction has been determined, an advantage of CT over other diagnostic imaging methods is the ability to frequently establish the cause. While bowel obstruction may be secondary to a wide variety of etiologies, two groups of patients deserve particular emphasis. The first group consists of patients with a known abdominal malignancy. In these patients, surgical versus conservative management is based on the cause of the obstruction (e.g., peritoneal carcinomatosis, radiation enteritis) (Level 11-3).[22] The percentage of cancer patients in whom bowel obstruction is due to adhesions ranges from 21% to 38% (Level II-3).[25] CT can be effectively utilized to determine the presence of peritoneal carcinomatosis by its ability to directly visualize the peritoneal surfaces (Level II-3).[26] The diagnosis of obstruction secondary to carcinomatosis is established by the demonstration of a mass or bowel-wall thickening evident along the serosa of the bowel at the transition zone. In the absence of a mass, adhesions would need to be considered as an etiology. In a series reported by Megibow, the correct diagnosis of malignant obstruction was made in 92% of patients (Level II-3).[22] The second group consists of patients in whom the obstruction is secondary to simple adhesions. This diagnosis is based on the absence of any other cause for the obstruction, as most simple adhesive bands cannot be seen. In the series reported by Megibow, successful characterization of the cause of obstruction on the basis of adhesions was made in 73% of cases (Level II-3).[24]

CT can also be used effectively in the assessment of complicated intestinal obstruction including strangulation, as well as closed-loop obstructions. Closed-loop or incarcerated obstructions of the small bowel result when a segment of bowel is occluded at two points along its course from a single constrictive lesion that occludes both the intestine and the small-bowel mesentery (Level II-3).[22] The two adjacent segments of bowel entrap and compromise the mesenteric attachments, which contributes to compromise of the vascular supply and drainage of the bowel and can result in ischemia and bowel necrosis. Adhesive bands and hernias are the most common causes of strangulating obstruction (Level II-3).[22]

As the mortality rates significantly increase from 5% in simple obstruction to 20% to 37% in patients with strangulation complicating the obstruction, the need for accurate diagnosis is underscored.[27] The CT findings in closed-loop obstructions include (1) evidence of a small-bowel obstruction; (2) a U-shaped or radial configuration of fluid-filled dilated bowel loops and associated mesenteric vessels converging toward the point of obstruction; and (3) a whirl sign, beak sign, triangular loop, or two adjacent collapsed loops at the site of obstruction.[2] In strangulating obstruction, the CT findings, in addition to evidence of obstruction, include (1) a circumferentially thickened loop with high attenutation within the wall, a target sign (thickened regionally enhancing bowel wall with submucosal edema), or evidence of pneumatosis; and (2) congestive changes or hemorrhage in the adjacent mesentery (Level III).[2] In cases of true infarction, moderate to large volumes of ascites, which in most cases will demonstrate higher attenuation than water, will be present.

The clinician has multiple diagnostic imaging choices in patients with suspected bowel obstruction. Certainly, conventional abdominal radiography remains the most reasonable initial examination and may be sufficient for clinical purposes in the majority of patients. When the plain abdominal examination is equivocal or normal and clinical concern persists, CT can be effectively utilized for rapid and definitive diagnosis. It may be particularly valuable in excluding complicated causes of obstruction (necessitating immediate intervention) when conservative therapy is otherwise being considered.

CT is particularly valuable in patients with a history of malignancy and clinical findings suggestive of obstruction. It has a more secondary role in postoperative patients without a history of malignancy in whom adhesive obstruction is overwhelmingly likely. Because of its ease and rapidity of performance, CT is increasingly being utilized in patients with suspected vascular compromise or palpable mass in association with signs of obstruction. Barium studies are most reasonably utilized in noncritically ill patients with histories of recurring obstruction or low-grade mechanical obstruction to help identify the obstructed segment as precisely as possible.

Abdominal and Pelvic Abscess

Despite improved surgical techniques and the use of perioperative antibiotics, abscesses continue to be encountered in the postoperative period. (Level II-3, Level III).[28–30] The ability to noninvasively and accurately evaluate patients with suspected abscess formation is of obvious importance. Imaging-guided percutaneous abdominal abscess drainage is becoming the preferred method of treatment. This section reviews the techniques useful for diagnosis and treatment of abdominal abscesses.

Diagnostic Imaging   Continuing advances in ultrasound and particularly CT have allowed these techniques to emerge and largely replace other diagnostic methods in the evaluation of suspected abdominal abscess (Level III).[28] Ultrasound is an extremely sensitive tool for the detection and localization of fluid collections in the abdomen and pelvis. The technique is rapidly accomplished and can be performed at the patient's bedside. It is important to recognize, however, that certain anatomic areas are better evaluated than others by ultrasound (right upper quadrant and pelvis) and the exam is best limited to evaluation of these areas.

With ultrasound, abscesses often appear as rounded or oval-shaped collections that contain internal echoes and debris and may have irregular walls. In the febrile postoperative patient, the demonstration of a fluid collection raises the question of whether the fluid is a simple postoperative collection (seroma, sterile hematoma) or abscess (Level III).[28] In a prospective ultrasound study of postoperative patients, Neff and colleagues found that 19% of asymptomatic postoperative patients had ultrasonically demonstrable fluid collections on the fourth postoperative day and that 80% of these collections conformed to peritoneal recessus (Level II-3).[29] Only 6% of these patients demonstrated persistence of the fluid by the eighth postoperative day, suggesting that simple fluid collections are common in the early postoperative period. The only collection in this series that proved to be an abscess increased in size over the observation period (Level II-3).[29] While certain collections can be highly suggestive for abscess on ultrasound, in many cases diagnostic uncertainty exists. In this setting, the collections can be percutaneously aspirated, allowing for a specific diagnosis.

Although a powerful technique, ultrasound is limited both by its nonspecificity and technical limitations, which do not allow for complete evaluation of the abdomen. Bowel gas, commonly encountered in postoperative patients with ileus, can limit the available acoustic windows for sonographic evaluation as can the presence of surgical dressings.

For many of these reasons, CT in most institutions has become the imaging technique of choice for the evaluation of patients with suspected abdominal abscess. As mentioned with ultrasound, the CT appearances of sterile and infected fluid collections frequently overlap and definitive diagnosis often requires aspiration. Most abscesses on CT are characterized by the presence of areas of low attenuation, either within parenchymal organs or in an extraluminal location within the peritoneal cavity (Level II-3).[28,30] Other useful features include the detection of gas, thick or irregular walls, and heterogeneous internal debris.

When performing CT scans to detect intra-abdominal abscess, it is essential that the study be performed using positive contrast agents to achieve bowel opacification and to avoid misdiagnosing fluid-filled bowel limits as possible abnormal fluid collections. A particular advantage of CT over ultrasound is in the assessment of the retroperitoneum and in the detection of abscesses located between bowel loops. It far exceeds ultrasound in the assessment of pancreatic inflammatory disease (see separate section).

The major limitation of CT relates to its nonspecificity, a weakness it shares with sonography. Even the presence of gas within a low-attenuation mass is not specific for abscess but may be seen with necrotic tumor and noninfected enteric fistulae. Additionally, in certain circumstances CT may not confidently differentiate between fluid collections and homogeneous solid masses.

Percutaneous Interventional Procedures As a result of the nonspecific nature of the information gathered on fluid collections using either ultrasound or CT, definitive diagnosis often awaits percutaneous aspiration and culture of the collection. Ultrasound can be readily employed for larger and more superficial locations, and CT can be reserved for smaller and more deeply located collections. The technique to be employed will in part reflect the experience and preference of the radiologist. If percutaneous drainage is being considered, care should be taken to aspirate only enough material for diagnostic purposes so as not to make subsequent placement of a larger-diameter drain more difficult. Selection of the access route is critical.

In contrast to biopsy of suspected solid tumor, for assessment of possible abscess it is critical that bowel not be traversed, even by a small-gauge needle. A sample that yields bacteria without white cells is most suggestive of bowel contents and mandates reassessment of the access route. If the patient is already receiving antibiotics, the presence of white cells without bacteria may represent a "sterile" abscess. Such collections should most likely be treated with catheter drainage (Level III).[28]

Percutaneous abscess drainage has become the preferred method for treatment of most abscesses located in the abdomen and pelvis (Level III, Level II-3).[28,30] Advances in technique have resulted in a procedure that is relatively safe, efficacious, and straightforward to perform. The technique is less invasive than surgical drainage and in most instances can be performed under regional anesthesia or conscious sedation. With developments in technique, the procedure is now most commonly performed in one stage utilizing either the modified Seldinger or trocar technique. This method has obviated the need for the patient to be moved to a fluoroscopic suite as was traditionally done when the procedure was performed in two stages. The pelvis is a common site of abscess formation, particularly in postoperative patients. Only a minority of these collections can be safely drained utilizing an anterior approach. Thus, alternative approaches include transgluteal, transrectal, and transvaginal, all of which have been done successfully.

Acute Renal and Urinary Tract Conditions

Patients with gynecological malignancies can present with acute urinary tract conditions that in many cases are relatively straightforward to diagnose and treat and thus do not require advanced imaging. Imaging studies are most valuable in patients who do not respond to antibiotic therapy and who may have complicating conditions such as pyonephrosis, perinephric abscess, or renal abscess. Additionally, postsurgical complications to the bladder and ureter commonly require diagnostic imaging. Most commonly, ultrasound and CT are utilized for diagnostic purposes. At times, intravenous urography and cystography are performed. Comments regarding the choice of appropriate procedure are given as each condition is considered.

Acute Infections   Acute renal infections are most commonly caused by hematogenous spread of organisms or by ascending infections from the bladder and are most commonly due to gram-negative organisms such as *Escherichia coli* (Level II-3).[31] Acute pyelonephritis is usually recognized clinically by the presence of fever, chills, flank pain, leukocytosis, and pyuria. The infection may be focal or diffuse. CT can be quite effective for diagnosis and should be performed with intravenous contrast administration (Level II-3).[31]

Acute focal pyelonephitris is characterized on CT by sharply marginated, wedge-shaped zones of decreased attenuation radiating from the collecting system to the renal capsule. When severe, the condition may progress to form a hypodense mass with bulging of the renal contour. When the condition is diffuse, it is manifest by poor renal contrast enhancement, delayed or nonexcretion of contrast material into the collecting system, and renal enlargement. On ultrasound, zones of acute pyelonephritis may appear normal or may manifest as focal areas of decreased or increased cortical echogenicity (Level II-3).[32] With severe infection, ultrasound may demonstrate hypoechoic, poorly marginated masses with scattered low-amplitude echoes and poor sound transmission (Level II-3).[33]

Emphysematous pyelonephritis is an acute complication and occurs most commonly in diabetic patients. The condition represents as a diffuse gas-forming parenchymal infection most commonly secondary to *E. coli*. CT is the most sensitive method for establishing the diagnosis and can distinguish between gas in the collecting system, with the parenchyma (required for diagnosis), and gas in the perinephric tissues (Level II-3).[34] If inadequately treated, small abscesses may form in areas of severe pyelonephritis. These are best imaged by CT.

Early in their evolution, prior to the development of necrosis, abscesses may be ill defined on CT and may manifest as zones of decreased parenchymal enhancement. The borders become increasingly well defined as the abscess encapsulates, and the area of infection is low in attenuation and typically does not enhance with contrast administration. With ultrasound, renal abscess is typically hypochoic or anechoic and demonstrates enhanced sound transmission. If the infection extends beyond the renal capsule, a perinephric abscess may result. This complication of renal infection is typically well defined by both CT and ultrasound, and if the collections are of sufficient size, they can be readily drained by percutaneous techniques.

Pyonephrosis, the accumulation of pus in the collecting system, represents a true urological emergency requiring relief of the obstruction. Ultrasound is the technique of choice for establishing the diagnosis, which is made by the demonstration of a dilated collecting system containing urine debris levels (Level II-3).[33] In some cases, however, pyonephrosis cannot be distinguished sonographically from simple hydronephrosis, and in these cases the diagnosis can be established by ultrasound guide aspiration of the collecting system. CT usually cannot reliably distinguish between infected and uninfected hydronephrosis, although the presence of gas in a dilated collecting system can strongly suggest the diagnosis (Level II-3).[35]

Acute Obstruction   Acute unilateral renal obstruction is most commonly caused by stone disease, but in the perioperative patient with gynecological malignancy the possibility of tumor or iatrogenic obstruction secondary to surgical intervention must be considered. Intravenous urography can be reliably utilized to diagnose obstruction and demonstrates the typical obstructive nephrogram characterized by both delayed onset and progressive increase in density. Urography also effectively demonstrates the level of obstruction in most cases.

Ultrasound is often utilized as the initial examination in assessing suspected acute renal obstruction and is especially useful in patients with compromised renal function and contrast allergies. Although ultrasound is highly sensitive in detecting the collecting system dilatation that accompanies obstruction, its value in acute obstruction is limited by the fact that up to 30% of acutely obstructed kidneys do not demonstrate pyelocaliectasis (Level II-3).[36] Therefore, some investigators have advocated the use of duplex Doppler examination of the small intrarenal arteries and determination of a resistive index.

Resistive index elevation may occur after 6 hours of clinical obstruction and may precede pyelocaliectasis. Some investigators have found that the resistive index in the acutely obstructed kidney usually exceeds .70 and is at least .10 higher than in the normal contralateral kidney (Level II-3).[36] Others, however, have disputed the usefulness of the resistive index and have found it insensitive for the diagnosis of acute urinary obstruction (Level II-3).[37]

CT may also assess acute renal obstruction. It is particularly valuable in the determination of the level and etiology of ureteric obstruction. Using sequential CT sections, a change in caliber of the ureter can be a reliable guide to the level of obstruction. Most stones are readily demonstrated secondary to their high attenuation values.

Acute Renal Vascular Disorders   Patients with major acute renal infarction often present with sudden onset of upper abdominal or flank pain, fever, and vomiting. If the main renal artery is occluded, global renal infarction occurs, and on contrast-enhanced CT the affected kidney shows lack of enhancement except for a high-density subcapsular cortical rim that reflects perfusion from collateral vessels (Level II-3).[33,38] If a major renal artery branch is occluded, global renal infarction occurs. Ultrasound may show no abnormality in acute infarction.

On CT, local infarctions are manifest as sharply marginated, wedge-shaped, low-attenuation lesions. The main CT differential diagnosis of acute focal infarction is acute pyelonephritis, as both manifest wedge-shaped low-attenuation lesions on CT. A subcapsular cortical rim should strongly suggest the diagnosis of acute renal infarction because it is usually not seen in acute pyelonephritis. Small renal infarctions may be difficult to differentiate from metastatic lesions on CT.

Patients with acute renal vein thrombosis usually complain of acute flank or abdominal pain and hematuria. Contrast-enhanced helical CT is an excellent method for diagnosis if renal function is normal (Level II-3).[39] Definitive diagnosis is based on the direct demonstration of a thrombus in the renal vein. Indirect CT signs include nephromegaly, ipsilateral prolonged corticomedullary enhancement, thickening of the renal fascia, and perinephric hemorrhage.

With ultrasound, patients with renal vein thrombosis manifest absent renal venous blood flow on Doppler examination and echogenic material in the main renal vein on gray-scale ultrasonography. Doppler study of the small intrarenal vessels may demonstrate a marked increase in resistive index. While the right renal vein is readily demonstrable utilizing the liver as an acoustic window, evaluation of the left renal vein is more problematic on ultrasound (Level II-3).[33]

THE CENTRAL NERVOUS SYSTEM

Whenever an oncology patient presents with a focal complaint in any part of the body, the first thought the patient and oncologist has is whether there is metastatic disease, especially in the brain and spine. In patients who present with neurologic symptoms with known central nervous system (CNS) metastasis, the question is usually if there is recurrence of treated tumor or complications from treatment. In those without known prior CNS disease, the issue is new tumor versus any of the other numerous diseases that affect the equivalent nononcology patient population.

A history and neurologic exam are key in performing the appropriate radiology work-up. Patients may present with a wide range of symptoms from the very nonspecific such as headache to a very localized symptom such as slurred speech. The neurologic exam can expose subtle findings such as a slight ataxia or a visual field deficit that are not always detected by the patient.

In the acute setting, where there is an abrupt change in the patient's neurologic status, an emergent study is essential. In this situation, a CT scan is the only front-line imaging modality for the brain. These are patients who present with altered mental status, severe headache, focal neurologic signs, or new onset of seizures (Table 4.1). A CT scan identifies life-threatening situations that require immediate neurosurgical decompression or treatment such as intracranial hemorrhage, mass lesions with impending herniation, and cerebral infarction. In the spine, magnetic resonance imaging (MRI) has replaced CT myelography and is used for patients with symptoms of cord compression who may require emergent radiation therapy or surgical intervention (Level II-2, II-3, II-3).[40–42]

Patients with subacute onset of symptoms will benefit most from MRI, including those who have progressive headaches, double vision, vomiting, slow

TABLE 4.1. Acute Indications for Central Nervous System Imaging

Altered mental state/decreased consciousness
Confusion
Focal neurologic deficit
  Aphasia
  Extremity weakness
Severe headache—"worst headache of my life"
Vertigo
Nausea/Vomiting
Ataxia
New onset seizures/status epilepticus
Visual disturbances
Accute radicular pain with loss of sensation or strength
Cord compression symptoms
  Bilateral loss of extremity sensation or strength
  Bowel/bladder dysfunction

onset of focal weakness, problems with memory, or back pain (Table 4.2). The advantage of MRI over CT is its multiplanar imaging capability and specialized imaging sequences that can define lesion tissue characteristics (Table 4.3). Contrast-enhanced CT or CT myelography can be used when MRI cannot be done (Table 4.4; Level II-3).[43]

Radiologists are often part of the oncology team and are the best resource in selecting the appropriate study in complicated cases as well as on a routine basis (Table 4.5). The following discussion gives an overview of the optimal imaging studies in the work-up of gynecologic oncology patients and the respective imaging findings, whether related to underlying tumor or to another disease process that affects the same population.

TABLE 4.2. Subacute Indications for Central Nervous System Imaging

Headaches—increasing in severity of frequency
Subacute onset of focal neurologic deficit
  Increasing extremity weakness
Memory loss
Vertigo
Visual disturbances
Back pain
  Generalized
  Focal
Radiculitis without weakness of decreased sensation
Paresthesias

TABLE 4.3. Common MR Imaging Sequences and Their Properties

T1-weighted sequence
  Demonstrates soft tissue structures
  Not very sensitive to pathology
  Sensitive to subacute hemorrhage
T2-weighted sequence
  Demonstrates pathology well by defining abnormal tissues/edema
  Can show characteristics that point to specific etiologies
T1-weighted sequence with gadolinium (intravenous contrast)
  Demonstrates pathology well by enhancing abnormal tissues
  Can show characteristics that point to specific etiologies
Fluid-attenuated inversion-recovery (FLAIR) sequence
  Extremely sensitive to abnormal tissues/edema
  Not usually specific as to etiology
Gradient-echo sequence
  Very sensitive to blood products, calcium, metallic deposits
  Not sensitive to other soft tissue structures or lesions
  Not specific as to etiology
Short inversion-recovery sequence (STIR)
  Excellent at defining abnormal bone marrow
  Not specific as to etiology
Magnetic resonance angiography (MRA)
  Demonstrates arteries from base of neck to Circle of Willis
  Defines focal stenosis, aneurysms and arterial malformations
  Not sensitive to vasculitis, distal vessel disease, small aneurysms (<4mm)
  Exaggerates degree of vessel stenosis
  Does not replace standard angiography when clinically indicated
Magnetic resonance venography (MRV)
  Demonstrates veins from base of neck to dural sinuses
  Defines occluded venous drainage
  Subject to marked normal variation in cerebral veins/sinuses

Brain Imaging in the GYN-Oncology Patient
Metastasis

In order of decreasing frequency, metastasis can be in one of three general locations: in the calvarium, in the brain parenchyma, or on the meningeal surfaces (Level II-3).[44] The calvarium, the most common location, is usually only part of generalized skeletal involvement and is addressed in other sections.

The brain parenchyma has the typical radiographic appearance of multiple enhancing soft-tissue lesions. CNS metastases are unusual at first presentation in most gynecologic cancers, but occur in patientswho have advanced or recurrent ovarian and uterine malignancies (Level II-3, Level III).[45–47] Gestational trophoblastic tumor and breast cancer are two exceptions and can initially present with CNS metastasis (Level II-3).[48,49] CNS involvement in cervical, vaginal, and vulvar cancers is almost never observed (Level II-3).[50,51]

TABLE 4.4. Contraindications to Magnetic Resonance Imaging[*]

Cardiac Pacemaker
Cerebral Aneurysm Clips
   If the clip has undergone and passed ex vivo testing the patient maybe scanned
Poppen-Blaylock Carotid Artery Clamp
   Other clamps are O.K.
Select breast tissue expanders
   Infall breast implant
   Tissue expander with metal port
Some Ocular Implants
Cochlear Implants
McGee stapes prosthesis (model recalled by manufacturer)
Intravascular coils, filters and stents that have been implanted less than 6 weeks
Some pellets/bullets, if they are located near a vital anatomic structure
Implanted magnetically activated or electronic devices

---

[*]From Pocket Guide to MR procedures and Metallic Objects: Update 1994. Frank G. Shellock. Raven Press 1995.

Patients with CNS metastasis generally have a subacute presentation with focal and/or generalized symptoms such as extremity weakness related to a lesion on the motor cortex, or memory loss and seizures related to a lesion in the temporal lobe. MRI is more sensitive than contrast-enhanced CT and often identifies more lesions (Level II-1, II-1).[52–54] The lesion(s) can enhance homogeneously, heterogeneously, or have a ring of peripheral enhancement. There is seldom a specific finding that can differentiate one type of metastasis from another, yet certain features such as calcification, melanin, and hemorrhage have very characteristic MRI signal properties and are very helpful if present (Level II-3).[44] Two such metastases are ovarian mucinous adenocarcinoma, which produces psammomatous calcifications, and choriocarcinoma, which commonly has foci of hemorrhage (Fig. 4.10).

TABLE 4.5. Modalities for Central Nervous System Imaging

Computed Tomography (CT)
   With or without iodinated intravenous contrast
Magnetic Resonance Imaging (MR/MRI)
   With or without contrast (Gadolinium)
Radionuclide Bone Scanning
   Used primarily in the spine
CT Myelography/Myelography
   Requires intrathecal injection of contrast material
Cerebral and Spinal Angiography
   Semi-invasive procedure with arterial catheterization, usually from groin site
   Potential life threatening complications such as stroke and hemorrhage
Ultrasound/Sonography
   Not used to evaluate the adult CNS

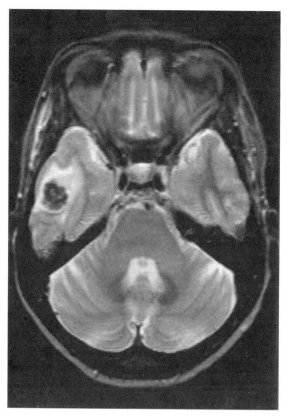

FIGURE 4.10. Metastatic mucinous ovarian carcinoma. (A) Axial T2-weighted MR image shows a focal lesion in the temporal lobe with a very dark signal consistent with calcification seen in ovarian CNS metastasis (arrow). Rim of very bright signal is peritumoral edema. (B) Axial T1-weighted postcontrast image shows homogeneous enhancement (arrow). Edema is not well defined in this type of image sequence.

Imaging must be combined with clinical information to make the correct diagnosis. Given just the imaging findings, other entities have identical appearances. For example, infections with ring-enhancing lesions may not be distinguishable from metastases. In the oncology patient, who may be immunocompromised, opportunistic infection is in the clinical and radiologic differential. Biopsy is occasionally needed to distinguish between the two.

The least common metastases involve neoplastic spread to the meningeal surfaces. Focal metastasis can be on the leptomeninges, on the dura, or both. Patients have nonspecific symptoms such as headache, rather than focal neurologic findings, in contrast to those with parenchymal involvement.

Meningeal metastases lie on the meningeal surfaces around the brain and spine, or intrathecally in the lumbosacral region (Fig. 4.11). On contrast-enhanced MRI there is one of three patterns: nodules of enhancement on the sur-

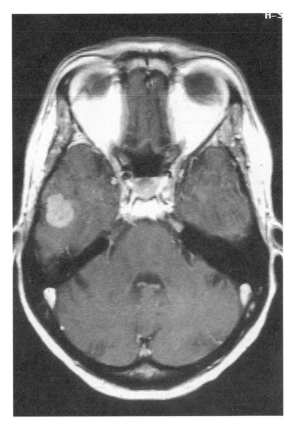

FIGURE 4.10. (*Continued.*)

face of the brain/dura, more subtle diffuse dural enhancement (leptomeningeal carcinomatosis), or a combination of the two (Level II-3).[54] Leptomeningeal carcinomatosis is a rare form of diffuse meningeal metastatic disease; however, it is seen in metastatic adenocarcinoma, particularly in the gynecologic oncology patient with a primary ovarian or breast neoplasm (Level II-3).[43,44] Gadolinium-enhanced MRI is optimal for imaging carcinomatosis; contrast-enhanced CT can be used if MRI is contraindicated, but it is much less sensitive (Level II-3).[55] MRI reveals subtle tumor interdigitating between the gyri and around the brain stem. The most useful clinical adjunct is positive spinal fluid for malignant cells. Spread of tumor to the dural surfaces of the brain can be a component of parenchymal disease, in which case the imaging findings are diagnostic. Meningeal metastasis involving the brain has the potential for spread to the surface of the spine.

Other "benign" causes of dural enhancement in oncology patients include infectious and chemical meningitis. Often the clinical picture of headache, nuchal rigidity, convulsions, altered mental status, and a "toxic" state help

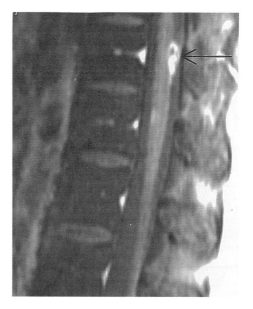

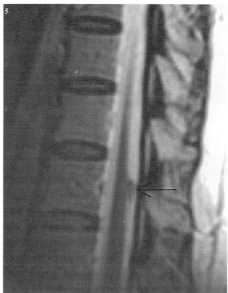

FIGURE 4.11. Intradural metastasis of the lumbar spine. (A) Sagittal postcontrast T1-weighted images with fat suppression show a very conspicuous focus of nodular enhancement along the conus medullaris (arrow). (B) Sagittal T2-weighted image—the lesion is almost invisible. (C) Sagittal postcontrast T1-weighted image in the same patient shows a larger lesion(s) at the sacral level (arrow). (D) Sagittal T2-weighted image detects the larger lesion(s) (arrow).

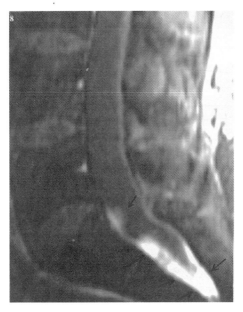

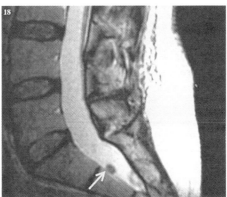

FIGURE 4.11. (*Continued.*)

to differentiate metastasis from infectious meningitis. Meningitis is discussed more thoroughly in the CNS infections section. Chemical meningitis is seen in patients who have had intrathecal administration of chemotherapy or recent subarachnoid hemorrhage.

Stroke

Gynecologic oncology patients are predominantly middle-aged to elderly and are not only at risk from complications related to their cancers but also from other diseases that are prevalent in this age group. Therefore, in the acute setting of altered mental status, especially with a focal neurologic finding such as weakness or slurred speech, stroke is an important consideration. CT scanning without contrast is the first choice in imaging acute stroke (Level II-3).[56] One exception is if the suspected stroke patient has symptoms that localize to the brain stem or cerebellum—the vascular distribution of the vertebral and basilar arteries. CT has decreased visualization of this area because of two factors, both caused by the thick skull base: There is decreased penetration of the X rays through the skull and "beam hardening artifact," which is essentially increased energy of the X-ray beam, resulting in loss of soft-tissue contrast. In this case, noncontrast MRI is exquisite in evaluating the posterior fossa.

There are myriad causes of stroke including emboli from carotid artery disease, cardiac sources, and hypercoagulable states. CT is excellent at showing the arterial distribution of infarction that may involve all or part of the anterior, middle, or posterior cerebral artery territories. Up to 12 hours following the ictus, the CT scan can remain normal (Level II-3).[56] After 12 hours, imaging reveals loss of the normal differentiation between gray and white matter, which is caused by edema in the infarcted brain tissue.

Large strokes have significant mass effect and often display small foci of hemorrhage. The CT appearance of a stroke in evolution is typical, and MRI is rarely needed (Level II-3).[57,58] MRI is reserved for cases in which there is either an atypical/nonvascular distribution of edema or clinical data that suggest an etiology other than stroke (Level II-3).[58] Currently, if the patient presents within 3 to 6 hours after ictus and the CT shows no evidence for infarction/hemorrhage, thrombolytic therapies should be implemented to lyse the clot and possibly reverse the stroke (Level I).[59]

Venous infarction is less common and occurs secondary to thrombosis of a major venous drainage, particularly the deep cerebral veins or dural sinuses. Thrombosis of the superior sagittal sinus results in obstruction of blood flow within the cortical and subcortical areas, causing infarction (Level II-3).[60] Venous sinus thrombosis is differentiated from arterial thrombosis in that it has a bilateral but not necessarily symmetric distribution, affecting the cortex and subcortical regions. Additionally, there is often a diffuse hemorrhagic component. Deep venous thrombosis affects the basal ganglia and thalami, but it is not common in adults (Level II-3).[61] MRI with MR venography (MRV) is the best noninvasive diagnostic tool. In addition to showing the classic cortical and subcortical distribution of brain edema with petechial hemorrhage, MRV demonstrates the occluded sinuses. Standard angiography may still be needed in patients who have equivocal MR findings related to a congenitally hypoplastic or a partially thrombosed sinus.

Brain Hemorrhage

Nontraumatic hemorrhage in the brain can be of three locations: parenchymal, subarachnoid, or subdural. Epidural hematomas are not included as they are almost exclusively seen in the context of trauma. In almost all instances, CT should be the first imaging study performed for suspected intracranial hemorrhage. Blood has the exceptional property of being "bright" on CT, and can easily be differentiated from the normal "gray" soft-tissue attenuation of the brain parenchyma. MRI is also exquisitely sensitive to parenchymal and subdural hemorrhage, especially if gradient echo sequences are performed.

MRI determines the stage of a blood clot: acute, subacute, or chronic. Standard spin-echo MRI is relatively insensitive to subarachnoid hemorrhage (SAH); however, a new sequence known as fluid attenuated inversion recovery (FLAIR) can identify SAH with better sensitivity to CT scanning (Level II-1).[62,63] The most common cause of spontaneous SAH is rupture of an aneurysm. Patients classically present with the worst headache they have ever experienced. However, CT imaging is still the study of choice followed by standard angiography if subarachnoid hemorrhage is seen (Fig. 4.12). Subacute blood or a small amount of hemorrhage may not be detected on the CT scan; if clinical suspicion is high for SAH, a spinal tap should be performed.

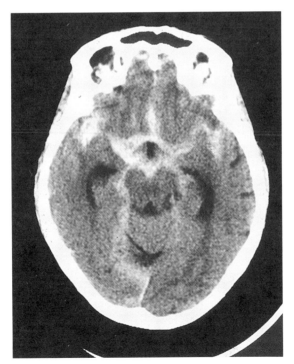

FIGURE 4.12. Subarachnoid hemorrhage. Axial CT scan of the brain shows the white density of blood all around the brain stem, extending into the suprasellar cistern and gyri of the temporal lobes (short arrows). Enlargement of the temporal horns of the lateral ventricles indicates early hydrocephalus caused by the hemorrhage (long arrows).

The most frequent cause of a focal parenchymal blood clot in the gyneco-logic oncology patient population is a hemorrhagic infarction; these infarctions are typically seen in chronically hypertensive patients and are located in the basal ganglia/thalamus (Level II-3).[64] The CT appearance ranges from a small focus of blood to a large parenchymal clot, but with the epicenter in the thalamus, putamen, or globus pallidus. An unusual type of cerebral hemorrhage caused by amyloid angiopathy is located peripherally in the cerebral hemisphere in patients past the seventh decade (Level II-3).[65] Less common in this population is parenchymal hemorrhage related to an underlying vascular malformation because this abnor-mality is unlikely to be quiescent and is present at a much earlier age.

Subdural hematomas (SDH) are common and can be spontaneous in the anti-coagulated patient; cancer patients are often anticoagulated pharmacologically, or secondarily from chemotherapy. Elderly patients who have had even minor head trauma can get SDH. The clinical presentation is classically insidious, but is frequently acute. CT is the imaging study of choice, but MRI can be equally useful. Both techniques will accurately identify a subdural hematoma. MRI provides information regarding the age of the clot and whether there has been rebleeding into an already existing hematoma (Level II-3).[66]

CNS Infections

Just as metastasis to the brain can be categorized into compartments, so can infections. Most infections are meningeal, some are localized to the brain parenchyma, and some are classified as both. Most intracranial infections are secondary to either systemic infection or extension from an adjacent site such as the paranasal sinuses. Oncology patients are subject to the same CNS infec-tions as those occurring in the general population; in addition, they may be susceptible to opportunistic infection because of an underlying immunocom-promised state related to chemotherapy or bone-marrow transplantation. The imaging characteristics are, in general, similar in the two groups. However, some salient differences are discussed.

Meningitis is usually a clinical diagnosis based on symptoms of fever, headache, altered mental status, seizures, nuchal rigidity, and abnormal cere-bral spinal fluid (CSF; Level II-3).[67] Imaging is helpful in diagnosing cases where the clinical picture is atypical or the CSF is indeterminate. Typically these patients are either immunocompromised or already on antibiotics and therefore do not have a clear clinical picture. In this case, contrast-enhanced MRI is the imaging modality of choice. The findings are characteristic with enhancement of the meninges—specifically the leptomeninges.

Imaging is also required in patients with suspected complications related to meningitis such as hydrocephalus, ventriculitis, cerebritis, venous sinus throm-bosis, or abscess formation. If there is associated cerebritis, a focal area of brain edema in the underlying cortex and white matter is seen, which is best demon-strated on T2-weighted images; cerebritis may not enhance with contrast. It is unusual to see a brain abscess in the setting of meningitis. It is very important to note that MRI may be normal in up to 70% of patients with meningitis (Level II-3).[68] In those patients in whom MRI is contraindicated, contrast-enhanced CT is a good alternative. Lastly, imaging is used to identify potential sources of intracranial infection such as paranasal sinusitis and mastioditis. In this case, CT scanning is optimal because it exquisitely demonstrates bone erosion in the setting of aggressive infection.

Brain abscesses have a fairly uniform appearance, regardless of etiology. MRI is the imaging study of choice, but CT is front line in the acute setting, especially in patients presenting with new onset of seizures or focal neurologic deficits. Brain abscesses occur but are infrequent in immunocompetent patients; when they do occur, they are secondary to an aggressive pathogen acquired in the community, mostly bacterial. Predominantly, brain abscesses are seen in the immunocompromised and there are a few pathogens that are worth discussion besides the classical bacterial abscesses.

Toxoplasmosis is the most commonly encountered opportunistic CNS infection and tends to affect the central portions of the brain (Level II-3).[68] MRI is the imaging study of choice, showing 1 to 2 centimeter ring-enhancing foci scattered in the basal ganglia, thalami, and periventricular regions. Lesions can be seen peripherally, but are less common (Level II-3).[69] Multifocal abscesses are common with nosocomial infections such as Nocardia or fungi (Level II-3).[69,70] Community-acquired bacterial abscesses such as those caused by staphylococcus species are usually solitary/multiple ring–enhancing lesions with marked surrounding edema (Fig. 4.13).

Less common CNS infections include cerebritis and encephalitis. Cerebritis is either a primary focal infection of the brain that can progress to abscess or the result of an aggressive meningitis that has extended into the underlying brain parenchyma. Encephalitis is a primary diffuse infection of the brain almost exclusively caused by viruses or unusual pathogens (Level II-3).[68,69] Contrast-enhanced MRI is the imaging modality of choice for these entities. The inflammatory changes are exquisitely demonstrated on the T2-weighted images, while the enhancement characteristics help define the extent of disease and exclude other differential possibilities. In particular, herpes simplex encephalitis warrants special mention; it can affect any host and is very aggressive. Morbidity and mortality are high if not treated promptly; early treatment can result in complete recovery (Level II-3).[70,71] A high index of suspicion along with early CSF studies and MRI are key in the work-up. MRI classically shows bilateral but not necessarily symmetric temporal lobe edema. Hemorrhagic necrosis is also seen, but this is a late finding, heralding a poor outcome (Level II-3).[72]

Although not often thought of as an infection, progressive multifocal leukoencephalopathy (PML) is the result of reactivation of a papova virus in the CNS of immunocompromised hosts (Level II-3).[73] This entity was originally described in patients who were being treated for leukemia, but now is a common pathogen in acquired immune deficiency syndrome (AIDS) patients. PML, however, is still seen in oncology patients, yet often the diagnosis is only considered based on the imaging findings. Patients present with both focal and

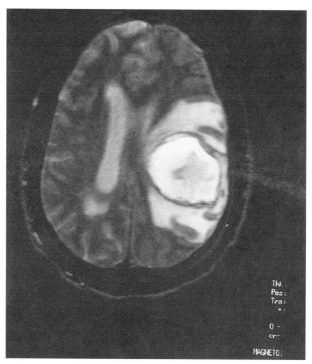

FIGURE 4.13. Brain abscess. (A) Axial T2-weighted image shows bright abscess cavity in the frontal-parietal region (long arrow). Marked edema is indicated by a bright signal surrounding the lesion. Notice the mass effect with compression of the lateral ventricle and effacement of the overlying sulci when compared to the "normal" side (short arrows). (B) Sagittal T1-weighted postcontrast image shows classical ring of enhancement around the abscess cavity (arrow).

global neurologic deficits. MRI is key in demonstrating multiple areas of abnormal white matter that do not have mass effect or enhancement. Large white-matter tracts such as the cerebellar peduncles and radial fibers of the cerebrum are the target areas affected by the virus (Level II-3).[74]

Aspergillus, Mucor, Candida, Cryptococcus, and other fungi are especially important to keep in mind when dealing with patients who are immunocompromised. Fungi are especially common in patients receiving chemotherapy or who have had bone-marrow transplantation. Their appearance on MRI is similar to other infectious agents causing meningitis, cerebritis, or abscesses (Level II-3).[68,69]

Iatrogenic Disorders

Many of the chemotherapeutic agents used today have CNS complications (Table 4.6). Mostly there is no need to image these patients, as the clinical

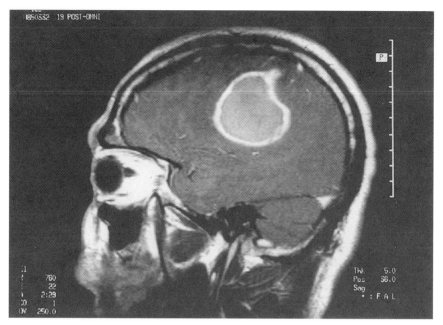

FIGURE 4.13. (*Continued.*)

picture is adequate. There are, however, some patients in which the presentation is atypical and imaging is useful. MRI is the primary imaging modality, as the onset of symptoms is subacute. Imaging shows an abnormal signal in the white matter that is diffuse or symmetric and can involve the gray matter, unlike PML (Level II-3).[69,74] The changes can be reversible pending the withdrawal of the offending agent.

Patients who have had radiation to the brain for metastatic disease are at risk for acute radiation edema, which is transient, followed by chronic changes including radiation necrosis, leukomalacia, and atrophy. Acutely, MRI shows either focal or diffuse edema. Later changes include focal or diffuse atrophy

TABLE 4.6. Chemotherapeutic Agents That Can Cause Imaging Findings*

Actinomycin D
Cis-Platinum
Cytosine arabinoside
Adenine arabinoside
Cyclosporine
Methotrexate

*From: Grossman RI, Yousem DM. Neuroradiology: the requisites. St. Louis: Mosby; 1994. Page 217.

with extensive white-matter gliosis extending to the subcortical area (Level II-3).[75,76,77] Patients who have had whole-brain radiation are at highest risk, while those who have had focal radiation treatments with a gamma knife or focused-beam radiation are generally spared complications. Pathology specimens subjected to whole-brain radiation show a diffuse arteritis/microangiopathy resulting in necrosis and then gliosis (Level II-2).[78] Patients can present with a wide range of symptoms, from focal neurologic deficits, to a progressively decreasing mental status.

Other CNS Neoplasms

While about 50% of CNS neoplasms are metastatic, the other 50% are primary to the brain (Level 11-3).[44] The peak incidence of these tumors, namely gliomas, is in the same population as the gynecologic oncology patients—the six and seventh decades. Clinically there is no differentiating factor, and the diagnosis of a primary neoplasm is suggested by the imaging findings, MRI being essential. A few points help to distinguish the two: Multiple lesions suggest metastatic disease, whereas a large solitary lesion suggests a glioma. Lesions that involve the corpus callosum are almost certainly either a glioblastoma multiforme (GBM) or primary CNS lymphoma. One pitfall is that GBM can be multicentric. Unfortunately, enhancement characteristics and edema patterns cannot discern between metastasis and a primary neoplasm. Posterior fossa lesions, especially when multifocal, are almost certainly metastasis. Occasionally, a solitary mass in the brain will require biopsy.

SPINE IMAGING IN THE GYN-ONCOLOGY PATIENT

General Modalities for Imaging the Spine

Ninety-eight percent of the general population will experience an acute episode of back pain in their lives, and many will have a recurrent problem. The situation in oncology patients is different: Their pain can be related to an underlying neoplasm; therefore, imaging is performed at the onset of acute symptoms. Plain radiography is still the initial imaging modality, as it is quick, easy, and the least expensive. Multiple lytic/sclerotic lesions or an acute abnormality such as a compression fracture can be identified. Even when plain films identify a "simple" noncomplicated fracture or diffuse metastases are seen, imaging is often required to assess for underlying pathology or to evaluate the extent of diffuse disease. Moreover, when there are symptoms of cord compression or the clinical picture is not concordant with plain films, additional imaging studies are required.

If symptoms are localized, such as a lumbar radiculitis or focal thoracic pain, then MRI with an inversion recovery sequence (a sequence that is very sensitive to bone lesions) is most appropriate. If the patient has a clinical picture that suggests diffuse skeletal disease, then radionuclide bone scan is the imaging study of choice. Bone scans are particularly useful, as they evaluate the entire skeleton at one time; if multiple (asymptomatic) lesions are seen elsewhere in the skeleton, the diagnosis of metastasis is made. Often the two studies are complimentary, as both the clinical and radiologic pictures can be complicated.

There is a separate group of patients who present with symptoms of cord compression or bowel/bladder dysfunction. These patients need to have MRI focused on the level of suspected abnormality; gadolinium enhancement has a role in these cases where there may be a paravertebral soft-tissue mass, epidural extension, or an intramedullary lesion (Level II-3).[79,80]

CT and CT myelography are reserved for those patients in whom definition of a bone lesion/fracture is critical or in patients who cannot have an MRI (Table 4.3). Specifically, MRI is suboptimal at defining bone fracture fragments that have been retropulsed and may be impinging upon the spinal cord. The addition of intrathecal contrast helps to evaluate the integrity of the spinal cord and roots.

Metastasis

Focal bone metastases are very common compared to lesions of the dural surfaces or the spinal cord itself (extremely rare). As discussed, plain films, MRI, and bone scans are performed, depending on the clinical picture. Plain films may be normal, even in patients with diffuse bone disease. However, the identification of focal lytic or sclerotic lesion is very helpful. A bone scan is done to evaluate the burden of disease on the entire skeleton. Both MRI and bone scans are very sensitive to metastasis. MRI demonstrates focal areas of abnormal signal consistent with soft-tissue replacement of the marrow. Bone scans show increased uptake of radionuclide related to increased bone turnover.

In general, bone and intradural metastases to the spine are unusual in gynecology-oncology patients during initial work-up. The exceptions are patients with gestational trophoblastic disease or breast cancer, in which CNS metastasis can be seen at initial presentation (Level II-3),[48,49] or patients with uterine or ovarian cancer who have recurrent or stage IV disease (Level II-3).[45,46,92] Intradural metastases are difficult to diagnose both clinically and radiographically. Often the patients have an insidious onset of nonspecific symptoms and/or radicular complaints. A high index of suspicion is required, and the neuroradiologist should be advised of the possibility; in this situation, contrast must be used, or the diagnosis can be missed. MRI is by far the best, although CT myelography can be done in patients who cannot go in the scanner.

MRI will show anywhere from very subtle enhancement of the surface of the cord—so-called sugarcoating of the spinal cord (Fig. 4.14)—to larger nodular soft-tissue masses clinging to the cord, nerve roots, or dural sac (Fig. 4.11; Level II-3).[81,82] CT myelography can show the nodular dural masses, but it is relatively insensitive to "sugarcoating." Metastases to the cord parenchyma are extremely rare and are best known to occur in breast cancer patients.[81,82] MRI

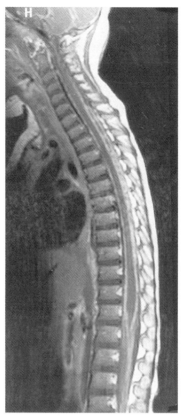

FIGURE 4.14. Metastatic disease "sugarcoating" the spinal cord. Sagittal postcontrast T1-weighted image of the spinal cord shows abnormal enhancement of the entire surface of the spinal cord, conus, and lumbar nerve roots (arrows). The T2-weighted images (not shown) were normal.

is optimal and shows a focal-enhancing lesion within the cord surrounded by edema.[82] These patients usually have quite marked neurologic deficits related to the location of the lesion.

Compression Fractures

The main issue to be addressed is how a benign compression fracture can be differentiated from a malignant one. Generalized bone metastases are discussed above and a compression fracture in this situation is assumed to be pathologic. However, in the setting of an isolated compression fracture in which the remaining spine/skeleton is normal, the situation is different. MRI is needed to differentiate between benign and pathologic fractures; if MRI clearly shows replacement of the normal marrow outside the fractured area, it is a reliable

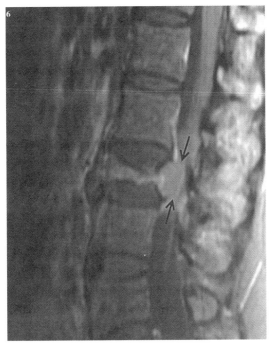

FIGURE 4.15. Pathologic compression fracture in lumbar spine. All sequences show that the normal marrow has been completely replaced. This is in conjunction with soft tissue extending beyond the confines of the vertebral body, which is diagnostic of a pathologic fracture/metastasis. (A) Sagittal T1-weighted postcontrast images show compression fracture with soft-tissue extension into the epidural space (arrow). There is complete replacement of the bone marrow by abnormal enhancement. (B) Sagittal T2-weighted images also show marrow replacement and soft tissue mass. Seen to better advantage is the compression of the cauda equina by the epidural mass (arrows).

sign of metastatic involvement (Fig. 4.15). If normal marrow is identified in the fractured vertebra, then it is more likely a benign process (Level II-3).[83,93] In cases where MRI is equivocal, a percutaneous biopsy using fluoroscopic or CT guidance should be done. Alternatively, follow-up imaging in 3 to 6 months is done; this is reserved for patients in whom imaging points to a benign fracture, they are at high risk for complications related to biopsy, and treatment can be delayed.

Disk Disease

A complete discussion of degenerative disk disease is beyond the scope of this section, yet a few important points can be made. It is one of the most common ailments affecting the adult spine and will therefore be common in the gynecology-oncology patient. There are two major categories of disease: The

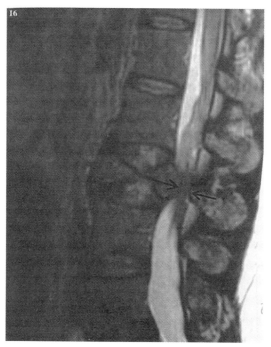

FIGURE 4.15. (*Continued.*)

first is related to disk material that has extended beyond the confines of the annulus to compromise nerve roots (Fig. 4.16). The second is spinal stenosis, which is congenital but becomes symptomatic when there is concomitant disk degeneration and osteophyte formation. The problem oncologists have is differentiating between common back ailments and complications from the patient's underlying neoplasm. As already discussed, MRI is the imaging study of choice and can define extruded disk material compressing a nerve root, the severity of a spinal stenosis upon the thecal sac, or the metastatic lesion compressing the cauda equina.

Infection

Infections of the spine can be broken down into five locations; in order of frequency, they are the vertebral body, the disk space, the epidural space, the meninges, and the spinal cord (Level II-3).[86] Infection of the spinal cord is extremely rare and is beyond the scope of this discussion. Osteomyelitis and diskitis are common and are a result of hematogenous seeding of pathogens. Clinically, patients complain of back pain, which is not radicular but can be severe. They may or may not have fever or an elevated white blood cell count, but do have elevated sedimentation rates (Level II-3).[87] Diskitis often spreads to adjacent vertebrae,

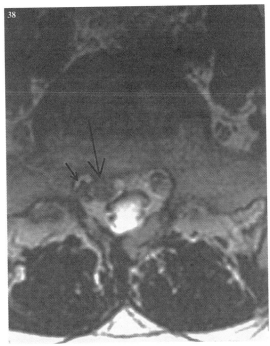

FIGURE 4.16. Extruded disk compromising nerve root. (A) Axial T2-weighted image shows 7 mm extruded disk fragment (long arrow) compressing the first right sacral root (short arrow). Sagittal proton density–weighted image shows the same fragment sequestered behind the first sacral vertebra (arrows). (B) Sagittal T2-weighted images also show marrow replacement and soft-tissue mass. Seen to better advantage is the compression of the cauda equina by the epidural mass (arrows).

causing osteomyelitis and vice versa. Spinal meningitis is similar in presentation and imaging to intracranial meningitis and is discussed above.

Osteomyelitis of vertebrae is best imaged with MRI. Although bone scans and plain films may be positive, they are less specific. MRI shows an abnormal edematous signal in the bone marrow that enhances with contrast material. There may even be a paravertebral abscess, at which point the diagnosis is made; percutaneous aspiration can be done (usually under CT guidance) to obtain cultures. Infection from neoplasm can also be defined when two adjacent vertebral bodies are abnormal and the disk space is spared; this situation is almost certainly metastasis, as infection does not "obey" the disk space, eroding through it. However, there may be difficulty in differentiating a solitary bone metastasis from osteomyelitis. In this case, depending on the clinical suspicion, the physician can either treat for injection empirically or biopsy/culture the vertebra. This can be done percutaneously with either CT or fluoroscopic guidance (Level II-3).[88,89]

Diskitis is easily differentiated from metastatic involvement of the spine with

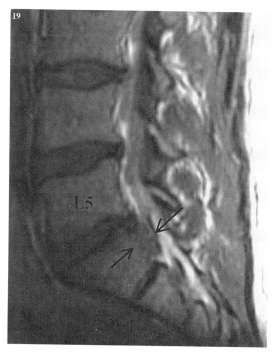

FIGURE 4.16. (*Continued.*)

MRI. The inflamed disk shows an edematous signal on the T2-weighted images, with rim-of-contrast enhancement. The adjacent vertebral endplates can be edematous, indicating extension of the infection into the vertebra (Fig. 4.17).[86] Blood cultures are almost invariably negative, but the sedimentation rate is elevated. Percutaneous aspiration using CT or fluoroscopy can be used to obtain cultures, but unfortunately will be negative in up to 70% of cases (Level II-3).[90]

The epidural space is an uncommon location for infection, but is seen more frequently in diabetics and immunocompromised patients. Epidural abscesses, however, can compress the spinal cord, causing paralysis or death, and are therefore a neurosurgical emergency. Patients who present with symptoms of cord compression need emergent MRI, preferably with contrast if infection or epidural tumor is suspected. MRI exquisitely demonstrates the epidural fluid collection/abscess with an enhancing rim (Level II-3).[91] The presence or absence of spinal cord compression is also evaluated. For patients who cannot undergo MRI, CT myelography should be done.

Paranasal Sinuses

Paranasal sinus infection is common in the general community. Infection in this location can be the cause of headaches, nasal drainage, and persistent cough.

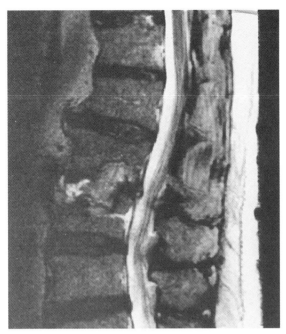

FIGURE 4.17. Diskitis in the lumbar spine. (A) Sagittal T2-weighted image of the lumbar spine shows abnormal bright signal centered about the disk space, but with extension into the vertebral endplates, indicating associated osteomyelitis (arrows). (B) Sagittal T1-weighted image of the same area shows abnormal dark signal (arrows). The involvement of the adjacent vertebral bodies is more extensive than suggested by the T2-weighted image.

Sinus infection is usually diagnosed clinically and treated with appropriate anti-biotic therapy. If symptoms persist, imaging is done to evaluate the extent of disease and any obstruction to the pathways for sinonasal drainage. Coronal CT imaging is optimal and exquisitely demonstrates air fluid levels, obstructed mea-tus, and complications of sinusitis, such as extension outside of the sinus cavity (Level II-3).[92] Importantly, immunosuppressed and diabetic patients are known to have very aggressive fungal infections, such as Mucor and Aspergillus, that can erode into the brain and skull base if not recognized early and treated. MRI is used in this setting, as fungi have the unusual characteristic of being black on T2-imaging sequences. Additionally, invasion into the brain and skull base are better detected by MRI (Level II-3).[92,93]

Metastatic disease involving the sinonasal region from neoplasms originat-ing below the clavicles is very rare and, if present, is part of very extensive, systemic disease. This author could not find specific reference of metastasis to the sinuses from gynecologic neoplasms except for breast cancer (Level II-3).[92]

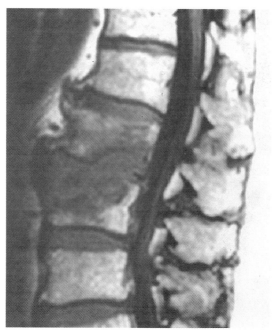

FIGURE 4.17. (*Continued.*)

REFERENCES

1. Cho KC, Baker SR. Extraluminal air: diagnosis and significance. *Rad Clin North Am* 1994;32:829–846.

2. Samuel E, Duncan JG, Philip T, et al. Radiology of the postoperative abdomen. *Clin Radiology* 1963;14:133.

3. Miller RE, Nelson SW. The roentgenological demonstration of tiny amounts of free intraperitoneal gas. Experimental and clinical studies. *AJR* 1971;112:574.

4. Menuck L, Siemers PT. Pneumoperitoneum: importance of right upper quadrant features. *AJR* 1976;127:753.

5. Stapakis JC, Thickman D. Diagnosis of pneumoperitoneum: abdominal CT versus upright chest film. *J Comput Assist Tomogr* 1992;16:713.

6. Federle MP, Chun G, Jeffrey RB, et al. Computed tomographic findings in bowel infarction. *AJR* 1984;142:91.

7. Bomelburg T. vonLengerke JH. Intrahepatic and portal venous gas detected by ultrasonography. *Gastrointestinal Radiol* 1992;17:237.

8. Baker SR. Plain film radiology of the peritoneal and retroperitoneal spaces. In *The Abdominal Plain Film*. East Norwalk, CT: Appleton and Lange, 1990.

9. Weltman DI, Zeman RK. Acute disease of the gallbladder and biliary ducts. *Radiol Clin N Am* 1994;32(5):933–949.

10. Ralls PW, Coletti PM, Lapin SA, et al. Real time sonography in suspected acute cholecystitis. *Radiology* 1985;155:767–771.

11. Jeffrey RB, Nin-Murcia M, Ralls PW, et al. Color Doppler sonography in acute cholecystitis. *Radiology* 1993;1989(P):311.

12. Kim CK, Juweid M, Woda A, et al. Hepatobiliary scintigraphy: morphine-augmented versus delayed imaging I patients with suspected acute cholecystitis. *J Nucl Med* 1993;34:506–509.

13. Halpert RD, Goodman P. *Gastrointestinal Radiology: The Requisites.* St. Louis: Mosby, 1993.

14. Mirvis SE, Vainright JR, Nelson AW, et al. The diagnosis of acute acalculous cholecystitis: a comparison of sonography, scintigraphy and CT. *AJR* 1986;147:1171–1175.

15. Strohl EL, Diffenbaugh WG, Baker JH, et al. Collective reviews: gangrene and perforation of the gallbladder. *Int Obstet Surg* 1962;114:1–7.

16. Kavin H, Jonas RB, Chowdry L. Acalculous cholecyctitis and cytomegalovirus infection in the acquired immunodeficiency syndrome. *Ann Intern Med* 1986;104: 53–54.

17. Rubesin SE, Levine MS, Glick SN, et al. Psuedomembranous colitis with rectosigmoid sparing on barium studies. *Radiology* 1989;170:811.

18. Cho KC, Morehouse HT, Alterman DD, et al. Sigmoid diverticulitis: diagnostic role of CT—comparison with barium enema studies. *Radiology* 1990;176:111.

19. Birnbaum BA, Balthazar EJ. CT of appendicitis and diverticulitis. *Radio Clin N Am* 1994;32:885–898.

20. Puylaert JBCM. Acute appendicitis: U.S. evaluation using graded compression. *Radiology* 1986;158:355.

21. Mucha P. Small intestinal obstruction. *Surg Clin N Am* 1987;67:597–620.

22. Megibow AJ. Bowel obstruction: evaluation with CT. *Radiol Clin N Am* 1994;32:861–870.

23. Fukuya T, Hawes DR, Lu CC, et al. CT diagnosis of small bowel obstruction: efficacy in 60 patients. *AJR* 1992;158:765–769.

24. Megibow AJ, Balthazar EJ, Cho KC, et al. Bowel obstruction: evaluation with CT. *Radiology* 1991;180:313–318.

25. Osteen R, Guyton S, Steele GJ, et al. Malignant intestinal obstruction. *Surgery* 1980;87:611–615.

26. Walkey MM, Friedman AC, Sohotra P, et al. CT manifestations of peritoneal carcinomatosis. *AJR* 1988;150:1035–1041.

27. Laws H, Aldtrete J. Small bowel obstruction: a review of 465 cases. *South Med J* 1976;69:733–744.

28. Gazelle GS, Mueller PR. Abdominal abscess: imaging and intervention. *Radiol Clin N Am* 1994;32(5):913–932.

29. Neff CC, Simeone JF, Ferrucci JF, et al. The occurrence of fluid collections following routine abdominal surgical procedures: sonographic survey in asymptomatic postoperative patients. *Radiology* 1983;146:463.

30. Haaga JR, Weinstein AJ. CT detection and aspiration of abdominal abscesses. *AJR* 1977;123:465–474.

31. Soulen MC, Fishman EK, Goldman SK, et al. Bacterial renal infection: role of CT. *Radiology* 1989;171:703m.

32. Bjorgvinsson E, Majd M, Eggli KD. Diagnosis of acute pyelonephritis in children: comparison of sonography and 99m Tc-DMSA scintigraphy. *AJR* 1991;157: 539.

33. Levine E. Acute renal and urinary tract disease. *Radiol Clin N Am* 1994;32(5): 989–1004.

34. Gold RP, McClennan BL, Rottenberg RR. CT appearance of acute inflammatory disease of the renal interstitium. *AJR* 1983;141:343.

35. Fultz PJ, Hampton WR, Totterman SRS. Computed tomography of pyonephrosis. *Abdom Imag* 1993;18:82.

36. Platt JF, Rubin JM, Ellis JH. Acute renal obstruction: evaluation with intrarenal duplex Doppler and conventional ultrasound. *Radiology* 1993;186:685.

37. Tubin ME, Dodd GD, Verdile VP. Acute urinary obstruction: accuracy of diagnosis with duplex Doppler US. *Radiology* 1992;185(P)105.

38. Glazer GM, Francis IR, Brady TM, et al. Computed tomography of renal vein thrombosis: clinical and experimental observations. *AJR* 1983;140:721.

39. Glazer GM, Francis IR, Gross BH, et al. Computed tomography of renal vein thrombosis. *J Comput Assist Tomogr* 1984;8:288.

40. Carmody RF, Yang DJ, Seeley GW, Seeger JF, Unger EC, Johnson JF. Spinal cord compression due to metastatic disease: diagnosis with MRI imaging versus myelography. *Radiology* 1989;173:225–229.

41. Smoker WRK, Godersky JC, Nutzon RK, et al. Role of MR imaging in evaluating metastatic spinal disease. *AJNR* 1987;8:901–908.

42. Beltram J, Noto AM, Chakeres DW, Christoforidis AJ. Tumors of the osseous spine: staging with MR imaging versus CT. *Radiology* 1987;162:565–569.

43. Atlas SW (Ed). *Magnetic Resonance Imaging of the Brain and Spine*, 2nd ed. Philadelphia: Lippincott-Raven, 1996, p. 409.

44. Russell DS, Rubinstein LJ. *Pathology of Tumors of the Nervous System*, 5th ed. Baltimore: Williams & Wilkins, 1989.

45. Aalders JG, Abeler V, Kolstad P. Recurrent adenocarcinoma of the endometrium: a clinical and histopathological study of 379 patients. *Gynecol Oncol* 1984;17:85–103.

46. Dauplat J, Hacker NF, Nieberg RK, Berek JS, Rose TP, Sagae S. Distant metastasis in epithelial ovarian cancer. *Cancer* 1987;60:1561–1566.

47. Ricke J, Baum K, Hosten N. Calcified brain metastases from ovarian carcinoma. *Neuroradiology* 1996;38:460–461.

48. Bakri Y, Berkowitz RS, Goldstein DP, Subhi J, Senoussi M, von Sinner W, Jabbar FA. Brain metastases of gestational trophoblastic tumor. *J. Reprod Med* 1994;39:179–184.

49. Athanassiou A, Begent RHJ, Newlands ES, Parker D, Rustin GJ, Bagshawe KD. Central nervous system metastasis of choriocarcinoma: 23 years experience at the Chaing Cross Hospital. *Cancer* 1983;52:1728–1735.

50. Berek JS (Ed), Adashi EY, Hillard PA (Assoc Eds). *Novak's Gynecology*, 12th ed. Baltimore: Williams & Wilkins, 1996.

51. Holland JF, Bast RC, Morton DL, Frei E, Kufe, DW, Weichselbaum RR. *Cancer in Medicine*, 4th ed. Baltimore: Williams & Wilkins, 1997.

52. Healy ME, Hesselink JR, Press GA, Middleton MS. Increased detection of intracranial metastases with intravenous Gd-DTPA. *Radiology* 1987;165:619–624.

53. Russell EJ, Geremia GK, Johnson CE, et al. Multiple cerebral metastases: detectability with Gd-DTPA-enhanced MR imaging. *Radiology* 1987;165:609–617.

54. Lee Y-Y, Glass JP, Geoffray A, Wallace S. Cranial computed tomographic abnormalities in leptomeningeal metastasis. *AJR* 1984;143:1035–1039.

55. Davis PC, Friedman NC, Fry SM, Malko JA, Hoffmann JC Jr, Braun IF. Leptomeningeal metastasis: MR imaging. *Radiology* 1987;163:449–454.

56. Marks MP. CT in ischemic stroke in "CT in Neuroimaging Revisited." *Neuroimag Clin N Am* 1998;8(3):515–523.

57. McAlister FA, Fisher BW, Houston SC. The timing of computed tomography in acute stroke: a practice audit. *Can Assoc Radiol J* 1997;48(2)123–129.

58. Mohr JP, Biller J, Hilal SK, Yuh WT, Tatemichi TK, Hedges S, Tali E, Nguyen H, Mun I, Adams HP, et al. Magnetic resonance versus computed tomographic imaging in acute stroke. *Stroke* 1995;26(5):807–812.

59. Hacke W, Kaste M, Fieschi C, Toni D, Lesaffre E, von Kummer R, Boysen G, Bluhmki E, Hoxter G, Mahagne MH, et al. Intravenous thrombolysis with recombinant tissue plasminogen activator for acute hemispheric stroke. The European Cooperative Acute Stroke Study (ECASS). *JAMA* 1995;274(13):1017–1025.

60. Zimmerman RD, Ernst RJ. Neuroimaging of cerebrovenous thrombosis. *Neuroimag Clin N Am* 1992;2:463–485.

61. Sandu AS, Johns D, Albertyn LE. Deep cerebral vein thrombosis. *Neuroradiology* 1991;33(suppl):241–243.

62. Singer MB, Atlas SW, Drayer BP. Subarachnoid space disease: diagnosis with fluid-attenuated inversion-recovery MR imaging and comparison with gadolinium-enhanced spin-echo MR imaging—blinded reader study. *Radiology* 1998;208(2):417–422.

63. Noguchi K, Ogawa T, Seto H, Inugami A, Hadeishi H, Fujita H, Hatazawa J, Shimosegawa E, Okudera T, Uemura K. Subacute and chronic subarachnoid hemorrhage: diagnosis with fluid-attenuated inversion-recovery MR imaging. *Radiology* 1997;203(1)257–262.

64. Lee KS, Bae HG, Yun IG. Recurrent intracerebral hemorrhage due to hypertension. *Neurosurgery* 1990;26:586–590.

65. Glenner GC, Murphy MA. Amyloidosis of the nervous system. *J Neurol Sci* 1989;94:1–28.

66. Fobben ES, Grossman RI, Atlas SW. MR characteristics of subdural hematomas and hygromas at 1.5 T. *AJNR* 1989;10:687–693.

67. Adams RD, Victor M, Ropper AH (Eds). *Principles of Neurology*, 6th ed. New York: McGraw-Hill, 1997. pp. 700–701.

68. Sze G, Zimmerman RD. The magnetic resonance imaging of infections and inflammatory diseases. *Radiol Clin N Am* 1988;26:839–859.

69. Atlas SW (Ed). *Magnetic Resonance Imaging of the Brain and Spine*, 2nd ed. Philadelphia: Lippincott-Raven, 1996, pp. 707–772.

70. Haimes AB, Zimmerman RD, Morgello S, et al. MR imaging of brain abscesses. *AJR* 1989;152:1073–1085.

71. Adams RD, Victor M, Ropper AH (Eds). *Principles of Neurology*, 6th ed. New York: McGraw-Hill, 1997, pp. 751–754.

72. Jordan J, Enzmann DR. Encephalitis. *Neuroimag Clin N Am* 1991;1:17–38.

73. Padget BL, Walker DL, ZuRhein GM, et al. Cultivation of papova-like virus from human brain with progressive multifocal leukoencephalopathy. *Lancet* 1971;1257–1260.

74. Whiteman MLH, Post MJD, Beger JR, et al. Progressive multifocal leukoencephalopathy in 47 HIV-seropositive patients: neuroimaging with clinical and pathologic correlation. *Radiology* 1993;187:233–240.

75. Brown MS, Simon JH, Stemmer SM et al. MR and proton spectroscopy of white matter disease induced by high-dose chemotherapy with bone marrow transplant in advanced breast carcinoma. *AJNR* 1995;16:2013–2020.

76. Rabin BM, Meyer JR, Berlin JW, Marymount MG, Palka PS, Russell EJ. Radiation-induced changes in the central nervous system and head and neck. *Radiographics* 1996;16:1055–1072.

77. Wang PY, Shen WC, Jan JS. Serial MRI changes in radiation myelopathy. *Neuroradiology* 1995;37:374–377.

78. Hecht-Leavitt C, Grossman RI, Curran SJ, et al. MR of brain radiation injury: experimental studies in cats. *AJNR* 1987;8:427–431.

79. Sze G. Gadolinium-DTPA in spinal disease. *Radiol Clin N Am* 1988;26(5):1009–1024.

80. Sze G. Magnetic resonance imaging in the evaluation of spinal tumors. *Cancer* 1991;15(67; suppl 4):1229–1241.

81. Mayer RJ, Berkowitz R, Griffiths T. Central nervous system involvement by ovarian carcinoma: a complication of prolonged survival with metastatic disease. *Cancer* 1978;41:776.

82. Atlas SW (Ed). *Magnetic Resonance Imaging of the Brain and Spine*, 2nd ed. Philadelphia: Lippincott-Raven, 1996, pp. 1339–1385.

83. Costigan DA, Winkelman MD. Intramedullary spinal cord metastases. A clinicopathological study of 13 cases. *J Neurosurg* 1985;62:227–233.

84. Algra PR, Bloem JL, Tissing H, et al. Detection of vertebral metastases: comparison between MR imaging and bone scintigraphy. *Radiographics* 1991;11:219–232.

85. Warnock NG, Yuh W. Magnetic resonance imaging in the discrimination of benign from malignant disease of the lumbosacral vertebral column. *Neuroimag Clin N Am* 1993;3(3):609–623.

86. Post MJ, Bowen BC, Sze G. Magnetic resonance imaging of spinal infection. *Rheum Dis Clin N Am* 1991;17(3):773–794.

87. Adams RD, Victor M, Ropper AH (Eds). *Principles of Neurology*, 6th ed. New York: McGraw-Hill, 1997, pp. 209–210.

88. Haddad MC, Sharif HS, Aideyan OA, et al. Infection versus neoplasms in the spine: differentiation by MRI and diagnostic pitfalls. *Eur Radiol* 1993;3–5:439.

89. Hovi I, Lamminen A, Salonen O, et al. MR imaging of the lower spine: differentiation between infectious and malignant disease. *Acta Radiol* 1994;35:532–540.

90. Atlas SW (Ed). *Magnetic Resonance Imaging of the Brain and Spine*, 2nd ed. Philadelphia: Lippincott-Raven, 1996, pp. 1207–1264.

91. Sandhu FS, Dillon WP. Spinal epidural abscess: evaluation with contrast-enhanced MR imaging. *AJNR* 1991;12:1087–1093.

92. Som PM, Curtain HD (Eds). *Head and Neck Imaging*, 3rd ed. St. Louis: Mosby, 1996, pp. 126–185.

93. Blitzer A, Lawson W. Fungal infections of the nose and paranasal sinuses. Part I. *Otolaryngol Clin N Am* 1993;26:1007–1035.

CHAPTER 5

RADIOLOGY OF POSTOPERATIVE PULMONARY COMPLICATIONS

STEFAN HEINZE, M.D., ROBERT SUH, M.D., and DENISE ABERLE, M.D.

Pulmonary complications are an important consideration in any postoperative patient. This is particularly true following gynecologic surgery, as these patients sustain inevitable, albeit transient, declines in lung function due to the effects of anesthesia, immobilization, and postoperative pain. These factors limit voluntary breathing and cough. The aim of this chapter is to describe the major postoperative pulmonary complications and their diagnoses, emphasizing the radiological components in each.

ATELECTASIS

Atelectasis, meaning the collapse of normally inflated lung, is the most common postoperative respiratory complication. Factors that promote atelectasis include upper abdominal, colonic, or gastroduodenal surgeries; obesity; perioperative hospitalization greater than 4 days; and advanced age. Interestingly, although they increase the risk of respiratory failure after surgery, smoking and chronic obstructive pulmonary disease (COPD) appear not to increase the risk of postoperative atelectasis.[15,44,77,78]

The pathophysiology is typically mucus plugging in postoperative lung in which significant collapse has already been caused by general anesthesia.[68] Decreased mucociliary clearance and decreased diaphragmatic excursion from pain promote stasis of airways secretions.[51,68] These inspissated secretions occlude the airways, and resorption of air distal to the plug causes lung collapse. Atelectasis is often clinically silent, although patients may experience dyspnea, chest pain, low-grade fever, or cough. The major laboratory finding is hypoxia.

Perioperative and Supportive Care in Gynecologic Oncology: Evidence-Based Management, Edited by Steven A. Vasilev.
ISBN 0-471-24788-X   Copyright © 2000 by Wiley-Liss, Inc.

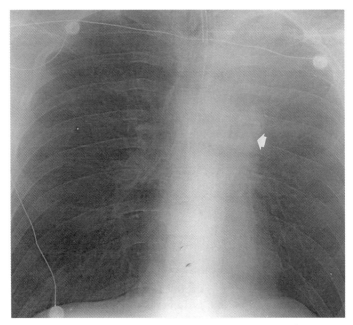

FIGURE 5.1. Veil-like left upper lobe opacity, raised left hilum (⟁), and crowding of ribs in a 36-year-old postoperative patient. Left upper lobe collapse.

Chest radiographs show discoid, subsegmental, segmental, lobar, or whole-lung collapse, depending on the severity and level of bronchial occlusion. In recumbent postoperative patients, atelectasis is an almost invariable occurrence in the lung bases. The cardinal radiographic sign of atelectasis is a loss of volume of the affected lung, as evidenced by displacement of the interlobar fissures, diaphragmatic elevation, depression of the ipsilateral hilum, mediastinal shift to the affected side, and ipsilateral rib crowding.[30] Increased opacity of the affected lung is also typical and is the result of postobstructive pneumonia or fluid transudate within the collapsed alveoli. The presence of volume loss and opacification of lung in a postoperative patient confirms the presence of atelectasis, but does not exclude concomitant causes of consolidation such as pneumonia. Examples of atelectasis are given in Figures 5.1, 5.2, and 5.3.

NOSOCOMIAL PNEUMONIA

Nosocomial pneumonia refers to lung infection occurring after 48 hours from admission and is exclusive of infection incubating at the time of admission. Nosocomial pneumonia is the leading cause of mortality from hospital-acquired infections, with reported mortality rates between 13% and 55%, particularly in patients in the intensive care unit.[14,18,19,27,59,93]

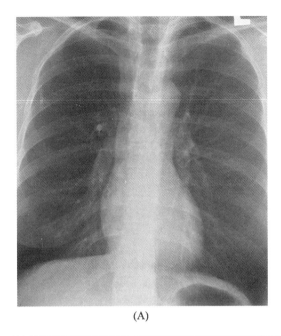

(A)

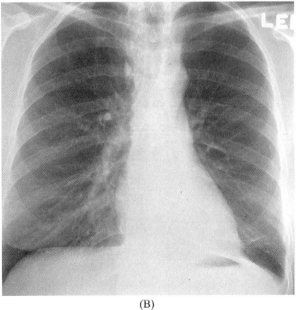

(B)

FIGURE 5.2. A preoperative film is normal (A). Postoperative PA film shows new retrocardiac opacity and loss of the medial aspect of the left hemidiaphragm (B). Lateral film (C) shows loss of the normal posterior outline of the left hemidiaphragm and ill-defined postero-inferior opacity (↺). Left lower lobe collapse.

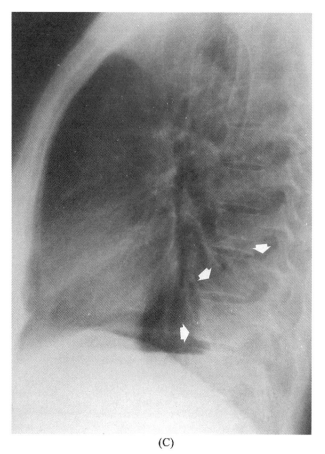

(C)

FIGURE 5.2. (*Continued.*)

Despite minor variations between centers, the most common nosocomial pathogens are aerobic gram-negative organisms and *Staphylococcus aureus.* Gram-negative organisms have become ubiquitous in intensive care units (ICU); oropharyngeal colonization occurs rapidly in the elderly, critically ill, or intubated patient and has been observed prospectively in the majority of patients admitted to the ICU, particularly if intubated. *S. aureus* remains a major nosocomial pathogen; methicillin-resistant strains are associated with a considerably increased mortality risk. Fungi, *Aspergillus,* and Mucor species are more typical in patients with diabetes or other immunocompromised hospitalized hosts.[61] Organisms typically seen with community-acquired pneumonia may also be nosocomial pathogens, including *Streptococcus pneumoniae,* *Haemophilus influenzae,* and *Legionella* species (Fig. 5.4).[4,5,14,56,60]

A number of factors are presumed to contribute to the development of nosocomial pneumonia. In most patients, nosocomial pathogens colonize the orophar-

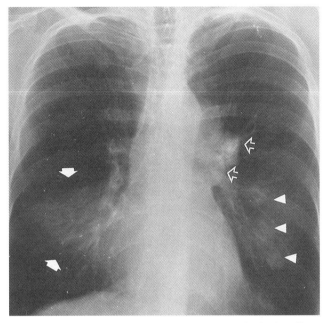

FIGURE 5.3. A 54-year-old patient postsurgery for gynecological malignancy. Wedge-shaped opacity adjacent to and obscuring the right heart border consistent with right middle lobe collapse (◊. Left hilar and aortopulmonary window metastatic lymph-adenopathy (⟹) and multiple left lower lobe metastases are also seen (▷).

ynx and stomach prior to the development of pneumonia. The normally acidic gastric milieu prevents bacterial growth; however, in patients given antacids or histamine-2 blockers, and in patients with achlorhydria, elevations of gastric pH > 4 promote bacterial overgrowth and the risk of nosocomial pneumonia.[22,23,32,48,49] Nasogastric intubation provides a conduit for the retrograde colonization of the oropharynx. In bypassing the lower esophageal sphincter, gastric reflux and aspiration are facilitated.[60] In addition, intubation circumvents the normal upper airway defenses, traumatizes the tracheal epithelium, promotes sinus stasis and colonization, allows leakage of pharyngeal flora around the cuff, and promotes contamination of the lower respiratory tract.[20,24,31,48,60]

Blood-borne infection is a less critical factor in nosocomial pneumonia, although bowel ischemia following abdominal and pelvic surgery may allow the direct bacterial invasion of the lymphatics and portal circulation from the intestinal lumen, with subsequent dissemination.[28] Colonization of water sources such as nebulizers, humidifiers, or water condensation in ventilator tubing may also be implicated in colonization of the lung, particularly in patients in the critical care setting. Finally, poor hand-washing techniques among hospital workers provide a conduit for cross-contamination between patients.[61]

The three mainstays of the clinical diagnosis of nosocomial pneumonia are

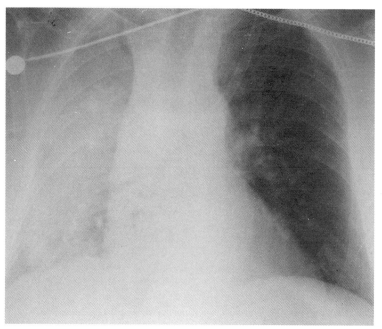

FIGURE 5.4. Dense opacification of the right hemithorax with air bronchograms in a postoperative patient. Nosocomial pneumonia due to *Legionella*.

(1) fever and a change in white cell count, (2) new opacities on chest radiographs greater than 48 hours after hospitalization (Figs. 5.5 and 5.6), and (3) the isolation of pathogenic bacteria from tracheal or other airway secretions.[56,60,69] The diagnosis is often obscured by the presence of edema, atelectasis, lung hemorrhage, pulmonary infarction, or other radiographic consolidations.[61] In hospitalized patients, clinical deterioration may prompt radiographic tests before consolidation has been able to develop, particularly in neutropenic patients.[99] Moreover, tracheobronchial colonization without true infection is common. Bronchoscopy with protected specimen brushing or bronchoalveolar lavage are more accurate than expectorated sputum samples, but are invasive and less commonly performed in nonintubated patients.[56,60,93]

In a previous autopsy study,[101] three radiographic signs were found to be relatively specific for nosocomial pneumonia: (1) airspace consolidation abutting a fissure (specificity 96%); (2) air bronchograms, especially when single; and (3) cavitation. Unfortunately, these signs are uncommon. Rapidly changing opacities, particularly in a basilar distribution, are often the results of atelectasis rather than pneumonia, but are also typical of aspiration pneumonia. Although parenchymal consolidations are no more specific on computerized tomography (CT) than chest radiography, cavitation and pleural collections such as empyema are often better visualized on CT, and may confirm the suspicion of nosocomial pneumonia.[10]

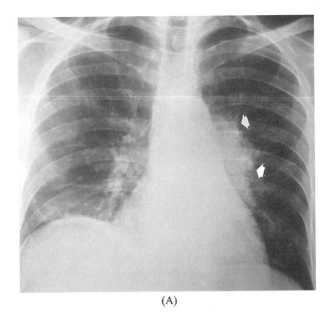

(A)

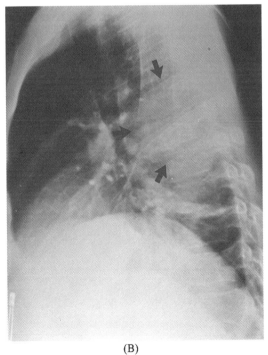

(B)

FIGURE 5.5. Rounded opacity in the superior segment of the left lower lobe on (A) PA (⇕) and (B) lateral radiographs (→). Nosocomial pneumonia.

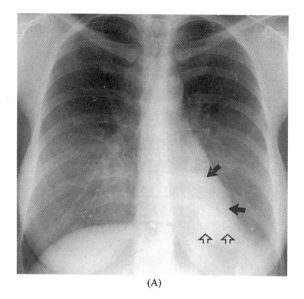

(A)

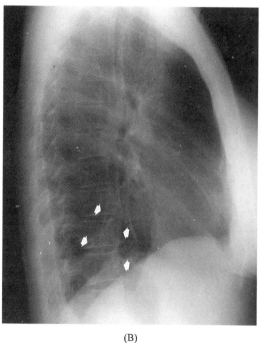

(B)

FIGURE 5.6. (A) A left lower lobe consolidation in a 36-year-old female patient. Retrocardiac opacity (→) and loss of the normal medial aspect of the left hemidiaphragm (⇒) are seen on the PA view. Nosocomial pneumonia. (B) Lateral view better shows ill-defined triangular lower lobe opacity (◊).

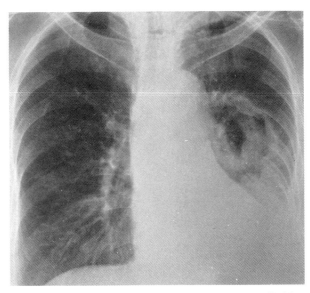

FIGURE 5.7. Complication of nosocomial pneumonia. Thick-walled lung abscesses in the superior segment of the left lower lobe following anaerobic left lower lobe pneumonia.

The initial choice of antibiotic coverage is institution specific, depending on the most prevalent nosocomial organisms, and is ultimately directed by bacterial susceptibilities. Despite the initiation of appropriate antibiotic therapy, the radiographic appearance of nosocomial pneumonia will not likely improve within the first 48 hours and rarely may progress, particularly with pneumonias due to *Legionella* or *Pseudomonas* species.[60] Following initial clinical improvement, recurrent fevers or leukocytosis (Fig. 5.7) should prompt evaluation for superimposed pathogens or complications such as lung abscess or empyema.

ASPIRATION PNEUMONIA

Aspiration pneumonia involves the inhalation of gastric material into the lungs. The severity of the insult is proportional to the amount of material aspirated as well as its physico-chemical composition.[30,81] The injury may be due to (1) chemical pneumonitis (usually with gastric pH < 2.5),[26,80] (2) particulate matter, or (3) contamination by nosocomial organisms.

Acidic gastric contents are highly irritating to the bronchoepithelium and effect the most severe injury. Liquid material is often diffusely distributed due to violent inhalation and coughing, with spread to the peripheral small airways. Damage to the bronchial and bronchiolar epithelium promotes increased alveolar capillary permeability and airspace edema with hemorrhage, eventuating in the adult respiratory distress syndrome (ARDS) and its functional sequelae.

Particulate matter can occlude the airways, prompting collapse and postobstructive consolidations. The aspirated particulate matter incites a granulomatous response, generally most marked in the terminal and expiratory bronchioles.[30,81]

In the immediate postoperative period, the risk of aspiration is heightened by the depressant effects of anesthesia on mental status, cough, gag, and swallowing reflexes. These effects are further magnified in patients with endotracheal or nasogastric intubation.[24] Bowel obstruction and emergency surgery also increase the risk of aspiration.

Clinical manifestations vary widely from minor symptoms to life-threatening respiratory compromise. Three general patterns may be seen: (1) self-limited respiratory compromise with rapid improvement; (2) rapid radiographic and clinical progression; (3) or transient stabilization followed by inexorable worsening, often with superimposed diffuse lung injury or nosocomial pneumonia.[12,13,82]

There are three basic radiological patterns of aspiration: (1) extensive bilateral airspace consolidation with confluent alveolar opacities; (2) widespread but discrete alveolar opacities; and (3) irregular opacities unlike either of the other patterns.[30,57] The radiographic distribution is influenced by the nature and volume of the contents aspirated as well as gravity. Purely liquid contents cause widespread changes because of reflex deep inspiration and coughing and also tend to lead to gravity-dependent changes. With particulate matter, changes are often segmental (Fig. 5.8) and involve at least one of the posterior segments

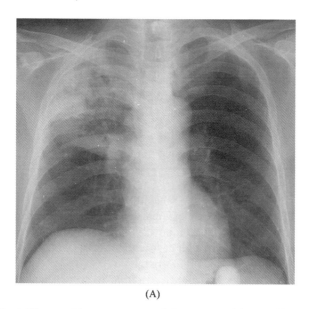

(A)

FIGURE 5.8. A 50-year-old woman post–pelvic surgery with consolidation of the right upper lobe on plain X ray (A) and CT (B). Focal aspiration pneumonitis. An incidental area of segmental atelectasis is seen on the PA film. Follow-up 3 months later (C) shows linear opacities in the right upper lobe (⟡) consistent with scarring.

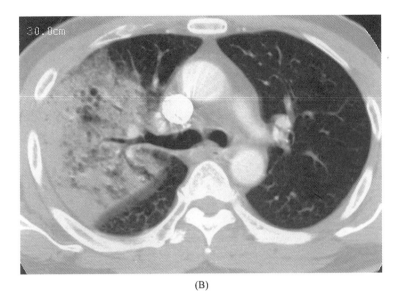

(B)

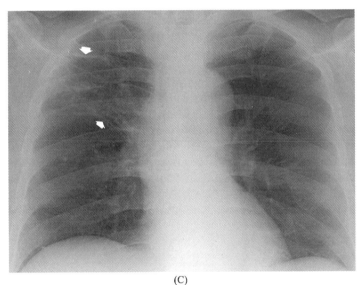

(C)

FIGURE 5.8. (*Continued.*)

of the upper or lower lobes, or the superior segments of the lower lobes. Posterior abnormalities predominate in critical care or postoperative patients, the majority of whom are supine when aspiration occurs. Unilateral consolidations on the right are common, and are ascribed to the more vertical orientation of the right mainstem bronchus as compared to the left.

The classic appearances described in Mendelson's syndrome (which involves

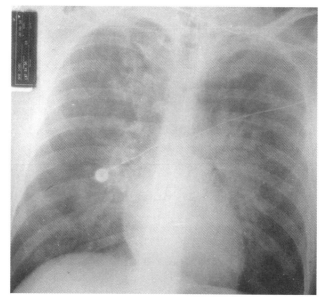

FIGURE 5.9. Widespread bilateral opacities with perihilar predominance in a patient who aspirated a large volume of liquid gastric contents. Mendelson's syndrome.

aspiration of a large volume of low-pH liquid secretions) are of bilateral widespread patchy airspace consolidation (Fig. 5.9). Aspiration pneumonia may be very difficult to distinguish from hydrostatic edema (e.g., cardiac, renal, or overhydration edema), although the absence of vascular redistribution and cardiomegaly are helpful in excluding the latter. Similarly, it may be impossible to differentiate aspiration pneumonia, nosocomial pneumonias, and ARDS due to other etiologies.[81] The interpretation of the radiograph is heavily influenced by the specific clinical context. Finally, the initial X-ray appearances do not necessarily correlate with the eventual outcome.[12,13]

PULMONARY EDEMA

Pulmonary edema is defined as an abnormal increase in extravascular lung water.[88] Pulmonary edema can be divided into two broad categories: hydrostatic and increased permeability types.[30,88] Increased permeability edema is discussed under ARDS (see below). Hydrostatic edema may be further divided based on etiology: cardiac and overhydration or renal edema. Cardiogenic edema results from left ventricular failure, usually within the context of ischemia, cardiomyopathy, valvular heart disease, or pericardial pathology. Renal or overhydration edema results from an increase in circulating blood volume due either to renal impairment or vigorous intravascular volume replacement.

Hemodynamic measurements have become standard practice in critical care units and are commonly used to support the diagnosis of edema and to distinguish hydrostatic and capillary leak etiologies. In otherwise normal subjects, a pulmonary capillary occlusion pressure greater than 15 mmHg is associated with pulmonary venous hypertension and hydrostatic edema. Hemodynamic monitoring is not a prerequisite for diagnosis and has the potential for error depending on the location of the pressure transducer relative to the heart. Other tests include radioisotope techniques[21] and single-pass multiple-indicator dilution techniques.[1,83] The measure of the edema protein to plasma protein concentration in the early stages of edema has been used to characterize edema in the experimental setting; however, chest radiography is probably the most commonly used noninvasive method of assessing pulmonary edema.[1,88] The pathophysiological changes of pulmonary edema, including the anatomical distribution of fluid accumulation, changes in the systemic and pulmonary venous circulations, and the mechanisms of edema clearance, are the basis for the radiographic findings.

Cardiac enlargement is present in a majority of patients with cardiogenic edema.[40,88] Cardiomegaly is a cardiothoracic ratio >0.55, where cardiac diameter is the largest sum of the most rightward and leftward margins of the cardiac shadow from midline; and thoracic diameter is the largest diameter of the thorax measured from the inner margins of the ribs.[50] Widening of the superior mediastinum (also called the vascular pedicle) may result from engorgement of the central systemic veins; however, its usefulness is limited due to considerable influences of supine versus upright positioning, patient obliquity, and lung volumes on the appearances of the superior mediastinum.

Pulmonary vascular changes are also an important physiologic index in patients with hydrostatic edema. There is normally a gravity-dependent, superior-to-inferior gradient of increasing pulmonary perfusion and vessel distension in the upright human. With hydrostatic edema of cardiac etiology, pulmonary venous hypertension results in pulmonary vascular redistribution, visible as distension of the upper lobe vessels. This appears as a relative increase in size of apical versus basal vessel caliber.[3,58] Vascular redistribution may also be inferred by an increase in the pulmonary artery to bronchus diameter ratio, in which the arteries become larger than their corresponding bronchi as seen end-on. The distinction between edema of renal (or overhydration) and cardiac etiologies is often not possible, although with renal edema the artery-to-bronchus ratio in both upper and lower lobes is increased, whereas in left ventricular failure the ratio is increased in the upper lobes only.[100] Obviously, these patterns are much less reliable with bedside radiography.

Interstitial edema normally develops with pulmonary venous hypertension greater than 19 mmHg (Figs. 5.10 and 5.11), as measured with pulmonary artery occlusion catheters. At this pressure, fluid leaks from the vascular compartment into the lung interstitium. Interstitial edemia of the bronchovascular interstitium produces peribronchial cuffing and obscuration of the normally sharp margins of the arteries.[16] Edema of the interlobular septa is visible as septal lines. The

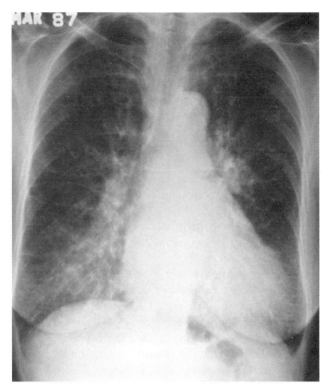

FIGURE 5.10. A 60-year-old female patient with CXR signs of cardiomegaly, upper lobe venous diversion, and Kerley B lines. Cardiogenic interstitial pulmonary edema.

interlobular septa form the interstitial envelope through which run pulmonary venules and lymphatics. Septal edema is most evident in the lung periphery as short subpleural lines perpendicular to the pleural surface; the more central septal architecture is less well developed but appears as lines 3–4 cm long radiating from the hila.[40] Lastly, edema around the hilar vessels results in subtle hazy opacification known as perihilar haze.[58,82]

Frank *airspace consolidation* (Figs. 5.12 and 5.13) occurs when the fluid capacity of the interstitial compartment is exceeded, usually at pulmonary capillary wedge pressures greater than 25 mmHg.[72] The classic distribution is bilateral and basal or perihilar ("bat wing" appearance).[30,88] Preexisting lung or pulmonary vascular disease as well as patient positioning can produce atypical patterns. A characteristic finding of right upper lobe edema has been seen in severe mitral regurgitation, presumably as a result of the direct orientation of the right superior pulmonary veins with respect to the regurgitant blood flow within the left atrium.[42]

Pleural effusions commonly accompany hydrostatic edema.[62,96] There is a strong association between presence of pleural effusion and elevated left atrial pressures, with one study suggesting a critical threshold of left atrial hyper-

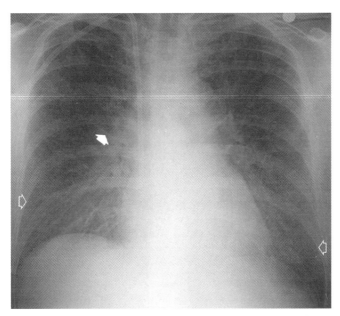

FIGURE 5.11. Plain X ray demonstrating interstitial opacities including Kerley A (◆) and Kerley B lines (◇). Cardiogenic interstitial pulmonary edema.

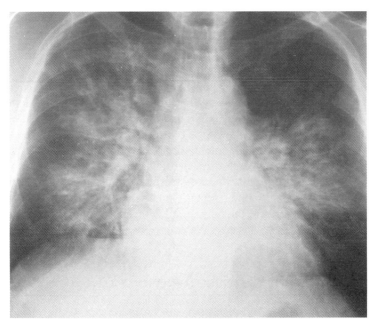

FIGURE 5.12. Plain CXR showing alveolar (airspace) opacities in "bat-wing" distribution, considered a classic finding of cardiogenic alveolar pulmonary edema.

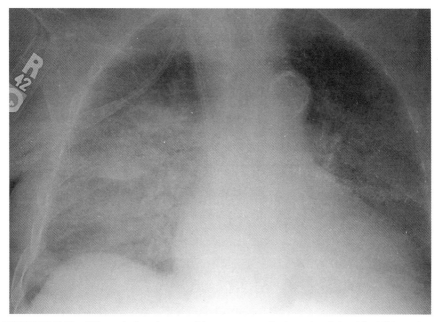

FIGURE 5.13. Bilateral alveolar opacities, more marked on the right side. This patient had been lying in right lateral decubitus position for some hours before this image was recorded. Asymmetric alveolar edema.

tension necessary for the formation of pleural effusions.[97] The pleura is also a major route for the resolution of pulmonary edema.

CT is not necessary for the diagnosis of hydrostatic pulmonary edema, but familiarity with CT appearances may be important to distinguish edema from other cardiopulmonary processes. CT signs parallel projectional radiography. Cardiomegaly is often evident, with CT offering a more accurate determination of specific chamber enlargement. Enlargement of nondependent arteries and veins, as well as an increase in size and number of small centrilobular vessels, reflects vascular redistribution.[29,87] Interstitial edema is evidenced by peribronchovascular, interlobular septal, and fissural thickening,[9,87] as well as ground glass opacification of the lung. Frank airspace consolidation occurs with severe edema.[88]

ADULT RESPIRATORY DISTRESS SYNDROME

The adult respiratory distress syndrome (ARDS) is a complex clinical and physiological syndrome characterized by severe respiratory failure. The clinical definition usually includes the following:[79,88] hypoxemia refractory to supplemental oxygen, chest radiographic consolidations, and the absence of pulmonary edema from cardiac or renal etiologies. The significant primary pathological event in ARDS is diffuse lung injury resulting from interruption of the alveolar capillary membrane,[2,79] either directly from blood-borne mediators and toxins or indirectly from the activation of inflammatory cells and mediators. Increased permeability of the endothelium results, with leakage of fluid from the intravascular space into the lung interstitium and airspaces. ARDS may be considered as incremental stages of evolution from the acute injury with destruction of Type 1 pneumocytes and edema, to a proliferative stage with formation of hyaline membranes and proliferation of Type 2 pneumocytes, culminating in a chronic stage in which collagen deposition may result in irreversible fibrosis. Although there are a number of conditions associated with ARDS, patients with gynecologic malignancies or those post-abdomino-pelvic surgery may be predisposed within the setting of sepsis, aspiration or other pneumonia, or postoperative pancreatitis.

Clinical manifestations may develop immediately after the inciting event or after a variable delay of hours. Clinical signs include progressive tachypnea, tachycardia, and hypoxia that is usually rapidly progressive and culminates in intubation with positive pressure ventilation and supplemental oxygen. Characteristic radiographic findings are seen in the sequential stages of ARDS.[1,88] Stage 1, early lung injury (Fig. 5.14), occurs within the first few hours of the inciting event and is often radiographically occult. Unless the inciting injury involves the lung, as with aspiration, chest radiographs may be normal or show decreased lung volumes due to diffuse microatelectasis from deranged surfactant metabolism. Proliferative ARDS, or Stage 2 (Figs. 5.15 and 5.16), occurs within 24 hours of injury. At this stage, multifocal airspace consolidations reflect the outpouring of edema and hemorrhage into the airspaces across the damaged alveolar epithelial-capillary endothelial membrane. In the absence of hydrostatic edema (e.g., left ventricular failure or high circulating intravascular volume), pleural effusions are not prominent. Stage 3 (Figs. 5.17 and 5.18) heralds the chronic stage of ARDS and is usually seen 3 or more days postinjury. At this stage, airspace consolidations become less confluent and ground glass and interstitial opacities may develop, corresponding to hyaline membrane deposition, hyperplasia of Type II pneumocytes, and the accumulation of fibroblasts and fibrous connective tissue. In this stage, the lung is noncompliant and the risk of barotrauma from mechanical ventilation is greatest.[88] Recovery from Stage III ARDS is variable: Patients may be left with residual fibrosis and architectural distortion or may experience near complete radiographic and functional recovery.

Barotrauma is common in ARDS and often presents as pneumothorax.[91,92] In many cases, the inciting event is pulmonary interstitial emphysema with retrograde dissection of extraalveolar air along the bronchovascular interstitium to the mediastinum. Ischemic foci of peripheral lung are relatively more compliant than edematous lung and may become cystic under the influence of positive pressure ventilation. These regions are vulnerable to high pressure and can rupture directly into the pleural space to cause pneumothorax. Pulmonary inter-

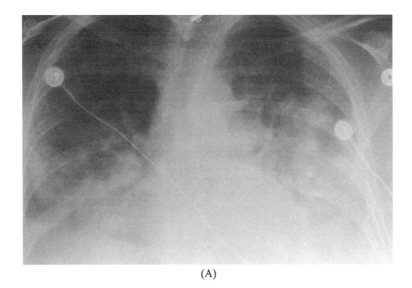

(A)

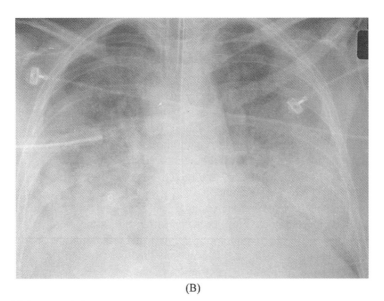

(B)

FIGURE 5.14. (A) Film taken shortly after aspiration shows bibasal ill-defined airspace opacities, consistent with aspiration. (B) Film taken 10 hours after A, showing increasing opacification of both hemithoraces, including the upper lobes. ETT and NGT have been inserted. (C) Film 4 days later shows development of ground glass opacity consistent with Stage 3 ARDS. Aspiration leading to ARDS.

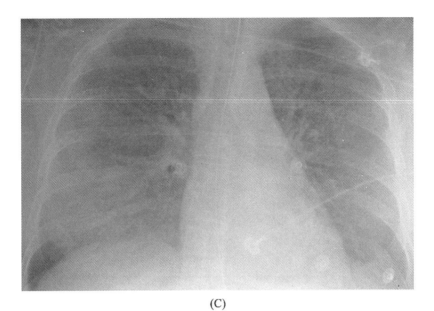

(C)

FIGURE 5.14. (*Continued.*)

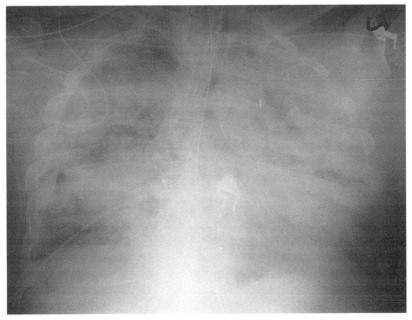

FIGURE 5.15. Confluent bilateral airspace opacities, consistent with Stage 2 ARDS.

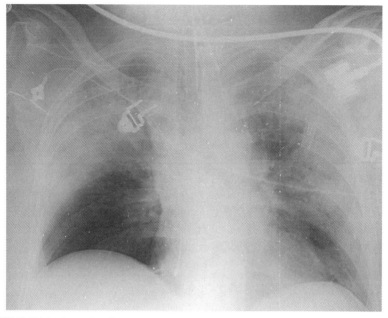

FIGURE 5.16. A predominantly peripheral pattern of opacity is occasionally seen in ARDS, also referred to as "reverse bat-wing" appearance.

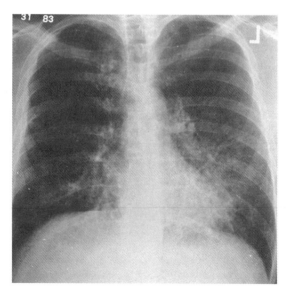

FIGURE 5.17. Film 5 weeks after development of ARDS shows bilateral coarse irregular opacities reflecting fibrosis. Stage 3 ARDS.

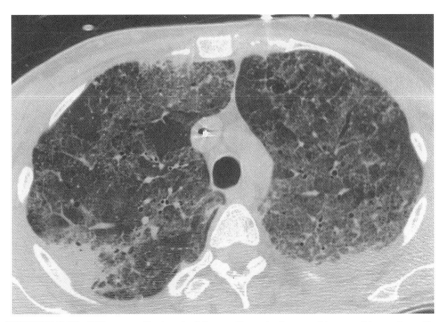

FIGURE 5.18. CT scan at the level of the aortic arch shows widespread irregular reticular opacities, ground glass opacity, traction bronchiectasis, and a confluent peripheral area of consolidation. Stage 3 ARDS.

stitial emphysema is notoriously difficult to detect on radiographs, but is suggested by the development of a "salt-and-pepper" texture of lung parenchyma, the presence of lucent halos surrounding intrapulmonary vessels, or nontapering streaks of air within the lung. This complication is ominous in that lung compliance is further compromised by interstitial air, despite the fact that lung volumes and consolidations may appear to improve.

CT findings in ARDS parallel those of projectional radiography.[35] With CT, the consolidations of ARDS migrate to dependent lung regions depending on patient positioning. Given the relatively viscous nature of the pulmonary edema, these positional changes in the distribution of consolidation have been ascribed to dependent atelectasis of noncompliant lung rather than true fluid migration. Pleural effusions are more commonly seen with CT, as are barotraumatic complications.

In clinical practice, it may be difficult to distinguish ARDS form hydrostatic edemas.[35,88] The presence of airspace consolidations within the context of a normal heart size, the absence of systemic venous distention (involving the superior vena cava or azygous vein), and the absence of pulmonary vascular congestion favor ARDS.[62,100] Unfortunately, in clinical practice, complicating factors such as preexisting cardiopulmonary disease, supine patient positioning, or combined hydrostatic and capillary leak edemas may make the distinction very difficult.[1] All radiographic findings must be interpreted within the context of available clinical information, including laboratory, hemodynamic, and ventilatory data.

PULMONARY EMBOLISM

Pulmonary embolism (PE) is the lodgment of thrombus within the pulmonary vascular bed. In 80% of cases or more, the thrombus originates from the systemic venous circulation of the pelvis or lower extremities, although the upper extremity is increasingly a source of thrombi due to the use of indwelling central venous catheters. Rarely, primary thrombus may form directly in the pulmonary circulation, typically in the setting of disseminated malignancy (Trousseau's syndrome).

Pulmonary embolism is associated with a number of congenital and acquired risk factors. Among the acquired risks are age greater than 40 years, previous thromboembolism, recent surgery, prolonged immobilization, malignancy, obesity, pregnancy or recent childbirth, and use of oral contraceptives. Congenital hypercoagulable states such as deficiencies of protein-C, protein-S, and antithrombin-3 are increasingly recognized, as are factor-5 mutations and antiphospholipid antibodies in patients with connective tissue diseases.[17,45,64,65,71] Of note is that between 6% and 26% patients have only subsegmental emboli. Treatment of this entity is controversial, especially given the only moderate sensitivity of most imaging modalities for detecting these small emboli.[34,41,66,89]

The clinical manifestations of PE are highly variable and nonspecific. The prevalence of high-probability radionuclide ventilation-perfusion (VQ) scans in asymptomatic patients with deep vein thrombosis (DVT) would suggest that 20% to 50% of patients are asymptomatic. In the PIOPED (Prospective Investigation of Pulmonary Embolism Diagnosis) study, the most common symptoms were dyspnea (80%), pleuritic chest pain (60%), cough (40%), and apprehension.[89] The classic triad of hemoptysis, pleuritic chest pain, and dyspnea are observed in a minority of patients,[98] typically those with peripheral thrombi in whom there is distal lung infarction.[67] Massive central thrombi may present as syncope, resulting from a dramatic decrease in cardiac output. Age does not appear to influence the clinical presentation.[84,86]

The most common clinical signs of PE are tachypnea (92%), tachycardia (44%), a prominent P2 or pulmonary component of the second heart sound (53%), and fever (43%).[8] As with symptoms, these signs are nonspecific and do not permit the confident diagnosis of PE. Hull and colleagues reported 85% sensitivity and 37% specificity of these signs for PE.[52]

A number of laboratory tests are helpful in suggesting the diagnosis of PE, but none has sufficient sensitivity or specificity to be conclusive. Patients are commonly hypoxemic acutely; arterial blood gases may also show respiratory alkalosis, hypocapnea, and a widened A-a gradient. Interestingly, 8% to 10% of patients with angiographically proven PE had a normal A-a gradient in the

PIOPED study. ECG changes range from normal (23% of cases) to sinus tachycardia, other supraventricular tachyarrhythmias, and nonspecific ST-T changes. The classic findings of right heart strain (e.g., S1Q3T3, right axis shift, and right bundle branch block) are relatively uncommon. However, the electrocardiogram (ECG) is also important in distinguishing PE from myocardial infarction (MI), with which it may be confused clinically.

In recent years, the D-dimer assay has begun to appear in diagnostic algorithms for suspected PE.[63] D-dimer is a breakdown product of cross-linked fibrin and therefore a marker of coagulation and thrombolysis. D-dimer is elevated in many situations, including MI, disseminated intravascular coagulation, surgery, malignancy, infection, cardiac failure, and age, and is therefore nonspecific. However, it is highly sensitive for thrombosis and has a high negative predictive value (80%–97%), making it valuable in excluding PE.[6,64] The reliability of D-dimer depends on the specific assay. Whereas the enzyme-linked immunosorbent assay (ELISA) has the highest specificity, it is not usually available in the acute setting. Agglutination tests are less sensitive, but can be completed within an hour.

THE RADIOLOGY OF THROMBOEMBOLISM

Chest Radiographs

Although nonspecific, many chest radiographic findings have been described, including the presence of atelectasis, consolidation, Westermark's sign (focal oligemia), enlargement of the affected central pulmonary artery, and pleural effusion. Chest radiographs in patients following gynecologic surgery commonly show some degree of basilar volume loss with effusions, which reduces the significance of these observations. The wedge-shaped pleural-based opacity, Hampton's hump (Fig. 5.19), represents peripheral infarction; although uncommon, this finding is more specific for PE than other findings.[45,84,94] The chest radiograph is important in excluding other conditions with similar presentations, such as pneumonia or pneumothorax, and in directing the diagnostic algorithm in patients with suspected PE (see below).[30]

Radionuclide Ventilation-Perfusion Scans

Since its introduction in the mid-1960s, the VQ scan has been the mainstay in the diagnostic work-up of PE. The PIOPED data were important in showing that the VQ scan is reliably diagnostic in two settings: (1) to exclude PE in patients in whom clinical suspicion is low and the VQ scan is normal or of very low probability; and (2) to diagnose PE in patients in whom there is high clinical suspicion and a high-probability VQ scan (Fig. 5.20). Under these conditions, no further work-up is necessary. Unfortunately, less than 30% of hospitalized patients fall neatly into one of these categories. In most patients, particularly those with underlying cardiopulmonary disease or abnormal chest radiographs,

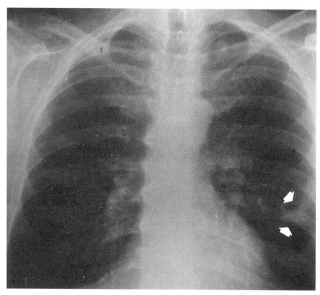

FIGURE 5.19. A 55-year-old postoperative patient with chest pain. Peripheral wedge-shaped opacity (◊) in left midzone consistent with Hampton's hump. Proven pulmonary embolus.

there is discordance between clinical suspicion and VQ result or the VQ scan is of intermediate probability (Fig. 5.21). In these patients, more definitive testing with classical angiography is necessary.[11]

Pulmonary Angiography

The pulmonary angiogram remains the reference standard for the diagnosis of PE,[70] and, unlike VQ scinitigraphy, it allows the direct visualization of emboli. Thrombus appears as a partial or complete intravascular filling defect (Fig. 5.22). Detection of clot in subsegmental or more distal vessels is possible, although interobserver variability limits the diagnostic accuracy of angiography for peripheral thrombi. Despite the low reported morbidity (3%) and mortality (<1%) of classical angiography,[85] it remains heavily underutilized in patients with a presumptive but unproven diagnosis of PE. The performance and interpretation of classical pulmonary angiograms require highly trained staff and careful hemodynamic monitoring of patients during the procedure, which contribute to its underutilization.

Ultrafast CT, Helical CT, and MR Pulmonary Angiography

With the advent of electron beam and helical technology, the use of comptuerized tomography (CT) for the diagnosis of PE has become possible. These tech-

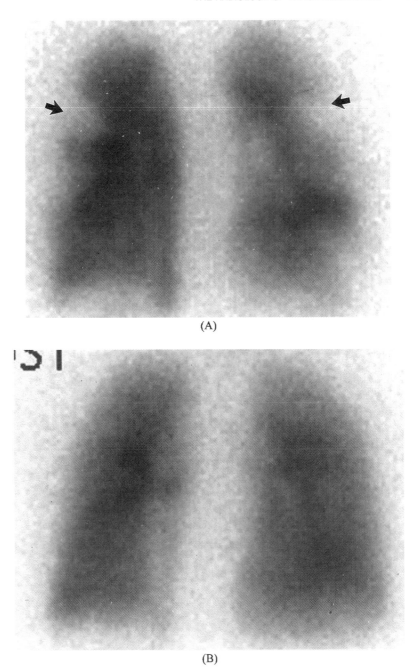

(A)

(B)

FIGURE 5.20. A 64-year-old postoperative patient. Perfusion scan (A) demonstrates multiple segmented areas of absent activity ($\rightarrow$). (B) Ventilation scan demonstrates uniform activity. High-probability VQ scan for pulmonary embolus.

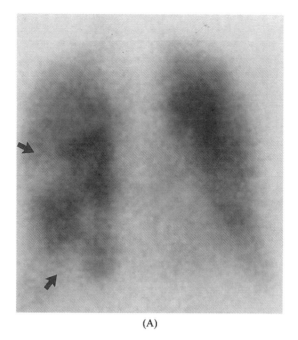

(A)

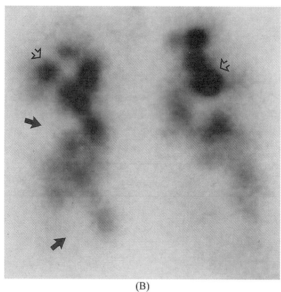

(B)

FIGURE 5.21. Ventilation-perfusion scan. 73-year-old female patient. (A) Perfusion scan shows right mid- and lower-zone segmental defects (→). (B) Ventilation scan demonstrates matched defects (→). Central pooling of inhaled radionuclide is seen on the ventilation images, consistent with dilated airways in COPD (⇒). Intermediate probability scan, requiring further work-up.

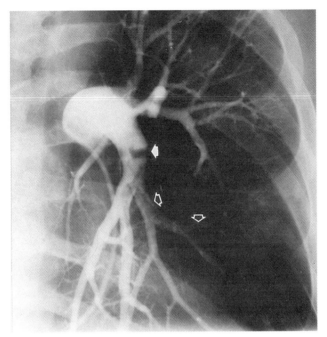

FIGURE 5.22. Selective left pulmonary angiogram on the patient in Fig. 5.1 reveals filling defects within the descending left pulmonary artery (⬧) and several segmental and subsegmental branches (⬦).

nologies provide fast image acquisition, allowing for relatively high spatial resolution sequences that cover the central pulmonary circulation within a single breath hold and with a minimum of motion unsharpness.[73,74] Several prospective studies with CT pulmonary angiography (CTPA) have reported high sensitivity (75%–100%) and specificity (80%–100%) for the diagnosis of segmental or more proximal thrombus (Figs. 23–25).[33,34,37,75,90,95]

The role of MR angiography (MRA) for PE is still evolving. MRA offers a number of theoretical advantages over CTPA, including the lack of ionizing radiation, the potential to demonstrate velocity changes associated with the cardiac cycle using cine angiographic techniques, and the assessment of the pelvic and lower extremity venous circulation in the same setting. Comparative studies with MRA report diagnostic accuracies comparable to that of CTPA (Fig. 5.26).[25,39] However, both CT and MR angiography are limited to the segmental or more proximal vascular generations. Although the PIOPED data suggest that isolated subsegmental thrombus occurs in only a minority of patients (6%), the significance of peripheral clot is controversial and is likely influenced by such individual factors as the degree of residual lower extremity clot burden and the presence or severity of underlying cardiopulmonary disease. Finally, both CT and MR angiography require considerable technical and diagnostic expertise,

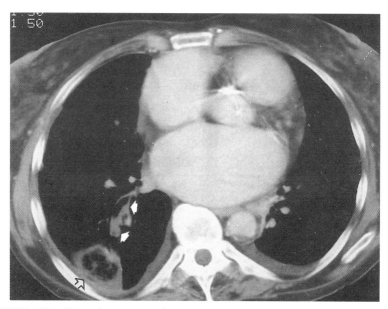

FIGURE 5.23. CT pulmonary angiogram demonstrates thrombus within segmental right lower lobe arteries (⇕) and a pulmonary infarct (⇒).

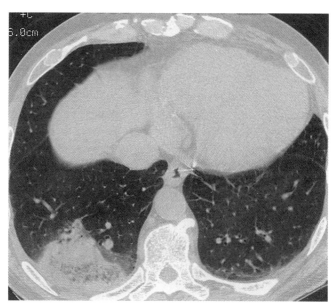

FIGURE 5.24. CT chest demonstrates a wedge-shaped peripheral right lower lobe opacity with "bubbly" areas of low attenuation. Classic CT appearance of a pulmonary infarct.

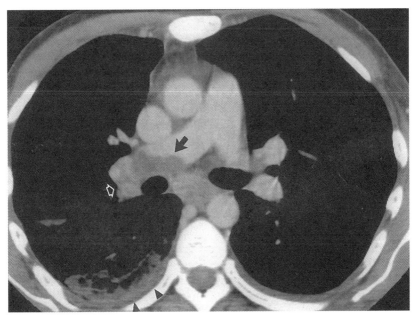

FIGURE 5.25. CT pulmonary angiogram demonstrates low-attenuation filling defects in the contrast-enhanced right main pulmonary artery ($\rightarrow$) and right intemediate pulmonary artery ($\lozenge$). A low-attenuation crescentic peripheral area is seen, consistent with pulmonary infarction ($\blacktriangleright$).

which will limit their application for thromboembolism to those institutions with the requisite expertise and resources.

Deep Venous System Imaging

In PE, the embolic source is generally the systemic veins of the pelvis and lower extremities. The intention of treatment for PE is to prevent recurrences that could incur morbidity or death. Imaging of the deep venous system is therefore important to the investigation of pulmonary embolus. Doppler ultrasound of the lower extremities has largely replaced classical venography for this purpose because it is noninvasive, requires no contrast, and has been shown to have high sensitivity and specificity for the diagnosis of thrombus within the veins of the thigh (Fig. 5.27).[76] Technical expertise in scanning is required for accurate studies of the calf, although the significance of venous thrombosis limited to the calf is debatable. A suggested algorithm for the imaging of suspected DVT is given (Fig. 5.28).

IMAGING ALGORITHM

In the postoperative patient with suspected PE, the variety of diagnostic tests is multiple, albeit individually less than perfect. Different algorithms will apply to

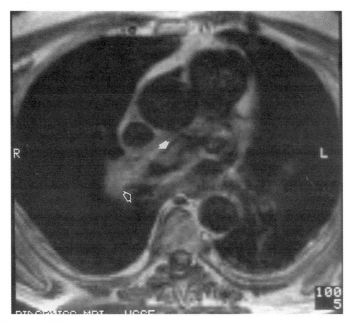

FIGURE 5.26. MRI thorax (gated T1-weighted spin-echo sequence) shows pulmonary embolus within the right main (◊) and right descending pulmonary arteries (◊).

different centers based on the availability of technologies, physician expertise, and the clinical index of suspicion. At most institutions in which CT pulmonary angiography is available, it has become the primary screening *and* diagnostic tool for suspected PE. A reasonable algorithm in Fig. 5.29 is supported by available evidence from experienced centers. The algorithm assumes expertise in CT angiography, but takes into account several factors, including the level of clinical suspicion for PE, the high incidence of indeterminate VQ scans in patients with abnormal chest radiographs or underlying cardiopulmonary disease, and the high diagnostic accuracy of CTPA for PE to the segmental arterial level. Although often elevated in postoperative patients, a negative D-dimer provides high negative predictive value. Where CTPA is not available, the evaluation of suspected PE will require VQ scanning. Patients with the unresolved suspicion of PE should be further investigated using either classical angiography, or in patients with unilateral leg symptoms, lower extremity Doppler ultrasound to search for a possible source of thrombi.

COMPLICATIONS OF CRITICAL CARE ADMISSION

Tubes and Catheters

The important anatomical landmarks in endotracheal tube placement are the carina and the vocal cords. An ideally positioned endotracheal tube (ETT) tip

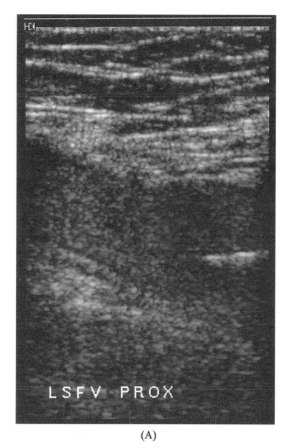

(A)

FIGURE 5.27. (A) Ultrasound image of left superficial femoral vein shows the lumen entirely filled with hyperechoic material consistent with thrombus. (B) Doppler examination of the same region shows no significant venous flow in the superficial femoral vein. Acute deep vein thrombosis of left lower limb.

lies in the midtrachea 3–6 cm above the carina with the patient's head in a neutral anatomical position. This allows for changes in the position of the tube tip in flexion or extension of the head and neck, which can change the tube tip position by up to 2 cm in either direction.[46,47] Malposition of the ETT occurs in up to 10% to 15% of patients.[7,11,36,38,54] The most common malposition is intubation of the right main bronchus due to the more obtuse angle it makes with the carina compared to the left main bronchus.

The tip of a tracheostomy tube should lie between one-half to two-thirds the distance between the tracheal stoma and carina at about the level of the T3 vertebral body.[46,47] The lumen of the tube should be approximately two-thirds the tracheal diameter under normal circumstances; the cuff should fill the tracheal lumen without distending the walls. Neck flexion and extension does not affect

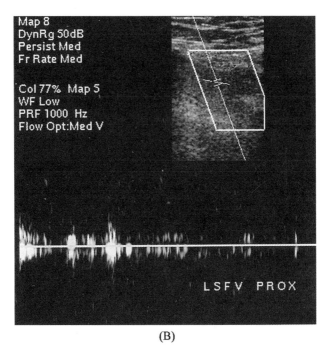

(B)

FIGURE 5.27. (*Continued.*)

the position of the tracheostomy tube. A small amount of subcutaneous emphysema is normal after tracheostomy tube insertion. Large amounts of subcutaneous air result from ectopic tube position or a cuff leak. Subcutaneous air may dissect directly into the mediastinum, if mechanical ventilation is used in this setting.

In an ICU setting, most central venous catheters (CVC) are inserted by subclavian or internal jugular approaches. The ideal position of the tip of the catheter in these cases is within the superior vena cava (SVC)[43,53] Radiographically, this corresponds to the space between the anterior ends of the first and third ribs. Anatomically, this places the catheter tip between the right atrium and the last venous valves of the subclavian and internal jugular veins, potentially allowing accurate pressure measurements. A peripherally inserted central catheter (PICC) may be used for longer-term intravenous therapy. The ideal placement of the tip of this catheter is within the SVC or brachiocephalic veins.[43,53]

Complications of subclavian or internal jugular central venous catheters include malposition, fracture (Fig. 5.30), rupture, and pneumothorax.[55] Malposition of the tip of the catheter in the ipsilateral or contralateral subclavian or internal jugular vein may compromise venous return from the upper extremity or central nervous system, respectively. Placement of the tip within the right atrium can cause cardiac perforation, although this is rare; placement within the right ventricle predisposes to cardiac arrhythmias. Rupture of the catheter tip into the mediastinum may occur. Radiological signs include widening of

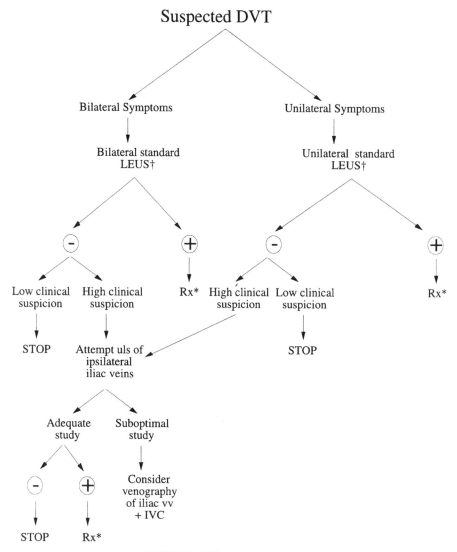

FIGURE 5.28. Suspected DVT.

the superior mediastinum (Fig. 5.31), apical pleural capping, and hemothorax. Neuropraxis of the phrenic nerve rarely occurs, causing elevation of the ipsilateral hemidiaphragm. Pneumothorax occurs in approximately 5% of patients following insertion of jugular or subclavian central venous catheters; hence the normal practice of obtaining an erect chest X ray (CXR) following catheter placement.[7,47] However, a low diagnostic yield is gained from follow-up chest radiographs for catheter placement.[47] CXR is recommended only when there is clinical suspicion of complications.

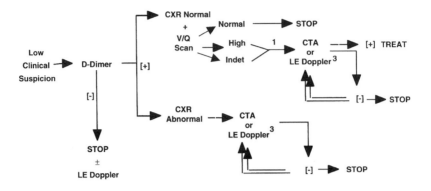

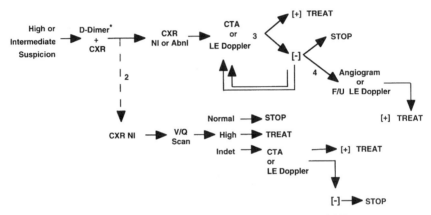

FIGURE 5.29. Clinical algorithms for suspected PE.

The ideal position of a Swan–Ganz pulmonary artery catheter is in the right or left main pulmonary arteries; the tip should not extend beyond the proximal interlobar pulmonary artery seen on CXR. Complications associated with insertion of Swan–Ganz catheters include pneumothorax, arrhythmias, and knotting or shearing during withdrawal or insertion of the catheter. Retained catheter segments predispose to sepsis, pulmonary embolism, cardiac arrhythmias, and vascular perforations. Pulmonary artery perforation or pulmonary infarction following balloon inflation may occur when the catheter tip lies too far distally. About 20% of Swan–Ganz catheters are found to be malpositioned on initial chest X ray.[47]

A specific complication of intra-aortic counterpulsation devices is distal or proximal malposition, resulting in occlusion of carotid and subclavian arteries or the renal arteries, respectively.[47] Otherwise, the complications for these and transvenous pacing devices are similar to those for Swan–Ganz catheters.

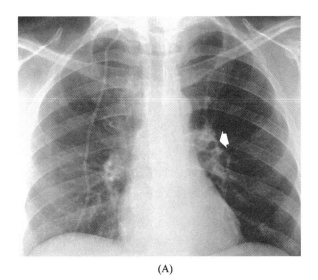

(A)

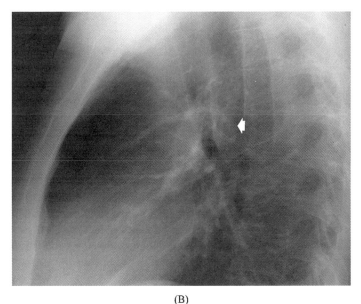

(B)

FIGURE 5.30. Fractured central venous catheter. Ectopic catheter frament is seen in the main and left pulmonary arteries on PA (A) and lateral (B) views (♭).

A nasogastric tube (NGT) inserted for gastric decompression should lie within the body of the stomach, with the proximal side hole (usually within 10 cm of the tip) in the stomach rather than the esophagus. Smaller-bore NGTs used for feeding should lie at least in the distal stomach but ideally within the duodenum. The incidence of clinically important complications from NGT mis-

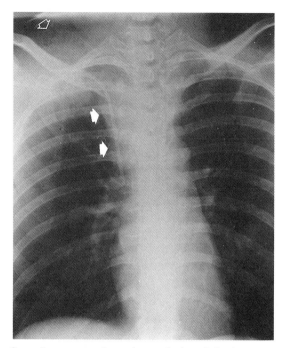

FIGURE 5.31. Central venous catheter inserted via subclavian approach with associated widening of the superior mediastinum (◆). Pre-CVC X ray was normal. Findings are consistent with mediastinal hematoma secondary to CVC insertion. A small amount of subcutaneous gas in the soft tissue of the right side of the next (◊) was likely introduced at the time of the procedure.

placement, such as placement of the tube within the airway, is approximately 1%[47] (Fig. 5.32). Of note, endotracheal and tracheostomy tubes do not necessarily protect the airway from endotracheal intubation with an NGT; in fact, the risk of feeding tube misplacement may even be increased in these patients. Pulmonary complications include pneumonia, abscess, empyema, and pneumothorax. Confirmation of the position of the tube within the stomach radiologically is recommended in all cases.

Barotrauma

Positive pressure ventilation, especially in the setting of acute lung disease such as ARDS, predisposes to barotrauma. It manifests in the pulmonary compartment as pulmonary interstitial emphysema (PIE) that results from rupture of noncompliant alveoli into the interstitium of the lung. "Salt- and -pepper" stippled opacity is produced in the consolidated lung, as well as perivascular lucent streakiness or halo formation. Later sequelae include dissection of air centrally along the bronchovascular bundles, resulting in pneumomediastinum, and air cyst formation, either subpleural or intraparenchymal.

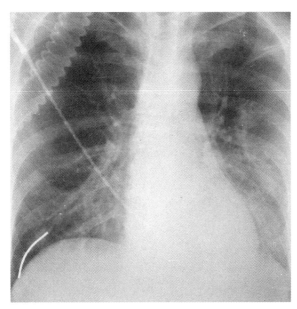

FIGURE 5.32. Nasogastric tube inserted into right main bronchus with tip lying periph-erally in the right lung. A subsequent film showed development of a right-sided pneu-mothorax.

Pneumothorax is another major feature of barotrauma[91,92,102] and is defined as air outside the lung, between the visceral and the parietal pleura. Risk factors for the development of pneumothorax in the critical care/postoperative setting include positive pressure ventilation, placement of intravenous lines such as central venous catheters, lung disorders such as ARDS that "stiffen" the lung, and bronchoscopy. Whatever the cause, mechanical ventilation tends to per-petuate an air leak once it has developed. It often leads to a rapid increase in size and severity of a pneumothorax, which if untreated, may go on to tension pneumothorax.[102] The size of the pneumothorax correlates poorly with clinical significance; a small pneumothorax, which in an otherwise healthy patient may be left untreated, may require drainage in a patient with severe cardiopulmonary compromise.[91,92]

The position of the air in the pleura depends on the posture of the patient and the condition of the pleura. An erect chest X ray typically results in an apical pneumothorax, which is seen as a thin white line beyond which no pulmonary vessels can be seen. Differentiation from skin folds, rib margins, lung bullae, and overlying catheters is important.

In the supine and semierect positions, only a minority (about 20%) of pneu-mothoraces will manifest in the apex or lateral aspect of the lung. More often, the pleural air, seeking the most anterior portion of the lung, will collect in the anterior costophrenic sulcus, resulting in hyperlucency over the involved

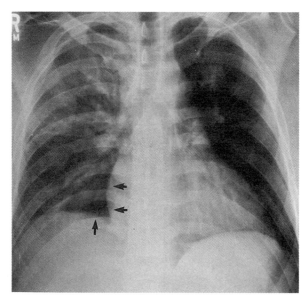

FIGURE 5.33. Supine CXR demonstrating sharp definition of right heart border by pleural air, which seeks the most anterior portion of the hemithorax (→). Supine pneumothorax.

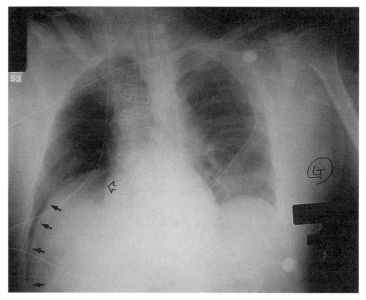

FIGURE 5.34. Supine plain X ray showing prominent right costophrenic sulcus (deep sulcus sign) (→) and sharp definition of the right heart border (◊). Supine pneumothorax.

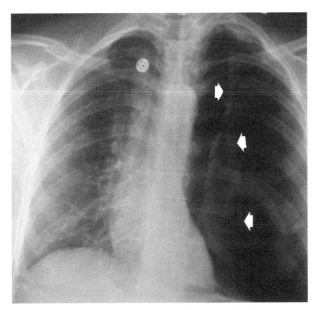

FIGURE 5.35. Markedly hyperlucent left hemithorax with diaphragmatic depression and mediastinal shift away from the side of the pneumothorax. Faint triangular opacity (⚐) represents the collapsed left lung. Left tension pneumothorax.

hemidiaphragm and upper abdomen, deepening of the costophrenic sulcus, and sharp demarcation of the cardiophrenic angle on the involved side (Figs. 5.33 and 5.34). The subtlety of these findings results in a low diagnostic rate of supine pneumothorax and a significant number of subsequent tension pneumothoraces (Fig. 5.35).

Tension pneumothorax results when air collects under pressure in the pleural space via a ball-valve mechanism. This causes mediastinal and diaphragmatic shift away from the affected side and marked cardiovascular compromise. Mediastinal shift is not necessarily present in patients on positive end-expiratory pressure (PEEP) ventilation; in this setting, diaphragmatic depression is a better indicator of tension. The presence of a chest tube on the side of the pneumothorax does not exclude the diagnosis of tension pneumothorax, as tube blockage, malposition, or noncommunication with a loculated tension pneumothorax can occur. Previous or current pleural disease can cause loculation of a pneumothorax.

REFERENCES

1. Aberle DR, Wiener-Kronish JP, Webb WR, Matthay MA. The diagnosis of hydrostatic versus increased pulmonary edema based on chest radiographic criteria in critically ill patients. *Radiology* 1988;168:73–79.

2. Albertine K. Histopathology of pulmonary edema and the acute respiratory distress syndrome. In Matthay M, Inghow D (Eds), *Pulmonary Edema*, Lung Biology in Health and Disease, vol. 116. Marcel Dekker, Inc., 1998.

3. Armstrong P, Wilson AG, Dee P, Hansell DM. *Imaging of Diseases of the Chest*, 2nd ed. St. Louis: Mosby, 1995, pp. 15–47.

4. Bartlett JG, Finegold SM. Anaerobic infections of the lung and pleural space. *Am J Respir Crit Care Med* 1974;110:56–77.

5. Bartlett JG, O'Keefe, P, Tally FP, Louie TJ, Gorbach SL. Bacteriology of hospital-acquired pneumonia. *Arch Intern Med* 1986;146:868–871.

6. Becker DM, Philbrick JT, Bachhuber TL, et al. D-dimer testing and acute venous thromboembolism. A shortcut to accurate diagnosis? *Arch Int Med* 1996;156:939–946.

7. Bekemeyer WB, Crapo RD, Calhoun S, et al. Efficacy of chest ratiography in a respiratory intensive care unit. *Chest* 1985;887:691.

8. Bell WR, Simon TL, DeMets DL. The clinical features of submassive and massive pulmonary emboli. *Am J Med* 1977;62:355–360.

9. Bessis L, Callard P, Gotheil C, Biaggi A, Grenier P. High-resolution CT of parenchymal lung disease: precise correlation with histologic findings. *Radiographics* 1992;12:45–58.

10. Beydon L, Saada M, Liu N. et al. Can portable chest x-ray examination accurately diagnose lung consolidation after major abdominal surgery? A comparison with computed tomography scan. *Chest* 1992;102:1697–1703.

11. Brunel W, Coleman D, Schwartz D, et al. Assessment of routine chest roentgenograms and the physical examination to confirm endotracheal tube position. *Chest* 1989;96:1043.

12. Cameron JL, Anderson RP, Zuidema GD. Aspiration pneumonia: a clinical and experimental review. *J. Surg Res* 1967;7:44–53.

13. Cameron JL, Mitchell WH, Zuidema GD. Aspiration pneumonia: clinical outcome following documented aspiration. *Arch Surg* 1973;106:49–62.

14. Celis R, Torres A, Gatell JM, et al. Nosocomial pneumonia: a multivariate analysis of risk and prognosis. *Chest* 1988;93:318–324.

15. Coleman DL. Control of post operative pain: nonnarcotic and narcotic alternatives and their effect on pulmonary function. *Chest* 1987;92:520–528.

16. Conway D, Johnson R. The nature and significance of peribronchial cuffing in pulmonary edema. *Radiology* 1977;125:577–582.

17. Coon WW. Venous thromboembolism: prevalence, risk factors, and prevention. *Clin Chest Med* 1984;5:391–401.

18. Craven DE, Kunches LM, Kilinsky V, Lichtenberg DA, Make BJ, McCabe WR. Risk factors for pneumonia and fatality in patients receiving continuous mechanical ventilation. *Am Rev Respir Dis* 1986;133:792–796.

19. Craven DE, Kunches LM, Lichtenberg DA, et al. Nosocomial infection and fatality in medical and surgical intensive care unit patients. *Arch Intern Med* 1988;148:1161–1168.

20. Cross AS, Roup B. Role of respiratory assistance devices in endemic nosocomial pneumonia. *Am J Med* 1981;70:681–685.

21. Dauber IM, Weil JV. Noninvasive radioisotropic assessment of pulmonary vascular protein leak: experimental studies and potential clinical applications. *Clin Chest Med* 1985;6:427–437.

22. Donowitz LG, Page MC, Mileur GL, Guenther SH. Alterations of normal gastric flora in critical care patients receiving antacid and cimetidine therapy. *Infect Control* 1986;7:23–26.

23. DuMoulin GC, Patterson DG, Hedley-Whyte J, Lisbon A. Aspiration of gastric bacteria in antacid patients: a frequent cause of post-operative colonization of the airway. *Lancet* 1982;1:242–245.

24. Elpern EH, Jacobs ER, Bone RC. Incidence of aspiration in tracheally intubated adults. *Heart Lung* 1987;16:427–531.

25. Erdman W, et al. Magnetic resonance imaging of pulmonary embolus. *Semin Ultrasound, CT and MRI* 1997;18(5):338–348.

26. Exharos ND. The importance of pH and volume in tracheobronchial aspiration. *Chest* 1965;47:167–169.

27. Fagon JY, Chastre J, Domart Y, et al. Nosocomial pneumonia in patients receiving continuous mechanical ventilation: prospective analysis of 52 episodes with use of a protected specimen brush and quantitative culture technique. *Am Rev Respir Dis* 1989;139:877–884.

28. Fiddian-Green RG, Baker S. Nosocomial pneumonia in the critically ill: product of aspiration or translocation. *Crit Care Med* 1991;19:763–769.

29. Forster BB, Müller NL, Mayo JR, Okazawa M, Wiggs BJ, Paré PD. High-resolution computed tomography of experimental hydrostatic pulmonary edema. *Chest* 1992;101:1434–1437.

30. Fraser D, Paré, PD. *Diagnosis of Diseases of the Chest.* W.B. Saunders Company, Philadelphia 1990.

31. Gastinne H, Wolff M, Delatour F, et al. A controlled trial in intensive care units of selective decontamination of the digestive tract with nonabsorbable antibiotics. *N Engl J Med* 1992;326:594–595.

32. Gianella RA, Broitman SA, Zamcheck N. Influence of gastric acidity on bacterial and parasitic enteric infections: a perspective. *Ann Intern Med* 1973;78:271–276.

33. Goodman LR, Curtin JJ, Mewissen MW, et al. Detection of pulmonary embolism in patients with unresolved clinical and scintigraphic diagnosis: helical CT versus angiography. *Am J Roentgenology* 1995;164:1369–1374.

34. Goodman LR, Lipchik RJ. Diagnosis of acute pulmonary embolism: time for a new approach. *Radiology* 1996;199:25–27.

35. Goodman LR. Congestive heart failure and adult respiratory distress syndrome: new insights using computed tomography. *Radiol Clin N Am* 1996;34:33–46.

36. Gray P, Sullivan G, Ostryzniuk P, et al. Value of postprocedural chest radiographs in the adult intensive care unit. *Crit Care Med* 1992;20:1513–1518.

37. Greaves SM, et al. CT of pulmonary thromboembolism. *Semin Ultrasound, CT and MRI* 1997;18(5):323–337.

38. Greenbaum DM, Marshall KE. The value of routine daily chest x-rays in intubated patients in the medical intensive care unit. *Crit Care Med* 1982;10:29.

39. Grist TM, Sostman HD, MacFall JR, et al. Pulmonary angiography with MR imaging: preliminary clinical experience. *Radiology* 1993;189:523–530.

40. Gropper MA, Wiener-Kronish JP, Hashimoto S. Acute cardiogenic pulmonary edema. *Clinics in Chest Med* 1994;15:501–515.

41. Gurney JW. No fooling around: direct visualization of pulmonary embolism (editorial). *Radiology* 1993;188:618–619.

42. Gurney JW, Goodman LR. Pulmonary edema localized in the right upper lobe accompanying mitral regurgitation. *Radiology* 1989;171:397–399.

43. Hadaway LC. An overview of vascular access devices inserted via the antecubital area. *J Intravenous Nurs* 1990;13:297–305.

44. Hall JC, Tarala RA, Hall JL, Mander J. A multivariate analysis of the risk of respiratory complications after laparotomy. *Chest* 1991;99:923–927.

45. Hampson N, et al. Clinical aspects of pulmonary embolism. *Semin Ultrasound, CT and MRI* 1997;18(5):314–322.

46. Henschke CI, Pasternack GS, Schroeder S, et al. Bedside chest radiography: diagnostic efficacy. *Radiology* 1983;149:23–26.

47. Henschke CI, et al. Accuracy and efficacy of chest radiography in the intensive care unit. *Radiol Clin N Am* 1996;34:21–31.

48. Heyland D, Mandell LA. Gastric colonization by gram-negative bacilli and nosocomial pneumonia in the intensive care unit patient: evidence for causation. *Chest* 1992;101:187–193.

49. Heyland DK, Cook DJ, Jaeschke R, et al. Selective decontamination of the digestive tract: an overview. *Chest* 1994;105:1221–1229.

50. Higgins CB. *Essentials of Cardiac Radiology and Imaging*, 1st ed. Philadelphia: Lippincott, 1992, pp. 1–48.

51. Hoffman RB, Rigler LG. Evaluation of left ventricular enlargement in the lateral projection of the chest. *Radiology* 1965;85:93–100.

52. Hull RD, Raskob GE, Carter CJ, et al. Pulmonary embolism in outpatients with pleuritic chest pain. *Arch Int Med* 1988;148:838–844.

53. James L, Bledsoe L, Hadaway L. A retrospective look at tip location and complications of peripherally inserted central catheter lines. *J Intravenous Nurs* 1993;12(2):104–109.

54. Janower ML, Jennas-Nocera A, Markai J. Utility and efficacy of portable chest radiographs. *Am J Roentgenology* 1984;142:265.

55. Kazerooni E, et al. The cardiac ICU. *Soc Thoracic Radiol: Thoracic Imag* 1998;613–626.

56. Kollef M, et al. Ventilator-associated pneumonia: clinical consideration. *Am J Roentgenology* 1994;163:1031–1035.

57. Landay MJ, Christensen EE, Bynum LJ. Pulmonary manifestations of acute aspiration of gastric contents. *Am J Roentgenology* 1978;131:587.

58. Lange S, Stark P. *Radiology of Chest Diseases*, 1st ed. Stuttgart, Germany: Thieme, 1990, pp. 149–163.

59. Leu HS, Kaiser DL, Mori M, Woolson RF, Wenzel RP. Hospital acquired pneumonia: attributable mortality and morbidity. *Am J Epidemiol* 1989;129:1258–1267.

60. Lipchik R, et al. Nosocomial pneumonia. *Radiol Clin N Am* 1996;34(1):47–58.

61. Lowenkron SE, Niederman MS. Definition and evaluation of the resolution of nosocomial pneumonia. *Semin Respir Infect* 1992;7:271–281.

62. Milne ENC, Pistolesi M, Miniati M, Giuntini C. The radiologic distinction of cardiogenic and noncardiogenic edema. *Am J Roentgenology* 1985;144:879–894.

63. Morpurgo M, Marzegelli M. D dimer in pulmonary embolism. In Morpurgo M (Ed), *Pulmonary Embolism.* New York: Dekker, 1994, pp. 107–114.

64. Moser KM. Diagnosing pulmonary embolism: D-dimer needs rigorous evaluation. *Br Med J* 1994;309:1525–1526.

65. National Institutes of health Consensus Conference. Prevention of venous thrombosis and pulmonary embolism. *JAMA* 1986;256:744–749.

66. Oser RF, et al. Anatomic distribution of pulmonary emboli at pulmonary angiography. Implications for cross-section imaging. *Radiology* 1996;199:31–35.

67. Palevsky M. Current approaches to the clinical diagnosis of pulmonary embolism. *Soc Thoracic Radiol: Thoracic Imag* 1998;205–216.

68. Platell C, et al. Atelectasis after abdominal surgery. *J Am Coll Surg* 1997;185:584–590.

69. Polk H, et al. Pneumonia in the surgical patient. *Curr Prob Surg* 1997;34:122–200.

70. Quinn MF, Lundell CI, Klotz TA, et al. Reliability of selective pulmonary arteriography in the diagnosis of pulmonary embolism. *Am J Roentgenology* 1987;149:469–471.

71. Raskob GE, Hull RD. Diagnosis and management of pulmonary thromboembolism. *Q J Med* 1990;76:787–797.

72. Ravin Ce. Pulmonary vascularity: radiographic considerations. *J Thorac Imag* 1988;3:1–13.

73. Remy-Jardin M, Remy J, Wattine L, Giraud F. Central pulmonary thromboembolism: diagnosis with spiral volumetric CT with single breath-hold technique: comparison with pulmonary angiography. *Radiology* 1992;185:381–387.

74. Remy-Jardin M, Caurain O, Remy J, Beregi J, Petyt L, Wannebroucq J. Diagnosis of central pulmonary embolism with spiral CT. *Radiology* 1994;193(P):262.

75. Remy-Jardin M, Remy J, Deschidre F, et al. Diagnosis of pulmonary embolism with spiral CT: comparison with pulmonary angiography and scintigraphy. *Radiology* 1996;200:699–706.

76. Rosen M, et al. Controversies in the use of lower extremity sonography in the diagnosis of acute deep vein thrombosis and a proposal for a unified approach. *Semin Ultrasound, CT and MRI* 1997;18(5):362–368.

77. Rothen H, Sporre B, Engberg G, et al. Prevention of atelectasis during general anaesthesia. *Lancet* 1995;345:1387–1391.

78. Roukema JA, Carol EJ, Prins JG. The prevention of pulmonary complications after upper abdominal surgery in patients with non-compromised pulmonary status. *Arch Surg* 1988;123:30–34.

79. Sachdeva R, et al. Acute respiratory distress syndrome. *Crit Care Clin* 1997;13(3):503–521.

80. Schwartz DJ, Wynne JW, Gibbs CP, et al. The pulmonary consequences of aspiration of gastric contents at pH values greater than 2.5. *Am J Respir Crit Care Med* 1980;121:119–126.

81. Shifrin R, et al. Aspiration in patients in critical care units. *Radiol Clin N Am* 1996;(34(1):83–96.

82. Short DS. Radiology of lung in left heart failure. *Br Heart J* 1956;18:233–240.

83. Staub NC. Clinical use of lung water measurements: report of a workshop. *Chest* 1996;90:588–594.

84. Stein PD, Gottschalk A, Saltzman HA, Terrin ML. Diagnosis of acute pulmonary embolism in the elderly. *J Am Coll Cardiol* 1991;81:1452–1457.

85. Stein PO, Athanasoulic C, Alvi A, et al. Complications and validity of pulmonary angiography in acute pulmonary embolism. *Circulation* 1992;85:462–468.

86. Stern PD, Terrin ML, Hales CA, et al. Clinical, laboratory roentgenographic, and electrocardiographic findings in patients with acute pulmonary embolism and no pre-existing cardiac or pulmonary disease. *Chest* 1991;100:598–603.

87. Storto ML, Kee ST, Golden JA, Webb WR. Hydrostatic pulmonary edema: high-resolution CT findings. *Am J Roentgenology* 1995;165:817–820.

88. Suh R, et al. Radiographic manifestations of pulmonary edema. In Matthay M, Inghow D (Eds), *Pulmonary Edema*, Lung Biology in Health and Disease, vol. 116. Marcel Dekker, Inc., 1998.

89. PIOPED Investigators. Value of the ventilation-perfusion scan in acute pulmonary embolism: results of the prospective investigation of pulmonary embolism diagnosis (PIOPED). *JAMA* 1990;263:2753–2759.

90. Teigen CL, Maus TP, Sheedy PF II, Stanson AW, Johnson CM, Breen JI, McKnside MA. Pulmonary embolism: diagnosis with contrast enhanced electron beam CT and comparison with pulmonary angiography. *Radiology* 1995;194:313–319.

91. Tocino I, et al. Barotrauma. *Radiol Clin N Am* 1996;34(1):59–81.

92. Tocino I. Pneumothorax in the supine patient: radiographic anatomy. *RadioGraphics* 1985;5(4):559–586.

93. Torres A, Anzar R, Gatell JM, et al. Incidence, risk, and prognosis factors of nosocomial pneumonia in mechanically ventilated patients. *Am Rev Respir Dis* 1990;142:523–528.

94. Urokinase Pulmonary Embolism Trial: A cooperative study. *Circulation* 1973;47 (suppl II):1–108.

95. van Rossum AB, Treurniet FEE, Kieft GJ, et al. Role of spiral volumetric computed tomographic scanning in the assessment of patients with clinical suspicion of pulmonary embolism and an abnormal ventilation/perfusion lung scan. *Thorax* 1996;51:23–28.

96. Weiner-Kronish JP, Matthay MA, Callen PW, Filly RA, Gamsu G, Staub NC. Relationship of pleural effusions to pulmonary hemodynamics in patients with congestive heart failure. *Am Rev Respir Dis* 1985;132:1253–1256.

97. Weiner-Kronish JP, Matthay MA. Pleural effusions associated with hydrostatic and increased permeability pulmonary edema. *Chest* 1988;93:852–858.

98. Wenger NK, Stein PD, Willis III PW. Massive acute pulmonary embolism: the deceivingly nonspecific manifestations. *JAMA* 1972;220:843–844.

99. Winer-Muram HT, Rubin SA, Ellis JV, et al. Pneumonia and ARDS in patients

receiving mechanical ventilation: diagnostic accuracy of chest radiography. *Radiology* 1993;188:479–485.

100. Woodring JH. Pulmonary artery-bronchus ratios in patients with normal lungs, pulmonary vascular plethora, and congestive heart failure. *Radiology* 1991;179:115–122.

101. Wunderink RG, Woldenberg LS, Zeiss J, et al. The radiologic diagnosis of autopsy-proven ventilator-associated pneumonia. *Chest* 1992;101:458–463.

102. Zimmerman J, et al. Effect of mechanical ventilation and positive end-expiration pressure (PEEP) on chest radiograph. *Am J Roentgenology* 1979;133:811–815.

CHAPTER 6

PERIOPERATIVE CARDIORESPIRATORY MONITORING AND MANAGEMENT

STEVEN A. VASILEV, M.D., M.B.A.

Technological advances have tremendously enhanced the ability to accurately monitor patients in the perioperative period, in the intensive care unit or on the ward. An in-depth discussion of physiology, ventilators, and the vast array of critical care management options is well beyond the scope of this book. However, the essentials are included to generally enable management of the perioperative patient and to provide specific evidence-based information for limiting unexplained practice variance. Much of the material in this chapter is considered axiomatic. Evidence-based levels, especially in those areas supported by Level I data sets, are noted for clinical decision-making subject matter.

Care of the complicated patient with underlying cardiopulmonary dysfunction should optimally include critical care/intensivist consultation. Available data suggest team-based, protocol-driven, full-time intensivist coordinated critical care unit outcomes are superior, from both medical and economic perspectives.[1,2] If a full-time appropriately trained intensivist is not available, surgeons may be required to care for their own critically ill postoperative patients, at least initially. This of course also depends on appropriate training and skill base of the surgeon and other consultants.

PHYSIOLOGY OF OXYGEN DELIVERY AND CARBON DIOXIDE ELIMINATION

Oxygen transport to the cells depends on circulating blood oxygen content, arterial oxygen delivery, and uptake at the cellular level. The basic oxygen deliv-

Perioperative and Supportive Care in Gynecologic Oncology: Evidence-Based Management,
Edited by Steven A. Vasilev.
ISBN 0-471-24788-X   Copyright © 2000 by Wiley-Liss, Inc.

ery (D_{O_2}) equation and its variables help break this process down into components that are clinically useful for determining interventions. Oxygen delivery (D_{O_2}) to the peripheral tissues depends on two variables: cardiac output and total oxygen content in the blood. In turn, total oxygen content is made up of the dissolved plasma oxygen (minor) and oxygen bound to hemoglobin (major). Cardiac output is a product of heart rate (HR) and stroke volume (SV), and is indexed according to body surface area. Finally, the oxygen-carrying capacity constant represents 1.34 ml O_2 bound by each gram of hemoglobin. Some have advocated 1.39 as a constant, but this takes into account hemoglobin fractions that do not bind oxygen. In order to convert the units for oxygen delivery to ml/min/m^2, a factor of 10 may be used such that the constant becomes 13.4.

Oxygen Delivery Equation

$$O_2 \text{ delivery} = (O_2 \text{ content})(\text{cardiac output}/m^2)$$
$$O_2 \text{ delivery} = (HR \times SV/m^2)(Hb \times O_2 \text{ saturation} \times 1.34) + (0.0031 \times pO_2)$$

Since plasma-dissolved oxygen represents a minor part of total oxygen content if pO_2 is less than 100mmHg and hemoglobin exceeds 7 g/dl, the equation can be simplified to

$$O_2 \text{ delivery} = (HR \times SV/m^2)(Hb \times O_2 \text{ saturation} \times 1.34)$$

Thus, there are seven variables that derive from the above relationships and influence tissue perfusion and D_{O_2}: (1) hemoglobin, (2) hemoglobin saturation, (3) oxygen-carrying capacity, (4) heart rate, (5) preload or intravascular volume status, (6) myocardial contractility, and (7) afterload. Each factor may be manipulated in preventing or treating shock states, which at their root are disorders of tissue oxygenation.

Oxygen uptake (V_{O_2}) by tissues is a function of the difference between arterial and venous blood oxygen content. Abnormally low levels may be the single best indicator that a shock state is present.

$$V_{O_2} = (\text{cardiac index}) \times (C_{aO_2} - C_{VO_2})$$

Finally, the oxygen extraction ratio (O_2ER) describes the amount of oxygen delivered to the peripheral microvasculature, which is actually taken up by the tissue, otherwise expressed as

$$O_2ER = V_{O_2}/D_{O_2}$$

O_2ER varies as a function of oxygen delivery. Under normal resting conditions, only a small portion (20–30%) of the oxygen delivered to the periphery is taken up. This represents a very large reserve. Under increased stress requirements (e.g., exercise) or decreased oxygen delivery, extraction can increase to 60% to 80%. Ideally this homeostatic mechanism is designed to maintain constant oxygen uptake under variable oxygen delivery conditions. However, at a critical point, denoted the "critical D_{O_2}," cellular metabolism becomes oxygen supply dependent. Such supply dependence usually requires a strategy aimed at improving the delivery of oxygen (D_{O_2}) by influencing the variables already noted.[3,4]

Carbon Dioxide Transport and Elimination

Carbon dioxide (CO_2) represents the oxidative metabolic end product of cellular respiration.[5] CO_2 readily dissolves into all fluid compartments in total body water. Its transport and elimination is far more complex than oxygen due to various transport and buffering reactions.

Initially CO_2 is hydrated and forms carbonic acid (H_2CO_3), with only a small fraction remaining in dissolved CO_2 form. This reaction occurs preferentially in the erythrocyte, where the enzyme carbonic anhydrase, which is absent in plasma, accelerates the hydration process. This results in a CO_2 gradient into the red cell. Once in the red cell, additional dissociation and buffering reactions take place that essentially create a "sink" for CO_2 within the erythrocyte. Caution should be exercised when administering acetozolamide diuretics (carbonic acid inhibitors), especially in patients with pulmonary disease and CO_2 retention. Marked and rapid pH decrease can occur.

Total circulating hemoglobin mass is far in excess of that required to transport oxygen. Instead, the hemoglobin pool is largely required to buffer and transport the acid ion equivalents of CO_2.[6] Via the *Haldane effect*, which represents the greater buffering capacity of desaturated hemoglobin, venous blood has a higher CO_2 content than arterial blood. The CO_2 equivalents are then carried to and reconstituted in the lung capillaries. Addition of O_2 to hemoglobin in lung capillaries increases CO_2 release and it is eliminated.

Elimination of volatile acid, which is equivalent to CO_2 metabolic production in steady state, is measured directly and expressed as V_{CO_2} = Cardiac Index × ($CvCO_2$ – $CaCO_2$). The latter portion of the equation represents the difference between venous and arterial CO_2 content. At an average of 15,000 mEq/24 hours, the lung is the primary organ excreting volatile acid. As a comparison benchmark, the kidneys excrete an average of only 70 mEq of acid per day.[6]

The first part of the V_{CO_2} equation denotes that CI has a major role in CO_2 clearance and acid base homeostasis. In the presence of pathologically high cellular metabolism and decreased CI, the decrease in pH can be 0.30 or more—that is, arterial venous pH difference rises rapidly as CI falls.

Minute ventilation (V_E) is the product of inspired tidal volume (V_T) and respiratory rate. In turn, part of the inspired V_T is lost to dead space (V_D). The following equation represents the relationship between V_E and $PaCO_2$:

TABLE 6.1. Body Surface Area Indexed Normal Values for Oxygen and Carbon Dioxide Transport

Oxygen delivery (D_{O_2})	520–720 ml/min/m^2
Oxygen uptake (V_{O_2})	120–160 ml/min/m^2
Oxygen extraction (O_2ER)	20–30%
Carbon dioxide elimination (V_{CO_2})	100–140 ml/min/m^2
Respiratory quotient (RQ)	0.80

$$PaCO_2 = 0.863 \ [V_{CO_2}/V_E(1 - V_D/V_T)]$$

The V_{CO_2} in the numerator underscores the fact that $PaCO_2$ is determined not by the minute ventilation alone but by the relationship between metabolic rate and ventilation.[7] The equation also states that not all breathed air (V_E) is available for CO_2 exchange, only that fraction that remains after allowing for dead space (V_D/V_T).

Respiratory Quotient

The relationship between oxygen uptake (VO_2) and carbon dioxide elimination (V_{CO_2}) is known as the respiratory quotient (RQ), the value of which depends on which type of fuel (carbohydrate/protein/lipid) is primarily being metabolized. On average, RQ = 0.8, meaning CO_2 is being eliminated at a rate (volume/time) of 80% of oxygen uptake. Stated another way, 0.8 ml of CO_2 is released from the pulmonary capillaries for every 1.0 ml of O_2 taken up. Under normal circumstances in the healthy adult, this relationship does not carry a major clinical significance. However, in the postoperative or critically ill patient, especially if ventilator dependent, the CO_2 load and pulmonary capacity to clear it may be significantly influenced by hypermetabolism and/or "overfeeding." This may in turn require ventilator adjustments and explains why seemingly appropriate minute ventilation settings (rate or V_T) are not adequate to clear CO_2. Body surface area indexed normal values for oxygen and carbon dioxide transport are summarized in Table 6.1.

ARTERIAL BLOOD GAS SAMPLING

Blood gas sampling for oxygenation assessment is often performed 30 minutes after any change in FIO$_2$ is made. However, if the clinical situation requires more rapid analysis, 90% equilibration occurs within 6 minutes.[8,9]

Blood gas samples should be immediately placed on ice in order to minimize in vitro oxygen consumption by neutrophils. Even though the measurements are subsequently undertaken at a rewarmed 37°C, the laboratory will report temperature corrected values if the patient's temperature is provided.[10]

In clinical practice, interpretation of blood gas analysis should occur within the context of changes in patient condition. Arterial pO$_2$ can vary by as much as

36 mmHg and pCO$_2$ by 12 mmHg without any change in patient condition.[11,12] Routine monitoring of gases in a stable patient is costly, may be morbid and misleading, and may lead to unnecessary and costly further diagnostic and therapeutic interventions where none were indicated. Acid base disorders are addressed in Chapter 7.

HYPOXEMIA AND HYPERCARBIA

A ventilation-to-perfusion (VQ) ratio equal to 1.0 at the alveolar capillary unit represents a benchmark perfect match in gas exchange. When VQ < 1, an intra-pulmonary shunt to ventilated nonperfused alveoli exists, usually representing a venous admixture rather than a true anatomic shunt in the perioperative gyne-cologic patient. In normal patients, up to 10% of the cardiac output (Qt) is shunted (Qs). Therefore, normal Qs/Qt < 0.10.

When VQ > 1, dead-space ventilation is increased, represented by perfused but nonventilated alveoli. In normal patients, up to 30% of total ventilation at the upper airway entry (Vt) is used for dead-space ventilation (Vd). Therefore, normal Vd/Vt = 0.3. Table 6.2 represents some common etiologies and conse-quences for these conditions.

The above discussion regarding the ventilation-perfusion relationship carries clinical importance for interpreting arterial blood gases and adjusting inspired oxygen (FIO$_2$) or minute ventilation in the presence of hypoxemia or hyper-capnia. In the presence of an increasing but low shunt fraction (Qs/Qt = 10–50%), increasing FIO$_2$ will decrementally improve PaO$_2$. However, once Qs/Qt exceeds 50%, increasing FIO$_2$ above "nontoxic" levels of 50% will no longer improve PaO$_2$. Other methods for improving PaO$_2$ have to be sought, such as increasing positive end-expiratory pressure (PEEP), discussed later. For-tunately, shunt fraction has to exceed 50% to 60% before it has a clinical impact on CO$_2$ clearance as measured by increasing PaCO$_2$.

Clinical determination of dead space and shunt fraction is possible using the following relationships:

TABLE 6.2. Ventilation-Perfusion Mis-match

VQ > 1	VQ < 1
PaO$_2$ decreased	PaO$_2$ decreased
PaCO$_2$ increased	PaCO$_2$ decreased or normal
Pulmonary embolism	Atelectasis
Cardiac failure	Pulmonary edema
Extracorporeal tubing excessive	Pneumonia/pneumonitis
Excessive positive end-expiratory pressure (PEEP)	Asthma/bronchitis

$$Vd/Vt = P_{arterial}CO_2 - P_{expired}CO_2/P_{arterial}CO_2$$

$$Qs/Qt = \frac{\text{Pulmonary capillary } O_2 - \text{arterial } O_2}{\text{Pulmonary capillary } O_2 - \text{mixed venous } O_2}$$

Expired CO_2 can be measured at the airway via infrared analyzer equipment and the shunt estimate should be calculated at an FIO_2 of 100%, with an assumption set that pulmonary capillary O_2 = 100%.

Ventilation perfusion mismatches can be assessed clinically by calculation of the alveolar-arterial pO_2 gradient:

$$P_{alveolar}O_2 = P_{inspired}O_2 - (P_{arterial}CO_2/RQ)$$

Given that $P_{inspired}O_2 = FIO_2 (P_{barometric} - P_{H2O})$. At humidified room air, on average, the equation simplifies to:

$$P_{alveolar}O_2 = 0.21(760mmHg - 47mmHg) - (40mmHg/0.8)$$
$$= 100mmHg$$

In a healthy patient, with an arterial pO_2 = 90 mmHg, the A-a gradient would be 10 mmHg. However, with increasing age and increasing FIO_2, the A-a gradient increases. At room air, average A-a gradient rises from 15 mmHg at age 40 to 30 mmHg by age 70. Additionally, a normal A-a gradient rises an average 6 mmHg for every 10% increase in FIO_2. Lastly, if a patient is ventilator dependent, the mean airway pressure (MAP) should ideally be added to the ambient barometric pressure, resulting in an additional small calculated adjustment in A-a gradient.

CARDIOVASCULAR MONITORING

Manometer

Normal blood pressure ranges were established using noninvasive data with cuff manometry. Essentially, the five phases of Korotkoff's sounds are formed by the passage of a jetstream of blood in a variably compressed artery as the cuff pressure is released. With the caveats described below, the systolic pressure may be more accurately determined than the diastolic pressure. For rapid patient assessment, a value that correlates well with the mean arterial pressure is just below the point of maximal oscillation of the gauge. In general, the pitfalls in reliability of this commonly used test are due to extremes of patient body habitus and hemodynamic instability.

In the presence of larger extremities, regular blood pressure cuffs will have pressure dissipated by the soft tissue, decreasing the accuracy, usually leading to falsely elevated values. In thin patients, the value may be falsely low. Using the right size of seven standard cuffs minimizes errors.[13–15] Size guidelines dictate that 40% of the circumference and 60% of the length of an extremity be covered. Bedside evaluation of cuff size is simple, requiring only that the cuff bladder encircle at least half the circumference of the upper arm. Small cuffs on large limbs produce the vast majority of clinically significant errors when compared to use of large cuffs on small limbs. In very large individuals, blood pressure should be measured in the thigh or the forearm.

Since Korotkoff's sounds are produced by ausculatation of blood flow, low-flow states due to hemodynamic compromise such as shock will lead to error as the sounds become faint. Systolic pressures may be markedly underestimated.[16]

Significant variability between auscultatory and direct invasive measurements is documented. Accuracy, as defined by 5 mmHg variability between direct and indirect measures, is poor. Up to 70% of hypotensive patients have a systolic blood pressure variance of more than 20 mmHg between direct and cuff measurements.[16,17] Plethysmographic methods such as the Dinamap are somewhat more reliable. However, in the hypotensive patient, the overall accuracy compared to direct measurement is still limited.

In short, the following recommendations apply. In the relatively normotensive/normovolemic perioperative patient, not at the extremes of body habitus, noninvasive cuff techniques may be used. Readings should be taken with the arm at heart level in order to limit intra-arterial blood collumn effect. In the hypoperfused critically ill patient, invasive direct measurement is much more accurate and reproducible, and should be used.

Arterial Line Pressure

Direct measurement of arterial pressure has its own limitations. As the pulse pressure waveform moves outward from the heart, the systolic pressure tends to increase. This increase from the heart to the extremity arteries can range from 10 to 20 mmHg.[18]

Pitfalls in measurement are based on the differential speed of travel from center to periphery of the pressure wave and flow wave. The pressure wave at the periphery can precede the flow wave of the delivered stroke volume by several seconds.[19] Additionally, the pressure wave is accompanied by systolic pressure increases as it moves toward peripheral circulation, due to reflection of distal pressure waves. As the circulation becomes inelastic and noncompliant in the elderly, the systolic pressure wave is further amplified. These mechanisms make the peripheral systolic pressure a poor indicator of actual stroke volume flow to the periphery.

Equipment-related artifact can distort the already inaccurate pressure waveform via several mechanisms. First, the fluid-filled transducer system can resonate spontaneously and the resulting oscillations can distort waveforms. This may be the result of a system that is excessively stiff in comparison to the patient's vascular compliance. Second, air or clot in the system can result in overdamping of the signal, which can be reduced by flushing the system thoroughly. Usually systems will tend to be underdamped, producing systolic pressure amplification. Next to a well-matched system, an underdamped system is preferred, since it can be damped as needed by insertion of circuit intermediaries. Finally, if the catheter moves within the vascular lumen, "catheter whip" will result, distorting the waveform.[19] This situation usually occurs more often in arteries larger than the commonly used radial artery. At the bedside, over- or underdamped systems may not be easily recognized, and hence the inaccuracy of systolic pressure measurement.

The "flush" or "snap" test can be performed at the bedside and can help assess system match to the patient's vasculature.[20] It is performed by flushing or rapidly opening the flow control valve in the system, allowing an abrupt square wave of high-pressure saline into the system. If a normal tracing returns immediately, the system is well matched. If it is hyporesonant, the system is overdamped or excessively compliant. If there is an overshoot, the system is hyperresonant or excessively stiff.

Mean arterial pressure (MAP), directly measured by computer from the monitor, is a more accurate reflection of central pressures and stroke volume flow to the periphery than systolic pressure. The systolic pressure increase toward the periphery is offset by a narrowing of the waveform, making the mean arterial pressure constant.[21] It is also not distorted by the mechanisms already noted. *Calculated* MAP is less accurate than *direct* measurement because the calculation (MAP = diastolic pressure + 1/3 pulse pressure) is based on a normal heart rate during which diastole represents two-thirds of the cardiac cycle. Since tachycardia is common in the postoperative patient, the calculation becomes incrementally inaccurate with heart rates above 60 per minute.

Central Venous Pressure

In general, central venous/right atrial (CVP = RAP) or filling pressure measurements are only accurate and useful when it is certain that any cardiovascular abnormalities are confined to the right heart circulation. In a healthy younger postoperative patient, these measurements may be adequate to assess preload and fluid status. However, in the compromised or elderly patient, right heart function and information gained from measuring right atrial pressure is a poor predictor of left heart function. Thus, the true hemodynamic state and contributory factors may not be accurately reflected.

Optimal measurements of right atrial pressure require the following: (1) A transducer with oscilloscope readout is used, not a manometer or digital readout, which are less accurate.[22] (2) Measurements are taken at end-expiration. (3) Measurements are taken supine and zeroed at the midaxillary line.[23] Normal variation is considered to be ±4 mmHg. More importantly, a single reading is far less significant than progressive changes, which mirror clinical status changes.

If the patient is ventilator dependent, the practice of taking the patient off the vent to get an accurate reading does not accurately reflect the true pressure dynamics the patient faces. Additionally, withdrawing a patient from PEEP for even a short period (e.g., 1 minute) may reverse any alveolar recruitment that had been obtained.[24] This practice may lead to inappropriate decisions, although it may be the only method by which to obtain an interpretable reading. If the patient is removed from the ventilator, it should be for the shortest possible period. If measured on the ventilator, the PEEP level should be subtracted from the measured end-expiratory right atrial pressure.[25,26]

Since the majority of complications associated with central venous pressure (CVP) measurement are associated with central venous puncture and placement of the percutaneous introducer itself, assessment of risk/benefit may lead to the conclusion that a pulmonary artery catheter is the better choice in patients who are severely compromised.

Pulmonary Artery Catheter

The flow-directed Swan–Ganz catheter, introduced in the mid-1970s, is largely responsible for the field of critical care, even though users have occasionally been labeled as a "cult."[27] The pulmonary artery catheter is not a therapy or a panacea, and potential for overuse has been passionately described.[28] Used judiciously, it is a good monitoring device, providing a number of useful parameters that can be either directly measured or easily derived. Although numerous features have been added over the years, most of the required data for perioperative management can be obtained from the basic dual-lumen thermodilution catheter. Clinically, several key perioperative pathophysiologic states can be differentiated by interpreting a profile of data, manually or with computer assistance.[29]

Unfortunately, several studies have documented the variability and prevalent deficiencies in physician understanding regarding proper use and interpretation of pulmonary artery catheter–derived data.[30,31] In most cases, trained intensivist consultation should be considered for optimal care. The basic information presented herein is intended to familiarize the gynecologic surgeon with the basics, such that profile interpretation by an intensivist can take potentially modifying surgical and oncologic disease factors into consideration. Additionally, the first hours of critical care may rest completely with the surgeon if consultants are not immediately available.

Some general indications for perioperative pulmonary arterial catheters are listed in Table 6.3. The original basic pulmonary catheter is double

TABLE 6.3. General Indications for Pulmonary Arterial Catheters

Any severe cardiopulmonary derangement: complicated MI, cardiogenic shock
Hypovolemia not responsive to volume administration
Systemic inflammatory response syndrome (SIRS)/sepsis
Cardiogenic/fluid overload, pulmonary edema vs. noncardiogenic (ARDS)
Prolonged surgical procedures with cardiopulmonary compromise
Coexistent pulmonary and renal organ system dysfunction
Multiple-organ dysfunction syndrome (MODS)

lumen for purposes of pressure monitoring and distal balloon inflation only. Catheters with additional features have been developed. The most common is a quadruple-lumen 5–7 Fr pulmonary artery catheter that allows measurement of both right atrial and pulmonary artery pressures, and assesses cardiac output via thermodilution/thermistor, while allowing concurrent drug infusion. Care should be taken in infusing vasocative or inotropic agents via proximal ports while cold injectate boluses are being administered via the same port for thermodilution cardiac output determination. Inadvertent vasoactive/inotropic boluses can result in patient destabilization. The most commonly used central hemodynamic measures can be stratified into *directly measured* and *derived* parameters, summarized in Table 6.4 along with normal ranges.

Complications of pulmonary artery catheter use include those found with CVP monitoring, specifically central venous catheterization and cordis placement. Less common complications include valvular damage, intracardiac knotting, pulmonary infarction, pulmonary artery perforation, and arrhythmias.[25] Right bundle branch block can complicate insertion, usually with transient and benign outcomes. However, in the presence of a preexisting left bundle branch block, complete heart block can result. These complications can be minimized by correcting electrolyte disturbances, limiting long-term use of the catheter, close observation for distal tip migration and permanent wedge pattern, and smooth, rapid introduction with the balloon inflated. The latter minimizes knotting and arrhythmias due to smooth passage and less myocardial irritation. The appearance of hemoptysis is an ominous finding, possibly signaling cardiovascular collapse due to pulmonary artery perforation. Emergency thoracotomy and lobectomy or pneumonectomy can salvage some patients.

Hemodynamic Profiles of Pathophysiologic States

The measured and derived parameters previously noted can be organized into distinct hemodynamic profiles as noted in Table 6.5.

Mean arterial pressure (MAP) <60 mmHg is reflective of a shock state and is a function of (1) preload or effective circulating blood volume filling pressure, reflected by the right atrial pressure (RAP), (2) myocardial function/contractility as evidenced by adequate SV and CI, and (3) systemic vascular resistance index (SVRI). In other words, is there adequate intravascular space volume, is it being pumped effectively, and against how much resistance?

Hypotension and shock classically are grouped by hypovolemic, cardiogenic, obstructive, and distributive or septic etiologies. *Hypovolemia*, whether by dehydration or hemorrhage mechanism, results in low filling pressures, and thus low stroke volume. In an attempt to maintain adequate MAP, the peripheral vasculature constricts as reflected by an elevated SVRI. Much of the cardiac output is supported by an increased heart rate instead of adequate stroke volume.

Once the V_{O_2} decreases, a hypovolemic, hypotensive state becomes a shock state, reflecting poor tissue oxygenation at the cellular level. At this point, oxy-

TABLE 6.4. Hemodynamic Measures and Normal Ranges

Directly Measured Parameters	Normal Ranges
Pressure Related	
Central venous = right atrial pressure (CVP = RAP)	2–10 cm H_2O
Pulmonary artery occlusion pressure (PAOP)	5–12 mmHg
Mean pulmonary artery pressure (MPAP)	11–15 mmHg
Diastolic pulmonary artery pressure	5–15 mmHg
Systolic pulmonary artery pressure	15–25 mmHg
Flow Related	
Cardiac index (CI)	2.8–4.2 ml/min/m$_2$

N.B. Normal RAP and PAOP variation is ± 4 mmHg
N.B. RAP (cm H_2O)/1.36 = RAP (mmHg)

Derived Parameters	Normal Ranges
Resistance	
Systemic vascular resistance index (SVRI)	80 (MAP − CVP)/CI = 1700–2600 dynes.sec.m^2/cm^5
Pulmonary vascular resistance index (PVRI)	80 (MPAP − PAOP)/CI = 150–300 dynes.sec.m^2/cm^5
Flow Related	
Stroke volume index (SVI)	CI/HR = 30–50 ml/beat/m^2
Left ventricular stroke work index (LVSWI)	SVI (MAP − PAOP) 0.014 = 44–68 g.m/m^2
Right ventricular stroke work index (RVSWI)	SVI (MPAP − CVP) 0.014 = 7–12 g.m/m^2
Tissue Oxygenation	
Mixed venous oxygen saturation (SVO2)	70–75%
Oxygen delivery (D_{O_2})	CaO2 × CI × 10 = 520–720 ml/min/m^2
Oxygen uptake (V_{O_2})	C(a − v)O2 × CI × 10 = 120–160 ml/min/m^2
Oxygen extraction (O2ER)	(CaO2 − CvO2)/CaO2 = V_{O_2}/D_{O_2} = 20–30%

TABLE 6.5. Hemodynamic Profiles

Profile	RAP	PAOP	CI	SVRI	PVRI	VO2
Right heart failure	high		low		high	normal
Left heart failure		high	low	high		normal
Hypovolemia	low	low	low	high		normal
Hypovolemic shock	low	low	low	high		low
Cardiogenic shock	high	high	low	high		low
Obstructive shock	low/normal	low/normal	low	high		low
Septic shock	normal/high	normal/high/low	high	normal/low/high		low
Cardiogenic pulmonary edema	high	high	low	high		
Capillary leak pulmonary edema (ARDS)	normal/high	normal	high	low		

gen delivery is exhausted, the critical DO_2 is exceeded, and oxygen delivery becomes supply dependent. Low VO_2 is present in all shock states, regardless of underlying etiology.

Cardiogenic shock, in the postoperative setting, usually is a result of a massive myocardial infarction. Most often, a left ventricular infarct comprising over 40% of the myocardium is involved.[32,33] A secondary life-threatening problem is development of lethal arrhythmias. Severe systolic cardiac performance depression occurs as reflected by a low cardiac index in the presence of high filling pressures (RAP and PAOP [pulmonary artery occlusion pressure]). Severe myocardial depression can also occur during sepsis, due to a circulating myocardial depressant factor, which creates a similar hemodynamic profile in the latter phases.[34]

Extracardiac obstructive shock in the postoperative pelvic surgery patient should always raise the suspicion of massive pulmonary embolism and resulting acute cor pulmonale. Commonly referred to as a *saddle* embolus, this life-threatening condition reflects more than 60% blockage of the pulmonary vasculature. Pericardial tamponade is the other form of obstructive shock, also usually diagnosed late in a crisis stage. Common signs are pulsus paradoxus and the presence of an electrocardiographic rhythm with no discernible pulse. Etiologies may include pericardial infectious effusion, malignant effusion, hemopericardium due to ventricular rupture, or excessive anticoagulation. Finally, tension pneumothorax may occur, for example, due to high intraoperative inspiratory pressures generated during laparoscopy while in steep Trendelenburg position. Clinical findings include absent or severely reduced breath sounds on one side of the chest.

The most complex shock state is that due to *systemic sepsis*. First and foremost, it may be insidious in onset and is often not recognized early at the most treatable phase. The hemodynamic profile changes through several discernible yet overlapping phases, reflecting a progressive systemic inflammatory response syndrome (SIRS). Initially, a hypovolemic state exists due to fluid transudation outward across capillary beds or due to venous pooling, both of which reduce effective preload/filling pressures. Myocardial contractility and stroke volume are progressively compromised by circulating depressant factors. Thus, the "hyperdynamic" state often described in sepsis is really an elevated CI supported by an increased heart rate, rather than an increased SVI. Initial peripheral vasodilatation may occur in the "warm shock" phase as reflected by a low/normal SVRI. An incrementally hypodynamic vasoconstricted phase then ensues in the "cold shock" phase. While the "warm" and "cold" shock phases are classic teaching descriptors, there is substantial overlap and variability in physiologic response and clinical presentation.

Evaluation of both *right and left heart function and failure* centers on key relationships between (1) filling pressures as reflected by the RAP and PAOP, (2) contractility as reflected by the SVI and CI, and (3) right and left outflow vascular bed resistance as reflected by the PVRI (pulmonary vascular resistance index) and SVRI, respectively.

Cardiogenic pulmonary edema is one of the end results of cardiogenic shock or left heart failure, thus sharing some profile similarities. Essentially, left heart dysfunction or fluid overload is reflected by a high PAOP and low CI.

Capillary leak pulmonary edema or *adult respiratory distress syndrome* (*ARDS*) is an end result of a systemic inflammatory response syndrome, whether due to systemic sepsis or other causes. As in other organs, capillaries become "leaky" and exudative debris fills alveolar spaces, usually in the presence of a normal PAOP. Computerized tomography (CT) studies demonstrate that lung injury occurs in stages and is usually diffuse but not uniform, as it is in cardiogenic pulmonary edema.[35–37] The hemodynamic profile usually reflects septic shock in one of its phases. Further discussion of ARDS and pulmonary edema can be found in Chapter 5.

NONINVASIVE CARDIOVASCULAR MONITORING

Noninvasive Cardiac Output

In rare postoperative settings, central venous catheterization or placement of a pulmonary artery catheter may be precluded or ill advised. For example, introducing a Swan–Ganz catheter in the presence of left bundle branch block can be hazardous as complete heart block can result. Noninvasive techniques for hemodynamic assessment are available and are based on (1) ultrasound/Doppler, (2) bioimpedance, and (3) indicator dye dilution, measured peripherally.[38–41] These techniques require specialized equipment, and accuracy may vary considerably based on technical skill requirements. An initial evaluation with such techniques may be suitable when central venous access and invasive monitoring are precluded. This may be appropriate to facilitate the initial decision making. Up to 85% of intensive care unit (ICU) patients can be accurately monitored on a continuous noninvasive basis. Cost analysis is situation specific.[41]

Echocardiography

In the perioperative and critical care setting, emergency transthoracic echocardiography can help diagnose suspected cardiac tamponade. Hemodynamic measures and clinical findings may resemble cardiogenic shock due to a massive myocardial infarction. Indeed, the two may coexist. However, unlike the high cardiogenic shock mortality rate that derives from ventricular failure or arrhythmias, pericardiocentesis can be immediately lifesaving in obstructive shock.

Pulse Oximetry

Clinical pulse oximetry is based on the spectrophotometric differences between oxyhemoglobin and reduced hemoglobin. Light diodes emit infrared (940 nm) and red (660 nm) wavelengths, which are transmitted through pulsatile arterioles at the fingertip. The device is designed such that only the pulsatile flow signal is recognized. The ratio of absorbance at these two wavelengths is calibrated against direct blood gas analysis of oxygen saturation in normal volunteers. Accuracy and precision of pulse oximeter saturation (SpO_2) is better than 97% when directly measured saturation (SaO_2) is greater than 75%.[11,42,43] Inaccuracies may also result when Hb is less than 3 g/dl, meth-hemoglobin or carboxyhemoglobin is present, or blood pressure drops below 30 mmHg.[44–46] The greatest reliability and safety is in steady-state conditions, where this technology safely and cost-effectively replaces routine invasive blood gas sampling. Target values of 92% (light skin) to 95% (dark skin) reflect adequate oxygenation.[42,47,48] Dark nail polish may lead to inaccurate readings.[49] Values in the high 80s reflect seriously low oxygenation. In the presence of unstable oxygenation and/or poor peripheral perfusion, readings can be unpredictable or slow to reflect acute changes.[44,45,50–52]

Capnometry

End-expiratory or end-tidal CO_2 ($P_{ET}CO_2$) is quantitatively measured via infrared transmission analysis at the expiratory end of ventilator tubing. The $P_{ET}CO_2$ and arterial $PaCO_2$ are almost equivalent under steady-state normal conditions, but a gradient can be as high as 5 mmHg ($PaCO_2 > P_{ET}CO_2$) in healthy subjects. If pulmonary gas exchange is compromised, the

$P_{ET}CO_2$ decreases faster, increasing the gradient. Rarely the gradient can be reversed with $P_{ET}CO_2 > PaCO_2$, and is usually associated with excessive CO_2 production.[53] However, under steady-state conditions, the $P_{ET}CO_2$ reliably mirrors $PaCO_2$ changes. In the presence of cardiopulmonary compromise, an initial correlating blood gas can help set the baseline gradient. Reliability may be compromised by conditions that alter the normal capnograph, which has a recognizable end expiratory plateau. Such conditions include airway obstruction, partial endotracheal tube (ETT) obstruction, malfunctioning ventilator circuit, or increased dead space.[54]

A primary clinical application for infrared capnometry is monitoring for ventilator–patient interface problems during mechanical ventilation and during weaning. A decrease in $P_{ET}CO_2$ may signify disconnection from the ventilator or migration of the ETT into the right main stem.[55,56] A rising $P_{ET}CO_2$ may reflect increased work of breathing or increased CO_2 production due to overfeeding as causes of difficult weaning.[56]

INITIAL MANAGEMENT OF PERIOPERATIVE SHOCK STATES

Although the etiology of shock states differs, a common thread exists at the cellular level for initial recognition and management of perioperative shock. Often there is a clinically mixed picture (Fig. 6.1), and evolution to death can occur

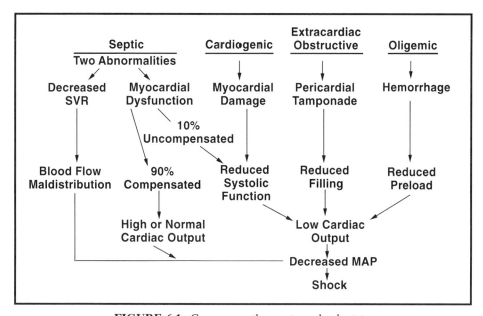

FIGURE 6.1. Common pathways to a shock state.

TABLE 6.6. Initial Therapy of Shock States

Think *rapid* initiation of therapy while determining etiology
Large-bore intravenous line or two and diagnostic blood tests
Fluid resuscitation based on history/findings: crystalloid, blood products
Pressors and inotropes as needed *after* fluid resuscitation
Arterial and central invasive monitoring
Bedside echocardiogram if cardiogenic or obstructive shock suspected: possible
    effusion, possible left ventricular dysfunction

within minutes, requiring diagnostic and therapeutic efforts to be simultaneous. Once a clear etiology is established, additional specific treatment modifications may apply. For example, extracardiac obstructive shock due to tamponade will initially respond to volume resuscitation, although pericardiocentesis will be required to complete effective treatment. Initial therapy should be based on the best rapid assessment of etiology for the given circumstance and can be modified at any point (Table 6.6). The key is to avoid irreversibility due to treatment delays.

At the cellular level, the common finding in shock states is impaired tissue perfusion and oxygenation. When oxygen uptake or consumption lags behind metabolic oxygen requirements, a shock state exists and is reflected by increasing serum lactate levels due to incomplete mitochondrial glucose oxidation and anaerobic metabolism.

As already noted, oxygen uptake (V_{O_2}) by tissues is reflected by the difference between arterial and venous blood oxygen content and, when low, is an excellent indicator that a shock state is present. Optimization of oxygen delivery and uptake by tissues is accomplished by manipulating the variables in the D_{O_2} and V_{O_2} equations, three of which are common to both (hemoglobin, arterial oxygen saturation, and cardiac output/index). The only difference between the D_{O_2} and V_{O_2} equations is that the oxygen content in the venous circulation, reflecting tissue oxygen consumption, is considered in the latter but not the former. Although this mathematical coupling leads to certain imprecision in oxygen transport monitoring, the point here is that clinical manipulation of these variables is required to improve both D_{O_2} and V_{O_2}. Additionally, when the V_{O_2} is measured directly rather than calculated, the mathematical coupling problem is minimized.[57,58]

$$D_{O_2} = (\text{cardiac index}) \times (\text{Hb} \times SaO_2 \times 13.4) \text{ in ml/min/m}^2$$

$$V_{O_2} = (\text{cardiac index}) \times (\text{Hb}) \times (SaO_2 - SvO_2) \times 13.4 \text{ in ml/min/m}^2$$

Homeostatic mechanisms allow tissue oxygen uptake to remain constant through a wide range of oxygen delivery under normal circumstances, reflected by an oxygen extraction ratio (O_2ER) adjustment. Normally O_2ER ranges between 20% and 30%, indicating a significant reserve. The threshold O_2ER appears to be approximately 50%, meaning 50% of oxygen delivered is consumed by tissues. After this point, VO_2 becomes supply dependent if DO_2 drops further. Any maneuver that improves DO_2 leads to improvements in VO_2 and a reduced O_2ER, even in critically ill patients who have a so-called pathologic supply dependency, which may be only artifactual in nature.[58]

Clinical signs and symptoms of impending shock are imprecise and may be as subtle as a slight tachypnea and pallor. Vital signs may reveal hypotension and tachycardia. None of these signs or symptoms accurately reflect the degree of tissue oxygen uptake impairment. For example, in the presence of hypovolemia due to 25% loss of circulating blood volume, sympathetic stimulation may compensate with a rise in heart rate and slight drop in blood pressure. After an acute 40% loss, the sympathetic compensatory mechanisms are overwhelmed and tissue dysoxia results. It is difficult to determine exactly when a true shock state develops within the above range of symptoms and signs. To help determine this state, objective measures that define the onset of shock include (1) measured VO_2 < 100 ml/min/m2, (2) O_2ER > 50%, and (3) arterial lactate > 4 mmol/L. As oxygen delivery (DO_2) drops, in the presence of normal or increased metabolism, the oxygen extraction increases (O_2ER), causing the VO_2 to drop below normal, reflecting shock. As the oxygen required to support aerobic metabolism drops further, glucose is incompletely metabolized and the arterial lactate increases. As such, an arterial lactate threshold level of 4 mmol/L is highly predictive of nonsurvival.[59,60] It should be noted that an elevated lactate level can also be due to hepatic insufficiency, alkalosis, and enteric microbial overproduction.

Prevention or correction of VO_2 deficit is a generic strategy regardless of shock etiology. Knowledge of shock-state etiology at the earliest possible moment will dictate which steps supersede others as discussed below. In general, each component of the DO_2 equation should be optimized:

$$D_{O_2} = (\text{cardiac index}) \times (\text{Hb} \times SaO_2 \times 13.4) \text{ in ml/min/m}^2$$

Cardiac index is determined by stroke volume and heart rate. Components of the former are preload, afterload, and myocardial contractility. Stroke volume enhancement is more energy efficient than heart rate in improving cardiac index. Therefore, the first order of intervention is to optimize cardiac index by ensuring adequate filling pressures and stroke volume. Central monitoring of right atrial pressure or wedge pressure is required. If filling pressures are low, volume resuscitation is the first line of treatment. If filling pressures are high, yet the cardiac index is low, inotropic support is indicated. The inotrope selected depends on blood pressure determination. If hypotension is evident, dopamine is indicated because it has a dose-dependent peripheral alpha-mediated vasoconstricting effect (dose > 10 mcg/kg/min) as well as central beta (inotropic and chronotropic) effects. Caution is warranted in the presence of suspected cardiogenic shock. The dopamine alpha effect will increase afterload and may result in a dose-dependent *decrease* in cardiac output. If blood pressure is acceptable, dobutamine is a stronger inotrope, produces less afterload, is less arrythmogenic, and is the drug of choice. Second, anemia should be corrected if Hb is less than 7–8 g/dl, especially in the presence of a persistently high O_2ER (>50%) despite normovolemia.[61]

Assessment of blood lactate levels helps determine if the VO_2 is adequate for a given metabolic rate. In the presence of a normal measured VO_2 and elevated lactate, attention should be given to decreasing metabolic rate by reducing hyper- or hypothermia (shivering), agitation, or feeding. Raising the VO_2 to "supranormal" may improve outcomes, but is very difficult to achieve and has not been substantiated as being effective by all investigators.[62–65]

Hypovolemic Shock

Hypovolemic etiology for shock is quite common in the perioperative setting and has been the best studied, with over 3,500 animal and human studies to date. Fortunately, it is the easiest shock state to treat with fluid resuscitation. The intravascular volume loss is usually either due to unrecognized or underestimated blood loss, prolonged emesis, or fluid third spacing. An acute 15% loss is usually well compensated via homeostatic mechanisms involving renin/angiotensin and increased sympathetic tone. With an acute 15% to 30% loss, signs and symptoms start to indicate decompensation as reflected by a decreased stroke volume, increased heart rate to support cardiac output, increased systemic vascular resistance to maintain pressure, and redistribution of blood flow to the brain and heart. Once an acute loss of 30% is realized, major hemodynamic changes and decreased urine output are evident. By the time an acute noncompensated loss of 40% is sustained, the ensuing shock state becomes potentially irreversible. To that end, rapid initiation of fluids is a major factor in survival. Multiple studies have documented lack of efficacy in attempting autotransfusion via Trendelenburg positioning.[66–68] MAST (military antishock trousers) suits have some efficacy in increasing systemic vascular resistance, but are also ineffective in increasing venous return.[69]

Vasopressors and inotropes are not usually part of initial therapy, since the first order of importance is fluid replenishment. However, in the presence of severe hypotension or depressed myocardial contractility, these agents may be required at the outset or if fluid resuscitation alone is inadequate. In these situations, they should be titrated down as soon as possible since they can give a false sense of security with "normalizing" blood pressure despite persistent hypovolemia. Tables 6.7 and 6.8 summarize the most common agents, their relative effects, indications, and dose ranges. Each clinical situation is different and may require combined agent support. Thus, this presentation represents a simplified overview for initial treatment selection.

TABLE 6.7. Common Inotropes and Vasopressors

Agent	Cardiac β_1	Vasodilate β_2	Vaso-constrict α	Dopa DA	Indication Shock: MAP < 60 mmHg; ±PCWP[a] > 15
Dopamine (low dose)	++	++	+	+++	May increase renal perfusion
Dopamine (>3–5 mcg)	++++	+	++++	0	Variable inotrope and pressor
Dobutamine	++++	++	0 to +	0	Stronger inotrope for decreased CO Inotrope > chronotrope Less $\alpha \rightarrow$ more CO; less afterload
Norepi	++	0	++++	0	Inotrope and pressor Dopamine failure in septic shock; add as second drug
Epi	++++	++	++++	0	Inotrope and pressor Norepi failure *Caution:* narrow safe therapeutic range
Phenylephrine	+ or –	0	++++	0	Pressor in presence of arrhythmias Mainly second agent with dopa/dobutamine
Isoproterenol	++++	+++++	0	0	Inotrope/chronotrope *Caution:* arrythmogenic as pure beta

[a]Pulmonary capillary wedge pressure.

+ = minimal effect

+++++ = major effect

TABLE 6.8. Common Hemodynamic Drug Dose Ranges

Agent	Usual Dose Range
Dopamine (renal)	1–3 mcg/kg/min
Dopamine (inotrope)	5–8 mcg/kg/min
Dopamine (pressor)	10–20 mcg/kg/min
Dobutamine	5–15 mcg/kg/min
Epinephrine	0.005–0.05 mcg/kg/min
Norepinephrine (Levophed)	2–8 mcg/min
Isoproterenol	1–4 mcg/min
Phenylephrine	0.04–0.08 mg/min

Initial infusion rates for most of the agents in Table 6.7 are calculated by the following formula and are convenient to express in microdrops/minute after adjustment for weight in kilograms:

$$\text{Infusion rate} = R/C \times 60$$

where R is the dose rate expressed in mcg/kg/minute and C is the drug concentration expressed in mcg/ml.

Extracardiac Obstructive Shock

Obstructive shock onset is rapid and the etiology is determined late, often during cardiopulmonary resuscitation in a crisis stage; the result is often fatal. Pericardial tamponade will initially respond to fluids but will require pericardiocentesis to effectively resuscitate a patient. Similarly, in the presence of a saddle pulmonary embolus, thrombolytics or embolectomy will be required. If tension pneumothorax is suspected, immediate angiocath decompression through the second intercostal space in the midclavicular line, followed by a chest tube thoracostomy, can be lifesaving.

Cardiogenic Shock

The most common cause of cardiogenic shock is massive left ventricular infarction, producing low-output hypervolemic symptoms, signs, and findings. Specific intervention depends on knowledge of the underlying cardiac pathology, which can be rapidly determined by bedside echocardiography and invasive monitoring.

Stroke volume reduction can occur due to abnormalities in (1) heart rate, (2) preload, (3) afterload, and (4) myocardial contractility. First, it is important to evaluate for abnormal rhythms, since ventricular dysrrhythmias occur often after infarction. While sinus tachycardia can develop as an appropriate physiologic response to shock states, ventricular arrhythmias can significantly alter stroke volume. Second, preload should be reduced with diuretics and venodilators (e.g., sodium nitroprusside [Nipride] or nitroglycerine). The resulting reduction of intracardiac pressure and coronary resistance also improves coronary blood flow, limiting ischemic spread. Third, carefully monitored afterload reduction will reduce the amount of work required to maintain cardiac output. Hypotension is a limiting factor and must be avoided. An intra-aortic balloon pump could be considered as a mechanical means of afterload reduction. Finally, inotropes may be required. However, due to the complexity of pump failure, special expertise with multiple-drug regimens is required to balance positive and negative effects of each agent.[70]

Septic Shock

If systemic sepsis is suspected, broad-spectrum antibiotics should be initiated and the source of infection sought. Today, gram-negative and gram-positive organisms are equally responsible for systemic sepsis.[71,72] Blood cultures may be negative 50% to 75% of the time and should not be the basis for treatment initiation decisions. False negative culture results are a function of the number and timing of cultures obtained with respect to episodic bacteremia.

Venous pooling or capillary leaks in the early stages produce a hypodynamic state and are responsive to aggressive fluid resuscitation.[73] Circulating myocardial depressant factor often reduces stroke volume such that cardiac output is supported by tachycardia. Thus, inotropic improvement in stroke volume should be a therapeutic goal once filling pressures are restored via fluid resuscitation.

The main disorder in septic shock is reduction in peripheral blood flow and increased peripheral resistance, leading to decreased D_{O_2} and V_{O_2}.[74] Care should be taken in selecting an inotropic agent and subsequent monitoring of peripheral and splanchnic circulation as the vasoconstrictive alpha effect may further worsen D_{O_2} and V_{O_2}.

Sepsis is a hypermetabolic state, thus increasing tissue oxygen requirements. In response, advocates have called for "supranormal" D_{O_2} stategies using dobutamine and volume resuscitation.[62,63,75,76] However, the data are conflicting in different patient subsets.[64,65] Such a strategy may still be worth considering in the presence of resuscitation failure, progressive organ dysfunction, and justification for heroic efforts (i.e., young patient with curable oncologic disease; Level I).[77]

Unfortunately, by the time it is clinically apparent, septic shock is often well along the inflammatory response cascade, is often not reversed by elimination of the initially offending infective vector, is resistant to hemodynamic interventions, and may progress to multiple-organ dysfunction syndrome (MODS).[64,65,71,77] The probability of this occurrence is related more to the host status than the virulence of an infective agent, which is reflected by mortality figures for septic shock; they were 40% in the early 1900s and remain in the 40% range, despite development of a myriad of antibiotics and hemodynamic support measures.[71,77] Although the acute hemodynamic instability may be better controlled today, the cause of patient mortality has shifted and is now due to ARDS and MODS.[71] In response, many agents have been investigated that counter known mediators of the inflammatory response cascade. Most research has focused on monoclonal antibody therapy directed toward endotoxins, interleukins, tumor necrosis factor, and various receptors.[77] Thus far, clinical trials have failed to produce improved outcomes using these modalities in systemic sepsis and septic shock (Level I).[78–81] However, the inflammatory response cascade is exceedingly complex, interaction between pathways is evident, and the inflammatory response to a certain extent may in fact be protective.[77] Thus, blockade of a single pathway in isolation (e.g., monoclonal antibody therapy)

TABLE 6.9. Inflammatory States

Term	Findings
SIRS	More than two signs of systemic inflammation, e.g., fever and leukocytosis
Sepsis	SIRS and infection
Severe sepsis	Sepsis and MODS
Septic shock	Severe sepsis and refractory hypotension

or of the entire inflammatory response (e.g., steroids) can be extremely counterproductive, worsening the course of shock (Level I to II-2).[82,83]

Systemic Inflammatory Response and Multiple-Organ Dysfunction

Systemic inflammatory response syndrome (SIRS) may be due to sepsis or other causes. It is important to note that inflammatory response per se does not mean a priori that an infection is present. However, when local host-protective mechanisms are overwhelmed, a common systemic inflammatory cascade ensues, representing progressive pan-endothelial disease, which leads to MODS and ARDS. Table 6.9 summarizes current nomenclature for these disorders.[84]

The most common organ failure due to runaway inflammatory response is ARDS. However, other organ systems commonly affected are the renal, cardiovascular, coagulation, and central nervous systems.[85] Mortality is related to the number of dysfunctional organ systems, exceeding 80% once four organ systems fail.[86]

PHYSIOLOGY OF VENTILATION AND OXYGENATION

During the immediate postsurgical period, patients often require respiratory, and in some cases ventilatory, support. This support ranges from simple intervention such as incentive spirometry and low-flow oxygen to prolonged mechanical ventilation. The degree of support required is influenced by factors such as age, incision site and length of procedure, body habitus, overall health, and the presence or absence of cardiopulmonary disease. Perioperative analgesics, which are central nervous system depressants, may further compromise spontaneous ventilation.

The dual insults of anesthetic inhalants and surgical visceral manipulation may have a deleterious effect on diaphragmatic function.[87-95] Whether this effect is caused by altered contractility of the diaphragm itself or by reflex disturbance of phrenic nerve output is unclear. Regardless of the root mechanism, the induction of anesthesia is followed by a cephalad shift of the diaphragm. The upward shift of the diaphragm produces decreases in vital capacity (VC), residual volume (RV), forced expiratory volume (FEV_1), and functional residual capacity (FRC).[87-90] This decrease in lung volumes may predispose the postoperative patient to complications such as atelectasis, blood gas abnormalities, and pneumonia. Atelectasis results in lung units that are perfused but not ventilated, producing arterial hypoxemia due to a right to left shunt. This type of hypoxemia is poorly responsive to supplemental oxygen administration since nonventilated alveoli are not available for partial pressure gradient–driven diffusion of O_2 across the alveolar capillary membrane.

Lung Volume Expansion

Hypoxemia caused by atelectasis and shunting responds well to volume expansion modalities such as deep breathing exercises (DBE), incentive spirometry (IS), and intermittent positive pressure breathing (IPPB). Although all three modalities appear to be equally effective in preventing or treating the complications arising from atelectasis, cost and safety considerations favor DBE or IS (Level I).[88] IPPB may be best reserved for those patients in whom active lung inflation is difficult or impossible due to altered neuromuscular physiology.

Changes in pulmonary function usually peak on the first postoperative day, with a return to 80% of normal within 3 days. However, complete resolution can take months. Smoking cessation begins to have positive effects with ciliary function improvement within 72 hours, sputum production decrease within 2 weeks, and improved pulmonary function testing within 4 weeks (Levels II-2 and I).[96,97] However, clinically significant reduction of postoperative pulmonary complications becomes statistically significant only at 8 weeks. Notwithstanding, whenever possible, patients should be advised to quit smoking and should be instructed in lung expansion exercises prior to surgery.

Oxygen Therapy

For patients who exhibit hypoxemia in spite of pulmonary volume expansion therapy, oxygen therapy is indicated. Although oxygen therapy is purely supportive and does not treat the underlying problem, it can prevent or reverse tissue hypoxia. The need for supplemental O_2 should be determined by either arterial blood gas analysis or pulse oximetry. These two measures should also be used to assess the effectiveness of the O_2 therapy once it is started. Once blood gas values and pulse oximeter readings have been obtained simultaneously, and have been found to correlate, pulse oximetry can be used to quickly and noninvasively follow the patient's oxygenation.

Oxygen therapy can cause complications such as ventilatory depression in patients with elevated $PaCO_2$, absorption atelectasis, and O_2 toxicity. In the gynecologic oncology patient, additional vigilance is necessary with a history of bleomycin exposure, as this can exacerbate O_2 toxicity.[98,99] Because of these potential complications, O_2 should be delivered at the lowest flow rate or concentration that will correct the arterial hypoxemia. As a patient's condition improves, O_2 flow rate/concentration should be reduced until weaning from oxygen is accomplished. Pulse oximetry is a valuable tool to aid in this weaning process.

Various devices are available to supply supplemental oxygen to patients.

They can be conveniently divided into two groups: low-flow systems and high-flow systems.

Low-Flow Systems As the name implies, low-flow systems deliver 100% O_2 to the patient at flow rates of 0.5–6.0 L/min. The remainder of ventilation is room air, which dilutes the oxygen delivered. Because the dilution ratio varies with such factors as tidal volume, minute ventilation, and breathing pattern, an exact FIO_2 is not possible using any of these devices.

Nasal Cannula This device is the most comfortable and versatile for administering supplemental O_2. Patients can eat, drink, and converse without interfering with the delivery of O_2. Flow rates of up to 6 L/min can be used. Patients receiving more than 4 L/min should have a humidifier added to the circuit in order to minimize mucosal desiccation.

Simple Oxygen Masks These devices are often used in the recovery room to deliver supplemental O_2. Flow rates in the 5–10 L/min range can be used. Flow rates below 5 L/min may allow exhaled CO_2 to be retained in the mask and should be avoided.

Non-Rebreathing Reservoir Masks These devices are usually used with 100% O_2 as the source gas at a flow rate sufficient to prevent the attached reservoir bag from collapsing during inspiration. Although an FIO_2 of 1.0 is theoretically possible, air leaks around the mask usually limit the maximum attainable FIO_2 to about 0.6.

High-Flow Systems High-flow devices are designed to provide a gas flow that exceeds a patient's ventilatory requirements while maintaining a constant FIO_2.

Air Entrainment Masks These masks, also known as jet-mixing masks or venturi-masks, can deliver O_2 concentrations in the 0.24–0.50 range. Total flow decreases as FIO_2 increases. Thus, at settings above an FIO_2 of 0.4, it is questionable if the total flow produced is adequate to meet the patient's ventilatory requirements. Since large volumes of room air are entrained, supplemental humidification is not required.

Large-Volume Aerosol Generators These devices, also sometimes called oxygen nebulizers, operate on the entrainment principle with the addition of water aerosol to the output gas. The FIO_2 produced ranges from 0.28 to 1.00. Like entrainment masks, total flow decreases as FIO_2 increases. Thus, patients with high-minute ventilations may not have their ventilatory needs met at high FIO_2 settings. The gas/aerosol produced can be delivered to patients via such devices as T-pieces, aerosol masks, tracheostomy collars, and face tents.

Blender/Heated Humidifier Gas from an oxygen-air blender is passed through a heated humidifier and delivered to the patient via large-bore corrugated tubing. Since blenders can provide gas at any concentration from 21% (air) to 100% oxygen at flow rates in excess of 100 L/min, this is the preferred method for patients with large-minute ventilation requiring a high FIO_2. The delivery devices are the same as those used with large-volume aerosol generators.

Mechanical Ventilation

While most postoperative patients do well with a minimum of respiratory support, some will require a period of mechanical ventilation. This is most likely to occur in patients who have preexisting chronic obstructive lung disease accompanied by a decreased arterial PaO_2. Use of routine postoperative mechanical ventilation after prolonged surgery in order to "optimize" cardiopulmonary status has not been tested prospectively. At the present time, there are no data to support this practice, and the harm is also unknown. Prospective trials are required.[100]

Although many types of machines exist that can provide mechanical ventilatory assistance to patients, this discussion is limited to the most common type employed in the postsurgical patient—namely, positive pressure volume or time-cycled ventilators. They allow the operator to control such variables as mode, tidal volume, respiratory rate, inspiratory flow rate, inspiratory:expiratory (I:E) ratio, FIO2, sensitivity, and positive end-expiratory pressure (PEEP). State-of-the-art ventilators also have alarms that can alert the operator to problems with the machine, the patient, or the machine/patient interface. The art and science of mechanical ventilation continue to advance rapidly. Unfortunately, controlled prospective trials are far outpaced by daily technological advances. Such detail and fine points are beyond the scope of this chapter, but the basic axioms of mechanical ventilation are well represented by a relatively recent consensus conference.[100]

Indications There are three general indications for initiation of mechanical ventilation: ventilation failure, oxygenation failure, and impending respiratory failure. In each case, the decision to initiate mechanical ventilation is determined *not* by a threshold value of a single measurement but by multiple factors and clinical judgment. Mechanical ventilation is purely supportive in nature and should not be viewed as therapeutic. The underlying pathology that precipitated the need for ventilatory assistance must be corrected before mechanical ventilation can be safely discontinued.

In most cases, sedation for postoperative and critically ill patients on a ventilator is preferable to paralysis. The exceptions are discussed within this chapter. Propofol and midazolam are commonly used sedatives in the ICU. Propofol unit dose is much more expensive than midazolam, but it is as safe and is associated with more rapid recovery of spontaneous respiration. Thus, propofol can shorten ICU length of stay and thereby has a more favorable cost-benefit ratio than midazolam.[101,102]

Ventilation Failure Ventilatory failure is characterized by the patient's inability to sustain an alveolar ventilation adequate enough to maintain a normal arterial pCO_2 and a normal pH. In the postoperative patient, depressed respiratory drive caused by pain medication or the use of paralyzing agents should always be suspected as the cause for an elevated $PaCO_2$. Anesthesia-induced diaphragm dysfunction in the presence of preexisting lung disease may also cause some patients to require a period of ventilatory assistance.

Oxygenation Failure Oxygenation failure requiring mechanical ventilation is characterized by hypoxemia that is not corrected by other means. The cause is often atelectasis and a resulting right to left shunt. Endotracheal intubation and the use of mechanical ventilation allows the clinician to use PEEP or continuous positive airway pressure (CPAP) to help reverse atelectasis and abolish the shunt.[100]

Impending Respiratory Failure This indication is characterized by patients who are maintaining adequate blood gases but at the expense of working very hard to breathe. These patients typically have respiratory rates >30 breaths per minute and are dyspneic. The continuously high work of breathing predisposes to ventilatory muscle fatigue, which leads to progressive hypercapnia and acidemia. Mechanical ventilation can relieve the respiratory muscles of all or part of the work of breathing while the underlying pathology, such as sepsis, is addressed.

Modes of Mechanical Ventilation There are several common modalities of ventilatory support. Machine settings may be unique to a specific mode or may be shared by several. There is no evidence that one particular mode is superior for management of the postoperative patient. The decision to use any particular mode generally relates to issues such as patient comfort and striving for better synchrony between machine and patient. Although the most frequently used mechanical ventilation mode has been volume cycled (inspiration is terminated when the preset tidal volume is delivered), it is possible on some machines to use pressure control (inspiration is terminated when a set airway pressure is reached). Various combinations of volume-limited and pressure-limited breaths have been proposed. The following modes are most commonly used.

Controlled Mechanical Ventilation (CMV) In continuous mandatory ventilation mode, all breaths are generated by the ventilator at a preset rate. This mode is often used in the paralyzed or heavily sedated patient, such as in the intraoperative setting. The patient cannot initiate any spontaneous or ventilator-assisted breaths. Thus, in the postoperative setting, this mode may lead to poor patient comfort due to no synchrony and fighting with the ventilator for spontaneous breaths.

Assist/Control (A/C)   In assist/control mode, every breath is a machine-delivered volume or pressure-limited breath. Typically, it is volume cycled with a preset V_T delivered at a preset rate. The patient will receive either the number of breaths/minute set on the rate control or the rate determined by inspiratory efforts, whichever is greater. Since no patient effort is required to initiate a breath, this mode can be used to ventilate narcotized patients with impaired respiratory drive. As such, A/C mode is often used as an initial setting, usually resulting in decreased work of breathing. If respiratory drive is intact, patient inspiratory effort and control rate may not be synchronized, thereby paradoxically increasing work of breathing as the patient fights with the ventilator.

Synchronized Intermittent Mandatory Ventilation (SIMV)   In SIMV mode, the patient receives the number of volume- or pressure-limited breaths set on the rate control (at a machine preset V_T) and can also take any number of additional "spontaneous" breaths between the machine-delivered breaths (at patient-generated V_T). The machine-delivered breaths are synchronized as much as possible with patient breathing efforts in order to minimize breath stacking.

Continuous Positive Airway Pressure (CPAP)   In CPAP mode, all breaths are "spontaneous" and none are machine delivered. Thus, it is not a mechanical ventilation mode per se. By applying positive pressure to the airway throughout the respiratory cycle, resting lung volume is increased with the goal of improving oxygenation. Like SIMV, CPAP is often used during the process of weaning from mechanical ventilation. Machine alarms are functional in CPAP mode, adding an element of safety to the weaning process.

Pressure Support Ventilation (PSV)   Pressure support is usually used in conjunction with either SIMV or CPAP to provide a preset pressure "assist" to those breaths that would otherwise be spontaneous. This mode can adjust the amount of respiratory work required to achieve a desired tidal volume (V_T). PSV is usually used during the weaning process to gradually transfer the work of breathing from the machine to the patient's respiratory muscles. Because patients can control respiratory rate and duration, tidal volume, and flow rates, they may find PSV more comfortable than the other modes of ventilation. However, a backup ventilation setting is mandatory in case of apnea.

Hemodynamic Considerations   Spontaneous respiration is associated with a negative intrathoracic pressure. When positive-pressure mechanical ventilation is initiated, the intrathoracic pressure becomes positive, which in turn bears hemodynamic consequences.[100] As pressure becomes positive, particularly as reflected by mean airway pressure, there is a progressive decrease in venous return and right heart filling pressures. Subsequently, stroke volume and cardiac output decrease. The degree of hemodynamic compromise depends on effective intravascular volume. Volume resuscitation can improve preload and minimize this complication of mechanical ventilation. Of all modes, CMV and A/C can lead to greatest compromise, since all or most breaths are machine initiated and are positive pressure. SIMV spontaneous breaths are initiated by negative inspiratory intrathoracic pressures and augment venous return, which results in higher cardiac output.

Ventilator Settings In addition to the general modes of ventilation, there are multiple settings that allow adjustment of the ventilator to best meet the needs of each patient. Although general guidelines exist, actual settings are often determined by such factors as arterial blood gas values, lung compliance, and airway resistance.

A critical consideration in ventilator management is assessment of lung compliance and airway resistance. How stiff are the lungs? Consider a normal spontaneously breathing adult, making reference to Figure 6.2. Normally, to breathe a spontaneous V_T of 500 cc from a baseline level at functional residual capacity (FRC) requires an alveolar inflation pressure of approximately 8 cm H_2O (Fig. 6.2: point A to point B). Periodically as all take a sigh, which fills the entire lung and prevents alveolar collapse, requiring a pressure of 30 cm H_2O (point B1). If alveoli collapse or are filled with fluid, FRC is decreased (point C). Dead-space volume V_D increases and oxygenation becomes a problem. Additionally, the pulmonary compliance curve (lung volume vs. alveolar inflation pressure) shifts to the right and flattens out. To deliver the same 500 cc V_T, an alveolar inflation pressure of 50 cm H_2O or more may be required (point C to point E). Essentially, the available alveoli are being overdistended with the same V_T, predisposing to barotrauma. Additional V_T will only increase this

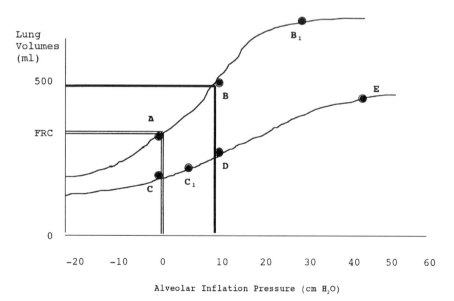

FIGURE 6.2. An illustrative volume-pressure pulmonary compliance curve.

risk. Thus, to "recruit" or gain back the atelectatic alveoli, PEEP is added at a level of 10 cm H_2O and the patient is ventilated at tidal breathing (from point C_1 to point D) with somewhat increased peak alveolar inflation pressures on the order of 20–30 cm H_2O (point D). With lung injury recovery, the compliance curve shifts back to the left and alveolar inflation pressures normalize, shunt decreases, and oxygenation improves.[103,104]

Tidal Volume   For most adults, an initial tidal volume setting of 8–12 ml/kg of ideal body weight is appropriate.[100,105–107] This generally corresponds to actual volumes ranging from 450 ml to 1000 ml. At a midrange setting of 10 ml/kg, the V_T delivered is approximately twice physiologic, which is required to minimize alveolar collapse. Barring other settings or alarms, this preset V_T is delivered regardless of peak inspiratory pressure. Therefore, risk of barotrauma increases with volume, especially in patients with decreased pulmonary compliance. The term *volutrauma* has been suggested as a better descriptor of alveolar hyperdistention.[108] This control is not functional (or not present) in pressure-controlled ventilation (PCV) mode, during which tidal volume is determined by such factors as preset pressure and respiratory system compliance. Therefore, PCV is risky in the unstable patient in whom lung compliance can change rapidly, leading to changes in V_T.[109]

Rate   Most adult patients without restrictive or obstructive lung disease will require rates in the range of 8–12 breaths per minute.[106] The product of V_T and rate is the minute ventilation (V_E). Patients with restrictive disease and small tidal volumes may require higher rates to achieve adequate-minute ventilation, while patients with obstructive disease may require lower rates. Generally, under normal circumstances the V_E should be delivered to maintain a pCO_2 of about 40 mmHg. Initially, the settings should be conservative to avoid over-ventilation and respiratory alkalosis, the most common ventilator complication. However, under aberrant acid base circumstances, the V_E should be adjusted to maintain normal acid base status, focusing on a target pH instead of pCO2.

Sensitivity   The sensitivity setting determines how much patient effort will be required to initiate a machine-delivered breath or to allow the patient to take a "spontaneous" breath. To minimize imposed work of breathing, the sensitivity should be set at the smallest possible value that does not result in the ventilator autocycling. This will generally be in the range of -0.5 to -1.5 cm H_2O[100]. Some ventilators have a flow-by feature in which an adjustable bias flow is delivered to the patient. When the patient begins to inspire and reaches a certain inspiratory flow rate (flow sensitivity), an inspiratory cycle is initiated. In this mode, the machine is flow triggered rather than pressure triggered, further reducing imposed work of breathing.

Inspired Oxygen Fraction (FIO2)   Due to potential oxidant lung damage caused by FIO_2 levels above 0.21 (room air), inspired oxygen should always be limited to the lowest level tolerated.[100] There is no universally safe FIO_2 level above 21%. Threshold level studies established that an FIO_2 of 0.60 for less than 48 hours is nontoxic in *healthy* adults. This was based on the finding that an FIO_2 at this level in the healthy individual will not cause tracheobronchitis or reduce vital capacity, which is ostensibly due to absorption atalectasis.[110] However, sick patients and those undergoing major stress secondary to surgery have variable levels of endogenous antioxidant depletion, which may lead to pulmonary oxidant injury in the presence of FIO_2 levels at any level above 0.21. Although exact cause-effect measurements are lacking, augmenting glutathione, selenium, and vitamin E in patients requiring prolonged supranormal oxygen support may be prudent.[111–113] With the above in mind, initial FIO_2 settings should be 50% to 100% and titrated down as rapidly as possible. At a 50% setting in most circumstances, more than adequate oxygenation is achieved while minimizing nitrogen depletion and absorption atelectasis.[100]

Inspiratory: Expiratory Flow Rates   During normal ventilation, the expiratory phase is approximately twice as long as the inspiratory phase. This ratio and flow rates can be adjusted in order to allow enough expiratory phase to clear the delivered V_T before the next inspiration. Normally, peak flow rates are set in the range of 40–100 L/min.[100] If the V_T is not allowed to clear, breath stacking occurs, along with progressive hyperinflation and high auto-PEEP, also known as occult PEEP. Auto-PEEP can be severe enough to cause hypotension and barotrauma. Patients with chronic obstructive pulmonary disease (COPD) are particularly predisposed to the latter. A common but not infallible way to detect auto-PEEP is to observe the ventilator manometer not decreasing to zero at end expiration. Increased flow rates shorten the inspiratory time and increase the expiratory phase, decreasing the risk of auto-PEEP.[100,114]

PEEP   The presence of a "physiologic" PEEP of 5 cm H_2O against a closed glottis in spontaneously breathing patients is controversial. Therefore, a routine setting of 5 cm H_2O PEEP, although widely utilized, carries no proof of benefit and is not recommended by many authorities.[109,115] It should primarily be used in euvolemic patients with evidence of decreased FRC.

The main indication for PEEP is recruitment of alveoli in diffuse or uniform lung injury (e.g., cardiogenic pulmonary edema), increasing FRC and decreasing shunt fraction. The settings should optimize MAP, optimize oxygenation, and minimize inspired FIO_2.[116] PEEP settings exceeding 15 cm H_2O should be avoided to minimize high peak inspiratory pressures, barotrauma, and a potential decrease in cardiac output. Titration should be in 2–3 cm H_2O increments, observing for adverse effects at each level. It is commonly felt that alveolar recruitment is not an immediate effect and can take hours or longer. However, with incremental PEEP adjustments, changes in cardiac output occur primarily within the first minute and are stabilized within 15 minutes. Arterial oxygenation effect is more gradual, but also stabilizes within 10 minutes. Therefore, the short-term cardiorespiratory effects of incremental PEEP can be reliably assessed in ventilated patients after 15 minutes (Level II-3).[117] Although apparently beneficial in early nonuniform lung injury such as ARDS, PEEP may worsen oxygenation and hasten barotrauma in later stages.[118] Overall, the risk-benefit of incremental PEEP becomes negative at approximately 12–15 cm H_2O.

Initial Ventilator Settings   The following represent general guidelines for initial ventilator settings and monitoring:

- FIO_2 of 50–100%: rapid decrease to lowest level required to maintain O_2 Sat >92%. Lower initial FIO_2 least likely to produce absorption atelectasis.
- Rate 10/min
- V_T 10 ml/kg

Assuming normal V_D/V_T, this rate and V_T result in V_E of 100 ml/kg/min. This translates into alveolar ventilation (V_A) of approximately 4 L/min, which should maintain a $PaCO_2$ of 40 mmHg. Adjust the rate and V_T to the target pH depending on the clinical scenario (i.e., COPD, metabolic acidosis, normal).

- Assist control mode: common initial mode setting that allows patient to set own rate. Trigger usually set low. If high spontaneous rate, may lead to respiratory alkalosis. Observe cardiac output effects.
- PEEP: Set as needed to maintain adequate oxygenation at lowest possible FIO_2. Main indication is diffuse lung injury and early ARDS.
- Alarm setting PIP max 40 cm H_2O: PIP is determined by V_T, flow rate, and PEEP, all of which can be adjusted, and lung compliance. Avoid auto-PEEP and breath stacking with flow rate and I:E ratio settings.

Worsening Respiratory Status   After mechanical ventilation has been initiated, one possible outcome is a worsening clinical picture. Assessment and intervention can be based on grouping into ventilation or oxygenation status.

Ventilation   The most common development is respiratory alkalosis, reflected by an elevated pH and low pCO_2. Adjustment rests with decreasing V_E via either rate or V_T reduction. If the patient is in A/C mode and the patient-activated rate is driving hyperventilation, a shift to SIMV mode may solve the problem.

An elevated pCO_2 despite an initial V_E setting of 100 ml/kg/min is usually the result of either excess metabolic CO_2 or low alveolar ventilation (V_A). Initial management should be a rate increase to 15 breaths/min. This may result in an increased mean airway pressure, requiring fluid resuscitation to maintain hemodynamic status. Further rate increases may reduce V_A. Thus, the next adjustment to consider is a V_T increase to a maximum of 15 ml/kg. Depending on pulmonary compliance, increases in peak pressures have to be observed carefully to avoid volu/barotrauma, becoming of major concern if peak alveolar pressures exceed 35 cm H_2O.[100,107,119]

If the preceding manipulation fails to resolve the problem, CO_2 excretion at the airway should be measured. If it exceeds 130 ml/min/m², the patient should be evaluated for excess CO_2 load, including (1) increased muscle activity/shivering, (2) sepsis, and (3) hyperalimentation overfeeding. At V_E exceeding 300 ml/kg/min, major complications can ensue. Considerations include paralysis to decrease muscle activity or sedation if the patient is simply bucking or fighting the ventilator.

Oxygenation If oxygenation remains poor despite an elevated FIO_2, a mismatch or right to left shunt must be suspected. FIO_2 increases beyond 60% are not effective in this setting and will eventually worsen oxgyenation via further absorption atelectasis.

Diffuse lung injury conditions such as pulmonary edema are best treated with alveolar recruitment via introduction of PEEP.[100] In order to minimize peak inspiratory pressure (PIP) increases, the V_T should be reduced somewhat and the rate increased to maintain the same V_E. Mean airway pressures may also increase, leading to decreased cardiac output and a resulting decrease in oxygen delivery (D_{O_2}) to the tissues. Fluids should be monitored to ensure adequate venous return. Of course, in the setting of severe cardiac depression, inotropes may be required as well.

A pulmonary artery catheter should be considered if PEEP > 5 cm H_2O is required. The "best PEEP" ensures adequate D_{O_2} at the tissue level, balancing increased V_A and pO_2 with adequate cardiac output as reflected by an SVO_2 > 70%. Taking all factors into consideration as discussed, D_{O_2} should be optimized via adequate hemoglobin levels, venous return, inotropes, and treatment of underlying disorders such as sepsis.

Ventilator Weaning

Weaning Parameters The postoperative patient requiring mechanical ventilation for at least 24 hours will often spend up to half of this time on the ventilator in a weaning mode.[120,121] Most often, the presence of comorbid conditions will exist that will require weaning or slow removal from, rather than immediate cessation of, mechanical ventilation postoperatively. Lengthy surgical procedures on their own do not warrant prolonged mechanical ventilation, nor should they warrant prolonged weaning efforts. The following general parameters must be met in order to initiate weaning, expedite the process, minimize failed extubation, and improve patient comfort while conserving valuable scarce ICU resources.

First, the patient must be normally conscious in order to follow directions and participate. Second, heavy sedatives and neuromuscular blocking agents must be completely withdrawn. Third, metabolic and electrolyte disorders must be corrected, especially hypophosphatemia and hypomagnesemia.[122,123] Fourth,

TABLE 6.10. Predictors of Weaning Success

Parameter	Required Value	Sensitivity	Specificity
Maximum inspiratory pressure $P_I$max	< -15 cm H_2O	1.00	0.11
Spontaneous tidal volume V_T	>325 ml	0.97	0.54
Spontaneous respirations RR	<38/minute	0.92	0.36
Spontaneous minute ventilation V_E	<15 L/minute	0.78	0.18
Respiratory rate/tidal volume RR/V_T	<105	0.97	0.64

there must be no ongoing reason for respiratory or cardiovascular failure, and no evidence of sepsis. Finally, the patient must have adequate arterial oxygenation ($PaO_2 > 60$ mmHg) at an $FIO_2 < 0.4-0.5$ with PEEP not exceeding 5 cm H_2O. Having met these general conditions, several objective parameters measurable at the bedside have commonly been used in predicting success (Table 6.10).

Several of the threshold values in Table 6.10 have greater practical utility with high positive and negative predictive values. (1) While exceeding a threshold PI_{max} value has a positive predictive value of 60%, predicting more successful weanings, this parameter has its greatest value is predicting those who will fail weaning. Fully 100% of those not achieving 20 cm H_2O PI_{max} will fail weaning. (2) Rapid and shallow breathing, a common finding in those patients who fail to wean, is reflected by a high RR/V_T ratio. A good threshold and breakpoint value is 105 breaths/min/L. If this threshold is exceeded, 95% fail to wean, whereas if the threshold is not reached, 78% wean successfully (Level II-1).[124]

Many other complex ratios and formulas, such as the CROP (compliance, rate, oxygen, pressure) index, have been proposed to facilitate weaning. None are more predictive than the parameters in Table 6.10.[124] While integrative indices are more predictive than single-component measures, they are generally more applicable to debilitated patients who have undergone protracted mechanical ventilation.

Methods of Weaning   In general, weaning involves either intermittent- and incremental-length spontaneous ventilation via a T-tube system or pressure support ventilation (PSV) mode, or gradual decrease of ventilator support via intermittent mandatory ventilation (IMV). None of these methods is clearly superior, and each case is individual. However, some recent evidence suggests that the simplest and fastest method is still T-piece trial weaning (Level I).[121]

T-piece Trial   weaning is the simplest and oldest method. In the postoperative patient, it may be the best option because the relatively uncomplicated patient can be weaned quickly. Although many different protocols have been proposed, the simplest, which leaves the patient on a T-piece as long as tolerated, probably makes the most sense. As such, the T-piece trial is really a trial of endurance. In an uncomplicated patient, 2 to 4 hours on the T-piece with no evidence of intolerance usually signifies a successful trial and extubation may be considered. If intolerance occurs, mechanical ventilation is reinstated and repeat trial within 24 hours is indicated. Earlier retrial attempts are usually not fruitful due to fatigue, although optimal timing data are lacking.[125] In the case of borderline trials, it should be noted that the endotracheal tube (ETT) and attached ventilator circuit may impose additional resistance and may increase work of breathing. However, when compared to the ETT alone, the work of spontaneous breathing after extubation may increase due to laryngeal edema.[126] A positive cuff-leak test, whereby the ETT cuff is deflated and an air leak around the ETT is sought as an indicator of laryngeal patency, may be reassuring but lacks specificity.[127]

Pressure Support Ventilation (PSV)   is a spontaneous mode of mechanical ventilation that can adjust the amount of respiratory work required to achieve a desired tidal volume (V_T). The patient initiates each breath; thus, the minute ventilation (V_E) is not directly affected. The respiratory work is thus shared to a variable and adjustable extent between the patient and the ventilator. Additionally, PSV removes the extra resistance load imposed by the endotracheal tube and ventilator circuitry. As the patient's ability to assume more work improves, or compliance increases, the level of PSV can be slowly adjusted by 2–4 cm H_2O decrements, weaning the patient. Although not conclusive, some clinical evidence suggests that PSV is more comfortable for patients than either IMV or A/C mode.[125] Goals for PSV weaning are an RR of <25/minute, V_T of 8–10 ml/kg, and pressure support of 8–10 cm H_2O. Upon achieving these levels, extubation can be considered. Since V_E is not regulated and is dependent on intrinsic respiratory drive, apnea alarms should be turned on and a backup mode of ventilation should be activated. Similarly, a given V_T is not ensured by PSV. Therefore, patients with decreased or worsening compliance should be monitored for inadequate alveolar ventilation (V_A).[125]

Intermittent Mandatory Ventilation (IMV)   delivers a predetermined number of preset controlled V_T breaths per minute, allowing spontaneous breaths in between. Synchronization to the best extent possible with the patient's inspiratory efforts via SIMV improves comfort. The weaning process simply decreases IMV by decrements of 2–4 breaths/min over a variable period of time. Data do not support any particular time interval as superior to another.[120,121] Goals for IMV weaning are tolerance of an IMV setting of 2–4 breaths/min. Unfortunately, spontaneous breaths are hindered by ventilator circuitry and the endotracheal tube, increasing the work of breathing between IMV breaths. For this reason, some degree of pressure support is often added to IMV weaning protocols.

Difficult Weaning   Difficult weaning is usually due to hypoventilation relative to the patient's CO_2 load. Oxygenation is rarely a problem in the absence
of severe cardiopulmonary compromise. Thus, there is either excess demand
on the system, a system failure, or both. The following are key questions to
consider in evaluating relative hypoventilation: (1) Is the patient in a state of
hypermetabolism/hyperthermia, perhaps due to sepsis? (2) Is there increased
CO_2 production due to overfeeding and lipogenesis?[128] (3) Is there a state of
respiratory muscle weakness due to metabolic factors such as low magnesium
or phosphorus? (4) Is anxiety producing rapid, shallow breathing? (5) Has cardiac output decreased due to the dynamics of changing from positive to negative
pressure ventilation, leading to decreased diaphragmatic contraction?[129,130] As
might be expected, weaning is far more difficult in the postoperative patient
in the presence of effusions, ascites, cardiac insufficiency, COPD, sepsis, and
ARDS.[120,121,125,131–133]

Extubation   Assessing the patient for extubation is the final and distinctly separate phase of ventilator weaning. The patient should have no evidence of intolerance off assisted ventilation as witnessed by a $PaCO_2 < 40$ mmHg, spontaneous respiratory rate $<20/min$, and pulse $<100–120/min$. Additionally, the
patient should possess a gag reflex, be able to clear secretions, and be alert in
order to minimize aspiration and mucus plugging. If these parameters are met,
the patient is generally ready for extubation.
   Unfortunately, there is no absolutely accurate way to predict successful
weaning and extubation. If all parameters are adequate, one-third will still fail.
This is mainly because a critical parameter, *endurance*, cannot be measured.
Usually these patients have underlying pulmonary pathology or have been on
prolonged ventilatory support. As noted, ventilatory failure after extubation can
occasionally occur due to laryngeal edema and increased work of breathing.
Conversely, one-third of patients with inadequate parameters will wean and
extubate successfully as highlighted by the large percentage of premature postoperative self-extubation cases not requiring reintubation. In the unlikely event
of severe laryngeal edema, as indicated by severe inspiratory stridor, threatening reintubation, aerosolized epinephrine has been proven effective in reducing
edema, whereas steroids have not (Level I).[125,134–137]

Tracheostomy   Patients who have been on extended ventilator support have
often been considered for tracheostomy in order to minimize laryngeal damage from endotracheal cuff pressure necrosis and thus minimize urgency for
extubation in the difficult-to-wean patient. Evidence is inconclusive.[138]

Marginal Analysis of Prolonged Ventilation in the ICU   It has been shown
that in elderly ICU patients requiring prolonged mechanical ventilation, each
additional life year saved is associated with very high direct costs when the sum
of age and days of mechanical ventilation is 100 or greater.[139] Additionally,
the incremental life years were not quality adjusted, making the cost-effective-

ness of prolonged ventilation in this age group even worse. Quality-adjusted life years (QALY) and marginal cost analysis should be considered in rational clinical and administrative decision making to avoid morbidity and high cost of futile care in any age population.[140–143]

ACKNOWLEDGMENTS

Kirk McClelland, RRT, former technical director of the Pulmonary Laboratory at the City of Hope National Medical Center, for valuable review and contribution to the pulmonary section.

REFERENCES

1. Pollock MM, Katz RW, Ruttimann UE, Getson PR. Improving the outcome and efficiency of intensive care: the impact of an intensivist. *Crit Care Med* 1988;16:11–17.

2. Fisher M. Intensive care: Do intensivists matter? *Intensive Care World* 1995;12:71–72.

3. Leach RM, Treacher DF. The relationship between oxygen delivery and consumption. *Dis Mon* 1994;30:301–368.

4. Dantzker DR, Foresman B, Guttierez G. Oxygen supply and utilization relationships. *Am Rev Resp Dis* 1991;143:675–679.

5. Nunn JF. *Nunn's Applied Respiratory Physiology*, 4th ed. Stoneham, MA: Butterworth, 1993, pp. 219–246.

6. Gattinoni L, Feriani M. Acid base derangements in acute renal failure. In Pinsky M, Dhainaut JF (Eds), *Pathophysiologic Foundations of Critical Care.* Baltimore: Williams and Wilkins, 1993.

7. Cunningham DJC, Robbins PA, Wolff CB. Integration of respiratory responses to changes in alveolar partial pressures of CO_2 and O_2 and in arterial pH. In Cherniack NS, Widdicombe JG (Eds), *Handbook of Physiology: Resiration*, vol. 2. Bethesda, MD: American Physiological Society, 1986, pp. 475–528.

8. Sasse SA, Jaffer MB, Chen PA, et al. Arterial oxygenation time after an FIO2 increase in mechanically ventilated patients. *Am J Respir Crit Care Med* 1995;152:148–152.

9. Solis R, Anselmi C. Lavietes M. Rate of decay or increment of PaO_2 following a change in supplemental oxygen in mechanically ventilated patients with diffuse pneumonia. *Chest* 1993;103:554–556.

10. Andritsch RF, Muravchick S, Gold MI. temperature correction of arterial blood gas parameters: a comparative review of methodology. *Anesthesiology* 1981;55:311–316.

11. Hess D, Agarwal NN. Variability of blood gases, pulse oximeter saturation, and end-tidal carbon dioxide pressure in stable, mechanically ventilated trauma patients. *J Clin Mon* 1992;8:111–115.

12. Sasse SA, Chen P, Mahutte CK. Variability of arterial blood gas values over time in stable medical ICU patients. *Chest* 1994;106:187–193.

13. Frolich ED, Grim C, Labarthe DR, et al. Recommendations for human blood pressure determination by sphygmomanometers: report of a special task force appointed by the steering committee, American Heart Association. *Hypertension* 1988;11:210a–221a.

14. Fifth annual report of the Joint National Committee on Detection, Evaluation and Treatment of High Blood Pressure. *Arch Intern Med* 1993;153:154–183.

15. American Society for Hypertension. Recommendations for routine blood pressure measurement by indirect cuff sphygmomanometry. *Am J Hypertension* 1992;5:207–209.

16. Cohn JN. Blood pressure measurements in shock: mechanisms of inaccuracy in auscultatory and palpatory methods. *JAMA* 1967;199:118–122.

17. Nystrom E, Reid KH, Bennet R, et al. A comparison of two automated indirect arterial blood pressure meters: with recordings from a radial artery catheter in anesthetized surgical patients. *Anesthesiology* 1985;62–67.

18. Karamanoglu M, O'Rourke MF, Avolio AP, et al. An analysis of the relationship between central aortic and peripheral upper limb pressure waves in man. *Eur Heart J* 1993;14:160–165.

19. Darovic GO, Vanriper S. Arterial pressure recording. In Darovic GO (Ed), *Hemodynamic Monitoring: Invasive and Noninvasive Clinical Application*, 2nd ed. Philadelphia: Saunders, 1995, pp. 177–210.

20. Gardner RM: Direct blood pressure measurement—dynamic response requirements. *Anesthesiology* 1981;54:227–231.

21. Darovic GO, Vanriper S, Vanriper J. Fluid filled monitoring systems. In Darovic GO (Ed), *Hemodynamic Monitoring: Invasive and Noninvasive Clinical Application*, 2nd ed. Philadelphia: Saunders, 1995, pp. 149–175.

22. Dobbin K, Wallace S, Ahlberg J, Chulay M. Pulmonary artery pressure measurement in patients with elevated pressures: effect of backrest elevation and method of measurement. *Am J Crit Care* 1992;2:61–69.

23. Kee LL, Simonson JS, Stotts NA, et al. Echocardiographic determination of valid zero reference leels in supine and lateral positions. *Am J Crit Care* 1993;2:72–80.

24. Craig KC, Pierson DJ, Carrico JC. The clinical application of PEEP in ARDS. *Respir Care* 1985;30:114–120.

25. Darovic GO: Pulmonary artery pressure monitoring. I Darovic GO (Ed), *Hemodynamic Monitoring. Invasive and Noninvasive Clinical Application*, 2nd ed. Philadelphia: Saunders, 1995, pp. 253–322.

26. Schmitt EA, Brantigen CO. Common artifacts of pulmonary artery and pulmonary artery wedge pressures. Recognition and management. *J Clin Monit* 1986;2:44–52.

27. Robin ED. The cult of the Swan–Ganz catheter. *Ann Intern Med* 1985;103:445–447.

28. Pesce RR. The Swan–Ganz catheter: It goes through your pulmonary artery and you pay through the nose. *Respir Care* 1989;34:785–789.

29. Viskocil JJ, Kruse JA. Hemodynamics and oxygen transport: using your computer to manage data. *J Crit Illness* 1994;9:447–459.

30. Iberti TJ, et al. A multicenter study of physicians' knowledge of the pulmonary artery catheter. *JAMA* 1990;264(22):2928–2932.

31. Wilson RF, et al. Pulmonary artery diastolic and wedge pressure relationship in critically ill and injured patients. *Arch Surg* 1988;123:933–937.

32. Alonso DR, Scheidt S, Post M, Killip T. Pathophysiology of cardiogenic shock: quantification of myocardial necrosis, clinical, pathologic and electrocardiographic correlations. *Circulation* 1973;48:588–596.

33. Harnarayan C, Bennett MA, Pentecost BL, Brewer DB. Quantitative study of infarcted myocardium in cardiogenic shock. *Br Heart J* 1970;32:728–732.

34. Parrillo JE. Pathogenic mechanisms of septic shock. *N Engl J Med* 1993;328: 1471–1477.

35. Suh R, et al. Radiographic manifestations of pulmonary edema. In Matthay M, Inghow D (Eds), *Pulmonary Edema*, Lung Biology in Health and Disease, vol. 116. New York: Marcel Dekker, 1998.

36. Gattinoni L, Pesenti A, Bombino M, et al. Relationships between lung computed tomography density, gas exchange and PEEP in acute respiratory failure. *Anesthesiology* 1988;69:824–832.

37. Gattinoni L, Pesenti A, Torresin A, et al. Adult respiratory distress syndrome profiles by computed tomography. *J Thoracic Imaging* 1986;3:25–30.

38. Ensing G, Seward J, Darragh R, et al. Feasibility of generating hemodynamic pressure curves from noninvasive Doppler echocardiographic signals. *J Am Coll Cardiol* 1994;23:434–438.

39. Belfort MA, Mares A, Saade G, et al. A re-evaluation of the indications for pulmonary artery catheterization in obstetrics: the role of 2D echocardiography and Doppler ultrasound. *Am J Obstet Gynecol* 1996;174:331–337.

40. Fromm RE Jr, Varon J. Invasive and noninvasive cardiac output determination. In Levine RL, Fromm RE Jr (Eds), *Critical Care Monitoring: From Pre-Hospital to the ICU*. St. Louis: Mosby Year Book, Inc., 1995, pp. 159–168.

41. Nishimura RA, Callahan MJ, Schaff HV, et al. Noninvasive measurement of cardiac output by continuous-wave Doppler echocardiography: initial experience and review of the literature. *Mayo Clin Proc* 1984;59:484–490.

42. Wahr JA, Tremper KK. Noninvasive oxygen monitoring techniques. *Crit Care Clin* 1995;11:199–217.

43. Webb KK, Ralston AC, Runciman WB. Potential errors in pulse oximetry. II. Effects of changes in saturation and signal quality. *Anaesthesia* 1991;96:207–212.

44. Severinghaus JW, Naifeh KH. Accuracy of response of six pulse oximeters to profound hypoxia. *Anesthesiology* 1987;67:551–558.

45. Severinghaus JW, Spellman MJ. Pulse oximeter failure thresholds in hypotension and vasoconstriction. *Anesthesiology* 1990;73:532–537.

46. Jay GD, Hughes L, Renzi FP. Pulse oximetry is accurate in acute anemia from hemorrhage. *Ann Emerg Med* 1994;24:32–35.

47. Ries AL, Prewitt LM, Johnson JJ. Skin color and ear oximetry. *Chest* 1989;96:287–290.

48. Jubran A, Tobin MJ. Reliability of pulse oximetry in titrating supplemental oxygen therapy in ventilator dependent patients. *Chest* 1990;97:1420–1425.

49. Rubin AS. Nail polish can affect pulse oximeter saturation. *Anesthesiology* 1988;68:825.

50. Clayton D, Webb RK, Ralston AC, et al. A comparison of the performance of 20 pulse oximeters under conditions of poor perfusion. *Anaesthesia* 1991;46:3–10.

51. Wiklund L, Hok B, Stahl K, et al. Postanesthesia monitoring revisisted: frequency of true and false alarms from different monitoring devices. *J Clin Anesthesiol* 1994;6:182–188.

52. Hutton P, Clutton-Brock T. The benefits and pitfalls of pulse oximetry. *Br J Med* 1993;307:457–458.

53. Moorthy SS, Losasso AM, Wilcox J. End-tidal PCO_2 greater than $PACO_2$. *Crit Care Med* 1984;12:534–535.

54. Jubran A, Tobin MJ. Monitoring gas exchange during mechanical ventilation. In Tobin MJ (Ed), *Principles and Practice of Mechanical Ventilation.* New York: McGraw Hill, 1994, p. 919.

55. Gandhi SK, Munshi CA, Bardeen-Henschel A. Capnography for detection of endobronchial migration of an endotracheal tube. *J Clin Monit* 1991;7:53–38.

56. Healey CJ, Fedullo AJ, Swineburne AJ, Wahl GW. Comparison of noninvasive measurements of carbon dioxide tension during weaning from mechanical ventilation. *Crit Care Med* 1987;15:764–767.

57. Hanique G, Dugernier T, Laterre PF, et al. Significance of pathologic oxygen supply dependence in critically ill patients: comparison between measured and calculated measures. *Intensive Care Med* 1994;20:12–18.

58. Archie JP Jr. Mathematical coupling of data: a common source of error. *Ann Surg* 1981;193:296–303.

59. Bakker J, Vincent JL, Gris P, Leon M, Coffernils M, Kahn RJ. Venoarterial carbon dioxide gradient in human septic shock. *Chest* 1992;101:509–515.

60. Aduen J, Bernstein WK, Khastgir T, et al. The use and clinical importance of a substrate-specific electrode for rapid determination of blood lactate concentrations. *JAMA* 1994;272:1678–1685.

61. Levy P, Chavez RP, Crstal GJ, et al. Oxygen extraction ratio: A valid indicator of transfusion need in limited coronary vascular reserve? *J Trauma* 1992;32:769–774.

62. Shoemaker WC, Appel PL, Kram HB, Waxman K, Lee TS. Prospective trial of supranormal values of survivors as therapeutic goals in high risk surgical patients. *Chest* 1988;94:1176–1186.

63. Shoemaker WC, Kram HB, Appel PL. Therapy of shock based on pathophysiology, monitoring and outcome prediction. *Crit Care Med* 1990;18:S19–25.

64. Gattinoni L, Brazzi L, Pelosi P, et al. A trial of goal-oriented hemodynamic therapy in critically ill patients. *N Engl J Med* 1995;333:1025–1032.

65. Hayes MA, Timmins AC, Yau EHS, et al. Elevation of systemic oxygen delivery in the treatment of critically ill patients. *N Engl J Med* 1994;330:1717–1722.

66. Amoroso P, Greenwood RN. Posture and central venous pressure measurements in circulatory volume depletion. *Lancet* 1989;99:258–260.

67. Sing R, O'Hara D, Sawyer MAJ, Parino PL. Trendelenburg position and oxygen transport in hypovolemic adults. *Ann Emerg Med* 1994;23:564–568.

68. Bivins HG, Knopp R, dos Santos PAL. Blood volume distribution in the Trendelenburg position. *Ann Emerg Med* 1985;14:641–643.

69. Ali J, Vanderby B, Purcell C. The effect of pneumatic antishock garment on hemodynamics, hemorrhage, and survival in penetrating thoracic aortic injury. *J Trauma* 1991;31:846–851.

70. Lawson N. Therapeutic combinations of vasopressors and inotropic agents. *Semin Anesthesia* 1990;9:270–287.

71. Brun-Buisson C, Doyon F, Carlet J, et al. Incidence, risk factors, and outcome of severe sepsis and septic shock in adults. *JAMA* 1995;274:968–974.

72. Pittet D, Tarara D, Wenzel RP. Nosocomial bloodstream infection in critically ill patients. *JAMA* 1994;271:1598–1601.

73. Rackow EC, Astiz ME. Mechanisms and management of septic shock. *Crit Care Clin* 1993;9:219–228.

74. Vincent JL, Van der Linden P. Septic shock: a particular type of acute circulatory failure. *Crit Care Med* 1990;18S:S70–74.

75. Tuchschmidt J, Fried J, Astiz M, Rackow E. Elevation of cardiac output and oxygen delivery improves outcome in septic shock. *Chest* 1992;102:216–220.

76. Boyd O, Grounds RM, Bennett ED. A randomized clinical trial of the effect of deliberate perioperative increase in oxygen delivery on mortality in high-risk surgical patients. *JAMA* 1993;270:2699–2707.

77. Natanson C, Hoffman WD, Suffredini AF, Eichacker PO. Selected treatment strategies for septic shock based on proposed mechanisms of pathogenesis. *Ann Int Med* 1994;120:771–783.

78. Dinarello CA, Gelfand JA, Wolff SM. Anticytokine strategies in the treatment of systemic inflammatory response syndrome. *JAMA* 1993;269:1828–1835.

79. McCloskey RV, Straube RC, Sanders C, et al. Treatment of septic shock with human monoclonal antibody HA-1A. *Ann Intern Med* 1994;121:1–5.

80. Abraham E, Wunderink R, Silverman H, et al. Efficacy and safety of monoclonal antibody to human tumor necrosis factor alpha in patients with sepsis syndrome. *JAMA* 1995;273:934–941.

81. Fisher CJ, Dhainaut JF, Opal SM, et al. Recombinant human interleukin 1 receptor antagonist in the treatment of patients with sepsis syndrome. *JAMA* 1994;271:1836–1843.

82. McGowan JR, Chesney PJ, Crossley KB, LaForce FM. Guidelines for the use of systemic glucocorticosteroids in the management of selected infections. *J Infect Dis* 1992;165:1–13.

83. Sprung CL, Caralis PV, Marcial E, et al. The effects of high dose corticosteroids in patients with septic shock: A prospective controlled study. *N Engl J Med* 1984;311:1137–1143.

84. American College of Chest Physicians/Society of Critical Care Medicine Consensus Conference Committee. Definition of sepsis and organ failure and guidelines for the use of innovative therapies in sepsis. *Chest* 1992;101:1644–1655 and *Crit Care Med* 1992;20:864–874.

85. Marshall JC, Cook DJ, Christou NV, et al. Multiple Organ Dysfunction Score: a reliable descriptor of a complex clinical outcome. *Crit Care Med* 1995;23:1638–1652.

86. Beal AL, Cerra FB. Multiple organ failure in the 1990s. Systemic inflammatory response and organ dysfunction. *JAMA* 1994;271:226–233.

87. Davies JM. Pre-operative respiratory evaluation and management of patients for upper abdominal surgery. *Yale J Biol Med* 1991;64:329–349.

88. Celli BR, Rodriguez K, Snider GL. A controlled trial of intermittent positive pressure breathing, incentive spirometry and deep breathing exercises in preventing pulmonary complications after abdominal surgery. *Am Rev Respir Dis* 1984;130:12–15.

89. Celli BR. What is the value of preoperative pulmonary testing. *Med Clin North Am* 1993;77:309–325.

90. Zibrak JD, O'Donnell CR, Marton K. Indications for pulmonary function testing. *Ann Int Med* 1990;112:763–771.

91. Meyers JR, Lembeck L, O'Kane H, et al. Changes in functional residual capacity of the lung after operation. *Arch Surg* 1975;110:576–583.

92. Ali J, Weisel RD, Layug AB, et al. Consequences of postoperative alterations in pulmonary mechanics. *Am J Surg* 1974;128:376–382.

93. Ford GT, Whitelaw WA, Rosenwal TW, Cruse PJ, Guenter CA. Diaphragm function after upper abdominal surgery in humans. *Am Rev Respir Dis* 1983;127:431–436.

94. Dureuil B. Viires N, Cantineau JP, Aubier M, Desmonts JM. Diaphragmatic contractility after upper abdominal surgery. *J. Appl Physiol* 1986;61:1775–1780.

95. Hall JC, Tarala RA, Hall JL, Mander J. A multivariate analysis of the risk of pulmonary complications after laparotomy. *Chest* 1991;99:923–927.

96. Warner DO, Offord KP, Warner ME, Lennon RL, Conover MA, Jansson-Schumacher U. Role of preoperative cessation of smoking and other factors in postoperative pulmonary complications: a blinded prospective study of coronary artery bypass patients. *Mayo Clin Proc* 1989;64:609–616.

97. Warner MA, Divertie MB, Tinker JH. Preoperative cessation of smoking and pulmonary complications in coronary artery bypass patients. *Anesthesiology* 1984;60:380–383.

98. Sostman H, Matthay R, Putnam C. Cytotoxicity induced lung disease. *Am J Med* 1977;62:608–610.

99. Comis RL. Detecting bleomycin pulmonary toxicity: a continued conundrum. *J Clin Oncol* 1990;8:765–767.

100. American College of Chest Physicians Consensus Conference on Mechanical Ventilation. *Chest* 1993;104:1833–1859.

101. Byatt CM, Lewis LD, Dawling S, et al. Accumulation of midazolam after repeated dosage in patients receiving mechanical ventilation in an intensive care unit. *Br Med J* 1984;289:799–800.

102. Carrasco G, Molina R, Costa J, Soler JM, Cabr L. Propofol vs midazolam in short-, medium-, and long-term sedation of critically ill patients: a cost-benefit analysis. *Chest* 1993;103:557–564.

103. West JB. *Pulmonary Pathophysiology—The Essentials*, 2nd ed. Baltimore: Williams and Wilkins, 1982.

104. West JB. *Respiratory Physiology—The Essentials*, 2nd ed. Baltimore: Williams and Wilkins, 1979.

105. Lee PC, Helsmortel CM, Cohn SM, et al. Are low tidal volumes safe? *Chest* 1990;97:425–428.

106. Kacmarek RM, Venegas J. Mechanical ventilatory rates and tidal volumes. *Respir Care* 1987;32:466–478.

107. Hickling KG, Henderson SJ, Jackson R. Low mortality associated with low volume, pressure limited ventilation with permissive hypercapnia in severe adult respiratory distress syndrome. *Intensive Care Med* 1990;16:372–377.

108. Dreyfus D, Saumon G. Barotrauma is volutrauma, but which volume is the one responsible? *Intensive Care Med* 1992;18:139–141.

109. Pilbeam SP. *Mechanical Ventilation: Physiologic and Clinical Applications*. St. Louis: Mosby-Yearbook, Inc., 1992, p. 149.

110. Lodato RF. Oxygen toxicity. *Crit Care Clin* 1990;6:749–765.

111. Hawker FH, Stewart PM, Switch PJ. Effects of acute illness on selenium homeostasis. *Crit Care Med* 1990;18:442–446.

112. Corbucci GG, Gasparetto A, Candiani A, et al. Shock induced damage to mitochondrial function and some cellular antioxidant mechanisms in humans. *Circ Shock* 1985;15:15–26.

113. Pincemail J, Bertrand Y, Hanique G, et al. Evaluation of vitamin E deficiency in patients with adult respiratory distress syndrome. *Ann NY Acad Sci* 1989;570:498–500.

114. Marini JJ, Ravenscraft SA. Mean airway pressure: physiologic determinants and clinical importance. Part 2: Clinical implications. *Crit Care Med* 1992;20:1604–1616.

115. Petty TL. The use, abuse, and mystique of positive end-expiratory pressure. *Am Rev Respir Dis* 1988;138:475–478.

116. Suter PM, Fairly HB, Isenberg MD. Optimum end expiratory airway pressure in patients with acute pulmonary failure. *N Engl J Med* 1975;292:284–289.

117. Patel M, Singer M. The optimal time for measuring the cardiorespiratory effects of positive end-expiratory pressure. *Chest* 1993;104:139–142.

118. Gattinoni L, Pesenti A, Baglioni S, et al. Inflammatory pulmonary edema and positive end-expiratory pressure: correlations between imaging and physiological studies. *J Thoracic Imaging* 1988;3:59–64.

119. Marini JJ. New approaches to the ventilatory management of the adult respiratory distress syndrome. *J Crit Care* 1992;87:256–257.

120. Esteban A, Alia I, Ibanez J, et al. Modes of mechanical ventilation and weaning. A national survey of Spanish hospitals. *Chest* 1994;106:1188–1193.

121. Esteban A, Frutcos F, Tobin MJ, Inmaculada A, et al. A comparison of four methods of weaning patients from mechanical ventilation. *N Engl J Med* 1995;332:345–350.

122. Aubier M, Murciano D, Lecoguic Y, et al. Effect of hypophosphatemia on diaphragmatic contractility in patientw with acute respiratory failure. *N Engl J Med* 1985;313:420–424.

123. Malloy DW, Dhingra S, Solven FS. Hypomagnesemia and respiratory muscle power. *Am Rev Respir Dis* 1984;129:497–498.

124. Yang KL, Tobin MJ. A prospective study of indexes predicting the outcome of

trials of weaning from mechanical ventilation. *N Engl J Med* 1991;324:1445–1450.

125. Lessard MR, Brochard LJ. Weaning from ventilatory support. *Clin Chest Med* 1996;17:475–489.

126. Kaplan JD, Schuster DP. Physiologic consequences of tracheal intubation. *Clin Chest Med* 1991;12:425–432.

127. Fisher MMcD, Raper RF. The "cuff-leak" test for extubation. *Anaesthesia* 1992;47:10–12.

128. Benotti PN, Bistrain B. Metabolic and nutritional aspects of weaning from mechanical ventilation. *Crit Care Med* 1989;17:181–185.

129. Nishimura Y, Maeda H, Tanaka K, et al. Respiratory muscle strength and hemodynamics in heart failure. *Chest* 1994;105:355–359.

130. Pinsky M. Cardiovascular effects of ventilatory support and withdrawal. *Anesthesiol Analg* 1994;79:567–576.

131. Brochard L, Rauss A, Benito S, et al. Comparison of three methods of gradual withdrawal from ventilatory support during weaning from mechanical ventilation. *Am J Respir Care Med* 1994;150:896–903.

132. Demling RH, Read T, Lind LJ, et al. Incidence and morbidity of extubation failure in surgical intensive care patients. *Crit Care Med* 1988;16:573–577.

133. Tomlinson JR, Miller KS, Lorch DG, et al. A propsective comparison of IMV and T-piece weaning from mechanical ventilation. *Chest* 1989;96:348–352.

134. Gaussorgues P, Boyer F, Piperno D, et al. Do corticosteroids prevent postintubation laryngeal edema? A prospective study of 276 adults. *Crit Care Med* 1988;16:649–652.

135. Nutman J, Brooks LJ, Deakins K, et al. Racemic versus 1-epinephrine aerosol in the treatment of postextubation laryngeal edema: results from a prospective, randomized, double blind study. *Crit Care Med* 1994;22:1591–1594.

136. Darmon JY, Rauss A, Dreyfuss D, et al. Evaluation of risk factors for laryngeal edema after tracheal extubation in adults and its prevention by dexamethasone: a placebo controlled, double blind, multicenter study. *Anesthesiology* 1992;77:245–251.

137. Stauffer JL, Olson DE, Petty DL. Complications and consequences of endotracheal intubation and tracheotomy—a prospective study of 150 critically ill patients. *Am J Med* 1981;70:65–76.

138. Colice C, Stukel T, Dain B. Laryngeal complications of prolonged intubation. *Chest* 1989;96:877–884.

139. Cohen IL, Lambrinos J, Fein IA. Mechanical ventilation for the elderly patient in intensive care: incremental charges and benefits. *JAMA* 1993;269:1026–1029.

140. Rosen RL, Bone RC. Economics of mechanical ventilation. *Clin Chest Med* 1988;9:163–169.

141. Fedullo AJ, Swinburne AJ. Relationship of patient age to cost and survival in medical ICU. *Crit Care Med* 1983;11:155–159.

142. Pesau B, Falger S, Berger E, et al. Influence of age on outcome of mechanically ventilated patients in an intensive care unit. *Crit Care Med* 1992;20:489–492.

143. Cullen DJ. Results and costs of intensive care. *Anesthesiology* 1977;47:203–216.

CHAPTER 7

FLUIDS, ELECTROLYTES, AND NUTRITION

HOWARD SILBERMAN, M.D.

FLUID AND ELECTROLYTE HOMEOSTASIS

In healthy persons, the fluid and electrolyte composition of the body is maintained by a variety of physiologic processes within a narrow range of normal, despite wide variation in consumption of salt and water. However, the homeostatic mechanisms involved frequently are disrupted by surgical illness as well as by operative therapy so that fluid and electrolyte balance becomes a key element in perioperative care.

Total body water (TBW) is distributed between the intracellular and extracellular compartments. The latter is subdivided into the interstitial and vascular (plasma) spaces. TBW as a proportion of body weight decreases with increasing body fat, since fat contains little water. The composition of the body fluid compartments is presented in Table 7.1. The distribution of water between the intracellular fluid (ICF) and extracellular fluid (ECF) compartments is determined by the concentration of osmotically effective particles within each of these compartments, which are separated by the functionally semipermeable cell membrane. Whereas all solutes contribute to body fluid osmolality, only those solutes whose movement is relatively restricted by cell membranes have the capacity to cause water to move from one body compartment to the other. This capacity to cause water to move is called *effective osmolality* or *tonicity*, and those solutes that contribute to tonicity are called *osmotically effective* solutes.[1]

The intracellular and extracellular compartments each have one primary solute, which is limited to that compartment and which therefore is the major determinant of its effective osmotic pressure (Fig. 7.1). In the extracellular

Perioperative and Supportive Care in Gynecologic Oncology: Evidence-Based Management,
Edited by Steven A. Vasilev.
ISBN 0-471-24788-X   Copyright © 2000 by Wiley-Liss, Inc.

TABLE 7.1. Body Fluid Compartments

Total Body Water	Percentage of Body Weight	Percentage of Total Body Water
	60	100
Intracellular	40	67
Extracellular	20	33
Intravascular	5	8
Interstitial	15	25

Source: From Greenfield LJ (Ed). *Surgery: Scientific Principles and Practice.* Philadelphia: JB Lippincott Company, 1993, p. 222.

space, sodium salts are the principal effective osmoles and, therefore, act to hold water in that compartment.[2] In contrast, potassium is the major intracellular ion, and thus it, with its associated anions, exerts the major osmotic force, tending to hold water within the cells. Although the cell membrane is in fact permeable to both sodium and potassium ions, these ions are able to act as effective osmoles because they are restricted to their respective compartments by the Na-K-ATPase pump in the cell membrane.[2] Whereas the movement of the major intracellular and extracellular ions, as well as protein, is restricted, water is freely diffusable. Thus, osmotic forces are the prime determinant of water distribution in the body, because they underlie the movement of water across cellular membranes in such a manner as to achieve osmotic equilibrium

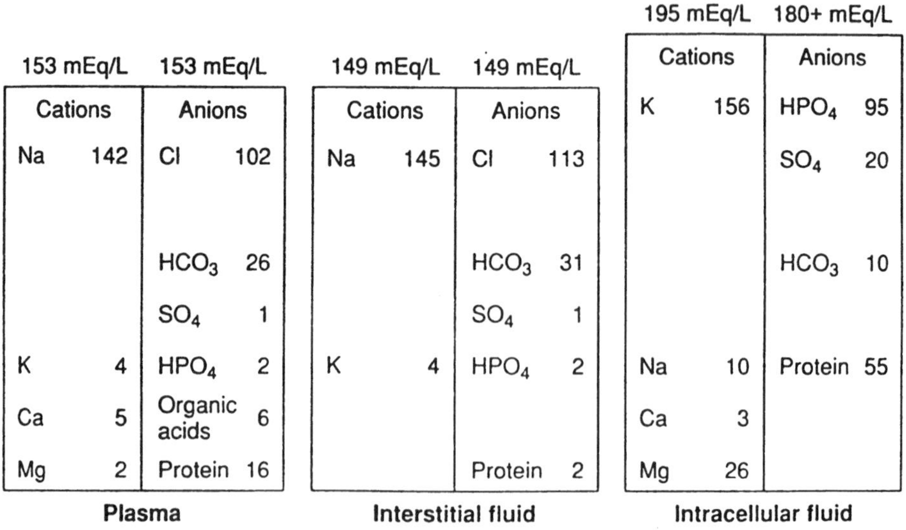

153 mEq/L	153 mEq/L		149 mEq/L	149 mEq/L		195 mEq/L	180+ mEq/L
Cations	Anions		Cations	Anions		Cations	Anions
Na 142	Cl 102		Na 145	Cl 113		K 156	HPO$_4$ 95
							SO$_4$ 20
	HCO$_3$ 26			HCO$_3$ 31			HCO$_3$ 10
	SO$_4$ 1			SO$_4$ 1			
K 4	HPO$_4$ 2		K 4	HPO$_4$ 2		Na 10	Protein 55
Ca 5	Organic acids 6					Ca 3	
Mg 2	Protein 16			Protein 2		Mg 26	
Plasma			**Interstitial fluid**			**Intracellular fluid**	

FIGURE 7.1. Electrolyte composition of the major fluid compartments. (From Levine et al. [Eds]. *Current Practice of Surgery.* New York: Churchill Livingstone, 1993, p. 4.)

(i.e., equal osmolalities) between all body compartments. If the tonicity of one fluid compartment changes, for example, by the addition of water or hypertonic saline solution to the extracellular compartment, water will move across the separating cellular membrane in an amount exactly necessary to reestablish osmotic equilibrium. The osmolality at the new equilibrium will be higher or lower than the normal body fluid osmolality of approximately 290 mOsm/kg H_2O, depending on the direction of water movement.

The addition of an osmotically *ineffective* solute, such as urea, to the ECF compartment results in an increase in *osmolality* of both the ECF and ICF compartments as urea permeates freely across cell membranes, but there is no change in body fluid *tonicity* and, therefore, no movement of water.

Tonicity is calculated from the measured concentration of all of the *effective* solutes in extracellular fluid.[1] ECF tonicity can be estimated from the following expression:

$$Tonicity(mOsm/kg) = (2 \times S_{Na}) + \frac{S_G}{18} \qquad (1)$$

where S_{Na} and S_G are the serum sodium and the serum glucose concentrations, respectively. S_{Na} (mEq/L or mmol/L) is multiplied by 2 to take into account the osmotic pressure exerted by the anions (largely chloride and HCO_3^-) that accompany sodium. S_G (mg/dL) is divided by 18 to convert to mmol/L. Thus,

$$Normal\ tonicity = (2 \times 140) + \frac{90}{18} = 285\ mOsm/kg \qquad (2)$$

In contrast to tonicity, body fluid osmolality is a function of all solutes, effective or ineffective. Plasma osmolality (P_{OSM}) can be calculated as follows:

$$P_{OSM}(mOsm/kg) = (2 \times S_{Na}) + \frac{S_G}{18} + \frac{BUN}{2.8} \qquad (3)$$

where BUN is the blood urea nitrogen (mg/dl); the latter is divided by 2.8 to convert to mmol/L. Thus,

$$Normal\ osmolality = (2 \times 140) + \frac{90}{18} + \frac{14}{2.8} = 290\ mOsm/kg \qquad (4)$$

Movement of water across cell membranes in response to a change in ECF tonicity (i.e., effective osmolality) results in a reciprocal change in cell volume. Thus, ECF hypertonicity leads to cell shrinkage or dehydration, and ECF hypotonicity leads to cell swelling or edema.[1] Similarly, deviations from normal tonicity produce a change in the volume of hypothalamic osmoreceptor cells, which in turn stimulates alterations in thirst, the major mechanism controlling

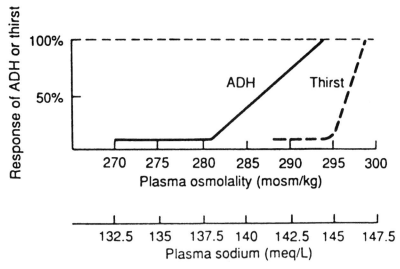

FIGURE 7.2. Comparative activities of ADH and thirst as a function of plasma osmolality and plasma sodium concentration. (From Cogan MG. *Fluid and Electrolytes.* Norwalk, CT: Appleton and Lange, 1991, p. 83.)

water intake, and antidiuretic hormone secretion, the major factor controlling water excretion. When the addition of impermeable solutes (effective osmoles) produces a rise in plasma osmolality above a threshold of approximately 280 mOsm/kg, the osmoreceptor cells shrink, resulting in a progressive stimulus to antidiuretic hormone (ADH) release. When plasma osmolality reaches about 290–292 mOsm/kg, an ADH level (5 pg/ml) is reached that causes the maximal renal antidiuretic effect, with resultant water reabsorption in the renal collecting tubules, yielding a maximum urine concentration of 1,000–1,200 mOsm/kg (Fig. 7.2).[3]

Sodium, as the primary extracellular effective solute, is the major osmotic stimulus to ADH release and, therefore, the major determinant of extracellular fluid volume in normal persons. The narrow range of plasma sodium concentration responsible for the spectrum of ADH response is 137–145 mEq/L (Fig. 7.2).[3] As ECF osmolality falls in response to water absorption, osmoreceptor cell volume increases, and the stimulus to ADH secretion decreases. ADH secretion is completely inhibited at an ECF osmolality of 280 mOsm/kg.

Osmoreceptors also regulate thirst, but compared to ADH release, higher thresholds for osmolality and sodium concentration (295 mOsm/kg and 145 mEq Na/L) are required to induce a response (Fig. 7.2). In clinical practice, it is important to recognize that the thirst response, the only physiologic mechanism that increases water intake, is abrogated in persons unable to drink because of illness, anesthesia, or postoperative ileus.

Whereas this osmoregulatory system is the homeostatic mechanism main-

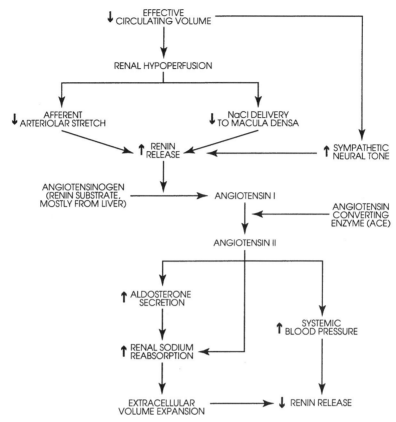

FIGURE 7.3. Renin-angiotensin-aldosterone system. (Modified after Rose BD. *Clinical Physiology of Acid-Base and Electrolyte Disorders*, 4th ed. New York: McGraw-Hill, Inc., 1994, p. 28.)

taining fluid balance in normal persons, large pathologic changes in volume generally produce a corresponding change in effective circulating volume, which in turn affects superior vena caval, atrial, arterial, and renal arteriolar baroreceptors. *Effective circulating volume (ECV)* is the portion of extracellular fluid within the arterial system that perfuses the tissues and generates the pressure that affects the baroreceptors. A reduction in effective circulating volume results in a fall in the perfusion pressure and a stretch in the region of the baroreceptors. This, in turn, results in a cascade of homeostatic events that tends to restore ECV and perfusion pressure. The intrarenal baroreceptors, located primarily in the juxtaglomerular apparatus of the afferent arteriole, affect volume by influencing the activity of the renin-angiotensin-aldosterone system (Fig. 7.3).[2] In contrast to the intrarenal baroreceptors, the extrarenal receptors respond to decreased ECV by stimulating the sympathetic nervous system (Fig. 7.4) and inhibiting release of atrial natriuretic peptide (ANP).

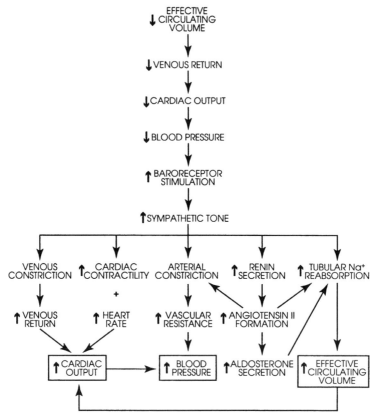

FIGURE 7.4. Hemodynamic responses induced by the sympathetic nervous system as a result of decreased effective circulating volume. (From Rose BD. *Clinical Physiology of Acid-Base and Electrolyte Disorders*, 4th ed. New York: McGraw-Hill, Inc., 1994, p. 244.)

Enhanced sympathetic tone tends to reverse the fall in perfusion pressure, and, as a result of renin and aldosterone release, tubular reabsorption of sodium and water increases circulating volume. Reduced atrial distention, or stretch, as a result of diminished ECV, removes the stimulus to increased urinary sodium and water loss normally induced by ANP, and thus renal sodium and water reabsorption is enhanced. Although ADH secretion is primarily controlled by the osmoreceptors, decreased ECV also stimulates ADH secretion by activating nonosmolal, volume-sensitive receptors for ADH release.[2]

Thus, the renal control of sodium and water excretion is the final common pathway by which homeostatic mechanisms maintain normal ECV. When ECV is low, renal sodium and water reabsorption increases, and when ECV is high, sodium and water diuresis ensues. ECV is not easily measured, but ECV depletion can be diagnosed by demonstrating renal Na^+ retention, as evidenced by

CAPILLARY DRIVING FORCES

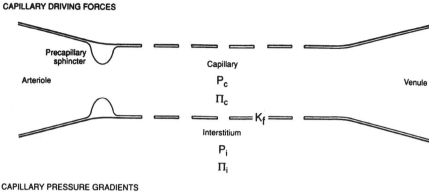

CAPILLARY PRESSURE GRADIENTS

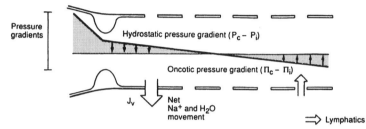

FIGURE 7.5. Forces governing transcapillary sodium and water distribution. (From Cogan MG. *Fluid and Electrolytes.* Norwalk, CT: Appleton and Lange, 1991, p. 5.)

a urinary Na^+ concentration below 15–20 mEq/L in the absence of diuretic therapy or intrinsic renal disease.[2]

In normal persons, ECV and ECF volume are directly proportional. In certain diseases, however, a dissociation between these two volumes occurs. For example, decreased ECV in the face of increased ECF volume is observed in congestive heart failure (decreased pressure at baroreceptors), arteriovenous fistulas (decreased pressure at baroreceptors), and advanced portal cirrhosis (ascites, arteriovenous fistulas). Low ECV despite elevated ECF is seen also in surgical patients with interstitial extravasation ("third-space" loss) due to peritonitis, intestinal obstruction (bowel-wall edema, transudation of fluid into bowel lumen), pancreatitis (retroperitoneal fluid extravasation), sepsis (capillary leak), extensive retroperitoneal dissection, major fractures, and thermal injuries.

The normal distribution of extracellular sodium, and the normal 3 : 1 ratio of water between the intravascular (plasma) and interstitial spaces (Table 7.1), is maintained as a result of the movement of these substances between the two spaces at the level of the capillaries and postcapillary venules. The forces (Starling forces) governing the net transcapillary sodium and water distribution (J_V) include the hydrostatic pressure within the capillary (P_C) and the interstitium (P_i), and the osmotic pressure in the capillary (Π_c) and the interstitium (Π_i) (Fig. 7.5).[3] In contrast to the cell membrane, the capillary wall is permeable to sodium salts and glucose so that the plasma proteins are the only effective osmoles, because they move across the capillary wall only to a limited degree. The *colloid osmotic pressure* or the *plasma oncotic pressure* denotes the sum of the contributions of the various fractions of the plasma proteins to osmotic pressure. Thus, 75% of the total colloid osmotic pressure results from the albumin fraction and 25% from the globulins. Fibrinogen makes a negligible contribution (Fig. 7.6).[4] The *Gibbs–Donnan effect* causes the colloid osmotic pressure of the plasma to be greater than that caused by the proteins alone. This results from the fact that at physiologic pH 7.4, proteins have a negative charge and therefore behave as anions. This electronegativity is balanced by cations, mainly sodium, which contribute to the total osmotic pressure.[4,5] The hydrostatic pressure within the capillary diminishes from the arterial end to the venous end. Consequently, fluid moves into the interstitium at the arterial end and reabsorption of about 90% of the filtrate occurs at the venous end. The net effect across the capillary is a small gradient (0.3 mmHg) favoring filtration into the interstitium. This interstitial filtrate is normally returned to the circulation by the lymphatics (Table 7.2).

In clinical practice, pathologic conditions may arise (e.g., increased capillary hydrostatic pressure), resulting in an increase in net filtration into the interstitium that exceeds the limit of lymphatic drainage, and edema supervenes (Table 7.3). Conversely, if the capillary pressure falls significantly, net reabsorption of fluid into the capillaries occurs (transcapillary filling), and the plasma volume increases at the expense of the interstitial compartment.[4,6,7]

ACID-BASE HOMEOSTASIS

Under normal conditions, the H^+ concentration, and therefore the pH of the extracellular fluid, varies little from the normal values of 40 nanomol/L and 7.4, respectively, despite the continuous addition of endogenously produced acids and bases. Thus, the daily metabolism of carbohydrates and fats generates 15,000 mmol of CO_2, from which carbonic acid is formed. In addition, noncarbonic acids and bases result from the metabolism of proteins and other substances. Noncarbonic acids are derived primarily from the oxidation of sulfur-containing amino acids (methionine and cysteine), cationic amino acids (arginine and lysine), and hydrolysis of dietary biphosphate, $H_2PO_4^{--}$. Metabolism of anionic amino acids (glutamate and aspartate) and organic anions (such as citrate and lactate) is the major source of alkali.[2]

Acid-base homeostasis involves three major processes: (1) chemical buffering by the extracellular and intracellular buffer systems, (2) regulation of the pCO_2 in the blood by alveolar ventilation, and (3) control of the plasma bicarbonate concentration by changes in renal hydrogen ion excretion.[2] Buffers are aqueous systems that tend to minimize changes in pH when small amounts of acid or base are added.[8] The body buffers are primarily a mixture of weak and therefore poorly dissociated acids and their salts. H^+ ions added in the form of a

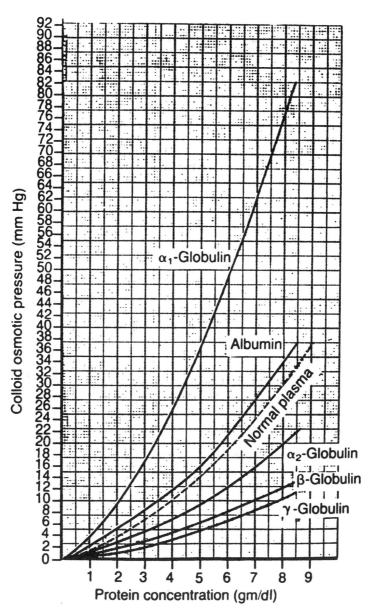

FIGURE 7.6. Colloid osmotic pressure in relation to the concentration of the various fractions of the plasma proteins. The dashed line shows the colloid osmotic pressure of normal plasma proteins, which are a mixture of the others. (From Guyton,[4] modified after Ott. *Klin Wschr* 1956;34:1079.)

TABLE 7.2. Exchange of Water Between the Intravascular (Plasma) and Interstitial Compartments

	Arterial End of Capillary	Venous End of Capillary	Mean
Forces Tending to Move Fluid out of Capillary (mmHg)			
Capillary hydrostatic pressure	30	10	17.3
Negative interstitial hydrostatic pressure	3	3	3.0
Interstitial colloid osmotic pressure	8	8	8.0
	41	21	28.3
Forces Tending to Move Fluid into Capillary (mmHg)			
Plasma oncotic pressure	28	28	28.0
Net Force			
	13 mmHg out of capillary	7 mmHg into capillary	0.3 mmHg out of capillary

Source: Modified after Guyton AC. *Textbook of Physiology*, 8th ed. Philadelphia: WB Saunders Company, 1991, pp. 178–179.

strong acid combine with anions from the salt component of the buffer to form a weakly dissociated acid that consequently yields fewer hydrogen ions than the strong acid originally added. As a result, the fall in pH is diminished.[9] The bicarbonate/carbon dioxide buffer system is the major extracellular buffer system. Other, quantitatively less important, buffers in the ECF include inorganic phosphate and the plasma proteins.[2]

The bicarbonate/carbon dioxide buffer system is described by the following equation:

$$H^+ + HCO_3^- \leftrightarrow H_2CO_3 \leftrightarrow H_2O + \underset{\substack{\text{aqueous} \\ \text{phase}}}{CO_2} \leftrightarrow \underset{\substack{\text{gas} \\ \text{phase}}}{CO_2} \qquad (5)$$

This buffer system is very effective because the pCO_2, reflecting the concentration of CO_2 in the gas phase, can be regulated by changes in alveolar ventilation.

The functions of this buffer system are quantitatively expressed in the Henderson–Hasselbach equation, which defines the pH in terms of the ratio of bicarbonate and carbonic acid present in the blood:[10]

$$pH = pK + \log \frac{HCO_3^-}{H_2CO_3} \qquad (6)$$

TABLE 7.3. Causes of Edema

I. Increased Capillary Pressure
  A. Excessive kidney retention of salt and water
  B. High venous pressure
    1. Heart failure
    2. Local venous block
    3. Failure of venous pumps
      (a) Paralysis of muscles
      (b) Immobilized parts of body
      (c) Failure of venous valves
  C. Decreased arteriolar resistance
    1. Excessive body heat
    2. Paralysis of sympathetic nervous system
    3. Effects of vasodilator drugs
II. Decreased Plasma Proteins
  A. Loss of proteins in urine (nephrosis)
  B. Loss of protein from denuded skin areas
    1. Burns
    2. Wounds
  C. Failure to produce proteins
    1. Liver disease
    2. Serious protein or caloric malnutrition
III. Increased Capillary Permeability
  A. Immune reactions that cause release of histamine and other immune products
  B. Toxins
  C. Bacterial infections
  D. Vitamin deficiency—especially vitamin C
  E. Prolonged ischemia
  F. Burns
IV. Blockage of Lymph Return
  A. Blockage of lymph nodes by cancer
  B. Blockage of lymph nodes by infection—especially with filaria nematodes
  C. Congenital absence of or abnormality of lymphatic vessels

Source: From Guyton AC. *Textbook of Medical Physiology*, 8th ed. Philadelphia: WB Saunders Company, 1991, p. 281.

where pK, the dissociation constant for this buffer system, has been measured to equal 6.1.

To maintain a normal body pH of 7.4, the ratio of bicarbonate to carbonic acid must remain 20:1, as depicted:

$$7.4 = 6.1 + \log \frac{27 \text{ mEq/L}}{1.35 \text{ mEq/L}}$$

$$7.4 = 6.1 + \log \frac{20}{1}$$

$$7.4 = 6.1 + 1.3$$

As long as the 20 : 1 ratio is maintained, regardless of the absolute values, the pH remains 7.4. When an acid, such as H_2SO_4, is added to the system, Equation 5 is driven to the right by mass action:

$$H_2SO_4 + 2NaHCO_3 \rightarrow Na_2SO_4 + 2H_2CO_3 \tag{7}$$

$$2H_2CO_3 \rightarrow 2H_2O + 2CO_2 \tag{8}$$

Thus, HCO_3^- concentration decreases, and aqueous CO_2 and hence alveolar CO_2 increase. The resultant rise in pCO_2 triggers an increase in alveolar ventilation that immediately eliminates CO_2 in an amount exactly necessary to restore the HCO_3^- : H_2CO_3 ratio to 20 : 1.[10]

These compensatory responses in the ECF compartment to minimize changes in pH are accompanied by analogous responses in the cells, since a portion of the H^+ ions added to the ECF enters the cells. To maintain electroneutrality, H^+ ions enter the cells in exchange for intracellular Na^+ and K^+. In erythrocytes, electroneutrality is maintained by the concomitant entrance of Cl^- and H^+ ions into the cells (Figure 7.7). Within cells the primary buffers are proteins and organic and inorganic phosphates; hemoglobin is the main buffer in erythrocytes.[2] In addition, bone represents an important site of acid-base buffering. Bone can take up excess H^+ ions in exchange for surface Na^+ and K^+, and pH is also controlled by the dissolution of bone mineral, which results in the release of buffer compounds into the ECF. These compounds include $NaHCO_3$ and $KHCO_3$ initially and then $CaCO_3$ and $CaHPO_4$.[2] It should be recognized that transcellular exchange of H^+ for K^+ observed in severe metabolic acidemia may result in clinically significant hyperkalemia.[2]

Although the various buffer systems minimize changes in pH consequent to the addition of acid or alkali to the ECF, the excess H^+ ions or HCO_3^- ions added must still be excreted by the kidney to prevent progressive depletion of the body buffers.[2] Thus, the renal contribution to acid-base balance consists mainly of reabsorption of normally filtered HCO_3^-, about 4,500 mEq/day, and the generation of new HCO_3^- to replace alkali lost in the stool or consumed in neutralizing acid produced by cellular metabolism or an exogenous acid load. These functions are accompanied by the tubular secretion of H^+. H^+ available for secretion is generated within the renal tubular cell from the reaction of CO_2 with H_2O to form H_2CO_3 and then $H^+ + HCO_3^-$. This reaction is catalyzed by carbonic anhydrase.[1]

Cell   Extracellular fluid

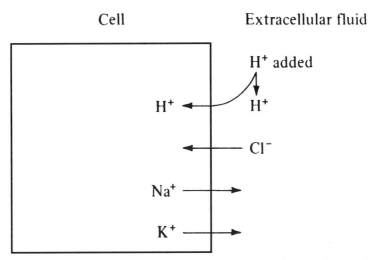

FIGURE 7.7. Effect of an HCl load on extracellular Cl^-, Na^+, and K^+. As H^+ enters the cells to be buffered, either Cl^+ follows H^+ into the cells or intracellular Na^+ and K^+ leave the cells and move into the extracellular fluid. These ion shifts are reversed when H^+ ions are removed from the extracellular fluid. (From Rose BD. *Clinical Physiology of Acid-Base and Electrolyte Disorders*, 4th ed. New York: McGraw-Hill, Inc., 1994, p. 291.)

The HCO_3^- ion formed in the reaction is reabsorbed into the peritubular blood. In the proximal tubular cells, H^+ is secreted into the tubular lumen (i.e., into the urine) in exchange for Na^+, and HCO_3^- moves from the tubular cells into the peritubular capillary blood accompanied by Na^+. In the cells of the collecting tubule, H^+ ion is secreted by active transport into the lumen (urine) or is secreted in exchange for K^+.[2] Here, HCO_3^- ions in the collecting tubule cell move into the peritubular capillary blood in exchange for Cl^- (Fig. 7.8).[2,4] In either case, the H^+ secreted into the tubular lumen may combine with filtered HCO_3^-, with NH_3, or with urinary buffers such as HPO_4^{--}, citrate, acetate, or creatinine,[1] forming titratable acid. If the secreted H^+ ions combine with filtered HCO_3^-, the net effect is HCO_3^- reabsorption; if the secreted H^+ ions combine with urinary buffers or NH_3, new HCO_3^- is added to the ECF, and the plasma HCO_3^- concentration rises (Fig. 7.9). These processes are reversed in the face of an alkali load.

The rate of tubular acid secretion is substantially regulated by the pH of the ECF. When pH < 7.4, hydrogen ion secretion can increase several fold with a concomitant increase in ECF HCO_3^- concentration. Conversely, at an ECF pH > 7.4, hydrogen ion secretion into the urine diminishes,[4] and sodium bicarbonate loss in the urine is increased as a result of secretion of bicarbonate and decreased reabsorption. These very efficient mechanisms available for the excretion of bicarbonate, however, are diminished in the presence of decreased effective circulating volume, chloride depletion, or hypokalemia. The latter are common clinical conditions most often associated with prolonged vomiting or loss of

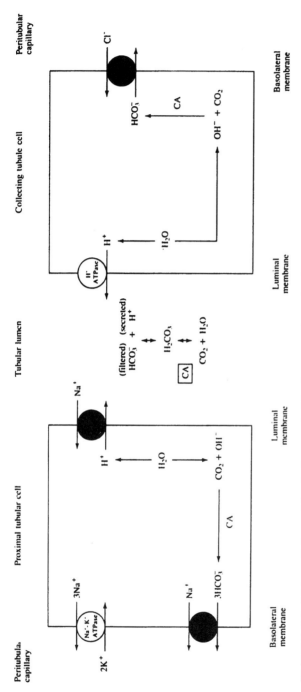

FIGURE 7.8. Major cellular and luminal events in bicarbonate reabsorption in the proximal tubule and the collecting tubules. Intracellular H_2O breaks down into an H^+ ion and an OH^- ion. The latter combines with CO_2 to form HCO_3^-, via a reaction catalyzed by carbonic anhydrase (CA). In the proximal tubule, the H^+ is secreted into the lumen by the Na^+–H^+ exchanger, whereas the HCO_3^- is returned to the systemic circulation primarily by a Na^+–$3HCO_3^-$ cotransporter. These same processes occur in the collecting tubules, although they are respectively mediated by an active H^+-ATPase pump in the luminal membrane and a Cl^-–HCO_3^- exchanger in the basolateral membrane. The secreted H^+ ions combine with filtered HCO_3^- to form carbonic acid (H_2CO_3) and then $CO_2 + H_2O$, which can be passively reabsorbed. This dissociation of carbonic acid is facilitated when luminal carbonic anhydrase (CA in box) is present, as occurs in the early proximal tubule. The net effect is HCO_3^- reabsorption, even though the HCO_3^- ions returned to the systemic circulation are not the same as those that were filtered. Although not shown, the collecting tubule cells also have H^+-K^+-ATPase pumps in the luminal membrane that are primarily involved in K^+ reabsorption. (From Rose BD. *Clinical Physiology of Acid-Base and Electrolyte Disorders*, 4th ed. New York: McGraw-Hill, Inc., 1994, p. 305.)

Tubular lumen
(Filtered)

Tubular Cell

Peritubular
Capillary

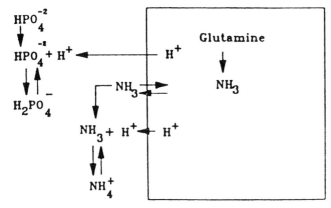

FIGURE 7.9. Formation of titratable acids and NH_4^+. (From Kelley WN [Ed]. *Textbook of Internal Medicine*, 2nd ed. Philadelphia: JB Lippincott Company, 1992, p. 689.)

gastric juice by nasogastric aspiration, producing metabolic alkalosis. Under these circumstances, the homeostatic mechanisms tending to restore volume prevail over those tending to relieve alkalosis.

Thus, decreased ECV triggers angiotensin and aldosterone release, which in turn stimulates reabsorption of urinary Na^+ and water. Angiotensin activates Na^+ reabsorption in exchange for H^+ secretion in the proximal renal tubule. Aldosterone promotes Na^+ reabsorption accompanied by Cl^- or in exchange for either K^+ or H^+.[10] In the face of hypokalemia, exchange for H^+ prevails. In addition, hypokalemia stimulates the movement of H^+ into cells in exchange for intracellular K^+, producing a fall in intracellular pH. Low pH in the renal tubular cells triggers renal urinary acidification, further enhancing Na^+ reabsorption in exchange for H^+. When Cl^+ depletion coexists, less Cl^- ion is available to accompany the renal Na reabsorption stimulated by low ECV. An increased proportion of Na^+ reabsorption must, therefore, be associated with exchange for H^+, to maintain electroneutrality. All of these responses enhance renal urinary acidification and explain the "paradoxical" aciduria observed in hypochloremic, hypokalemic alkalosis and the perpetuation of the alkalosis (contraction alkalosis) until ECV and plasma potassium and chloride levels are returned to normal.[2,3,5,10,11]

Analysis of Acid-Base Derangements

Acid-base derangements may be due to (1) disturbances that primarily affect alveolar ventilation, thereby producing abnormalities in arterial pCO_2 (Table 7.4), or (2) diseases that primarily affect the pH of the ECF and, therefore,

TABLE 7.4. Causes of Respiratory Disturbances

Acidosis (Hypoventilation)	Alkalosis (Hyperventilation)
Airway obstruction	Central nervous system disorders
Foreign body, pneumonia, emphysema, laryngospasm	Injury, tumor, stroke, anxiety
Central nervous system depression	Hypoxia
Narcotics, anesthetics, injury, tumor	Adult respiratory distress syndrome, pulmonary embolus, atelectasis, anemia
Thoracic injury	Mechanical ventilation
Pneumothorax, flail chest, tracheal tear	Exces tidal volume and/or rate
Mechanical ventilation	Hypermetabolism
Inadequate rate and/or tidal volume, increased dead space	Fever, injury, sepsis
Miscellaneous	Miscellaneous
Congestive heart failure, myopathy, severe obesity	Congestive heart failure, salicylate intoxication, cirrhosis

Source: From Sabiston DC Jr (Ed). *Textbook of Surgery: The Biological Basis of Modern Surgical Practice*, 14th ed. Philadelphia: WB Saunders Company, 1991, p. 63.

the plasma HCO_3^- concentration. Respiratory acidosis and respiratory alkalosis, characterized by high and low pCO_2 levels, respectively, can be partially compensated by renal mechanisms that produce secondary changes in plasma HCO_3^- concentration. Metabolic acidosis and metabolic alkalosis, characterized by low or high plasma HCO_3^- concentration, respectively, each trigger a sequence of compensatory responses over time, including secondary changes in alveolar ventilation and, hence, in arterial pCO_2 levels (Fig. 7.10, Table 7.5).

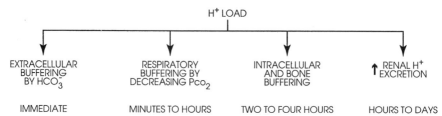

FIGURE 7.10. Sequential response to a H^+ load, culminating in the restoration of acid-base balance by the renal excretion of the excess H^+. (From Rose BD. *Clinical Physiology of Acid-Base and Electrolyte Disorders*, 4th ed. New York: McGraw-Hill, Inc., 1994, p. 337.)

TABLE 7.5. Summary of Acid-Base Disorders

	Defect	Common Causes	$\dfrac{BHCO_3}{H_2CO_3}$	Compensation
Respiratory acidosis	Retention of CO_2 (decreased alveolar ventilation)	Depression of respiratory center by morphine CNS injury Pulmonary disease: emphysema, pneumonia	↑Denominator Ratio less than 20:1	Renal Retention of bicarbonate, excretion of acid salts, increased ammonia formation Chloride shift into red cells
Respiratory alkalosis	Excessive loss of CO_2 (increased alveolar ventilation)	Hyperventilation: emotional disturbances, severe pain, assisted ventilation, encephalitis	↓Denominator Ratio greater than 20:1	Renal Excretion of bicarbonate, retention of acid salts, decreased ammonia formation
Metabolic acidosis	Retention of fixed acids or loss of base bicarbonate	Diabetes, azotemia, lactic acid accumulation, starvation Diarrhea, small bowel fistulas	↓Numerator Ratio less than 20:1	Pulmonary (rapid): increased rate and depth of breathing Renal (slow): as in respiratory acidosis
Metabolic alkalosis	Loss of fixed acids Gain of base bicarbonate Potassium depletion	Vomiting or gastric suction with pyloric obstruction Excessive intake of bicarbonate Diuretics	↑Numerator Ratio greater than 20:1	Pulmonary (rapid): decreased rate and depth of breath[a] Renal (slow): as in respiratory alkalosis

[a]Compensation limited by the fall in pO_2 associated with decreased ventilation.[13]

Source: Modified after Sabiston DC Jr (ed). *Textbook of Surgery: The Biological Basis of Modern Surgical Practice*, 14th ed. Philadelphia: WB Saunders Company, 1991, p. 62.

TABLE 7.6. Respiratory and Metabolic Components of Acid-Base Disorders

	Acute (Uncompensated)			Chronic (Partially Compensated)		
	pH	pCO$_2$ (respiratory component)	Plasma HCO$_3$ (metabolic component)	pH	pCO$_2$ (respiratory component)	Plasma HCO$_3$ (metabolic component)
Respiratory acidosis	↓↓	↑↑	N	↓	↑↑	↑
Respiratory alkalosis	↑↑	↓↓	N	↑	↓↓	↓
Metabolic acidosis	↓↓	N	↓↓	↓	↓	↓
Metabolic alkalosis	↑↑	N	↑↑	↑	↑?	↑

Source: Modified after Sabiston DC Jr (Ed). *Textbook of Surgery: The Biological Basis of Modern Surgical Practice*, 14th ed. Philadelphia: WB Saunders Company, 1991, p. 62.

In acute, uncompensated acid-base disturbances, determining the nature of the derangement is simplified because only the pCO$_2$ *or* the HCO$_3^-$ concentration is abnormal. In patients in whom there are changes in both the pCO$_2$ *and* the HCO$_3^-$ concentration, the abnormalities may reflect partial compensation for primary respiratory or primary metabolic illness (Table 7.6),[10] or may reflect separate, coexistent respiratory and metabolic disorders, producing a mixed acid-base derangement. Since treatment is based on the underlying pathology, it is necessary to determine the respiratory and metabolic components in a given patient. Arterial blood gas analysis, including pH, pCO$_2$, and HCO$_3^-$ concentration, gives the requisite information for diagnosis. Primary changes in pCO$_2$, acute or chronic, are associated with corresponding changes in pH and HCO$_3^-$ concentration (Table 7.7).[12] For example, for each acute 10 mmHg deviation of pCO$_2$ above or below a normal value of 40, the pH changes in the opposite direction by approximately 0.07 units. These relationships permit determination of pH and HCO$_3^-$ values that can be attributed exclusively to a given pCO$_2$ level. pH and HCO$_3^-$ values outside the range expected with this pCO$_2$ level reflect the metabolic component of the acid-base disturbance. For example, a patient with acute respiratory distress has the following arterial blood gases:

$$pCO_2 = 70 \text{ mmHg}$$
$$pH = 7.10$$
$$HCO_3^- = 21 \text{ mEq/L}$$

Respiratory acidosis alone producing a pCO$_2$ of 70 should be associated with a pH of 7.19–7.23 and an HCO$_3^-$ level of 26–29 mEq/L (Table 7.7). The lower actual values in this patient indicate a concomitant metabolic acidosis.[12]

The metabolic component of an acid-base derangement is often reported in

TABLE 7.7. Acute and Chronic Changes in pCO$_2$, Arterial Ph, and HCO$_3^-$

pCO$_2$ (mmHg)	Arterial pH		HCO$_3^-$	
	Acute	Chronic	Acute	Chronic
15	7.61–7.74		15–21	
20	7.55–7.66		18–23	10–14
25	7.49–7.59		20–24	13–16
30	7.45–7.53	7.38–7.51	21–26	17–23
35	7.40–7.48		22–27	
40	7.37–7.44	7.37–7.51	23–27	23–31
45	7.33–7.39		24–28	
50	7.31–7.36	7.35–7.47	24–28	27–35
60	7.24–7.29	7.33–7.44	25–28	31–40
70	7.19–7.23	7.30–7.42	26–29	33–44
80	7.14–7.18	7.28–7.39	26–29	
90	7.09–7.13		27–29	
100		7.24–7.35		42–54

Source: From Civetta JM, Taylor WW, Kirby RR (Eds). *Critical Care.* Philadelphia: JB Lippincott Company, 1988, p. 338.

blood gas analyses in terms of *base deficit* or *base excess*, indicating metabolic acidosis or metabolic alkalosis, respectively. In performing blood gas analysis, the respiratory component is eliminated by equilibrating the arterial blood sample at 38°C in a gas with a pCO$_2$ of 40 mmHg and a pO$_2$ of 100 mmHg. This allows calculation of the *standard bicarbonate*, and from this value the base excess or base deficit, representing the metabolic component of the abnormality, can be determined.[10,13] The various causes of acid-base disturbances are outlined in Tables 7.8–7.11.

The metabolic acidoses can be divided into two groups by determining the *anion gap*:

$$\text{Anion gap} = [Na^+] - ([Cl^-] + [HCO_3^-]) \tag{9}$$

The normal value is 10–15 mEq/L. The "gap" represents anions not routinely measured in blood electrolyte determinations and thus reflects the sum of the serum proteins, sulfate, inorganic phosphate, and organic acids present in low concentrations. Acidosis associated with a high anion gap is generally secondary to increases in endogenously produced acids (e.g., lactic acidosis or ketoacidosis), decreases in renal excretion of acids (e.g., renal failure), or ingestion of toxins (Table 7.10).[14]

TABLE 7.8. Causes of Respiratory Acidosis

Alveolar hypoventilation
  Central nervous system depression
    Drug induced
    Sleep disorders
    Pickwickian syndrome
    Cerebral ischemia
    Cerebral trauma
  Neuromuscular disorders
    Myopathies
    Neuropathies
  Chest-wall abnormalities
    Flail chest
    Kyphoscoliosis
  Pleural abnormalities
    Pneumothorax
    Pleural effusion
  Airway obstruction
    Upper airway
      Foreign body
      Tumor
      Laryngospasm
      Sleep disorders
    Lower airway
      Severe asthma
      Chronic obstructive airway disease
      Tumor
  Parenchymal lung disease
    Pulmonary edema
      Cardiogenic
      Noncardiogenic
    Pulmonary emboli
    Pneumonia
    Aspiration
    Interstitial lung disease
  Ventilator malfunction
Increased CO_2 production
  Large carbohydrate loads (enteral or parenteral nutrition)
  Malignant hyperthermia
  Intense shivering
  Prolonged seizure activity
  Thyroid storm
  Extensive thermal injury (burns)

Source: From Morgan GE, Mikhail MS. *Clinical Anesthesiology.* Norwalk, CT: Appleton & Lange, 1992, p. 499.

TABLE 7.9. Causes of Respiratory Alkalosis

Central stimulation
  Pain
  Anxiety
  Ischemia
  Stroke
  Tumor
  Infection
  Fever
  Drug induced
    Salicylates
    Progesterone (pregnancy)
    Analeptics (doxapram)
Peripheral stimulation
  Hypoxemia
  High altitude
  Pulmonary disease
    Congestive heart failure
    Noncardiogenic pulmonary edema
    Asthma
    Pulmonary emboli
  Severe anemia
Unknown mechanism
  Sepsis
  Metabolic encephalopathies
Iatrogenic
  Ventilation induced

Source: From Morgan GE, Mikhail MS. *Clinical Anesthesiology.* Norwalk, CT: Appleton & Lange, 1992, p. 503.

FLUID AND ELECTROLYTE THERAPY

A variety of crystalloid and colloid preparations for parenteral administration are available to maintain homeostasis in fasting individuals, to replace ongoing losses, or to treat existing derangements. Commonly used preparations are presented in Tables 7.12 and 7.13.

Maintenance Therapy

In order to preserve fluid and electrolyte homeostasis for brief periods (e.g., 7–10 days), patients receive infusions of water, sodium, and potassium, usually as the chloride salts, in amounts approximating losses measurable in the urine and stool and insensible losses from the lungs and skin. Urine volume averages 0.5–1.0 ml/kg/hour; stool water is approximately 250 ml/day. Insensible losses average about 10 ml/kg/day and are increased 10% for each degree of fever above 37°C.[15] The requirement for sodium is in the range of 1–2 mEq/kg/day

TABLE 7.10. Causes of Metabolic Acidosis

Increased anion gap
  Increased production of endogenous nonvolatile acids
    Renal failure
      Acute
      Chronic
    Ketoacidosis
      Diabetic
      Starvation
    Lactic acidosis
    Mixed
      Nonketotic hyperosmolar coma
      Alcoholic
    Inborn errors of metabolism
  Ingestion of toxin
      Salicylate
      Methanol
      Ethylene Glycol
      Paraldehyde
      Toluene
      Sulfur
    Rhabdomyolysis
Normal anion gap (hyperchloremic)
  Increased gastrointestinal losses of HCO_3^-
    Diarrhea
    Anion exchange resins
    Ingestion of $CaCl_2$, $MgCl_2$
    Fistulae (pancreatic, biliary, or small bowel)
    Ureterosigmoidostomy or obstructed ileal loop
  Increased renal losses of HCO_3^-
    Renal tubular acidosis
    Carbonic anhydrase inhibitors
    Hypoaldosteronism
  Dilutional
    Large amounts of bicarbonate-free fluids
  Total parenteral nutrition
  Increased intake of chloride-containing acids
    Ammonium chloride
    Lysine hydrochloride
    Arginine hydrochloride

Source: From Morgan GE, Mikhail MS. *Clinical Anesthesiology.* Norwalk, CT: Appleton & Lange, 1992, p. 499.

and for potassium approximately 0.5–1.0 mEq/kg/day. Because normal kidneys can conserve or excrete as necessary to preserve fluid and electrolyte balance, normal persons have an enormously broad tolerance for salt and water. Therefore, homeostasis can be maintained with a wide variety of fluid and electrolyte

TABLE 7.11. Causes of Metabolic Alkalosis

Chloride sensitive
  Gastrointestinal
    Vomiting
    Gastric drainage
    Chloride diarrhea
    Villous adenoma
  Renal
    Diuretics
    Posthypercapnic
    Low chloride intake
  Sweat
    Cystic fibrosis
Chloride resistant
  Increased mineralocorticoid activity
    Primary hyperaldosteronism
    Edematous disorders (secondary hyperaldosteronism)
    Cushing's syndrome
    Licorice ingestion
    Bartter's syndrome
  Severe hypokalemia
Miscellaneous
  Massive blood transfusion
  Acetate-containing colloid solutions (Plasmanate)
  Alkaline administration with renal insufficiency
    Alkali therapy
    Combined antacid and cation exchange resin therapy
  Hypercalcemia
    Milk-alkali syndrome
    Bone metastases
  Sodium penicillins
  Glucose feeding after starvation

Source: From Morgan GE, Mikhail MS. *Clinical Anesthesiology.* Norwalk, CT: Appleton & Lange, 1992, p. 503.

formulations. However, for practical purposes, administration of maintenance fluid volumes in accordance with body weight, as indicated in Table 7.14, simplifies order writing, since the calculations outlined in the table apply to patients from infancy to old age. If the volume calculated is provided as dextrose (glucose) 5% in sodium chloride 0.2% with the addition of potassium chloride, 20 mEq/L, then the infusion will meet the maintenance fluid and electrolyte requirements outlined here. Thus, a 70 kg patient would receive a daily infusion of 2,500 ml of D_5 0.2% NaCl containing 20 mEq/L of KCl, calculated as follows:

TABLE 7.12. Commonly Used Parenteral Infusion Solutions

	Approx pH	mOsm/L	kcal/L	Na mEq/L	K mEq/L	Ca mEq/L	Cl mEq/L	Lactate mEq/L
Dextrose 5% in water	4.3	253	170[a]					
Dextrose 10% in water	4.3	505	340[a]					
Dextrose 5% in sodium chloride 0.2%	4.4	320	170[a]	34			34	
Dextrose 5% in sodium chloride 0.45%	4.4	405	170[a]	77			77	
Dextrose 5% in sodium chloride 0.9%	4.4	560	170[a]	154			154	
Sodium chloride 0.45%	5.6	154	—	77			77	
Sodium chloride 0.9%	5.6	308	—	154			154	
Dextrose 5% in lactated Ringer's	5.0	530	170[a]	130	4	3	109	28
Lactated Ringer's	6.3	275	—	130	4	3	109	28

[a]Based on caloric value of 1 g of monohydrated glucose, 3.4 kcal.

Source: Data from Trissel LA. *Handbook on Injectable Drugs*, 8th ed. Bethesda: American Society of Hospital Pharmacists, pp. 1109–1111.

1st 10 kg of body weight	$1,000$ ml (100×10)
2nd 10 kg of body weight	500 ml (10×50)
Remaining 50 kg of body weight	$\underline{1,000 \text{ ml } (50 \times 20)}$
	$2,500$ ml

This regimen would deliver 85 mEq of sodium (34 mEq/L × 2.5 L = 85 mEq), providing 1.2 mEq/kg and 50 mEq of potassium (20 mEq/L × 2.5 L = 50 mEq), providing 0.7 mEq/kg. The electrolytes are provided in a 5% dextrose solution to avoid hypotonic infusions but, more importantly, to meet the energy requirements of the brain and the other glucose-dependent glycolytic tissues (erythrocytes, leukocytes, active fibroblasts, certain phagocytes, peripheral nerves). When insufficient glucose is prescribed, the required energy substrate is derived by means of protein catabolism and gluconeogenesis. This protein-spar-

TABLE 7.13. Plasma Expanders and Colloid Preparations

	Approx pH	mOsm/L	kcal/L	Na mEq/L	Cl mEq/L
Human Albumin					
1. Human Albumin, 25%				130–160	
2. Human Albumin, 5%				130–160	
Plasma Protein Fraction, 5%					
1. Plasmanate (Cutter)				130–160	
2. Plamatein (Alpha Therapeutic)				130–160	
3. Plasma-Plex (Armour)				130–160	
4. Protenate (Hyland)				130–160	
Dextrans and Starch					
Dextrans and Starch					
1. Dextran 75, 6% in dextrose 5%	4	253	170		
2. Dextran 75, 6% in sodium chloride 0.9%	4.5	309		154	154
3. Dextran 70, 6% in sodium chloride 0.9%	4.5–7	300	—	154	154
4. Dextran 40, 10% in dextrose 5%	3–7	309	170		
5. Dextran 40, 10% in sodium chloride 0.9%	3.5–7	317		154	154
6. Hetastarch, 6% in sodium chloride 0.9%	3.5–7	310	—	154	154

ing effect of glucose is maximally achieved with about 100–150 g of glucose providing about 400 kcal. No further benefit in protein economy accrues, even with higher caloric intake in the absence of dietary protein.[16]

The maintenance fluid and electrolyte regimen outlined here is satisfactory for most surgical patients who must fast for up to 7–10 days. If oral intake must

TABLE 7.14. Maintenance Fluid Requirements

Body Weight	Fluid Required
For the 1st 10 kg (0–10 kg)	100 ml/kg/day
For the 2nd 10 kg (11–20 kg)	Add 50 ml/kg/day
For each kg over 20 kg	Add 20 ml/kg/day[a]

[a]For elderly patients or patients with cardiac disease, reduce this amount to 15 ml/kg/day.

be withheld for more than 7–10 days, a complete nutritional program should be considered in order to provide additional energy, a protein source, vitamins, essential fatty acids, and sufficient macro- and micronutrients so that energy, protein, and mineral balance can be achieved (infra vide).

Fluid Resuscitation

The fluid preparation chosen to replace ongoing volume losses or replete existing deficits depends on the nature and composition of the loss as well as its rapidity and hemodynamic consequences. Despite years of study, controversy remains concerning the relative merits and drawbacks of crystalloid and colloid infusions.

Restoration of intravascular volume deficits due to moderate blood loss or third-space extravasation associated with acute peritonitis, bowel obstruction, sepsis, burns, or extensive operative dissection can be achieved with available crystalloid or colloid preparations (Tables 7.12 and 7.13). In contrast to colloid infusions, crystalloids are rapidly equilibrated throughout the *entire* ECF compartment, and consequently volumes three- to fourfold greater than colloid infusions are necessary to achieve equivalent *intravascular* volume expansion. This rapid equilibration has the apparent benefit of restoring interstitial space deficits that accompany intravascular losses, but excess interstitial water may result in peripheral edema, depending on the amount of the crystalloid infusion. In addition, reabsorption of the excess interstitial space fluid into the vascular space as the acute illness resolves may result in pulmonary congestion, in the absence of careful hemodynamic monitoring. In response to clinical concerns that fluid resuscitation with large, rapid infusions of crystalloid solutions will increase the incidence of cardiopulmonary dysfunction, adult respiratory distress syndrome, and the requirement for ventilatory support, advocates of crystalloid resuscitation cite data indicating no increased incidence of these problems when the fluid therapy is appropriately monitored by hemodynamic parameters.[6,17]

In contrast, colloid infusions have the theoretical advantage that much smaller volumes can replete the intravascular space and, therefore, resuscitation is more rapid. This advantage is based on the fact that colloid preparations have a greater capacity to remain in the intravascular space unless the underlying disease is associated with increased microvascular permeability. In addition, as a result of increased plasma colloid oncotic pressure, interstitial fluid may be drawn into the intravascular space, thereby reducing interstitial edema and producing an amount of volume expansion that may actually exceed the quantity of colloid infused. However, in the presence of increased microvascular permeability (as in severely traumatized patients with sepsis), extravasation of intravascular colloid into the pulmonary interstitium may result in increased, rather than decreased, interstitial edema, thereby causing or aggravating the adult respiratory distress syndrome.[18,19]

Commercially available colloid preparations include blood-derived products (albumin and plasma protein fraction), products from bacterial sources (the dextrans), and synthetic products (hetastarch) (Table 7.13). Albumin and plasma protein fraction are heated to 60°C for at least 10 hours to minimize the risk of transmitting the hepatitis viruses. Plasma protein fraction contains about 88% albumin and 12% globulins. Dextrans are colloid preparations of glucose polymers that are produced by the bacterium *Leuconostoc meserentoides*. The two most widely used products are dextran 70 (average molecular weight 70,000) and dextran 40 (average molecular weight 40,000). Dextran 70 is generally preferred for volume expansion because dextran 40 is more rapidly eliminated.[17] These agents are associated with a dose-related hemostatic defect resulting from a decrease in platelet aggregation and adhesiveness. Infusions exceeding 20 ml/kg/day can interfere with blood typing and have been associated with renal failure. Anaphylactic reactions have also been described.[14,17] Hetastarch (hydroxyethyl starch) is an artificial colloid composed almost entirely of amylopectin. Sporadic cases of coagulopathy have been described, but coagulation studies are usually unaffected by infusions of 1–2 L.[14] The volume-expanding capacity of the various colloids appears to be comparable.

In 1989, Velanovich[19] published a meta-analysis of then-available randomized trials comparing mortality rates associated with crystalloid and colloid resuscitation (Level I evidence). In this analysis, a 12.3% difference in mortality rate in favor of crystalloids was observed among the trauma patients in the study population. In contrast, when nontrauma patients were pooled from the various studies, the meta-analysis revealed a 7.8% difference in mortality rate in favor of colloid therapy. Despite these trends, this meta-analysis evidently was not statistically significant at the 95% confidence interval.[17]

In 1998, Schierhout and Roberts[20] conducted a more extensive meta-analysis based on mortality data for 1,315 patients from 19 randomized or quasi-randomized trials in which critically ill patients who required fluid resuscitation were assigned to receive either colloid or crystalloid infusions (Level I evidence). Enrolled patients had sepsis, burns, trauma, or major surgery. The data from this meta-analysis revealed that mortality rates were similar between the groups receiving colloid or crystalloid solutions for volume replacement and did not support the benefit of colloid resuscitation in nontrauma patients reported by Velanovich.

Various investigators have reported successful resuscitation using hypertonic saline in patients suffering hemorrhage, endotoxic shock, trauma, and burns.

A survival benefit has been observed in some but not all studies comparing this form of therapy with isotonic fluid resuscitation.[6,17] Hypertonic solutions have greater volume-expanding capacity than isotonic crystalloid solutions, and volume expansion is probably enhanced at the expense of the intracellular fluid compartment.[17] In their review of the current status of resuscitation, Shires et al.[6] state that patients resuscitated with hypertonic saline require especially close monitoring of serum electrolytes to prevent hypernatremia and hyperosmolar coma. Thus, the safety and efficacy of hypertonic saline resuscitation remain to be determined.[6,18]

Replacement of Gastrointestinal Losses

Patients with abnormal losses of fluids and electrolytes from the gastrointestinal tract require fluid and electrolytes in amounts necessary to meet maintenance requirements, replete deficits, and replace ongoing losses. Modest volume losses extending over brief periods may be treated with standard fluid preparations with an electrolyte composition that approximates losses. Normal kidneys will adjust to compensate for minor disparities in electrolyte composition between the infusate and the gastrointestinal loss. The volume and electrolyte content of the various gastrointestinal secretions are presented in Table 7.15. Gastric losses can be managed with a solution of 0.45–0.9% NaCl in 5% dextrose containing 20 mEq KCl/L. Bicarbonate-containing secretions generally

TABLE 7.15. Volume and Electrolyte Content of Gastrointestinal Fluid Losses[a]

	Na^+ (mEq/L)	K^+ (mEq/L)	Cl^- (mEq/L)	HCO_3^- (mEq/L)	Volume (ml)
Gastric juice, high in acid	20 (20–30)	10 (5–40)	120 (80–150)	0	1,000–9,000
Gastric juice, low in acid	80 (70–140)	15 (5–40)	90 (40–120)	5–25	1,000–2,500
Pancreatic juice	140 (115–180)	5 (3–8)	75 (55–95)	80 (60–110)	500–1,000
Bile	148 (130–160)	5 (3–12)	100 (90–120)	35 (30–40)	300–1,000
Small-bowel drainage	110 (80–150)	5 (2–8)	105 (60–125)	30 (20–40)	1,000–3,000
Distal ileum and cecum drainage	80 (40–135)	8 (5–30)	45 (20–90)	30 (20–40)	1,000–3,000
Diarrheal stools	120 (20–160)	25 (10–40)	90 (30–120)	45 (30–50)	500–17,000

[a]Average values/24 hr with range in parentheses.

Source: From Way LW (Ed). *Current Surgical Diagnosis and Treatment*, 10th ed. Norwalk, CT: Appleton & Lange, 1994, p. 134.

can be replaced with lactated Ringer's solution in 5% dextrose; 10–20 mEq KCl should be added to each liter. When losses are sustained or massive, more precise replacement is required. In such patients, an aliquot of draining fluid is analyzed for electrolyte content, and additions to a standard preparation are made in the pharmacy so that the infusate matches the electrolyte content of the draining secretions. Excessive replacement should be avoided not only to prevent pulmonary congestion and edema but also because the additional fluid infused may actually further stimulate digestive secretions, the so-called third kidney effect of the gastrointestinal tract.[21] In this situation, a positive feedback cycle is initiated in which excessive parenteral infusion leads to increased gastrointestinal secretions, which in turn are replaced by ever greater parenteral volumes. This vicious cycle is identified by progressively increasing gastrointestinal secretions accompanying a concomitant diuresis. Although oliguria may occur, usually an increasing urine output is the cue to reduce the replacement volume.

Analysis of Fluid and Electrolyte Status

Assessment of fluid and electrolyte status is based on history, physical examination, serum electrolyte levels, urine values including volume, concentration, and sodium content, and, if necessary, hemodynamic parameters such as central venous pressure, pulmonary capillary wedge pressure, and cardiac output. Important features in establishing a diagnosis of hypovolemia or dehydration include a history of external losses such as vomiting, profuse diarrhea, tube or fistula drainage, or polyuria; the presence of acute conditions associated with third-space extravasation such as acute peritonitis or pancreatitis; or the use of diuretics or vigorous purging as in surgical bowel preparation. In addition, patients with complex problems often undergo a series of diagnostic tests requiring them to refrain from eating or drinking for a period of time preceding the test. A prolonged sequence of such tests is a subtle and often unrecognized basis for hypovolemia. The magnitude of the deficit can be estimated from such physical findings as tachycardia, hypotension, peripheral vasoconstriction, and oliguria, which occur promptly when there are large acute fluid losses. Decreased tissue turgor and intraocular pressure are manifestations of more chronic, ongoing negative fluid balance (Table 7.16). Laboratory findings in dehydration include rising hematocrit, increasing serum urea concentration, high urinary specific gravity, and low urinary sodium level (see below). Low central venous and pulmonary capillary wedge pressures confirm the diagnosis. The effect of dehydration on acid-base status is determined from serum electrolyte and arterial blood gas values, as discussed previously.

Volume overload is also an important finding in surgical patients and is manifest by cardiac gallop, dyspnea, rales, and dependent edema. A history of cardiac, renal, or liver disease may establish the etiology of the hypervolemia.

TABLE 7.16. Signs of Hypovolemia

Sign	Fluid Loss (Expressed as Percentage of Body Weight)		
	5%	10%	15%
Mucous membranes	Dry	Very dry	Parched
Sensorium	Normal	Lethargic	Obtunded
Orthostatic changes in pulse or blood pressure	Mild	Present	Marked
Urinary flow rate	Mildly decreased	Decreased	Markedly decreased
Pulse rate	Normal or increased	Increased	Markedly increased
Blood pressure	Normal	Mildly decreased	Decreased

Source: From Morgan GE, Mikhail MS. *Clinical Anesthesiology.* Norwalk, CT: Appleton & Lange, 1992, p. 478.

Preoperative Fluid Management

Anesthetic and operative risk is increased among patients arriving in the operating room with fluid or electrolyte derangements. For example, hypotension is frequently observed in dehydrated patients on the induction of general anesthesia. The effect of hypovolemia is magnified by the vasodilatation and myocardial depression associated with inhalation anesthetics. The interruption of normal baroreceptor reflexes by anesthesia abruptly reverses the increased vascular resistance and tachycardia that compensates for volume depletion in the awake patient.[18] Therefore, patients must be assessed preoperatively and appropriate treatment prescribed to render the patient euvolemic.

Many patients undergoing elective surgery do not require any preoperative intervention; refraining from eating or drinking for 12 hours prior to surgery has no discernible adverse consequences. On the other hand, patients with significant fluid and electrolyte abnormalities should be treated preoperatively; the time devoted to such resuscitative therapy depends on the urgency of the proposed operation. Patients undergoing diagnostic studies or treatments such as surgical bowel preparation, known to predispose to negative fluid balance, should receive parenteral infusions on the preoperative day to avoid fluid and electrolyte deficits. Lactated Ringer's solution or a solution of 0.45% NaCl and 5% dextrose, each containing 20 mEq of KCl/L, in volumes necessary to meet maintenance requirements as well as to replace losses, is generally satisfactory.

Intraoperative Fluid Management

The goals of intraoperative fluid therapy are to correct any remaining preexisting deficits, supply maintenance fluids and electrolytes, and replace blood loss, evaporative losses, and third-space extravasation. Patients with normal hemoglobin concentrations prior to operation can sustain losses of 10–20% of their blood volume (approximately 500–1,000 ml) without transfusions; crystalloid or colloid replacement suffices. Blood is administered for greater losses or when the hemoglobin level or the hematocrit falls below 7–10 g/dl or 21–30%, respectively. In elderly patients or those with significant cardiac disease, blood transfusion is recommended when the Hgb concentration falls below 10 g/dl.[14]

Evaporative losses are proportional to the size of the operative wound, the surface area of the body cavity exposed, and the duration of the surgical procedure.[14] In addition, evaporative losses are aggravated by the peripheral vasodilatation associated with regional and general anesthesia.[17] Third-space extravasation represents an internal redistribution of fluids, resulting in a decrease in the functional volume of the ECF compartment but not a loss of fluid from the body. Interstitial fluid increases in areas of surgical dissection, trauma, or inflammation. In abdominal surgery, fluid collects in the lumen and in the wall of the small bowel, and transudation of fluid across serosal surfaces results in the accumulation of free fluid in the peritoneal cavity. Again, the decrease in functional ECF volume is proportional to the magnitude of tissue injury, inflammation and surgical dissection, and the surface area of the affected tissues.

Evaporative and third-space losses are estimated and replaced continuously during the operation. Shires et al.[10] recommend replacement with a balanced salt solution such as lactated Ringer's solution, 500–1,000 ml/hour to a maximum of 2–3 L during a 4-hour major abdominal procedure. Morgan and Mikhail[14] have estimated requirements in relation to the magnitude of the operation (Table 7.17). Overaggressive fluid treatment is to be avoided because of the risk of fluid overload and pulmonary congestion in the postoperative period.

Intraoperative fluid management is monitored in the usual way, measuring hemodynamic parameters such as pulse and blood pressure, and urine output. Invasive monitoring with central venous or Swan–Ganz catheter is indicated when major fluid shifts are anticipated or occur unexpectedly intraoperatively.

TABLE 7.17. Evaporative and Third-Space Surgical Fluid Losses

Degree of Tissue Trauma	Additional Fluid Requirement
Minimal (eg, herniorrhapy)	0–2 ml/kg/hr
Moderate (eg, cholecystectomy)	2–4 ml/kg/hr
Severe (eg, bowel resection)	4–8 ml/kg/hr

Source: From Morgan GE, Mikhail MS. *Clinical Anesthesiology.* Norwalk, CT: Appleton & Lange, 1992, p. 481.

Postoperative Fluid Management

Considerations in the 24-hour period immediately following operation include maintenance therapy, treatment of any residual deficits, and replacement of ongoing losses (e.g., nasogastric suction, drainage tubes) and continuing third-space extravasation. The latter is most commonly observed in patients with massive peritonitis or extensive retroperitoneal dissection, as in ruptured aortic aneurysm. Potassium supplements are generally withheld on the operative day because a mild hyperkalemia is routinely observed after operation, due in part to release of potassium from dissected or injured tissues.[7,10,18] More importantly, potassium is withheld because the status of kidney function is unknown in the first hours following operation, even when urine volume is apparently normal. In the event of impaired renal function, hyperkalemia is a life-threatening abnormality. The likelihood of renal impairment correlates with the magnitude of the operation, the amount of blood loss, and the occurrence of episodes of hemodynamic instability and hypotension. Occasionally, however, potassium supplements are required, primarily when marked hypokalemia occurs or when borderline low potassium levels are observed in patients receiving digitalis preparations. If postoperative renal function is normal, potassium supplements may be started on the first or second postoperative day.

In the immediate postoperative period, measurement of urinary output is the primary method of monitoring fluid status. The goal of fluid therapy is to achieve urinary output of at least 0.5 ml/kg/hour.

Later in the postoperative course, as inflammatory conditions resolve and areas of injury and dissection heal, third-space sequestered fluid is reabsorbed into the vascular space. This autotransfusion, which often begins as early as the third postoperative day, may result in significant fluid overload with pulmonary congestion, tachycardia, gallop rhythm, and edema. In patients with conditions associated with large third-space extravasation, reabsorption should be anticipated by restricting fluids; diuretics are occasionally indicated.

Analysis of Oliguria

Low urine volume in the early postoperative period is a common clinical problem, usually but not always due to volume depletion. The differential etiology is presented in Table 7.18. The intraoperative record of fluid administration and estimated losses may or may not be helpful in the analysis. History, physical examination, electrocardiogram, arterial blood gases, and irrigation of the urinary catheter to establish patency can readily eliminate most of the causes of postoperative oliguria except hypovolemia and renal failure. Tachycardia, hypotension, and peripheral vasoconstriction with cold extremities support the diagnosis of volume depletion. A low hemoglobin concentration or hematocrit level is consistent with unreplaced blood loss, but these indices do not reliably reflect the extent of acute hemorrhage. An unexpectedly high hemoglobin or hematocrit level suggests unreplaced crystalloid losses.

TABLE 7.18. Etiology of Postoperative Oliguria or Anuria

A. Prerenal Causes

1. Volume depletion
   a. Unreplaced or ongoing blood loss
   b. Unreplaced or ongoing external loss of body fluids
   c. Unreplaced or ongoing third-space extravasation
2. Other causes of decreased effective circulating volume
   a. Congestive heart failure
   b. Myocardial infarction
   c. Pericardial tamponade
   d. Acute pulmonary embolism
   e. Advanced hepatic cirrhosis
   f. Arteriovenous fistula
   g. Hypotension:
      (1) Hypovolemia (See A1)
      (2) Anesthetic agents
      (3) Narcotics or other drugs
   h. Peripheral vasodilation due to bacteremia
3. Increased renovascular resistance
   a. Anesthesia
   b. Surgical operation
   c. Hepatorenal syndrome
4. Bilateral renovascular obstruction
   a. Embolism
   b. Thrombosis

B. Renal Causes: Acute Renal Failure

C. Postrenal Causes: Obstructive Uropathy

1. Bilateral ureteral obstruction or injury
2. Prostatic hypertrophy or other cause of bladder outlet obstruction
3. Pelvic hematoma
4. Urethral obstruction
5. Malfunctioning urinary catheter

In clinical practice, the most common diagnostic (and therapeutic) approach to differentiate hypovolemia from renal failure is to rapidly administer a fluid challenge of 250–500 ml of balanced salt solution, or transfuse blood, if indicated. Increased urine output establishes the diagnosis of volume depletion, but a failure to respond may reflect a residual large volume deficit unaffected by only 250–500 ml of fluid or, alternatively, acute renal failure. In this setting, another fluid challenge may be ordered if the lungs remain clear. Blood chemistry and urine studies are also helpful in distinguishing oliguria due to hypovolemia or renal failure (Table 7.19). When the diagnosis remains in doubt, central pressure monitoring is useful. When filling pressures are low, fluid admin-

TABLE 7.19. Laboratory Values in the Analysis of Oliguria

	Prerenal	Renal
Urine Specific Gravity[a]	>1.020	1.010
Urine Osmolality[a] (mOsm/kg)	>500	<400
Urine Sodium (mEq/L)	<20	>40
BUN/Serum Creatinine	>15	<10
Urine/Plasma Creatinine	>40	<20
Urine/Plasma Urea	>8	<3
Fractional Excretion of Filtered Sodium (FE$_{Na}$)[b]	<1	>2

[a]Interpretation invalid in presence of glucosuria or proteinuria.
[b]FE$_{Na}$ = (U/P Na) (100)/(U/P Cr).

istration is continued until values are normalized. Hypovolemia and acute renal failure can coexist initially, since hypovolemia, especially when associated with hypotension, may be the etiologic background for the development of intrinsic renal injury. Under these circumstances, oliguria will persist despite volume repletion, and fluid restriction must then be prescribed (see below).

Fluid and Electrolyte Management of Postoperative Renal Failure

In the presence of renal failure, fluid and electrolyte administration is markedly restricted. Dextrose, 5% in water, is provided at a daily maintenance rate of 10 ml/kg to cover insensible losses. Additional fluid and electrolytes are infused to replace other significant ongoing losses, including any urine output, but potassium is withheld. Central venous or left atrial pressure monitoring is invaluable in the assessment of fluid requirements when significant fluid shifts are anticipated. Restriction of fluid and potassium is of utmost importance since it is frequently desirable to delay hemodialysis in the newly postoperative patient as long as possible because of the dangers inherent in the use of heparin usually required for the extracorporeal circuit. On the other hand, surgical operations produce a catabolic state, resulting in accelerated azotemia and hyperkalemia, so dialysis is generally required by the second postoperative day. Marked hyperkalemia is the most common reason for earlier dialysis, but fluid overload, often manifest by hypertension, is another important indication.[22] Life-threatening hyperkalemia must be treated emergently while dialysis is being arranged. The pharmacologic management is presented in Table 7.20.

Analysis and Management of Hyponatremia

Low serum sodium concentration may be due to a variety of causes (Fig. 7.11). Hyponatremia can occur in patients with increased, near-normal or decreased ECF volume; increased, near-normal or decreased total body sodium;[23] and it may be associated with hypotonic, isotonic, or hypertonic serum. Never-

TABLE 7.20. Emergency Treatment of Hyperkalemia

Method/Agent	Dose	Onset of Effect
1. Antagonism of Membrane Actions of Potassium		
A. Calcium	10 ml of calcium gluconate infused IV over 2–3 minutes with EKG monitoring. Can repeat after 5 minutes if EKG changes of hyper-kalemia persist.	Within 5 minutes
B. Hypertonic saline (if hyponatremic)	As needed to increase serum sodium	—
2. Increased Potassium Entry into Cells		
A. Glucose and Insulin	IV administration of 10 units of regular insulin and 50 g glucose. Also may use continuous infusions of glucose and insulin: 500 ml 10% glucose with 10 units of regular insulin.	Within 30 minutes
B. Sodium bicarbonate	1 ampule (44.6 mEq) of 7.5% $NaHCO_3$ infused IV over 5 minutes. May repeat in 30 minutes	Within 30–60 minutes
C. β_2-adrenergic agonists	Albuterol, 10–20 mg by nebulizer or 0.5 mg IV	Within 30 minutes
D. Hypertonic saline (if hyponatremic)		
3. Removal of the Excess Potassium		
A. Cation-exchange resin (Kayexalate)	20 mg Kayexalate orally with 100 ml of 2% sorbitol solution; or retention enema containing 50 g Kayexalate, 50 ml of 70% Sorbitol, and 100–150 ml tap water. Can repeat orally every 4–6 hr. Can repeat enema every 2–4 hr.	Variable

Source: Modified after Rose BD. *Clinical Physiology of Acid-Base and Electrolyte Disorders*, 4th ed. New York: McGraw-Hill, Inc. 1984, p. 848.

theless, hyponatremia, defined as a plasma sodium concentration below 135 mEq/L, usually reflects hypotonicity. It is the latter condition that is primarily responsible for the neurologic manifestations of severe hyponatremia, since low-plasma tonicity induces the movement of water into cells, including brain cells, and water intoxication.[2]

Despite a wide array of potential conditions that may underlie hypotonic

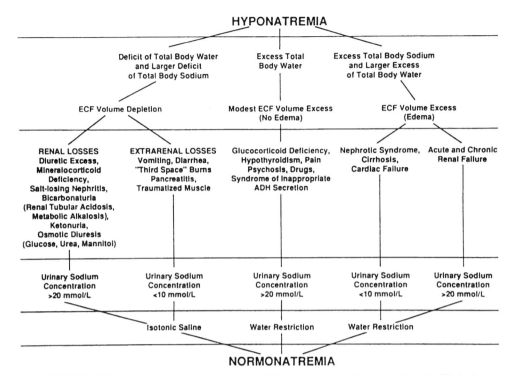

FIGURE 7.11. Analysis and management of hyponatremia. (From Berl et al. Clinical disorders of water metabolism. *Kidney Int* 1976;10:117.)

hyponatremia in surgical patients, the usual causes are (1) extrarenal losses such as vomiting, diarrhea, and third-space extravasation, producing ECF volume depletion; (2) the more subtle but perhaps more common condition of modest volume expansion due to free-water retention; or (3) volume expansion and sodium retention due to an edematous disorder, such as congestive heart failure, or portal cirrhosis. Distinguishing between these conditions is important since the treatments, volume repletion in the first and volume restriction, sometimes with concomitant loop diuretics, in the latter two, are diametrically opposed.

In volume-depleted patients, hyponatremia (hypotonic dehydration) usually reflects partial volume repletion due to oral water consumption induced by the thirst mechanism or, among hospitalized patients, parenteral infusion of hypotonic solutions. These patients have a low concentration of urinary sodium (<10 mEq/L). Treatment consists of volume and sodium repletion.

In contrast to these volume-depleted surgical patients with a deficit in total body sodium, hyponatremia may be observed in postoperative or trauma patients as a result of excessive free-water retention due to increased ADH secretion. Increased ADH secretion unrelated to the usual stimuli of hyperosmolality or hypovolemia is commonly observed for 2–5 days after major surgery.[2,18] The ADH response appears to be mediated by pain afferents that directly stimulate the hypothalamus. The hyponatremia observed under these circumstances may be aggravated by infusion of hypotonic solutions. These patients have high urinary sodium values (>20 mEq/L). The hyponatremia generally responds to fluid restriction.

Certain drugs have also been associated with free-water retention and antidiuresis, presumably by increasing ADH activity, just as seen in postoperative patients. Of particular interest for oncologists is the association of hyponatremia with the antineoplastic agents vincristine, vinblastine, and cyclophosphamide. It is particularly important to anticipate potential acute hyponatremia in patients receiving intravenous cyclophosphamide, because these patients are often vigorously hydrated to avert urologic complications, such as hemorrhagic cystitis.[2,23] Hyponatremia due to free-water retention likewise has been observed in patients with a wide array of tumors, including cancer of the lung, duodenum, pancreas, ureter, bladder, prostate; thymoma; lymphoma; and Ewing's sarcoma. The mechanism is thought to be tumor production of ectopic ADH.

Finally, oxytocin, a hormone synthesized in the hypothalamus and released from the neurohypophysis, as is ADH, also has significant antidiuretic activity. Infusion of oxytocin in dextrose and water, to stimulate labor in pregnant women, has resulted in water retention, severe hyponatremia, and seizures in both mother and fetus. These complications can be avoided by restricting water consumption and preparing the hormone infusion in isotonic saline rather than in dextrose and water.[2]

When severe clinical manifestations of hypotonic hyponatremia supervene, urgent therapy with hypertonic saline is required to raise ECF tonicity and thereby ameliorate cerebral edema, the major underlying pathology. The morbidity and mortality of this condition are influenced by several factors: the severity and rate of development of the hyponatremia, the age and gender of the patient, and the nature and magnitude of the underlying disease. The very young, the very elderly, women, and alcoholics appear to be at particular risk. Neurologic symptoms usually do not occur until body tonicity falls below 250 mOsm/kg, corresponding to a serum sodium concentration of 125 mEq/L. At this level of hypotonicity, anorexia, nausea, and malaise may develop. At sodium levels of 110–120 mEq/L, headache, lethargy, confusion, agitation, and obtundation can be seen. Seizures and coma may occur when serum sodium falls below 110 mEq/L.[24]

Symptomatic hypotonic hyponatremia that develops acutely, within several days, should be treated aggressively with 3–5% hypertonic saline infused at a rate necessary to increase serum sodium concentration about 1–2 mEq/L/hr, until a sodium level of 120–125 mEq/L is reached. Chronic hypotonicity that develops over many days or weeks is more safely treated by increasing serum sodium levels no more than 0.5 mEq/L/hr.[18,24] In patients at risk of developing pulmonary edema due to volume overload (such as those with congestive heart failure), loop diuretics are administered to achieve negative fluid balance, and 3% saline is infused concomitantly to replace urinary sodium losses while the fluid status is closely followed. In addition, careful monitoring during hypertonic saline infusion is mandatory because, despite the dangers of severe hyponatremia and hypotonicity, overly rapid correction may also be harmful, leading to a severe neurologic disorder, central pontine myelinolysis.[2]

To estimate the amount of sodium required to increase the serum concentration to a safe level of 125 mEq/L, the deficit per liter is multiplied by the total body water.[2] The latter is approximately 60% of body weight. Thus, the sodium required for a 70 kg patient with serum sodium of 110 mEq/L can be calculated as follows:

$$\text{Sodium required} = (125 - 110)(70 \times 0.6)$$
$$= 15 \times 42$$
$$= 630 \text{ mEq}$$

Isotonic hyponatremia is an artifactual reduction of plasma sodium concentration due to paraproteinemia or hypertriglyceridemia. These substances do not contribute to osmolality but produce an increase in plasma volume (but not plasma water). *Hypertonic hyponatremia* is associated with hyperglycemia or the administration of hypertonic substances, such as mannitol, which induces water movement out of the cells across a transcellular osmotic gradient. The initial effect is a dilutional hyponatremia. Later, when significant osmotic diuresis ensues, hypernatremia will develop.

Analysis and Management of Hypernatremia

Hypernatremia, defined as a serum sodium concentration greater than 145 mEq/L, may be due to a variety of causes (Fig. 7.12), but, regardless of etiology, hypernatremia always implies coexistent hypertonicity of all body fluids and intracellular volume contraction.[24] This condition may arise from a pure water deficit so that the total body sodium remains normal. Extracellular fluid contraction occurs, but clinical hypovolemia is unusual because the loss is significantly compensated by a shift of water from the intracellular space to the ECF compartment. Among cancer patients, this mechanism of hypernatremia is observed primarily in those with *secondary neurogenic diabetes insipidus* due to suprasellar and intrasellar tumors, primary or metastatic; or in those with *nephrogenic diabetes insipidus* due to hypokalemia or hypercalcemia (the major electrolyte abnormalities associated with a defect in renal concentrating capacity); or is due to various drugs such as the antineoplastic agents vinblastine, ifosfamide, cisplatinum; certain antibiotics such as amphoteracin, gentamicin, and methicillin; or angiographic dye.[2,23] Finally, essentially pure water deficits also are observed when insensible losses from the skin are increased by fever or exercise and in patients with a tracheostomy who are breathing unhumidified air.

Hypernatremia may also be caused by loss of sodium and water but with a

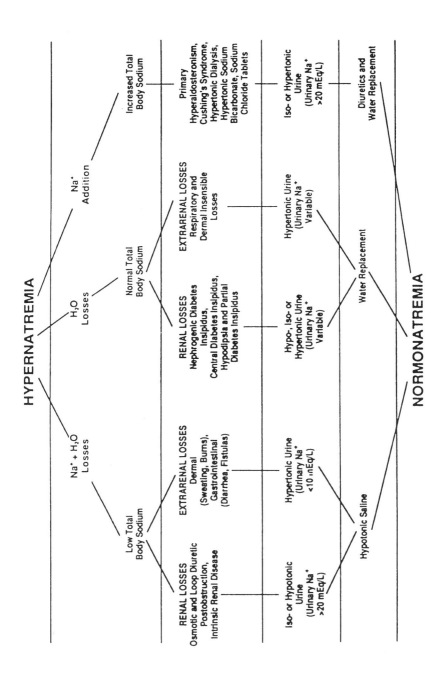

FIGURE 7.12. Analysis and management of hypernatremia. (From Berl et al. Clinical disorders of water metabolism. *Kidney Int* 1976;10:117.)

relatively greater loss of water. Total body sodium falls and symptomatic hypovolemia may supervene. Profuse sweating due to exercise or evaporative loss from burns may result in hypernatremia by this mechanism, but in oncologic patients the more common causes are gastrointestinal losses of hypotonic secretions, such as nasogastric tube drainage, vomitus, or diarrhea;[24] and osmotic diuresis due to mannitol, hyperglycemia, or, occasionally, urea.

Glucosuria, which develops when serum glucose levels reach 180–200 mg/dL, induces an osmotic diuresis resulting in an obligatory excretion of large volumes of salt-poor urine so that free water loss greatly exceeds sodium loss. As discussed previously, the initial increase in serum tonicity due to hyperglycemia will result in dilutional hyponatremia as intracellular water moves into the extracellular compartment. However, as osmotic diuresis continues, volume depletion and hypernatremia supervene. Sustained hyperglycemia with massive osmotic diuresis will eventually produce neurologic manifestations such as confusion, disorientation, lethargy, and finally hyperosmolar coma. Treatment is aimed toward reducing blood sugar and volume repletion with 0.45% sodium chloride solution.[10,16] Potassium supplements may be required as resuscitation proceeds.

Intake of high protein, hyperosmolar enteral or parenteral feeding solutions may induce a urea diuresis resulting in azotemia, hypernatremia, and low ECF volume. These effects, especially common in patients unable to drink or communicate thirst, can be averted when feedings provide at least 7 ml of free water per gram of dietary protein.[3,10,16]

The magnitude of free-water deficit when hypernatremia occurs with negligible or minimal sodium loss can be estimated by assuming that the total body osmoles remain unchanged.[2,24] For example, in a 60 kg patient with a serum sodium of 160 mEq/L, the water deficit can be estimated as follows:

(1) Normal total body water (TBW) = $(60 \times 60\%) = 36$ L

(2) Total body osmoles = $TBW \times P_{osm}$

Since the P_{osm} is primarily determined by the plasma Na^+ concentration and its accompanying anions,

$$(3) \text{ Total body osmoles} \cong TBW \times 2[Na^+]$$
$$\cong 36L \times 280$$
$$\cong 10080 \text{ mOsm}$$

$$(4) \text{ Current total body water} \cong \frac{10080}{2 \times 160} = 31.5 \text{ L}$$

$$(5) \text{ Water deficit} \cong 36 - 31.5 \simeq 4.5 \text{ L}$$

Rapid replacement of large water deficits carries the risk of acute cerebral edema. In general, no more than half the estimated deficit should be replaced during the first 24 hours.[24]

Management of Metabolic Acidosis

The causes of metabolic acidosis have been outlined previously (Table 7.10). In surgical patients, the common causes are gastrointestinal bicarbonate loss and lactate accumulation due to impaired tissue perfusion.

Significant gastrointestinal bicarbonate loss, which may be due to diarrhea (including that associated with most colonic villous adenomas) or pancreatic or biliary drainage or fistulas, produces a hypokalemic, hyperchloremic metabolic acidosis with a normal anion gap. Treatment is directed at reducing or eliminating the underlying problem and restoring volume with electrolyte solutions containing bicarbonate or bicarbonate-yielding anions, such as lactate. Potassium supplements are required since correction of the acidosis tends to decrease the plasma potassium concentration. Ongoing losses should be replaced with lactated Ringer's solution; saline infusions are inappropriate since they will aggravate the acid-based abnormality.

Lactic acidosis, with an increased anion gap, is usually the result of hypoxia due to inadequate tissue perfusion and circulatory failure. The primary therapeutic approach is to reverse shock and restore hemodynamic stability. Volume resuscitation alone may be sufficient to correct the acidosis in hemorrhagic shock. Bicarbonate administration alone without restoring tissue perfusion is generally unsuccessful. Use of vasopressors to treat hypotension in the face of volume depletion may worsen the acidosis.

Bicarbonate therapy is indicated for severe degrees of acidosis, when pH falls below 7.2, especially after cardiac arrest, when partial correction of pH may be essential to preserve or restore myocardial function. The goal is to increase pH to 7.2–7.3 by administering 1 or 2 ampules of bicarbonate (44.5–50.0 mEq/ampule) initially and basing the need for additional bicarbonate on serial blood gas analyses.[10,18]

Management of Metabolic Alkalosis

Vomiting or nasogastric suction, especially in the face of gastric outlet obstruction, is the common setting for the development of metabolic alkalosis in surgical patients. Hypokalemia and hypochloremia accompany the alkalosis. In addition, a small subset of patients with colonic villous adenomas produce an acidic hyperchloremic diarrhea resulting in alkalosis.

Until the underlying problem is corrected, reversal of the metabolic abnormality requires volume repletion with sodium chloride; potassium replacement is also a key feature of therapy. In the absence of sufficient supplemental potassium, paradoxic aciduria will develop, and alkalosis will persist.

Management of Ascites

Portal hypertension due to liver disease (such as alcoholic cirrhosis) or due to postsinusoidal obstruction (as in acute right-sided heart failure and Budd–Chiari syndrome) produces an increase in capillary hydrostatic pressure that may result in the transudation of fluid from the intravascular to the extravascular department and then into the peritoneal cavity from the surfaces of the liver, bowel, and mesentery, and hence the formation of ascites. Factors that promote the development of ascites in portal hypertension include hypoalbuminemia and a resultant reduction in plasma colloid osmotic pressure; renal sodium retention; and water retention. The pathogenesis of the sodium and water retention observed in cirrhosis is not firmly established, but vasodilatation, which results in reduced effective circulating volume and, therefore, resultant activation of the renin-angiotensin system with increased aldosterone secretion, appears to be a major determinant.[25,26] Experimental data indicate that the hemodynamic abnormalities, including peripheral and splanchnic vasodilation, that characterize cirrhosis and the sodium and water retention that leads to ascites are mediated by nitric oxide. This conclusion is supported by the finding that inhibition of vascular nitric oxide production in cirrhotic rats with ascites results in increased renal sodium and water excretion and normalization of the decreased serum sodium concentration and serum osmolality. If these findings are confirmed in humans, modulation of nitric oxide synthesis could represent a new therapeutic approach to the management of the circulatory and renal dysfunction in patients with cirrhosis.[26a,26b]

Currently recommended clinical management of ascites due to portal hypertension consists of sodium restriction (0–50 mEq/day), fluid restriction (1 L/day), administration of an aldosterone antagonist such as spironolactone, and often a thiazide or loop diuretic. Potassium supplementation is frequently necessary. Close monitoring is required since hypokalemia, hypocalcemia, hypomagnesemia, and metabolic alkalosis may complicate therapy.

In oncology patients, ascites may develop as a result of massive liver metastases or peritoneal carcinomatosis. Massive liver metastases apparently produce intrahepatic portal hypertension, and thus the pathogenesis of ascites is similar to that seen in portal cirrhosis. Here the ascitic fluid is often cytologically negative for malignant cells, and the ascites responds to the same treatment found effective in cirrhotic patients. In contrast, malignant ascitic fluid elaborated from tumor-involved peritoneal surfaces generally has been regarded as resistant to diuretic therapy and to sodium and fluid restriction. Under these circumstances, lymphatic obstruction inhibits fluid reabsorption.[27] Pockros et al.[28] studied nine patients with ascites associated with peritoneal carcinomatosis. The patients received a diet providing 44 mEq sodium per day. Spironolactone, alone or in combination with furosemide, was given in increasing doses until a desired weight loss of 0.5 kg/day was achieved. Pretreatment renin and aldosterone levels were normal. No significant decrease in the volume of ascites was observed. Seven of the nine patients, however, had a decrease in plasma volume, producing symptomatic hypotension in one patient and renal dysfunction in two. The authors concluded that diuretics should not be used to treat malignant ascites.

In contrast to the findings of Pockros et al., Greenway and associates[29] reported clinical clearance of malignant ascites in 14 of 15 patients they treated with spironolactone in daily doses of 150–450 mg. Sodium intake was restricted in only 5 patients. All of the patients demonstrated sodium retention; spironolactone therapy produced an increase in urinary sodium excretion rates from less than 35 mEq/day before treatment to 50–245 mEq/day after treatment. Plasma renin and aldosterone levels were determined in 5 patients: Renin levels were elevated in all 5, whereas aldosterone was raised in only 3.

PARENTERAL AND ENTERAL NUTRITION

The crystalloid and colloid preparations already discussed are effective in maintaining or restoring fluid and electrolyte homeostasis indefinitely, and when they are supplied in 5% glucose solution, the energy requirements of the glycolytic tissues, primarily the brain, are met. However, such solutions do not provide the energy and protein sources necessary for metabolic processes, growth or homeostasis, tissue repair, maintenance of body temperature, immunologic responses, or physical activity. In fasting patients, energy requirements can be met temporarily from endogenous calorie stores, but protein requirements cannot, because there are no protein reserves; each molecule of protein serves a specific nonfuel function, either as an enzyme or as a contractile protein.[16]

Potential endogenous energy sources for fasting patients include glycogen, protein, and fat. Glycogen stores are limited and totally dissipated within the first 1–3 days of fasting. Body protein represents a large potential energy source, but protein catabolism to provide energy (gluconeogenesis) is associated with some functional or structural loss. Fat is the main fuel reserve, and the length of survival during starvation correlates with the quantity of fat stores present at the onset of the fast. In the initial stages of starvation, adipose triglycerides provide about 85% of energy requirements, but as starvation proceeds protein catabolism in both the skeletal and visceral compartments increases, with increasing compromise of body function as protein-fuel conversion continues. As lipid stores are depleted, protein catabolism will affect even the essential proteins of the heart, lungs, blood cells, other vital tissues, and the immune system.[16]

Among patients requiring surgical therapy, the presence of nutritional deficits is of clinical importance because a substantial body of information attests to a strong association between the existence of such deficits and the occurrence of postoperative morbidity and mortality.[30] In 1936, Studley[31] observed a 10-fold increase in postoperative mortality among patients undergoing gastrectomy for intractable peptic ulcer disease who had sustained a preoperative weight loss of 20% or more. In 1944, Cannon and associates[32] reported the etiologic relationship between protein malnutrition, immune deficiencies, and an increased incidence of infection in experimental animals. In 1955, Rhoads and Alexander[33] demonstrated an association between postoperative infections and poor nutritional status and depressed serum albumin levels in patients. More recent observations also indicate a correlation between parameters that are influenced by nutritional status and postoperative morbidity and mortality. Thus, Mullen and associates[34] found that serum albumin levels <3 g/dl and transferrin levels <220 mg/dl are associated with a significant increase in the incidence of postoperative complications.

Similar adverse effects are observed when patients exhibit impaired reactivity to a panel of standard skin test antigens. A nearly eightfold increase in postoperative mortality and a fourfold increase in postoperative sepsis were reported by Pietsch and associates[35] among surgical patients who failed to react to any of five antigens before undergoing operation. Furthermore, when sequential skin testing indicates an improvement in immune reactivity, a reduced incidence of complications is observed.

Smale and associates[36] have used a prognostic nutritional index (PNI) to quantify the probability that various deficits in putative nutritional indices will have an adverse effect on postoperative outcome. The PNI* is a computer-generated regression equation designed to predict the risk of postoperative complications, taking into account the serum albumin and transferrin concentrations, triceps skinfold thickness, and delayed hypersensitivity skin test reactivity. A group of 159 cancer patients scheduled for elective curative or palliative surgery were categorized according to their PNI values. Those deemed at high risk for the development of complications because of malnutrition (defined as PNI ≥ 40%) actually experienced a 5.7-fold increase in postoperative morbidity. Twenty-nine percent of high-risk patients died; there was no mortality among the low-risk group (PNI < 40%).

The influence of serum albumin concentration and body weight on the postoperative course of patients with operable colorectal cancer was studied by Hickman and associates.[37] Morbidity and mortality rates were significantly higher in patients with low albumin levels or low body weight. When both abnormalities were present, the complication rate exceeded 70%, and the mortality rate was 42%.

Generally, crystalloid solutions containing 5% glucose are appropriate to maintain fluid and electrolyte homeostasis in fasting, well-nourished patients when resumption of normal oral diet is anticipated in 5–10 days. Providing approximately 400 kcal as glucose will meet the energy requirements of the glycolytic tissues, thereby limiting gluconeogenesis and achieving maximal protein sparing until lipid stores are depleted. On the other hand, special nutritional

---

*PNI (%) = 158 − 16.6 (ALB) − 0.78 (TSF) − 0.20 (TFN) − 5.8 (DH), where ALB is the serum albumin concentration (g/dl); TSF is the triceps skinfold thickness (mm); TFN is the serum transferrin level (mg/dl); and DH is the delayed hypersensitivity skin test reactivity to any one of three recall antigens (mumps, *Candida*, streptokinase-streptodornase) graded 0 (nonreactive), 1 (<5 mm induration), or 2 (≥5 mm induration).

support, enteral or parenteral feedings, is indicated for the following groups of patients (Level III evidence):

1. Initially well-nourished patients unable to resume oral diets after 5–10 days of fasting
2. Initially well-nourished patients with clinical conditions known to preclude oral diets for 5–10 days (e.g., acute hemorrhagic pancreatitis, short-bowel syndrome, midgut fistulas)
3. Initially malnourished patients unable to meet colorie and protein requirements with oral diets

Patients unable to meet nutritional requirements by normal or enriched oral diets may receive enteral (tube) feedings or total parenteral nutrition using preparations formulated to replete deficits and provide all required nutrients.

Essential Components of Nutrient Solutions

The essential ingredients of enteral and parenteral preparations designed to meet all known nutritional requirements include nonprotein calories, utilizable nitrogen for protein synthesis, minerals, essential fatty acids, trace elements, and vitamins. Meeting the therapeutic goal of homeostasis (nitrogen equilibrium) or growth or nutritional repletion (positive nitrogen balance) is dependent on a variety of factors, most importantly the levels of energy and nitrogen consumption.[38] At any given level of protein or nitrogen intake, nitrogen balance progressively improves to some maximum level as caloric intake increases from levels below requirements to levels exceeding requirements.[39] Maximum protein sparing and optimal utilization of dietary protein is achieved when the energy sources include at least 100–150 g of carbohydrates daily. As previously discussed, the requirement for this minimum amount of carbohydrates is based on their unique ability to satisfy the energy requirements of glycolytic tissues, including the central nervous system, erythrocytes, leukocytes, active fibroblasts, and certain phagocytes. The remaining energy requirements of most individuals can be met equally effectively by additional carbohydrates, fats, or a combination of these two.

At any given level of energy intake, nitrogen balance improves as nitrogen consumption increases. This dose-response relationship is curvilinear, and the nitrogen balance plateaus at higher dosages of nitrogen intake.[39] To avoid the limiting effects of calories on nitrogen or of nitrogen on calories, nutrient solutions are prepared so that the nitrogen content bears a fixed relationship to the nonprotein calories provided. In studies of normal, active young men fed orally, optimal efficiency was achieved at a calorie : nitrogen ratio of approximately 300–350 kcal to 1 gram of nitrogen.[39,40] However, protein economy decreases during most serious illnesses, and nitrogen losses increase; therefore, dietary protein requirements rise. Nitrogen equilibrium or retention can usually be achieved by approximately doubling the quantity of nitrogen required by a normal man at any given level of caloric intake. Thus, a calorie : nitrogen ratio of 150 : 1 is thought optimal for seriously ill patients, although the ratio actually may range between 100 : 1 and 200 : 1.[39]

Minerals required in amounts exceeding 200 mg per day include sodium, potassium, calcium, magnesium, chloride, and phosphate. These macronutrients are essential for the maintenance of water balance; cardiac function; mineralization of the skeleton; function of nerve, muscle, and enzyme systems; and energy transformation. In addition, protein utilization is affected by the availability of sodium, potassium, and phosphorus in the diet; nitrogen accretion is impaired when any of these mineral nutrients is withdrawn. Nutritional repletion evidently involves the formation of tissue units containing protoplasm and extracellular fluid in fixed proportion and with fixed elemental composition.[41] Thus, the retention of 1 gram of nitrogen is characteristically associated with the retention of fixed amounts of phosphorus, potassium, sodium, and chloride.

Linoleic acid is the primary essential fatty acid for humans, and consequently it must be provided in order to avoid chemical and clinical evidence of deficiency. Linoleic acid requirements are generally met when a fat emulsion is used to provide at least 4% of calories as linoleic acid.[16]

Micronutrients, or trace elements, presently recognized as essential for humans include iron, iodine, cobalt, zinc, copper chromium, manganese, and possibly selenium. Cobalt is supplied as vitamin B_{12}, and iron is generally withheld because of poor marrow utilization in critical or chronic illness. The remaining trace elements are routinely supplied in the nutrient solution.

Finally, all the water-soluble and fat-soluble vitamins, except vitamin K, are also provided. Vitamin K is given on an individual basis depending on the prothrombin time and any clinical indication for anticoagulation.

Estimating Nutrient Requirements

The calorie requirement is usually estimated from simple formulas adjusted for activity and stress (Tables 7.21, 7.22, and 7.23). Protein requirements can likewise be estimated from balance studies measuring nitrogen losses in various illnesses (Fig. 7.13). It appears that the requirements for essential amino acids and protein for malnourished or hospitalized patients approximate those of a normally growing 10- to 12-year-old (Table 7.24). Hence, a protein intake of 1.0–1.5 g/kg of ideal body weight comprised of at least 25% essential amino acids has been recommended.[16] Requirements for trace elements and vitamins are outlined in Tables 7.25 and 7.26.

Formulating Nutrient Solutions

The specific nutrient requirements for a given individual depend on the initial nutritional and metabolic status of the patient and the underlying disease process. Although the precise requirements for each nutrient can be determined by

TABLE 7.21. Caloric Requirements: Estimation of Resting Metabolic Expenditure (RME) from Harris–Benedict Equations (HBE)[a]

For men:	RME(kcal/day) = 66.4730 + 13.7516(W) + 5.0033(H) − 6.7550(A)
For women:	RME(kcal/day) = 655.095 + 9.563(W) + 1.8496(H) − 4.6756(A)

Where W = body weight in kg; H = height in cm;
  A = age in years

[a]Predicts RME for *normal* men and woman. Correction factors must be applied for sick persons (Table 7.22).

Source: From Silberman H. *Parenteral and Enteral Nutrition*, 2nd ed. Norwalk, CT: Appleton & Lange, 1989, p. 91.

TABLE 7.22. Correction Factors for Estimating Caloric Requirements of Hospitalized Patients from Harris–Benedict Equations[a]

Clinical Condition	Correction Factor[b]
Nutritional status	
Normal	1.3[c]
Depleted	1.5[c,d]
Fever	1.0 + 0.13 per °C
Elective surgery	1.0–1.2
Peritonitis	1.2–1.5
Soft-tissue trauma	1.14–1.37
Multiple fractures	1.2–1.35
Major sepsis	1.4–1.8
Major head injury (with steroids)	1.4–2.0
Major head injury (without steroids)	1.4
Thermal injury[e]	
0–20%	1.0–1.5
20–40%	1.5–1.85
40–100%	1.85–2.05
Starvation (adults)	0.70

[a]Total nonprotein energy requirement is estimated from the product of correction factors × HBE.
[b]Correction factors apply to men and women: Figures represent maximal increases and must be adjusted as recovery and convalescence proceed.
[c]Provides allowance for minimal activity above resting.
[d]Estimates additional requirement to achieve anabolism when accompanied by optimal protein intake.
[e]Percent body surface burned.

Source: Adapted from Silberman H. *Parenteral and Enteral Nutrition*, 2nd ed. Norwalk, CT: Appleton & Lange, 1989, p. 94.

TABLE 7.23. Caloric Requirements: Empiric Method

Clinical Status	kcal/kg Ideal Body Weight
Basal state	25–30
Maintenance (ambulatory)	30–35
Mild stress and malnutrition	40
Severe injuries and sepsis	50–60
Extensive burns	80

Source: From Silberman H. *Parenteral and Enteral Nutrition*, 2nd ed. Norwalk, CT: Appleton & Lange, 1989, p. 95.

metabolic balance studies and direct or indirect calorimetry, such techniques are generally not employed in routine clinical practice. Instead, on the basis of data from clinical investigations applying such balance studies to patients with various diseases, injuries, and degrees of stress, requirements can be accurately estimated as presented in Tables 7.21 through 7.26. As a result of these estimates, it is possible to formulate basic nutrient solutions of essentially fixed composition that can be used to meet the needs of most patients by varying only the volume of the basic formulation and by making appropriate adjust-

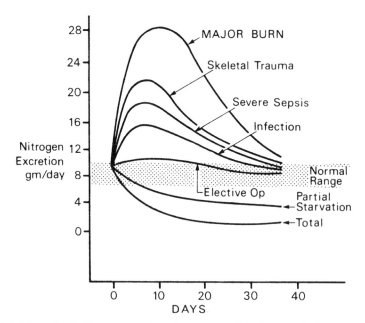

FIGURE 7.13. Catabolic response to serious illness. The increased nitrogen excretion and, therefore, the nitrogen requirement for homeostasis depend on the magnitude of the insult. (From Long CL. Energy and protein needs in the critically ill patient. *Contemp Surg* 1980;16:29–42.)

TABLE 7.24. Essential Amino Acids and Total Protein Requirements for Normal Persons

Amino Acid	Adults		Boys 10–12 yr	
	mg/kg	%TPR[a]	mg/kg	%TPR[a]
Histidine[b]	(12)	(1.6)	(19)	(1.9)
Isoleucine	10	1.3	28	2.8
Leucine	14	1.9	44	4.4
Lysine	12	1.6	44	4.4
Methionine + cystine	13	1.7	22	2.2
Phenylalanine + tyrosine	14	1.9	22	2.2
Threonine	7	0.9	28	2.8
Tryptophan	3.5	0.5	3.3	0.3
Valine	10	1.3	25	2.5
Total EAA[c] without histidine	83.5	11.1	216.3	21.8
Total EAA including histidine	95.5	12.7	235.3	23.8
Total protein requirement[d] (gm/kg)	0.75		1.0	

[a]%TPR, proportion of total protein requirement (high-quality protein) supplied as given amino acid.
[b]Estimated requirement for histidine, which apparently is essential for adults and children as well as infants.
[c]EAA, essential amino acids.
[d]The level of intake of high-quality protein that will meet the needs of nearly all normal persons.
Source: Based on data from *Energy and Protein Requirements*, World Health Organization, 1985. From Silberman H. *Parenteral and Enteral Nutrition*, 2nd ed. Norwalk, CT: Appleton & Lange, 1989, p. 99.

ments in electrolyte administration. Therefore, in clinical practice the caloric requirement is usually estimated from simple formulas adjusted for activity and stress. Although nitrogen requirements can likewise be determined or estimated, nitrogen needs are usually met as a consequence of the fixed calorie:nitrogen ratio, 100:1 to 200:1, of the nutrient solution. Thus, as the volume of solution

TABLE 7.25. Recommended Daily Allowances of Trace Elements[a]

	Oral	Intravenous
Zinc	10–15 mg	2.5–4.0 mg
Copper	1.2–3 mg	0.5–1.5 mg
Chromium	50–290 µg	10–15 µg
Manganese	0.7–5 mg	0.15–0.8 mg
Iodine	150 µg	1–2 µg/kg

[a]Chronically treated patients may require additional elements including iron, selenium, and molybdenum.
Source: From Silberman H. *Parenteral and Enteral Nutrition*, 2nd ed. Norwalk, CT: Appleton & Lange, 1989, p. 108.

TABLE 7.26. Recommended Daily Dosage of Vitamins

	Oral Dosage			Intravenous Dosage
Vitamin	Normal	Moderate Injury	Severe Injury	
A, as retinol (IU)[a]	3,300.0	5,000.0	5,000.0	3,300.0
D (IU)[b]	400.0	400.0	400.0	200.0
E, α-tocopherol (IU)	10.0	—	—	10.0
K (mg)[c]	—	2.0	20.0	—
Thiamine, B1 (mg)	1.5	2.0	10.0	3.0
Riboflavin, B2 (mg)	1.7	2.0	10.0	3.6
Niacin, B3 (mg)	19.0	20.0	100.0	40.0
Pantothenic acid, B5 (mg)	7.0	18.0	40.0	15.0
Pyridoxine, B6 (mg)	2.2	2.0	40.0	4.0
B12 (μg)	3.0	2.0	4.0	5.0
Ascorbic acid, C (mg)	60	75.0	300.0	100.0
Folic acid (μg)	400.0	1,500.0	2,500.0	400.0
Biotin (μg)	200.0	—	—	60.0

[a]One IU is equivalent to 0.3 mg of retinol.
[b]One IU is equivalent to 0.025 mg of vitamin D (cholecalciferol).
[c]No specific recommendation for normal persons because of the synthesis of vitamin K by intestinal bacteria. Vitamin K (phylloquinone), 2–4 mg once weekly, is recommended in parenteral form for patients receiving intravenous nutrition and who do not require anticoagulation.

Source: Adapted from Silberman H. *Parenteral and Enteral Nutrition*, 2nd ed. Norwalk, CT: Appleton & Lange, 1989, p. 111.

prescribed is increased to meet increased caloric demands, the additional nitrogen requirements, which generally parallel the rising caloric needs, are likewise met. Although such standard preparations can be used to satisfy the needs of most individuals, fluid-restricted patients, severely hypermetabolic patients, or those with renal or hepatic failure may require special nutrient formulations.

Enteral Nutrition (Tube Feedings)

The feasibility of enteral nutrition is dependent on the presence of sufficient functioning small bowel to allow the absorption of provided nutrients. Among patients meeting this criterion, suitable candidates include those in whom oral consumption is inadequate or contraindicated. Anorexia, weakness, lethargy, nausea, or oral inflammation are examples of factors contributing to poor oral intake. In addition, patients with diseases associated with markedly increased nutritional requirements, such as major burns, trauma, and sepsis, may be unable to eat enough to meet demands but often can be successfully nourished with the continuous administration of high-calorie, high-protein tube feedings. Patients in whom oral intake is contraindicated but who nevertheless may be candidates for enteral feeding include those who have certain neurologic disorders, including some patients following a cerebrovascular accident, and sometimes those who are comatose, stuporous, or extremely lethargic. Patients unable to eat because of oral, pharyngeal, esophageal, or proximal gastrointestinal conditions such as facial or jaw injuries, obstructing lesions, dysphagia, proximal enterocutaneous fistulas, or recent surgery may also be candidates for tube feedings delivered distal to the lesion. In addition, enteral nutrition may be indicated for patients with certain gastrointestinal disorders that may benefit from an elemental diet, because such a diet is often unpalatable when taken orally.

Enteral feedings are contraindicated in patients at high risk for pulmonary aspiration and in patients with peritonitis, intestinal obstruction, paralytic ileus, gastrointestinal hemorrhage, or intractable vomiting or diarrhea. In addition, enteral feedings are likely to produce a salutary effect in the management of only the most proximal and distal intestinal fistulas. In the treatment of other fistulas, parenteral nutrition is preferred, since enteral feedings will usually increase fistulous output with concomitant fluid and electrolyte disturbances and skin breakdown. In addition, enteral feedings are not recommended in the presence of severe malabsorptive states or in the early stages of short-bowel syndrome, because the adequate absorption of nutrients is unlikely in these circumstances. Finally, enteral nutrition is contraindicated when a properly managed trial of such therapy fails to meet the nutritional goals, aggravates the underlying condition, or is associated with pulmonary aspiration or unmanageable diarrhea.[16]

Formulation of Enteral Feeding Products A wide variety of liquid feeding preparations are presently available that differ in their content and source of protein, carbohydrate, and fat as well as in their osmolality, caloric density, sodium content, and residue. Amino acids may be derived from intact protein in the form of pureed meat, eggs, or milk; from intact protein provided as semipurified isolates from milk, soybean, or eggs; or from hydrolyzed protein with supplementary amino acids; or they may be provided as purified free amino acids.

Early formulations utilizing glucose or sucrose as the carbohydrate source were high in osmolality. The current use of starches, dextrins, and glucose oligosaccharides reduces the number of active chemical components and hence the osmolality, because the latter is a colligative property. The content of fat varies considerably among liquid feeding preparations; most contain long-chain fats, such as corn oil, soy oil, and safflower oil. However, some products contain medium-chain triglycerides (MCT), which are not dependent on pancreatic lipase or bile salts for digestion; they pass through the intestinal epithelium directly into the portal system as free fatty acids.

Commercially available, nutritionally complete formulations may be classified as follows:

1. Polymeric formulas containing lactose with nitrogen supplied as intact protein

2. Polymeric formulas without lactose with nitrogen supplied as intact protein and/or protein isolates

3. Lactose-free diets with nitrogen supplied as hydrolyzed protein or amino acids (peptide or elemental formulas)

These formulations are designed to be nutritionally complete and, therefore, supply essential fatty acids and all the minerals, including trace elements, and vitamins (except vitamin K) necessary to meet the requirements of *normal* persons when sufficient volume is provided to meet caloric and protein requirements. Products contain vitamin K in variable amounts, and its presence must be considered in patients who are receiving oral anticoagulants. Supplements of essential fatty acids, minerals, and vitamins may be required by patients with malabsorption, marked gastrointestinal losses, increased demands associated with critical illness, or a preexisting deficiency state.

Preparations providing intact protein require effective digestive and absorptive processes for utilization and are therefore suitable only for patients with sufficient gastrointestinal function. In contrast, formulations providing utilizable nitrogen in the form of free amino acids or di- or tripeptides plus amino acids (elemental or peptide diets) may be suitable for patients with a variety of disorders of the small intestine or with severe insufficiency of the exocrine pancreas, because these preparations demand no digestive effort on the part of the handicapped alimentary tract and require only a minimal mucosal surface for absorption.

Formulations low in lactose are frequently indicated because of a high incidence of lactase deficiency in normal adults. In addition, bowel disease, fasting, starvation, protein depletion, and total parenteral nutrition have been associated with the development of temporary lactase deficiency.[42] Lactose consumption by affected patients may result in osmotic diarrhea, bloating, gas, and abdominal cramps.[43]

Long-chain triglycerides require pancreatic lipase, bile salts, and an adequate absorptive mucosal surface for satisfactory assimilation. Consequently, formulations containing long-chain triglycerides as a major energy source should be restricted in patients with severe exocrine pancreatic insufficiency, cholestatic jaundice, severe mucosal abnormalities, or short-bowel syndrome.[44] In contrast, medium-chain triglycerides (MCT) may be beneficial as they are well absorbed in such patients. When prescribed, MCTs should be introduced into the diet slowly to avoid nausea, vomiting, and diarrhea. In addition, because they are ketogenic, administration to diabetic, ketotic, or acidotic patients may be undesirable.[45–47] MCTs do not provide essential fatty acids.[45]

Site of Nutrient Delivery Nutrients may be infused into the stomach, duodenum, or jejunum. *Intragastric feedings* have the advantage that the osmotic load reaches the duodenum in gradual fashion, limiting the incidence of the dumping syndrome. However, pulmonary aspiration is the major complication to be avoided, so candidates for intragastric feedings must be alert with gag and cough reflexes intact, and gastric emptying should be normal. Suitable patients should have conditions that allow them to assume the semi-Fowler position (30° upright) for the duration of tube feeding therapy. Thus, intragastric feedings are contraindicated in comatose, stuporous, or lethargic patients, in severely debilitated or weak patients, in those with endotracheal or tracheostomy tubes, and in those with persistently high gastric residual volumes. Candidates for enteral nutrition who have a condition making intragastric feeding inadvisable can often be successfully managed by introducing nutrient solutions more distally.

Duodenal feedings have the advantage that the pyloric sphincter is interposed between the nutrient solution and the tracheobronchial tree, so the incidence of aspiration is reduced although not eliminated. The disadvantage is that the symptoms of the dumping syndrome are more frequent.

Jejunal feedings are generally not subject to regurgitation, and therefore the risk of pulmonary aspiration is least associated with nutrients infused here. Jejunal feedings also enable patients with more proximal disease of the alimentary tract to receive enteral nutrition. In addition, the paralytic ileus associated with abdominal surgery affects primarily the stomach and colon; therefore, safe and effective enteral nutrition can sometimes be provided in the immediate postoperative period when the feedings are delivered directly into the jejunum. Finally, jejunostomy feedings induce less pancreatic stimulation than intragastric or intraduodenal diets, and therefore may have a specific advantage in patients with inflammatory diseases of the pancreas. In contrast to these advantages of jejunal feedings, symptoms of the dumping syndrome associated with hyperosmolar nutrient solutions are more common with this method than with intragastric delivery.

Access to the Alimentary Tract   Enteral feedings are infused through tubes placed in the stomach, duodenum, or jejunum. Intubation can be achieved using nasal, percutaneous, or surgical methods.

Nasal Intubation   Intubation of the stomach, duodenum, or occasionally the jejunum with a feeding tube of appropriate length passed through the nose is satisfactory for most hospitalized patients for whom the eventual resumption of oral feeding is anticipated. The correct position of the tube should be confirmed radiographically. When proper positioning is difficult, placement can be facilitated by direct endoscopic guidance.

Percutaneous Intubation   Percutaneous endoscopic gastrostomy (PEG) has become the intubation technique of choice for most patients requiring a prolonged or indefinite period of enteral feeding and for those requiring continued therapy at home. This method eliminates the less cosmetic and more irritating nasal tube and obviates the necessity for general anesthesia and celiotomy necessary for surgical construction of a gastrostomy. If duodenal or jejunal feedings are indicated, an additional tube may be attached to or passed through the gastrostomy tube. This second, longer tube may then be advanced endoscopically into the small intestine.

Surgical Intubation   A tube gastrostomy or jejunostomy is usually constructed in conjunction with another intra-abdominal operation. It is indicated when the need for enteral feeding is anticipated in the postoperative period. The common surgical techniques include those of Stamm and Witzel, and the newer technique of needle catheter jejunostomy. Celiotomy exclusively for the purpose of establishing access for feeding generally is indicated only in patients requiring enteral nutrition indefinitely or permanently when the percutaneous techniques are contraindicated or have been unsuccessful.

Access to the alimentary tract by means of cervical esophagostomy (or pharyngostomy) may be of value for patients requiring long-term or permanent tube feeding, because celiotomy is not required and the procedure can be performed using local anesthesia.[48–50] A tube esophagostomy is usually created, but a permanent stoma can be constructed, if indicated.

Prescribing Therapy   The specific nutrient formulation to be administered is chosen in relation to the patient's clinical status, the digestive and absorptive function of the small intestine, and the anatomic site selected for infusion. Additional considerations include the patient's caloric requirements and fluid and electrolyte status. The commercially available nutritionally complete products have a total caloric density, including both nonprotein and protein calories, varying between 1 and 2 kcal/ml. Fluid-restricted patients or those with high caloric requirements should receive a product with a high caloric density. Conversely, dehydrated patients or those with ongoing fluid losses require more fluid and therefore should receive more dilute formulations.

Expert opinions vary as to the optimal technique for initiating therapy. Patients commonly experience abdominal discomfort and diarrhea of varying severity during the initial phases of therapy. These symptoms have been attributed (without thorough study) to the rapid infusion of high osmolal solutions. Consequently, it has been customary to initiate enteral feedings with the continuous infusion of small volumes of diluted formula; others, however, recommend starting with full-strength formula.

At the University of Southern California, the volume of full-strength solution that will meet calorie and protein demands is determined. Then the enteral feeding formulation selected is diluted to one-third strength, placed in an enteral feeding container, and delivered continuously to the patient in the semi-Fowler position (30° upright). Infusion is begun at a rate of 50 ml/hr. Thereafter, the rate of administration is increased in increments of 25 ml/hr every 12 hours so that by 24 to 36 hours, a rate that will provide the predetermined volume generally has been attained. As therapy proceeds, the patient is observed for manifestations of intolerance, such as abdominal cramps, diarrhea, glucosuria, and in the case of intragastric feedings, gastric retention. The presence of any of these findings early in the course of therapy is an indication to slow the rate of advancement to allow a longer period of adaptation. Until sufficient volume of solution is tolerated, supplemental intravenous fluid may be required to maintain water and electrolyte balance. After the dilute solution is administered for 24 hours at full volume with no manifestations of intolerance, the concentration of the nutrient is increased to two-thirds strength for 12 to 24 hours, and finally to full strength without alteration in volume.

As previously discussed, hyperosmolar nutrient solutions may be associated with hypernatremic dehydration. Consequently, patients are allowed to freely consume clear liquids if feasible. In other patients, especially those unable to express thirst, free water should be given and can be provided with the tube feedings. Water is conveniently administered when the feeding bag is changed, usually every 8 hours. Thus, 100 to 200 ml of water can be administered over 30 minutes every 8 hours through the feeding tube. This arrangement has the advantage that the tube is flushed after each container of liquid formula is administered, thus reducing the incidence of tube occlusion.

Continuous around-the-clock delivery of liquid formula diets is generally preferred to intermittent bolus feedings. Greater total daily volumes are tolerated with less gastric retention and fewer manifestations of gastrointestinal intolerance.[16]

Complications Enteral nutrition is often prescribed without appropriate attention to technique or protocol because it is widely assumed that tube feedings are associated with few complications. In fact, complications are common, though often minor when promptly recognized and treated. The reported overall incidence of morbidity is quite variable, apparently reflecting the intensity of observation and care and the definition of terms. Cataldi-Betcher and associates[51] reported a complication rate of 11.7% among 253 patients studied, including an incidence of diarrhea (more than three liquid stools a day) of only 2.3%. In contrast, Heymsfield and associates[52] found that diarrhea occurred in up to 20% of patients. Silk and associates[44] reported that signs of gastrointestinal intolerance developed in 25% of their patients. Up to half of their patients developed metabolic abnormalities (hypokalemia, hypophosphatemia), and 40% had derangements of liver indices (alkaline phosphatase, transaminase) during the course of enteral nutrition.

Potential complications may be classified as mechanical, gastrointestinal, or metabolic and infectious (Table 7.27). Pulmonary aspiration of the feeding formula has emerged as the most common serious, potentially fatal complication of enteral nutrition.[16] Reported incidence is highly variable (0–95%) depending on the population of patients studied and the definition of aspiration. Chemical evidence of aspiration is more common than clinically significant aspiration. Factors that increase the risk of this complication include mental obtundation, poor cough or gag reflexes, feeding in the supine position, impaired gastric emptying, an artificial airway, and gastroesophageal reflux. The latter may be induced or aggravated by feeding tubes, especially those of large diameter, traversing the gastroesophageal junction.

TABLE 7.27. Potential Complications During Enteral Nutrition

Mechanical	Gastrointestinal	Metabolic and Infectious
Depressed cough	Abdominal	Congestive heart failure
Dysphagia	cramping	Disorder of calcium, magnesium,
Esophageal erosions	Abdominal	phosphorus
Esophageal reflux	distension	Essential fatty acid deficiency
Esophagitis	Aggravation of	Fluid and electrolyte disturbances
Increased airway	primary	Hypercapnia and respiratory failure
secretions	disease	Hyperglycemia and hypoglycemia
Otitis media	Diarrhea	Hyperosmolar dehydration
Nasopulmonary	Malabsorption	Hyperosmolar nonketotic coma
intubation	Nausea and	Hypoprothrombinemia
Parotitis	vomiting	Inadvertent intraperitoneal infusion
Pharyngitis	Pneumatosis	Inadvertent intravenous infusion
Pneumothorax	intestinalis	Liver abnormalities
Pulmonary aspiration		Microbial growth in formula
Rhinitis		Prerenal azotemia
Tube dislodgement		Vitamin deficiencies
Tube obstruction		Warfarin resistance
		Zinc and copper deficiency

Source: From Silberman H. *Parenteral and Enteral Nutrition*, 2nd ed. Norwalk, CT: Appleton & Lange, 1989, p. 147.

Total Parenteral Nutrition

Total parenteral nutrition (TPN) refers to a variety of methods by which all required nutrients can be provided intravenously independent of alimentary tract function. TPN is extremely effective, even lifesaving, therapy for patients with medical conditions in which alimentary tract nutrition, either by mouth or by feeding tube, is inadequate or inadvisable.

The efficacy of total parenteral nutrition was established in a series of now-classic, modern-day animal experiments in which Rhoads, Dudrick, Wilmore, Vars, and their associates at the University of Pennsylvania demonstrated normal growth and development of beagle puppies fed exclusively by vein after weaning.[53-56] The animals received a hypertonic infusate of glucose, protein hydrolysates, vitamins, and minerals through a central venous catheter. These investigators subsequently reported comparable results in humans: normal growth and development in children, nitrogen equilibrium in normal adults, and nutritional repletion in malnourished individuals.[53,54,56]

Formulating Nutrient Solutions In current practice, nutrient solutions designed for parenteral administration are based on either carbohydrates or lipids as the major caloric source. Solutions of synthetic crystalline amino acids are used to meet protein requirements. In the carbohydrate-based system, glucose is the carbohydrate of choice, since it is the normal physiologic substrate;

it naturally occurs in blood; and it is abundant, inexpensive, and readily purified for parenteral administration. Glucose can be given in high concentrations and in large amounts that are well tolerated by most patients after a period of adaptation. Other carbohydrates such as fructose, sorbitol, xylitol, and maltose have been evaluated experimentally, but each has disadvantages that preclude clinical application at the present time. Glucose for parenteral infusion is commercially available in concentrations from 5% to 70% and is provided as glucose monohydrate with a caloric density of 3.4 kcal/g. Although isotonic (5%) solutions of glucose are available, concentrated glucose solutions are necessary in parenteral nutrition protocols in order to provide required calories in physiologic volumes of fluid.[38]

Lipids are the alternative clinically useful major caloric source. Fat emulsions derived from soybean oil and safflower oil were approved for use in the United States in 1975 and 1979, respectively. The soybean oil emulsions had been used in Europe for nearly 20 years prior to their introduction in the United States. Currently available fat emulsions are derived from soybean oil or are mixtures of soybean oil emulsion and safflower oil emulsion. The use of lipid emulsions in intravenous feeding regimens is attractive because of the high caloric density of fat (9 kcal/g), and because they are made isotonic by the addition of glycerol, these products can provide many calories in relatively small volumes via peripheral veins. Although early experience with lipids using the cottonseed oil emulsion Lipomul was unsatisfactory because of the toxicity of that preparation, fat emulsions derived from soybean oil and safflower oil have proven safe for clinical use.

The infusion of fats is associated with an increase in heat production and oxygen consumption, a decrease in respiratory quotient, and the appearance of carbon-14 (^{14}C) in the expired air of patients receiving ^{14}C-labeled fat. These observations indicate that the infused fats are in fact used for energy. The fat emulsions are available in 10%, 20%, and 30% concentrations and are mixtures of neutral triglycerides of predominantly unsaturated fatty acids. The major component fatty acids are linoleic, oleic, palmitic, and linolenic. The total caloric value of the 10% emulsions, including triglyceride, phospholipid, and glycerol, is 1.1 kcal/ml, of which about 0.1 kcal/ml is derived from the added glycerol. The corresponding value for the 20% and 30% emulsions is 2 kcal/ml and 3 kcal/ml, respectively.[38]

The Glucose System   This is the original carbohydrate-based system developed by Dudrick and his associates.[55] Each liter of nutrient solution is prepared aseptically by the admixture of 500 ml of 50% glucose and 500 ml of 8.5% crystalline amino acids, and the addition of appropriate electrolytes, vitamins, and trace elements (Table 7.28). Such a solution provides 850 nonprotein kcal/L, and approximately 6.5 g of nitrogen, equivalent to 41 g protein. Consequently, the solution has a calorie : nitrogen ratio of about 131 : 1. The nitrogen content and the calorie : nitrogen ratio will vary slightly depending on the brand of amino acid solution used. Due to the osmolar contribution of each of the con-

TABLE 7.28. The Glucose System of Total Parenteral Nutrition
(Preparation of 1 Liter)[a,b]

8.5% Amino acids[c]	500 ml
50% Glucose	500 ml
Sodium (as acetate)	45 mEq
Potassium (as chloride)	35 mEq
Potassium (as acid phosphate)[d]	8.8 mEq
Phosphate (as potassium acid phosphate)[d]	6 mM
Magnesium (as sulfate)	8 mEq
Calcium (as chloride)	5 mEq

[a]Trace elements and vitamins are added to 1 L each day.
[b]Essential fatty acids and vitamin K are supplied separately.
[c]As FreAmine III, 8.5%. Contains 10 mEq/L of sodium and 20 mEq (10 mM)/L of phosphate. Comparable amino acid solutions have different electrolyte contents.
[d]Provided as potassium acid phosphate solution in which each ml contains 4.4 mEq potassium and 3 mm phosphate (equivalent to approximately 5.4 mEq assuming average valence of 1.8).

Source: From Silberman H. *Parenteral and Enteral Nutrition*, 2nd ed. Norwalk, CT: Appleton & Lange, 1989, p. 226.

stituents, this nutrient solution has a final concentration of approximately 2,000 mOsm/L. Such a solution can never be safely infused through peripheral veins. Consequently, the glucose system must be delivered into a *central vein* where the infusate is immediately diluted. Vascular access is usually through a percutaneously placed subclavian venous catheter. Other routes are used occasionally with variable success. The incidence of morbidity associated with establishing and maintaining central venous access is influenced by the site and technique of insertion of the venous cannula and the diligence with which the apparatus is managed during the course of nutrition therapy.

Because of the high concentration of glucose in this form of parenteral nutrition, therapy should begin gradually to allow adaption and thereby avoid hyperglycemia. Generally, on the first day, a patient receives 1 liter of nutrient solution, which is infused at a constant rate over the full 24-hour period. Blood and urine glucose levels are monitored frequently, and if this initial rate of infusion is well tolerated, the volume prescribed is increased from day to day until the volume infused meets the caloric requirement of the individual patient. Requirements for most patients are met by 2.5 to 3 L of the nutrient solution per day, providing 2,125 to 2,550 nonprotein kcal. Infusion of the glucose system at a constant rate is a critical feature of safe practice, since abrupt changes in the rate of delivery may be associated with marked alterations in blood sugar levels. The constant rate of infusion is most efficiently achieved by using an infusion pump. At the conclusion of therapy, the rate of infusion should be tapered gradually, over 1 to 2 days, to avoid hypoglycemia. When infusion must be abruptly terminated, a solution of 10% glucose is substituted for nutrient solution.

TABLE 7.29. University of Southern California Lipid System of Total Parenteral Nutrition (Preparation of 1 liter)[a]

10% fat emulsion	500 ml
50% glucose	100 ml
8.5% amino acids	350 ml
Sodium (as acetate)	45 mEq
Potassium (as chloride)	40 mEq
Magnesium (as sulfate)	8 mEq
Calcium (as gluconate)	5 mEq
Heparin	1,000 IU
Distilled water	qs.ad. 1,000 ml

[a]Trace elements and vitamins are added to 1 L each day. Vitamin K is supplied separately, as needed. Electrolyte additives listed here based on use of FreAmine III. Comparable amino acid products have different electrolyte contents. Phosphorus provided by FreAmine III (10 mm/L) and fat emulsion (approximately 15 mm/L).

Source: From Silberman H. *Parenteral and Enteral Nutrition*, 2nd ed. Norwalk, CT: Appleton & Lange, 1989, p. 266.

The Lipid System The system of total parenteral nutrition based on glucose as the major caloric source is simple in concept, but patients' glucose metabolism must be closely monitored, and administration of the infusate requires technical expertise to achieve and maintain the central venous access necessary for safe treatment. The use of lipid emulsions as the major caloric source is attractive because of the high caloric density and isotonicity of these products. Such considerations have logically led to the preparation of nutrient solutions based on fat as the major caloric source, with the goal of providing all required nutrients by *peripheral vein*. An example of such a lipid-based system of total parenteral nutrition is presented in Table 7.29. This formulation was devised with the aim of maximizing caloric and amino acid content without producing a solution with a concentration that would preclude safe peripheral venous administration.[57–59] Each liter provides 720 nonprotein kcal and 4.6 g of nitrogen, equivalent to 29 g of protein. The calorie : nitrogen ratio is 157 : 1. The nitrogen content of the solution will vary slightly, depending on the amino acid product used in its preparation.

The same careful attention to aseptic preparation in the pharmacy required for the glucose system is applicable in preparing the lipid system. As with the glucose system, sufficient volume is given to meet measured or estimated caloric requirements. As many as 5 L have been infused daily for weeks to months without apparent adverse effect.

Complications Morbidity associated with intravenous feedings may be related to drug toxicity, difficulties with vascular access, sepsis, or metabolic derangements.

Drug Toxicity Adverse reactions to the components of parenteral nutrition solutions are uncommon. Although glucose is virtually nontoxic, the hypertonic solutions employed in the glucose system of TPN may be associated with potentially serious complications usually related to alterations in blood glucose levels (see below). Currently used solutions of synthetic amino acids provide all of the nitrogen in the form of free L-amino acids and, in contrast to previously used protein hydrolysates, no potentially toxic ammonia or peptide products are present. Toxicity associated with the intravenous infusion of the currently available fat emulsions also has been minimal. The most frequent acute adverse reactions are fever, sensations of warmth, chills, shivering, chest or back pain, anorexia, and vomiting. Similarly, adverse reactions associated with chronic infusions of fat emulsions are quite uncommon. Anemia and alterations in blood coagulation have been observed during treatment, but the etiologic relationship to the lipid infusions has been unconfirmed. The most serious adverse effects have been observed in infants and children. The "fat overload" syndrome associated with the older cottonseed emulsion has rarely been observed with the newer current preparations. Nevertheless, several reports have been published in which children receiving fat emulsions have developed marked hyperlipidemia, gastrointestinal disturbances, hepatosplenomegaly, impaired hepatic function, anemia, thrombocytopenia, prolonged clotting time, elevated prothrombin time, and spontaneous bleeding. These findings resolved when the fat emulsion was withdrawn.[38,60]

Complications of Vascular Access The lipid-based system of parenteral nutrition can be infused through the ordinary venous cannulae used for the administration of crystalloid solutions. Local phlebitis and inflammation from infiltration and cutaneous extravasation occur with about the same frequency as that associated with the infusion of nonnutrient solutions. In contrast, hospitalized patients receiving the glucose system require a percutaneously introduced subclavian venous catheter. Complications that may occur during the placement of the catheter include improper advancement of the catheter tip into one of the jugular veins or the contralateral innominate vein, instead of into the superior vena cava. In addition, air embolization or cardiac arrhythmias may occur, or there may be an injury to an adjacent anatomic structure, such as the brachial plexus, the subclavian artery, the great vessels, or the thoracic duct. Pneumothorax, usually resulting from inadvertent entrance into the pleural cavity, is probably the most common complication of attempted subclavian catheterization and has been reported to occur in about 2% to 3% of attempts in large series. Late complications after successful insertion may include air embolism, catheter occlusion, central vein thrombophlebitis, and catheter-related sepsis.

Systemic Sepsis Sepsis attributable primarily to the administration of parenteral nutrition should be an infrequent complication in modern practice. A variety of factors may contribute to the development of this complication. Patients requiring TPN are often inordinately susceptible to infection because of serious illness, malnutrition, and chronic debilitation—all conditions associated with impaired immune responses. Patients receiving immunosuppressive therapy, cytotoxic drugs, or corticosteroids are likewise susceptible to infection. These drugs as well as prolonged administration of broad-spectrum antibiotics may subject patients to sepsis from unusual, ordinarily saprophytic, microorganisms.

In addition to these patient-related factors, several specific TPN-related factors contribute to the pathogenesis of sepsis. The various components of the nutrient solution can become contaminated during manufacture or at the time of component admixture in the hospital pharmacy. The ability of the nutrient solution to support microbial growth is well established; but with present techniques of solution preparation, sepsis from contamination should be rare. The subclavian catheter appears to be the most common source of TPN-associated sepsis. Contamination may take place when the catheter is inserted; when containers of the nutrient solution are changed; when intravenous tubing is replaced; when in-line filters are inserted; or when the intravenous cannula is used for measurement of central venous pressure, blood sampling, or the infusion of medication or blood products. Also, to-and-fro motion of the subclavian catheter due to inadequate fixation to the skin will allow exposed portions of the catheter to enter the subcutaneous tract leading to the vein, which may result in infection.

Hematogenous contamination of the catheter may occasionally occur following bacteremia secondary to a distant focus of infection. More commonly, however, catheter-related sepsis is due to contamination of the subclavian catheter by organisms colonizing the skin surrounding the catheter insertion site. The incidence of sepsis varies greatly in reported series, but in recent years TPN has been administered with very low rates of infection. This improving trend is evidently due to increasing experience with this relatively recent modality of treatment, adherence to rigid protocols of practice, and the development of the multidisciplinary team approach to parenteral nutrition. With this kind of proper management, TPN-related sepsis occurs in about 3% of patients receiving the glucose system. This complication is much less common among patients receiving the lipid-based system of parenteral nutrition through a peripheral vein.[16,38,58] Systemic sepsis due to bacterial translocation in patients receiving parenteral nutrition is discussed below.

Metabolic Complications   A variety of metabolic derangements have been observed during the course of total parenteral nutrition. These abnormalities may reflect preexisting deficiencies, or they may develop during the course of parenteral nutrition as a result of an excess or deficiency of a specific component in the nutrient solution. As would be expected, the standard solutions may not contain the ideal combination of ingredients for a given individual. Consequently, patients must be carefully monitored so that the content of the nutrient solution can be adjusted during the course of therapy. For example, minor alterations in electrolyte content are often necessary.

Abnormalities of blood sugar are the most common metabolic complications observed in patients receiving total parenteral nutrition. These abnormalities are largely confined to the population of patients receiving the glucose system rather than the lipid system, since the latter provides substantially less glucose. Hyperglycemia may be manifest when the full caloric dosage of the glucose system is inappropriately given initially and later when rates of infusion are abruptly increased. In addition, glucose intolerance may be a manifestation of overt or latent diabetes mellitus, or it may reflect reduced pancreatic insulin response to a glucose load, a situation commonly observed during starvation, stress, pain, major trauma, infection, and shock. Hyperglycemia also may be a reflection of the peripheral insulin resistance observed during sepsis, acute stress, or other conditions that are accompanied by high levels of circulating catecholamines and glucocorticoids.

The incidence of hyperglycemia can be minimized by initiating therapy with the glucose system gradually. Full dosage should be achieved over a 3-day period, during which time adaption to the glucose load takes place. In addition, careful metabolic monitoring during this period will disclose any tendency to hyperglycemia. Subsequently, a constant rate of infusion is maintained. An inadvertent decrease in the rate of the infusion should not be compensated by abrupt increases in rate; such "catching up" is not allowed. When hyperglycemia supervenes despite these precautions, the etiology is sought. The common cause of hyperglycemia after a period of stability is emerging sepsis, the overt manifestations of which may not appear for 18 to 24 hours after development of elevated glucose levels. Uncomplicated moderate hyperglycemia is controlled initially by subcutaneous or intravenous administration of insulin; the TPN infusion is continued at the usual rate. Subsequently, the appropriate amount of insulin is added to the TPN solution during its aseptic preparation in the pharmacy. Providing insulin in the TPN solution has the advantage that inadvertent alterations in the rate of glucose delivery are automatically accompanied by appropriate adjustments in the amount of insulin administered. Patients with hyperglycemia complicated by massive diuresis, dehydration, neurologic manifestations, or the syndrome of hyperosmolar nonketotic coma are managed by immediate termination of the TPN infusion, fluid resuscitation, and insulin administration.

In contrast to the problem of hyperglycemia, blood sugar levels may decrease significantly when the rate of infusion of the glucose system is abruptly reduced. Symptomatic hypoglycemia is most likely to occur when the reduction of the infusion rate is preceded by an increase in rate. When the glucose system is to be discontinued electively, the rate of delivery should be tapered gradually over 1 to 2 days. Patients who are hemodynamically unstable or who are undergoing surgery should not receive TPN, since fluid resuscitation may be inadvertently carried out using the TPN solution. Therefore, the TPN infusion is discontinued abruptly in such patients, and hypoglycemia is averted by infusing a solution of 10% glucose. Hypoglycemia may also reflect an excessive dosage of exogenous insulin. This most commonly occurs as a result of failure to recognize the resolution of peripheral insulin resistance and the associated decreased insulin requirement when the provoking condition responds to therapy.

Deficiencies of the major intracellular ions may occur in the catabolic state, since the protein structure of cells is metabolized as an energy source, intracellular ions are lost, and the total body concentration of these ions, including potassium, magnesium, and phosphate, is decreased. Furthermore, during nutritional repletion, these ions, derived from the serum, are deposited or incorporated in newly synthesized cells. When supplementation of these ions in nutrient solutions is insufficient, hypokalemia, hypomagnesemia, and hypophosphatemia ensue. Serum levels of these substances should be measured regularly during TPN, since such monitoring will disclose deficiencies before the clinical manifestations develop. Symptoms of hypokalemia are unusual when serum levels of potassium exceed 3.0 mEq/L. Asymptomatic hypokalemia can be managed by increasing the potassium supplement added to the nutrient solution at the time of preparation. When cardiac arrhythmias or other significant symptoms develop, the rate of TPN infusion should be tapered promptly while serum glucose levels are monitored closely, and an intravenous infusion of potassium chloride is begun.

Intracellular consumption of inorganic phosphate during the synthesis of proteins, membrane phospholipids, DNA (deoxyribonucleic acid), and ATP (adenosine triphosphate) may produce a striking deficit in the serum phosphate level after only several days of intravenous feedings devoid of or deficient in phosphate. Symptoms of hypophosphatemia may occur when serum phosphate levels fall to 2 mg/dl. However, severe manifestations are particularly apt to occur as levels fall below 1 mg/dl. These include acute respiratory failure, marked muscle weakness, impaired myocardial contractility, severe congestive cardiomyopathy, acute hemolytic anemia, coma, and death. Hypophosphatemic patients who are asymptomatic can be managed by increasing the phosphate supplement in the nutrient solution. Symptomatic patients or those with serum phosphate levels less than 1 mg/dl should be repleted intravenously through a separate infusion line. Parenteral nutrition should be stopped, and a 10% glucose solution should be infused to avert hypoglycemia. Since intracellular phosphate consumption is dependent on caloric intake, withdrawing TPN alone often results in an increase in serum phosphate levels within 24 hours.

Healthy or malnourished individuals who receive a constant parenteral infusion of a fat free but otherwise complete diet eventually develop clinical and biochemical manifestations that are completely reversed by the administration of linoleic acid. Thus, the syndrome of essential fatty acid deficiency in humans is due principally, if not exclusively, to a lack of *linoleic acid*. Exogenous linolenic acid is required by some species, but its essentially for humans is unproven. The most commonly recognized manifestation of linoleic acid deficiency is an eczematous desquamative dermatitis largely but not always confined to the body folds. Other clinical findings may include hepatic dysfunction, anemia, thrombocytopenia, hair loss, and possibly impaired wound healing. Growth retardation has been observed in infants. Fatty acid deficiency is treated by the administration of linoleic acid, usually by infusing one of the currently available fat emulsions. Patients receiving the glucose-based system of parenteral nutrition should be treated prophylactically by providing 4% of calories as linoleic acid. This requirement is usually met by infusing 1 L per week of a 10% fat emulsion.

Transient derangements of liver function indices occur in the majority of patients receiving parenteral nutrition of either type. The etiology of these changes is uncertain and probably multifactorial. One hypothesis is that calorie and protein infusions in amounts exceeding requirements may contribute to these changes. An infectious etiology also has been suggested, since oral metronidazole has been reported to reverse the changes. In any case, the clinical course associated with the liver changes is nearly always benign, so TPN need not be discontinued. Nevertheless, several patients receiving long-term TPN have developed severe or chronic liver disease, but the etiologic relationship is unclear.[16,38,61,62]

Finally, when nutritional repletion of chronically malnourished patients is undertaken, therapy must be gradual to avoid a series of "refeeding" syndromes including hypokalemia, hypophosphatemia, acute thiamine deficiency, and congestive heart failure.[16,63]

Comparison of Glucose and Lipid-Based Parenteral Nutrition Factors to be considered in comparing the glucose-based and lipid-based systems of parenteral nutrition include the composition and nutrient value of the two methods, the relative efficacy of glucose and lipid calories, the ease and safety of administration, and cost-effectiveness.

Composition of the Standard Glucose and Lipid Systems The glucose system has a caloric density of 0.85 nonprotein kcal/ml exclusively of carbohydrate origin, whereas the caloric density of the lipid system is 0.72 kcal/ml, of which nearly 70% is of lipid origin. The glucose system provides about 40% more nitrogen per liter, but its greater osmolarity requires central venous administration. The lesser concentration of the lipid system permits safe peripheral venous administration (Table 7.30).

Glucose Versus Lipids as a Caloric Source The relative impact of glucose and lipid calories on nitrogen retention or body composition has been the subject of some controversy. However, the preponderance of evidence now supports the conclusion that the two caloric sources are of comparable value in their effect on nitrogen retention in normal persons or in chronically ill, malnourished patients.[16,64,65] The major study supporting this conclusion is that of Jeejeebhoy and associates,[65] who observed that optimal nitrogen retention with the lipid system requires a period of about 4 days to establish equilibrium, after which nitrogen balance is positive to a comparable degree with both the glucose and lipid systems.

Ease and Safety of Administration The glucose system requires central venous administration. The central venous catheter must be placed by a physi-

TABLE 7.30. Comparison of Glucose and Lipid Systems

	Glucose System	Lipid System
Carbohydrate calories	850 kcal/L	220 kcal/L
Lipid calories	—	500 kcal/L
Caloric density	0.85 kcal/ml	0.72 kcal/ml
Nitrogen provided	6.5 g/L	4.6 g/L
Protein equivalent	41 g/L	29 g/L
Calorie:nitrogen ratio	131 : 1	157 : 1
Concentration (approximate)	2000 mOsm/L	900 mOsm/L

Source: From Silberman H. *Parenteral and Enteral Nutrition*, 2nd ed. Norwalk, CT: Appleton & Lange, 1989, p. 333.

cian under sterile conditions and may be associated with certain complications discussed previously that are not seen with the peripherally administered lipid system. In contrast, the ordinary venous cannulae used for infusion of the lipid system can be easily inserted and maintained by paramedical personnel. Whereas the central venous catheter requires special care and attention to prevent catheter sepsis, the cannulae used in the lipid system require the same simple care and need to be changed with about the same frequency as those used in the peripheral venous administration of crystalloid solutions. The peripherally infused lipid system is rarely associated with systemic sepsis.

Cost-effectiveness   At present, materials required for preparation of the lipid system are more costly than those required for isocaloric volumes of the glucose system.

Choosing the Glucose or Lipid System   For most patients, nutritional requirements are met equally well by either the glucose or lipid system. However, one system may have an advantage in some patients because of nonnutritional factors. For example, fluid-restricted patients currently receive the glucose-based system because of its higher caloric density.[16,66] For patients requiring greater fluid restriction, the standard glucose system presented here can be modified using 70% glucose (2.4 kcal/ml). The recently introduced 30% fat emulsion (3 kcal/ml) may offer a lipid-based alternative for such patients.

The glucose system is advisable in acute myocardial ischemia, because elevated free fatty acid levels, sometimes observed with lipid infusions, have been associated with arrhythmias and extension of ischemic damage.[67] The lipid system has an advantage in patients with hyperglycemia due to stress or diabetes mellitus.[68,69] In contrast, the lipid system is contraindicated in patients with abnormalities of lipid metabolism. Patients with thrombosed or fragile peripheral veins precluding satisfactory fluid therapy need a central catheter merely to achieve vascular access. Such patients generally receive the less costly glucose system.

Patients with a tracheostomy who receive the glucose system are at increased risk of subclavian catheter sepsis because of the adjacent tracheostomy stoma. The peripherally infused lipid system has an advantage in these patients. Percutaneous subclavian catheterization, associated with a 2% risk of pneumothorax in the general population, is best avoided in patients in whom the risk of pneumothorax is significantly increased (e.g., patients with bullous emphysema) or in whom the consequences of pneumothorax may be severe morbidity or even death (e.g., patients with severe pulmonary dysfunction or respiratory failure). The lipid system infused through a peripheral vein is a useful alternative in such patients.

A more subtle but evidently important advantage of the lipid-based system in patients with severe pulmonary dysfunction relates to the relative amounts of carbon dioxide produced by the metabolism of isocaloric quantities of glucose and fat. Stoichiometric analysis of fuel oxidation indicates that isocaloric substitution of glucose with lipids produces a 23% reduction in the amount of carbon dioxide produced (0.0069 vs. 0.009 m/kcal) and, therefore, needs to be eliminated by the lungs:[70]

$$0.0015\ C_6H_{12}O_6 + 0.009\ O_2 \rightarrow 0.009\ CO_2 + 0.009\ H_2O \qquad (10)$$
(1 kcal glucose)

$$0.00043\ CH_3(CH_2CH_2)_7COOH + 0.01\ O_2 \rightarrow 0.0069\ CO_2 + 0.0069\ H_2O$$
(1 kcal palmitic acid) $\qquad (11)$

The additional carbon dioxide production associated with glucose oxidation may produce hypercarbia in patients with pulmonary insufficiency. The amount of carbon dioxide produced during oxidation (or lipogenesis) is often erroneously correlated with the respiratory quotient (RQ). Carbon dioxide production is not linearly related to RQ, since oxygen consumption may vary disproportionately with carbon dioxide production.[58,70]

Thus, the choice of lipid-based or glucose-based TPN in a given patient is based on a clinical judgment that weighs the relative advantage and disadvantages of the various nutritional and nonnutritional features of the two systems. The applicable considerations in a variety of clinical entities are summarized in Table 7.31.

Parenteral Nutrition at Home The development of the cuffed silicone rubber catheter (Hickman catheter) and similar vascular access devices associated with low thrombogenicity and minimal tissue reaction has made it possible to provide parenteral nutrition on an ambulatory basis at home for patients with chronic alimentary tract dysfunction. Such patients generally receive a glucose-based system because it is less costly and because the long-term cardiovascular effects of lipid infusions are unknown.

TABLE 7.31. Factors in Prescribing Parenteral Nutrition

Clinical Setting	Relevant Considerations	References
Acute myocardial ischemia	Lipid infusions may induce high blood levels of free fatty acids, which may incite arrhythmias and extend area of infarction. Therefore, glucose system recommended.	65,67,68
Fluid restriction	Glucose-based systems have higher caloric density. Therefore, glucose system recommended.	16
Glucose intolerance	Blood glucose levels more easily managed with lipid system. Therefore, lipid system often advantageous.	68,69
Hyperlipidemia	Lipid system contraindicated.	16
Immunodepression	Malnutrition-related immunodepression reversed by both forms of TPN.	71
Hepato-biliary function	1. Both systems commonly associated with elevated liver indices, rarely of clinical significance in adults.	61,72
	2. Long-term TPN with either system associated with increased incidence of gallstones.	61,72
Pancreatitis	Lipid infusions do not stimulate the pancreas and can be prescribed in the absence of underlying hyperlipidemia.	73,74
Pregnancy	Both systems are safe and effective in the second and third trimesters; experience is limited in the first trimester.	75
Pulmonary insufficiency	1. Less carbon dioxide is produced with the lipid system.	
	2. Using the lipid system eliminates the small risk of a dangerous pneumothorax that may complicate central venous catheter insertion.	16,70
Tracheostomy	The glucose system requires a central catheter that is in close proximity in the stoma. This can be avoided with the lipid system.	16

Source: Adapted from Silberman H. Administration of lipids. In Vincent JL (Ed), *Update in Intensive Care and Emergency Medicine.* New York: Springer-Verlage, 1986, p. 329.

Given a period of adaption in the hospital to the high glucose loads, it is usually possible to meet nutritional requirements at home with cyclic infusion. For example, patients may receive the nutrient solution over an 8- to 16-hour period at night so that they can be free of the infusion apparatus during all or a portion of their waking hours.

Comparison of Enteral and Parenteral Nutrition

Nitrogen Balance The preponderance of data derived form controlled, prospective studies in humans (Level I evidence) indicates that the nitrogen economy is supported to the same extent when equivalent nutrients are provided intravenously or by continuous infusion into the gastrointestinal tract.[16] Although the nutrient value of enterally and parenterally administered diets may be comparable, several investigators found that the time necessary to reach nitrogen equilibrium was greater in enterally fed patients because initial gastrointestinal intolerance slowed the advancement of enteral feedings to full prescription. However, this delay in achieving nitrogen equilibrium may not be of clinical significance. In their study comparing TPN and jejunostomy feedings, Adams and associates[76] found that equivalent nitrogen balance could be attained if the volume of enteral feedings prescribed was increased 20% above that calculated to meet requirements. This increase in the rate of infusion was necessary to compensate for interruptions in enteral therapy necessitated by periods of gastrointestinal intolerance.

Effects on the Alimentary Tract Involutional changes, both morphologic and functional, occur in the gastrointestinal tract and the pancreas when nutrition is maintained exclusively by vein, but not when the same nutrients are provided orally or enterally. The changes observed during TPN include a significant reduction in the mass of the small and large intestine, and a marked decrease in mucosal enzyme activity. Enzymes affected include maltase, sucrase, lactase, and peroxidase. In addition, the production of secretory IgA is impaired during TPN. TPN is associated with retarded intestinal growth and development in growing animals and impaired adaptive hyperplasia of residual intestine after enteric resection.[16]

These changes are not a response to intravenous nutrition as such but reflect the need for luminal nutrients for growth, development, and maintenance of normal intestinal mass and function. The mechanism by which food exerts a trophic effect appears to be twofold: (1) a direct effect related to utilization of luminal nutrients to meet the metabolic needs of the absorptive cells and (2) an indirect effect related to release of enteric hormones that have a trophic effect on the proliferative cells. Thus, supplemental gastrin can restore and maintain intestinal mass in animals receiving TPN, and cholecystokinin and secretin have similar trophic effects. The action of the last two hormones may be related to their stimulation of pancreatic and biliary secretions, both of which stimulate intestinal hypertrophy. Hwang and associates[77] studied the effect of glutamine-enriched parenteral nutrition on the morphologic integrity of the jejunum. This amino acid is a major oxidative fuel for the small intestine, but it is not present in the commercially available amino acid solutions. Addition of glutamine to the TPN solution significantly retarded but did not completely reverse the jejunal atrophy observed in rats during intravenous nutrition with standard solutions.

In most patients, the involutional changes occurring during parenteral nutrition are of little clinical relevance, and they apparently are reversed when oral alimentation is resumed. In certain conditions, however, these changes have clinical implications. For example, the reduction in motility and secretory output of the small intestine associated with TPN is thought to be beneficial in the management of enterocutaneous fistulas. Similarly, TPN-induced pancreatic hyposecretion may be of therapeutic value in cases of acute pancreatitis and pancreatic fistula. On the other hand, in short-bowel syndrome the involutional changes associated with TPN are undesirable because maximal compensatory villous hypertrophy is achieved only when enteral nutrition is part of the therapeutic regimen.[16]

In addition, it is possible that enteric involution may have an important impact in critically ill patients suffering multiple-organ trauma or thermal injuries. Several lines of evidence have led to the hypothesis that the sepsis that often develops after severe trauma and burns is due, at least in part, to bacterial translocation, a process wherein enteric organisms spread systemically by crossing the intact gastrointestinal mucosal barrier. In a series of animal experiments by Deitch and associates,[78–83] it has been shown that conditions that promote bacterial translocation include trauma (especially in combination with retained necrotic tissue as in severe burns), endotoxemia, an immunosuppressed state, and an altered enteric microflora due to bacterial overgrowth or oral antibiotics. Translocation was not observed by these investigators when starvation or malnutrition was the sole experimental variable, but the transmural bacterial invasion seen after endotoxin administration was aggravated when malnutrition was also present.

It is thought that this systemic invasion by enteric organisms reflects an impairment of the normal gut mucosal defense system, the components of which include gastric acid, mucus, normal peristalsis, and secretory IgA. Because TPN is associated with impairment of these protective mechanisms, whereas enteral feedings can maintain the functional and morphologic integrity of the alimentary tract, it has been suggested that enteral, rather than parenteral, nutrition may be important in preventing sepsis in the critically ill.

Moore and associates[84] randomized 75 patients to receive either TPN or enteral feeding within 12 hours of laparotomy for major abdominal trauma. Fewer septic complications were observed in the enterally fed group, primarily due to a reduction in the occurrence of pneumonia. The basis for this difference is uncertain, since lung invasion by translocating bacteria is quite uncommon. In a similar study, Kudsk et al.[85] randomly assigned 98 patients to receive enteral or parenteral nutrition within 24 hours of sustaining blunt or penetrating abdominal trauma. Again a significant reduction in septic morbidity was observed in the enterally fed group. However, the clinical significance of this finding is uncertain, since the two treatment groups did not differ in length of hospital stay, in antibiotic requirements, in ventilator-hours, and most importantly in survival. Moore et al.[86] published a meta-analysis of eight randomized trials comparing early enteral or parenteral nutrition in high-risk surgical patients. Nitrogen balance and weight gain were superior in the TPN group, but more infectious complications were observed even when catheter sepsis was eliminated. Again there was no difference in mortality, length of hospital stay, or cost between the two groups.

Many clinicians have concluded from these studies that enteral feedings are superior to parenteral feedings, and there is considerable enthusiasm for providing early or even immediate postoperative enteral nutrition to patients sustaining abdominal trauma in the hope of reducing septic morbidity. However, additional data are emerging that fail to support these conclusions.[76,87–89] Based on this information, albeit inconclusive, enteral feeding is preferred when safe and feasible because such a regimen is less costly and may possibly be associated with fewer septic complications than TPN. A similar conclusion was reached by Lipman in his recent review of the literature comparing enteral and parenteral nutrition in humans: With the exception of decreased cost and probable reduced septic morbidity in acute abdominal trauma, the available literature does not support the thesis that enteral nutrition is better than parenteral nutrition.[90]

Nutritional Support in Cancer Patients

Malnutrition is a frequent accompaniment of malignant disease, and when it occurs, prognosis is adversely affected.[16] As previously discussed, Smale and associates[36] calculated the prognostic nutritional index (PNI) for a series of cancer patients requiring elective surgery. These authors documented a significant increase in postoperative morbidity and mortality among those deemed at high risk because of malnutrition. DeWys and associates[91] analyzed the effect of weight loss on the survival of patients scheduled to receive chemotherapy for various lesions. For patients with nearly every tumor type, weight loss was associated with a statistically significant reduction in survival.

The malnutrition observed in cancer patients is related not only to the tumor per se but also to the adverse nutritional consequences of the antineoplastic therapy prescribed, including paralytic ileus, nausea, vomiting, mucositis, and diarrhea. The foregoing observations have led to the evaluation of nutritional support of cancer patients undergoing surgery, chemotherapy, or radiation.

Parenteral Nutrition as an Adjunct to Surgery   Smale et al.[36] reported that 6 or more days of preoperative TPN was associated with a 2.1-fold reduction in all postoperative complications, a 2.9-fold reduction in major sepsis, and a 2.7-fold reduction in mortality among poorly nourished, high-risk cancer patients (PNI ≥ 40). However, preoperative TPN did not benefit the well-nourished low-risk group. The findings of this retrospective study are similar to those of the more recent randomized trial of perioperative parenteral nutrition conducted by the Veterans Administration.[92] In this latter study, patients requiring elective surgery for benign or malignant disease were randomized to a control group receiving no preoperative TPN or to an experimental group in which TPN was given for 7 to 15 days prior to operation. Overall, no benefits were observed among the TPN-treated patients; in fact, the incidence of infectious complications was significantly increased. In contrast, in the subset of severely malnourished patients receiving TPN, significantly fewer noninfectious complications were observed with no concomitant increase in infectious complications. It appears, therefore, that in addition to the usual indications for enteral and parenteral nutrition, 7 to 15 days of preoperative TPN will benefit severely malnourished patients requiring elective oncologic surgery.

Parenteral Nutrition as an Adjunct to Chemotherapy   Adjunctive TPN is often advisable in severely depleted patients because nutritional repletion may enable such patients to receive aggressive chemotherapy that would otherwise be contraindicated because of fear of complications from malnutrition and inanition.[93] Unfortunately, however, randomized trials have failed to demonstrate a survival benefit or a diminution of chemotherapy-associated toxicity attributable to adjunctive TPN.

Parenteral Nutrition as an Adjunct to Radiation Therapy   Malnutrition occurring in patients undergoing radiation therapy may be a result of the underlying malignant disease, but may also be associated with or aggravated by the treatment itself. Thus, radiation therapy may be associated with loss of taste, anorexia, and dysphagia; or nausea, vomiting, and diarrhea secondary to radiation enteritis. Some patients may obtain marked relief of symptoms when they receive nutrients intravenously and refrain from oral intake. In addition, adjunctive TPN is able to stabilize or improve body weight. TPN may also be useful in reducing delays in initiating or carrying out a planned course of radiotherapy because of inanition. However, the major finding in prospective, randomized trials is that adjunctive TPN does not enhance the efficacy of radiotherapy. No improvement has been demonstrated in antitumor response or local control, in tolerance to treatment, or in the incidence of complications of therapy.[16,94]

Indications for Enteral and Parenteral Nutrition in Cancer Patients   The efficacy of enteral nutrition in cancer patients has been less intensively studied than TPN. However, based on data from other groups of malnourished patients, it is assumed that enteral and parenteral nutrition are comparable in achieving the goals of nutritional support when the usual requirements for safe and effective enteral nutrition are met. Therefore, based on the foregoing discussion, enteral or parenteral nutrition is indicated in cancer patients primarily to treat or prevent malnutrition and its complications when effective antitumor therapy is available. Routine adjunctive nutrition therapy is not recommended because specific oncologic benefits have not been demonstrated. However, nutrition therapy has an indirect oncologic benefit in repleting patients with a degree of inanition so severe as to otherwise preclude administration of optimally aggressive antitumor therapy. In addition, adjunctive TPN or enteral feedings may be indicated to prevent malnutrition in patients receiving a course of therapy known to produce anorexia or other significant side effects that would preclude normal oral intake. Such aggressive nutritional support usually is not indicated for patients for whom no effective antitumor therapy is available.

REFERENCES

1. Humes HD, Cox M. Principles of the renal regulation of fluids and electrolytes. In Kelley WN (Ed), *Textbook of Internal Medicine*, 2nd ed. Philadelphia: JB Lippincott Company, 1992, pp. 684–690.

2. Rose BD. *Clinical Physiology of Acid-Base and Electrolyte Disorders*, 4th ed. New York: McGraw-Hill, Inc., 1994.

3. Cogan MG. *Fluid and Electrolytes: Physiology and Pathophysiology*. Norwalk: Appleton and Lange, 1991.

4. Guyton AC. *Textbook of Medical Physiology*, 8th ed. Philadelphia: WB Saunders Company, 1991.

5. Goodwin CW Jr. Fluid and electrolyte balance and disorders of acid-base balance. In Levine BA, Copeland EM III, Howard RJ, Sugarman H, Warshaw AL (Eds), *Current Practice of Surgery*. New York: Churchill Livingstone, 1993, pp. 1–27.

6. Shires GT, Barber AE, Illner HP. Current status of resuscitation: solutions including hypertonic saline. *Adv Surg* 1995;28:133–170.

7. Moore FD. *Metabolic Care of the Surgical Patient*. Philadelphia: WB Saunders Company, 1959.

8. Lehninger AL. *Principles of Biochemistry*. New York: Worth Publishers, Inc, 1982.

9. Cantarow A, Schepartz B. *Biochemistry*. Philadelphia: WB Saunders Company, 1962.

10. Shires GT, Canizaro PC. Fluid and electrolyte management of the surgical patient. In Sabiston DC Jr (Ed), *Textbook of Surgery*, 14th ed. Philadelphia: WB Saunders Company, 1991, pp. 57–76.

11. Halperin ML, Goldstein MB. *Fluid, Electrolyte and Acid-Base Physiology: A Problem-Based Approach*, 2nd ed. Philadelphia: WB Saunders Company, 1994, pp. 145–183.

12. Boysen PG, Kirby RR. Acid-base problem solving. In Civetta JM, Taylors RW, Kirby RR (Eds), *Critical Care*. Philadelphia: JB Lippincott Company, 1988, pp. 335–339.

13. Shoemaker WC. Fluids and electrolytes in the acutely ill. In Shoemaker WC, Thompson WL, Holbrook PR (Eds), *Textbook of Critical Care*. Philadelphia: WB Saunders Company, 1984, pp. 614–640.

14. Morgan GE, Mikhail MS. *Clinical Anesthesiology*. Norwalk CT: Appleton and Lange, 1992.

15. Hayes MA. Water and electrolyte therapy after operation. *N Engl J Med* 1968;278:1054–1056.

16. Silberman H. *Parenteral and Enteral Nutrition*, 2nd ed. Norwalk, CT: Appleton and Lange, 1989.

17. Ratner LE, Smith GW. Intraoperative fluid management. *Surg Clin N Am* 1993;73:229–241.

18. Wait RB, Kahng KU. Fluid and electrolytes and acid-base balance. In Greenfield LJ, Mulholland MW, Oldham KT, Zelenock GB (Eds), *Surgery: Scientific Principles and Practice.* Philadelphia: JB Lippincott Company, 1993, pp. 222–245.

19. Velanovich V. Crystalloid versus colloid fluid resuscitation: a meta-analysis of mortality. *Surgery* 1989;105:65–71.

20. Schierhout G, Roberts I. Fluid resuscitation with colloid or crystalloid solutions in critically ill patients: a systemic review of randomised trials. *Br Med J* 1998;316:961–964.

21. Berry REL. The "third kidney" phenomenon of the gastrointestinal tract: a complication of parenteral fluid therapy and intestinal trauma. *Arch Surg* 1960;81:193–204.

22. Silberman H. Renal failure and the surgeon. *Surg Gynecol Obstet* 1977;144:775–784.

23. Berl T, Schrier RW. Disorders of water metabolism. In Schrier RW (Ed), *Renal and Electrolyte Disorders*, 5th ed. Boston: Little, Brown and Company, 1992, pp. 1–87.

24. Weisberg LS, Szerlip HM, Cox M. Approach to the patient with altered sodium and water homeostasis. In Kelley WN (Ed), *Textbook of Internal Medicine*, 2nd ed. Philadelphia: JB Lippincott Company, 1992, pp. 839–848.

25. Atterbury CE, Groszmann RJ. Approach to the patient with cirrhosis and portal hypertension. In Kelly WN (Ed), *Textbook of Internal Medicine*, 2nd ed. Philadelphia: JB Lippincott Company, 1992, pp. 652–663.

26. Grieg PD, Langer B. Peritoneovenous shunts for intractable ascites. In Sabiston DC Jr (Ed), *Textbook of Surgery*, 15th ed. Philadelphia: WB Saunders Company, 1997, pp. 1104–1110.

26a. Kumar S, Berl T. Sodium. *Lancet* 1998;352:220–228.

26b. Martin P-V, Gines P, Schrier RW. Nitric oxide as mediator of hemodynamic abnormalities and sodium and water retention in cirrhosis. *N Engl J Med* 1998;339:533–541.

27. Baker AR, Weber J. Treatment of malignant ascites. In DeVita VT Jr, Hellman S, Rosenberg SA (Eds), *Cancer: Principles and Practice of Oncology*, 4th ed. Philadelphia: JB Lippincott Company, 1993, pp. 2255–2261.

28. Pockros PJ, Esrason KT, Nguyen C, et al. Mobilization of malignant ascites with diuretics is dependent on ascitic fluid characteristics. *Gastroenterology* 1992;103:1302–1306.

29. Greenway B, Johnson PJ, Williams R. Control of malignant ascites with spironolactone. *Brit J Surg* 1982;69:441–442.

30. Silberman H. The role of preoperative parenteral nutrition in cancer patients. *Cancer* 1985;55:254–257.

31. Studley HO. Percentage of weight loss: a basic indicator of surgical risk in patients with chronic peptic ulcer. *JAMA* 1936;106:458–460.

32. Cannon PR, Wissler RW, Woolridge RL, Benditt EP. The relationship of protein deficiency to surgical infection. *Ann Surg* 1944;120:514–525.

33. Rhoads JE, Alexander CE. Nutritional problems of surgical patients. *Ann NY Acad Sci* 1955;63:268–275.

34. Mullen JL, Gertner MH, Buzby GP, Goodhart GL, Rosato EF. Implications of malnutrition in the surgical patient. *Arch Surg* 1979;114:121–125.

35. Pietsch JB, Meakins JL, Maclean LD. The delayed hypersensitivity response: application in clinical surgery. *Surgery* 1977;82:349–355.

36. Smale BF, Mullen JE, Buzby GP, Rosato EF. The efficacy of nutritional assessment and support in cancer surgery. *Cancer* 1981;47:2375–2381.

37. Hickman DM, Miller RA, Rombeau JL, Twomey PL, Frey CF. Serum albumin and body weight as predictors of postoperative course in colorectal cancer. *JPEN* 1980;4:314–316.

38. Silberman H. Nutrition, parenteral. In Webster JG (Editor-in-chief), *Encyclopedia of Medical Devices and Instrumentation*, vol. 3. New York: John Wiley and Sons, 1988, pp. 2081–2090.

39. Wilmore DW. Energy requirements for maximum nitrogen retention. In Greene HL, Holliday MA, Munro HN (Eds), *Clinical Nutrition Update: Amino Acids*. Chicago: American Medical Association, 1977, pp. 47–57.

40. Calloway DH, Spector H. Nitrogen balance as related to caloric and protein intake in active young men. *Am J Clin Nutr* 1954;2:405–412.

41. Rudman D, Millikan WJ, Richardson TJ, Bixler TJ II, Stackhouse WJ, McGarrity WC. Elemental balances during intravenous hyperalimentation of underweight subjects. *J Clin Invest* 1975;55:94–104.

42. Levine GM, Deren JJ, Steiger E, Zinno R. Role of oral intake in maintenance of gut mass and disaccharide activity. *Gastroenterology* 1974;67:975–982.

43. Stephenson LS, Latham MC. Lactose intolerance and milk consumption: the relation of tolerance to symptoms. *Am J Clin Nutr* 1974;27:296–303.

44. Silk DBA. *Nutritional Support in Hospital Practice*. Oxford: Blackwell Scientific Publications, 1983.

45. Sucher KP. Medium chain triglycerides: a review of their enteral use in clinical nutrition. *Nutr Clin Prac* 1986;1:146–150.

46. Bach AC, Babayan UK. Medium chain triglycerides: an update. *Am J Clin Nutr* 1982;36:950–962.

47. Gorden EE, Duga J. Experimental hyperosmolar diabetic syndrome: ketogenic response to medium chain triglycerides. *Diabetes* 1975;24:301–306.

48. Meehan SE, Wood RAB, Cuschieri A. Percutaneous cervical pharyngostomy: a comfortable and convenient alternative to protracted nasogastric intubation. *Am J Surg* 1984;148:325–330.

49. Bucklin DL, Gilsdor RB. Percutaneous needle pharyngostomy. *JPEN* 1985;9:68–70.

50. Graham WP III, Royster HP. Simplified cervical esophagostomy for long term extraoral feeding. *Surg Gynecol Obstet* 1967;125:127–128.

51. Cataldi-Betcher EL, Seltzer MH, Slocum BA, Jones KW. Complications occurring during enteral nutrition support: a prospective study. *JPEN* 1983;7:546–552.

52. Heymsfield SB, Erbland M, Casper K, et al. Enteral nutritional support: metabolic, cardiovascular, and pulmonary interrelations. *Clin Chest Med* 1986;7:41–67.

53. Dudrick SJ, Wilmore DW, Vars HM. Long term total parenteral nutrition with growth in puppies and positive nitrogen balance in patients. *Surg Forum* 1967;18:356–357.

54. Dudrick SJ, Rhoads JE. New horizons for intravenous feeding. *JAMA* 1971;215:939–949.

55. Dudrick WJ, Wilmore DW, Vars HM, Rhoads JE. Long-term total parenteral nutrition with growth, development, and positive nitrogen balance. *Surgery* 1968;64:134–142.

56. Wilmore DW, Dudrick SJ. Growth and development of an infant receiving all nutrients exclusively by vein. *JAMA* 1968;203:860–864.

57. Silberman H, Freehauf M, Fong G, Rosenblatt N. Parenteral nutrition with lipids. *JAMA* 1977;238:1380–1382.

58. Silberman H. Total parenteral nutrition by peripheral vein: current status of fat emulsions. *Nutr Internat* 1986;2:145–149.

59. Silberman H. Fat emulsions as a major calorie source in total parenteral nutrition. *Nutrition* 1991;7:333–334.

60. Hansen LM, Hardie WR, Hidalgo J. Fat emulsion for intravenous administration: clinical experience with Inralipid 10%. *Ann Surg* 1976;184:80–88.

61. Wagner WH, Lowry AC, Silberman H. Similar liver function abnormalities occur in patients receiving glucose-based and lipid-based parenteral nutrition. *Am J Gastroenterol* 1983;78:199–202.

62. Bowyer BA, Fleming CR, Ludwig J, Petz J, McGill DB. Does long-term home parenteral nutrition in adult patients cause chronic liver disease? *JPEN* 1985;9:11–15.

63. Silberman H. Use and abuse of parenteral nutrition. *West J Med* 1991;155:405.

64. Wolfe BM, Culebras JM, Sim AJW, et al. Substrate interaction in intravenous feeding: comparative effects of carbohydrate and fat on amino acid utilization in fasting man. *Ann Surg* 1977;186:518–540.

65. Jeejeebhoy KN, Anderson GH, Nakhooda AF, et al. Metabolic studies in total parenteral nutrition with lipid in man: comparison with glucose. *J Clin Invest* 1976;57:127–136.

66. Silberman H. Parenteral nutrition in adults. In Rakel RE (Ed), *Conn's Current Therapy 1992*. Philadelphia: WB Saunders Company, 1992, pp. 531–535.

67. Free fatty acids and arrhythmias after acute myocardial infarction (editorial). *Lancet* 1975;1:313–314.

68. Meguid MM, Schimmel E, Johnson WC, et al. Reduced metabolic complications in total parenteral nutrition. Pilot study using fat to replace one third of glucose calories. *JPEN* 1982;6:304–307.

69. Kleinberger G, Druml W, Laggner A, Lenz K. Parenteral nutrition of diabetic patients with fat. *JPEN* 1981;5:579.

70. Silberman H, Silberman AW. Parenteral nutrition, biochemistry and respiratory exchange. *JPEN* 1986;10:151–154.

71. Wagner WH, Silberman H. Lipid-based parenteral nutrition and the immunosuppression of protein malnutrition. *Arch Surg* 1984;119:809–810.

72. Doty JE, Pitt HA, Porter-Fink V, et al. The effect of intravenous fat and total parenteral nutrition on biliary physiology. *JPEN* 1984;8:263–268.

73. Edelman K, Valenzuela JE. Effect of intravenous lipid on human pancreatic secretion. *Gastroenterology* 1983;85:1063–1066.

74. Silberman H, Dixon NP, Eisenberg D. The safety and efficacy of lipid-based system of parenteral nutrition in acute pancreatitis. *Am J Gastroenterol* 1982;77:494–497.

75. Seifer DB, Silberman H, Catanzarite VA, et al. Total parenteral nutrition in obstetrics. *JAMA* 1985;253:2073–2075.

76. Adams S, Dellinger EP, Wertz MJ, et al. Enteral versus parenteral nutritional support following laparotomy for trauma: a randomized prospective trial. *J Trauma* 1986;26:882–891.

77. Hwang TL, O'Dwyer ST, Smith RJ, Wilmore DW. Preservation of small bowel mucosa using glutamine enriched parenteral nutrition. *Surg Forum* 1986;37:56–58.

78. Deitch EA, Winterton J, Berg R. Effects of starvation, malnutrition, and trauma on the gastrointestinal tract flora and bacterial translocation. *Arch Surg* 1987;122:1019–1024.

79. Deitch EA, Winterton J, Berg R. The gut as a portal of entry for bacteremia: role of protein malnutrition. *Ann Surg* 1987;205:681–692.

80. Deitch EA, Bridges RM. Effect of stress and trauma on bacterial translocation from the gut. *J Surg Res* 1987;42:536–542.

81. Deitch EA, Berg R. Endotoxin but not malnutrition promotes bacterial translocation of the gut flora in burned mice. *J Trauma* 1987;27:161–166.

82. Deitch EA, Winterton J, Berg R. Thermal injury promotes bacterial translocation from the gastrointestinal tract in mice with impaired T-cell-mediated immunity. *Arch Surg* 1986;121:97–101.

83. Deitch EA, Maejima K, Berg R. Effect of oral antibiotics and bacterial overgrowth on the translocation of the GI tract microflora in burned rats. *J Trauma* 1985;25:385–392.

84. Moore FA, Moore EE, Jones TN, et al. TEN versus TPN following major abdominal trauma—reduced septic morbidity. *J Trauma* 1989;29:916–923.

85. Kudsk KA, Croce MA, Fabian TC, et al. Enteral versus parenteral feeding. Effects on septic morbidity after blunt and penetrating abdominal trauma. *Ann Surg* 1992;215:503–513.

86. Moore FA, Feliciano DV, Andrassy RV, et al. Early enteral feeding, compared with parenteral, reduces postoperative septic complications. The results of a meta-analysis. *Ann Surg* 1992;216:172–183.

87. Cerra FB, McPherson JP, Konstantinides FN, et al. Enteral nutrition does not prevent multiple organ failure syndrome (MOFS) after sepsis. *Surgery* 1988;104:727–733.

88. Eyer SD, Micon LT, Konstantinides FN, et al. Early enteral feeding does not attenuate metabolic response after blunt trauma. *J Trauma* 1993;34:639–644.

89. Watters JM, Kirkpatrick SM, Norris SB, et al. Immediate postoperative enteral feeding results in impaired respiratory mechanics and decreased mobility. *Ann Surg* 1997;226:369–380.

90. Lipman TO. Grains or veins: Is enteral nutrition really better than parenteral nutrition? A look at the evidence. *JPEN* 1998;22:167–182.

91. DeWys WD, Begg C, Lavin PT, et al. Prognostic effect of weight loss prior to chemotherapy in cancer patients. *Am J Med* 1980;69:491–497.

92. Buzby GP, and the Veterans Affairs Total Parenteral Nutrition Cooperative Study Group. Perioperative total parenteral nutrition in surgical patients. *N Engl J Med* 1991;325:525–532.

93. Copeland EM III, MacFadyen BV Jr., Lanzotti VJ, Dudrick SJ. Intravenous hyper-alimentation as an adjunct to cancer chemotherapy. *Am J Surg* 1975;129:167–173.

94. Donaldson S. Nutritional support as an adjunct to radiation therapy. *JPEN* 1984;8:302–310.

PART II

PERIOPERATIVE MANAGEMENT OF GYNECOLOGIC SURGERY

CHAPTER 8

PREOPERATIVE EVALUATION

PAUL S. LIN, M.D.

Preoperative assessment is an integral part of preparation for surgery and should be considered as important as the surgery itself. Unfortunately, the importance of attention to detail in such preoperative evaluation is underestimated. Instead, a battery of tests and evaluations are routinely and reflexively ordered without careful regard for the patient's history, cost, or discomfort and potential morbidity to the patient. As a result, more than $30 billion is spent per year in the United States on routine preoperative testing.[1] Up to 60% of these routine testing procedures could be eliminated without adversely affecting outcomes.[2–4]

Needless to state, a systematic history and physical should be performed on all patients scheduled for an operative procedure. Medical tests and evaluations should then be selectively obtained in order to determine which patients may have contraindications for surgery, to help anticipate possible adverse outcomes, and to guide postoperative management. This chapter reviews the necessity of routine preoperative laboratory studies including chemistries, coagulation studies, chest X rays, and preoperative pulmonary evaluation from an evidence-based point of view. Cardiac evaluation is addressed in Chapter 9. Although these recommendations are evidence based, they should serve only as guidelines; no recommendations should replace good clinical judgment.

CLINICAL SIGNIFICANCE OF LABORATORY TESTS

Various gynecology texts have differing recommendations as to routine preoperative testing. One widely used text recommends that a complete blood count (CBC), urinalysis, and chest radiograph (chest X ray) be obtained in all patients and an electrocardiogram (EKG) in patients over 40.[5] Another popularly used text agrees with a routine CBC and recommends electrolytes, chest X-ray, and EKG in patients older than 40.[6]

Perioperative and Supportive Care in Gynecologic Oncology: Evidence-Based Management,
Edited by Steven A. Vasilev.
ISBN 0-471-24788-X   Copyright © 2000 by Wiley-Liss, Inc.

At what level does the literature support specific evidence-based guidelines addressing preoperative studies? Firm evidence exists regarding the lack of clinical value for routine preoperative coagulation studies, specifically prothrombin time (PT) and partial thromboplastin time (PTT). In a prospective study of 282 patients, 4% of coagulation studies performed were abnormal. However, none of these abnormalities identified a clinically significant coagulopathy that altered patient management.[7] In a retrospective study of 480 patients who had PT and PTT performed without specific indications, 13 or 2.7% had abnormal results.[8] Only one of these patients had a bleeding complication; this patient underwent a second operation to control arterial bleeding. It is unclear whether this complication can be truly ascribed to the abnormal PTT. Others have similarly found no benefit.[9,10] Therefore, there is no benefit in obtaining PT and PTT as routine preoperative screening when a history and physical does not suggest a possible coagulopathy.

Studies regarding the necessity of other preoperative tests have not been as conclusive. Two large studies, one retrospective and the other prospective, have suggested that other routine preoperative laboratory evaluations, when done as routine without any specific clinical indications, are of little clinical value. However, both of these studies are limited by study design.

Kaplan et al. retrospectively reviewed preoperative labs done at a single teaching hospital at the University of California, San Francisco, to assess their necessity.[2] Routine preoperative lab tests including CBC, platelet count, differential, PT, PTT, electrolytes, creatinine (Cr), and glucose were retrospectively reviewed for medical indication, and whether an abnormal result altered surgical or anesthetic management. Of the 2,785 laboratory tests reviewed, 60% were ordered without any apparent specific medical conditions being present and therefore defined as "unindicated." The hemoglobin level as part of a CBC was deemed indicated in this study if the planned surgery was "potentially bloody" (i.e., vaguely defined as a procedure requiring preoperative crossmatching). Of these unindicated tests, there were only 4 (0.22% of all unindicated labs) abnormal laboratory tests that were judged to be of clinical significance, in which the result may possibly have altered surgical or anesthetic management. However, on further review of medical records, no alteration in management induced by these lab results was noted. Furthermore, Kaplan estimated that in his hospital, where approximately 8,600 procedures are performed each year, not performing this unindicated battery of preoperative labs would result in 1 death in 100 years, or in economic terms, $4.2 million would be spent on routine, unindicated labs to save one life.

However, this retrospective study only identified abnormal labs that may have delayed or canceled surgery, or altered anesthesia management. It did not or was not able to identify labs that may possibly have affected postoperative management. Such a retrospective study may have limitations in identifying such potential consequences.

Similarly, in a prospective study of 520 general, vascular, head and neck, and thoracic surgery patients, univariate and multivariate analyses were used in assessing the ability of electrolytes, glucose, blood urea nitrogen (BUN), creatinine (Cr), CBC, total protein/albumin/lymphocyte count (nutritional studies), coagulation studies, and urinalysis in predicting postoperative complications.[10] Overall, the routine preoperative labs studied were of no to minimal clinical value in predicting meaningful clinical complications. Although not confirmed by multivariate analyses, univariate analyses suggested correlation between abnormal nutritional tests (total protein/albumin/lymphocyte count) and postoperative death. This, however, should not be interpreted that such tests should be obtained preoperatively on all patients, since the incidence of death is low and there are usually clinical findings that suggest a severely malnourished state. Although this study addressed the likelihood that preoperative tests may predict postoperative complications, it did not determine whether the labs may have altered perioperative management in any other way.

Almost all agree that the hemoglobin/hematocrit portion of a preoperative CBC is prudent prior to a major surgery regardless of whether such a test could be predictive of a potential postoperative complication. The value of a CBC extends beyond the ability to predict postoperative complications, providing information for intraoperative planning. However, how to act on a hemoglobin level preoperatively or perioperatively is debatable. Traditional perioperative management dictated red blood cell transfusion for a hemoglobin level of less than 10 g/dl.[11,12] Modern practice suggests that most patients around 10 g/dl rarely need blood transfusions, and other conditions such as the presence of signs and symptoms of anemia, coronary vascular disease, and baseline hemoglobin level should enter into consideration. Moreover, evidence suggests that perioperative morbidity is not adversely affected by mild to moderate anemia if the patient remains normovolemic.[13]

With regard to preoperative preparation for possible blood product use, it is important to note that hospitals must maintain an inventory based on the amount of blood crossmatched (i.e., reserved) rather than the amount used. Therefore, some basic strategies should be considered for optimal resource utilization.[14,15] This should be based on the probability of significant bleeding, preoperative hemoglobin value, and the knowledge of how rapidly red cell blood products can generally become available.

Complete compatibility testing (ABO, Rh, antibody screen, and crossmatch) in the absence of unexpected red cell antibodies can generally be performed within 1 hour. If an antibody screen is positive, this process can take twice as long or longer. However, if a type-and-screen procedure is performed preoperatively, the ABO/Rh/antibody status is already known intraoperatively. Assuming no antibodies are isolated, in the event of unanticipated transfusion need, the blood can become available within 10 to 15 minutes.

If a type and screen is not ordered preoperatively, type-specific or emergency crossmatched blood can also rapidly become available. However, antibody screening is not performed in this circumstance, increasing transfusion reaction risk.

If preoperative antibody screening reveals the presence of complex antibodies, it may be prudent to crossmatch several units of blood even in patients who are at relatively low risk for significant blood loss. Generally, presence of antibodies in the recipient is more dangerous than in the donor, since any donor antibodies present are diluted within the recipient's circulation during transfusion, minimizing the reaction.

Preparation for autologous blood use deserves special comment. National trends reflect the perception that autologous blood is safer than allogenic blood during transfusion. Between 1989 and 1992, the overall transfusion rate decreased, but autologous blood donation increased by 60%.[17] Unfortunately, up to half of these units are never used. Additionally, transfusion is not risk-free, with an estimated overall transfusion risk of 1 in 15,000 to 50,000 units.[17] Thus, the benefits are not clear-cut. Cost analysis reveals that processing autologous blood is also significantly more expensive. Marginal analysis has demonstrated that costs range from $235,000 to $23 million per quality-adjusted life year (QALY) gained using autologous blood.[18] Given the low donated autologous unit utilization rates, preoperative strategy should be based on the likelihood of transfusion just as recommended for allogeneic blood product use.

A complete discussion of transfusion medicine is beyond the scope of this chapter and the reader is referred elsewhere.[19] Overall, given the evidence available, the following preoperative laboratory guidelines can be recommended:

1. CBC should be obtained in all patients undergoing major surgery with significant risk for hemorrhage.
2. A qualitative HCG (human chorionic gonadotropin) pregnancy test should be obtained on all patients of reproductive potential for medicolegal reasons, as well as for the concern that the procedure or anesthesia may potentially impact the pregnancy.
3. A PT/PTT should not be obtained routinely, and is indicated preoperatively when there is clinical concern for a coagulopathy.
4. Evidence suggests but is not conclusive that urinalysis, electrolytes, BUN/Cr, and other chemistries ordered preoperatively on a routine basis may be omitted if no clinical evidence of indication is discerned.
5. Preoperative type and crossmatch versus type and screen should depend on the anticipated need for blood product use.

Blery et al. proposed a protocol of selectively obtaining preoperative labs under certain guidelines and evaluated such a protocol prospectively at a teaching hospital in Paris, France.[20] Clinical indications suspected by history for ordering preoperative labs are as follows:

1. Type and screen for major surgical procedures
2. Hemoglobin for major surgical procedures
3. PT/PTT for malignancy, hepatobiliary and bleeding disorders, or use of anticoagulants

4. Electrolytes for age greater than 70, renal disorder, diabetes, use of diuretics, digitalis, or corticosteroids
5. BUN/Cr for age greater than 70, renal disorder, diabetes, or use of diuretics
6. Glucose for diabetes or use of corticosteroids
7. Chest X ray for cardiovascular or pulmonary disorders
8. EKG for age greater than 40, cardiovascular or pulmonary disorders

This protocol was employed over 1 year in which 3,866 patients were enrolled. Upon discharge or after an appropriate postoperative period had lapsed, anesthesiologists were asked to review the hospital course to determine whether any of the above evaluations not obtained would have been "potentially useful." No perioperative deaths were attributed to omission of an evaluation. Furthermore, only 0.2% of omitted labs were deemed to have been potentially useful upon review of the perioperative course.

One serious postoperative complication occurred in a 23-year-old man who was noted to have a cardiac arrhythmia and pulmonary edema after an appendectomy. A postoperative EKG revealed Wolff–Parkinson–White syndrome. Additionally, the authors felt that omission of tests may have hampered diagnosis or therapy in 10 other cases. However, half of these scenarios could have been avoided if a thorough history and physical were performed.

The protocol presented above served as a guideline, and in 18% of the cases, deviations from the guideline were made because of individual preferences of the attending physicians. No modification to this protocol was made during the prospective study. Nevertheless, the size of this study prevents concluding whether omission of any tests may have significantly increased perioperative morbidity. The authors felt their protocol was acceptable, but warned that it be used only as a guideline, and should not replace good clinical judgment.

CHEST RADIOGRAPH

A study that could definitively determine the value of routine preoperative chest X rays would be difficult to accomplish. Ideally, it would involve a prospective investigation in which patients were randomized to having a preoperative chest X ray or no chest X ray, followed by an analysis of health outcomes between the two groups. Such a definitive study would require large numbers of patients (>20,000).[21] Also contributing to the difficulty of such a study is the fact that clinical decisions based on chest X-ray findings are often subjective and individualized. For example, a particular chest X-ray finding may alter one surgeon's plan of management, whereas such a finding may have no effect on another's clinical plan. It would be virtually impossible for a prospective study to attempt to control or standardize widely different management styles.

Several retrospective studies, although limited by the adequacy of record charting as is common in retrospective chart reviews, have not been able to demonstrate much value of routine preoperative chest X rays in the general patient population. The largest study was conducted by the Royal College of Radiologists, a multicenter study that surveyed the practice of obtaining routine preoperative chest X rays in noncardiopulmonary surgical patients among eight hospitals in Great Britain.[22] Of 10,619 patients involved in this survey, only 30% had a routine preoperative chest X ray. Practice variance was wide among the various institutions, ranging between 12% and 54%.

The investigators in this study defined as their outcome the impact of an abnormal chest X ray on the decision to operate or on the type of anesthesia used. Findings in this study suggested that the preoperative chest X ray had little influence on either outcome. Regarding whether the preoperative chest X ray may have altered the decision to operate, 96% of patients with a normal chest X ray and 92% of patients with significant radiological abnormalities proceeded to surgery. The difference was not statistically significant. Similarly, chest X-ray findings did not seem to affect the anesthesia used with 96% of patients with normal chest X rays and the same percentage with abnormal chest X rays undergoing inhalational anesthesia. However, the study design limits conclusions regarding whether a preoperative chest X ray may have in any other way altered perioperative management.

Some have argued that preoperative chest X rays are of value in serving as a baseline to which subsequent postoperative chest X rays could be compared. Mendelson and colleagues attempted to address this question in a review of 369 general surgery patients.[23] Of this number, 65 underwent postoperative chest X rays. The authors reported that in approximately half of these cases (33 out of 65), a preoperative chest X ray was "essential" in making an accurate interpretation of the postoperative chest X ray. Unclear in this study is whether an increased accuracy in interpreting the postoperative chest X ray truly altered postoperative clinical management.

Another factor that could be evaluated is the likelihood of finding significant radiologic abnormalities on preoperative chest X rays done without any clinical indications. One study by Sagel revealed a 1% incidence of a serious radiological abnormality found on chest X rays in patients under 30 years of age.[24] In patients 50 to 60 years of age, the incidence of significant abnormalities increased to approximately 20% and attained an even higher percentage with increasing age (Table 8.1).

Tornebrandt and Fletcher reported a 37% rate of serious abnormal preoperative chest X-ray findings such as cardiomegaly, pulmonary venous hypertension, and emphysema in patients 70 years or older who had no other medical indications for having a chest X ray.[25] Rucker and colleagues proposed certain risk factors that could predict the likelihood of having an abnormal preoperative chest X ray (Table 8.2).[26] These risk factors include age greater than 60, history of cardiac or pulmonary disease, and signs and symptoms of chest disease. Using their criteria, 905 patients from various surgical services including gynecology and general surgery were studied. Of the 368 patients who had no

TABLE 8.1. Risk of Clinically Significant Chest Radiograph Abnormality By Age

Age	Number of Serious Abnormality	Percentage Abnormality
00–19	0/521	(0)
20–29	9/894	(1)
30–39	22/942	(2)
40–49	66/928	(7)
50–59	179/883	(20)
60–69	290/977	(30)
≥70	347/832	(42)

Source: Adapted from Sagel SS, Evens RG, Forrest JV, Bramson BE. Efficacy of routine screening and lateral chest radiographs in a hospital-based population. *N Engl J Med* 1974;291:1001–1004.

risk factors, only 1 patient had a significant abnormality (elevated diaphragm), and none of the patients in this low-risk group had any postoperative pulmonary or cardiac complications.

In summary, available studies in the literature have been unable to support the use of routine, preoperative chest X ray in the general patient population. Nevertheless, in certain patient populations at higher risk of having a clinically significant radiological abnormality on chest X ray, such as the elderly, a preoperative chest X ray may be of value. Certainly, patients with cardiopulmonary findings on history and physical should undergo a preoperative chest X ray. In these situations, chest X rays would not be considered routine, which implies chest X rays are obtained with no other indications other than as part of general presurgical preparation. There may be other reasons for obtaining a chest X ray before surgery, such as in the evaluation of a patient with a newly diagnosed gynecological malignancy. The finding of distant metastasis may dramatically change the surgery planned. It is not within the scope of this chapter to discuss these circumstances.

CLINICAL SIGNIFICANCE OF PULMONARY FUNCTION EVALUATIONS

Pulmonary complications, such as atelectasis or pneumonia, are a frequent and important group of complications postoperatively with a generally reported incidence ranging between 6% and 60%.[27] Abdominal incisions, especially in the upper abdomen, are frequently associated with pulmonary complications postoperatively.[27–31] No other class of surgery except for thoracotomies are associated with a higher frequency of pulmonary problems.

A major factor accounting for the pathophysiology behind pulmonary complications after abdominal surgery is the decrease in lung volumes and flow rates that occur postoperatively.[29–31] This is felt to be secondary to diaphragmatic dysfunc-

TABLE 8.2. Risk Factors for Abnormal Chest Radiographs

Medical History

Cancer at any site
Valvular heart disease
Stroke
Myocardial infarction
Angina
Asthma
Tuberculosis
Chronic obstructive pulmonary disease
Cigarettes
Occupational exposures: asbestos, fumes, or ores

Review of Systems

General: fever, chills, sweats, or weight loss
Paroxysmal nocturnal dyspnea
Orthopnea
Class 3 or 4 dyspnea
Angina

Physical Findings

Vital signs: fever, tachycardia, hypertension, or tachypnea
Chest: abnormal breath sounds, abnormal adventitial sounds,
    or dullness
Cardiovascular: severe murmurs, S3, or displaced point of
    maximum impulse

Source: Adapted from Rucker L, Frye EB, Staten MA. Usefulness of screening chest roentgenograms in preoperative patients. *JAMA* 1983;250:3209–3211.

tion from decreased phrenic nerve output. Other risk factors associated with post-operative pulmonary complications include history of cigarette smoking,[27,29–32] underlying respiratory disease,[33] obesity,[31] and prolonged anesthesia time >3–3.5 hours.[27,29] Increasing age has also been associated with pulmonary complications. However, age is not felt to be a major independent risk factor. The higher rate of complications seen in older patients is probably due to a higher prevalence of chronic pulmonary disease and decreased pulmonary function.[32]

Pulmonary function tests or spirometry is a common screening tool used in the evaluation of the respiratory system. The objective of this section is to review the literature assessing the value of spirometry in its ability to prevent or decrease pulmonary complications. Spirometry has been demonstrated to be of value in lung resection surgeries.[28] Due to the lack of studies specifically evaluating preoperative pulmonary function tests in gynecologic surgeries, this review is directed toward studies focused on abdominal surgeries.

One of the major difficulties in evaluating the role of spirometry is the subjectivity by which outcomes are assessed, which in this case would be pulmonary complications. The wide range of reported pulmonary complications ranging from 6% to as high as 80% underlies the lack of strict objective criteria by which pulmonary complications are defined and diagnosed.[27,33] Some authors have included as pulmonary complications clinically trivial situations such as the presence of atelectasis on chest X ray without regard to the clinical situation of the patient, or simply a temperature elevation of 1–2°F postoperatively. Others, recognizing the difficulty in strictly defining pulmonary complications, have instead used clinically meaningful outcomes such as length of hospital stay or mortality secondary to respiratory complications as surrogate measures of pulmonary complications.

In order for spirometry to be of clinical value as a screening tool, it must first accurately predict patients at risk for pulmonary complications. Second, there must exist some type of medical management that could be employed, depending on the results of the screening test, that could prevent those deemed at higher risk from developing pulmonary complications.

A widely cited study promoting the use of routine screening spirometry preoperatively in predicting patients at risk for pulmonary problems was a 1962 report by Stein and colleagues.[34] In this study, 63 patients scheduled for a variety of surgeries including dilatation and curettage, hysterectomy, bowel resection, and pneumonectomy underwent preoperative spirometry. Based on the results of spirometry, 33 patients were classified in the normal risk group and 30 were classified in the high-risk category. Among the normal patients, only 1 was deemed to have developed a postoperative pulmonary complication, whereas among the patients in the high-risk group, 21 were determined to have pulmonary complications. Considering only patients who had abdominal incisions, 9 patients had normal spirometry, none of whom developed pulmonary complications. Of the 14 patients who had abnormal spirometry, 11 developed pulmonary complications.

Unfortunately, major criticisms of this study include the lack of objective information regarding the diagnosis and severity of pulmonary complications, and that assessors of pulmonary complications were not blinded to the preoperative spirometry result. Both of these conditions may have introduced significant potential for bias. Other subsequent papers addressing patients undergoing abdominal surgeries have similarly concluded that preoperative pulmonary function tests are of value as a screening tool.[33,35,36] However, all of these studies have methodological flaws that preclude drawing any firm conclusions.

Postoperative pulmonary complications ranged between 14% and 76% in these reports. This wide range was due not only to differences in patient populations but also to differences in types of outcomes assessed and varying definitions of pulmonary complications. For example, one study of 46 patients with only upper abdominal surgeries reported a 76% incidence of postoperative pulmonary complications, including the presence of atelectasis on chest X ray.[33] Another study, a retrospective chart review, which defined outcomes of pulmonary complications as respiratory failure or death, reported spirometry was predictive of pulmonary complications. However, other factors such as simply the patient's age, serum albumin level, or PaO2 were even more predictive than spirometry in this report.[36]

One prospective study examined 100 "apparently normal" clinical subjects who underwent preoperative spirometry.[35] Among the 14% of patients who developed pulmonary complications, a higher percentage (57%) had an abnormal FEV1/FVC ratio compared to only 8% of the group of patients who did not develop complications. However, there were other confounding factors in the complications group, such as higher average age and higher frequency of upper abdominal incisions, which preclude drawing the conclusion that spirometry alone could accurately predict those at risk.

The second requirement before a screening test could be of clinical value is that clinical approaches or techniques exist that could be implemented to decrease the pulmonary complication rate. In a follow-up to his 1962 study on the predictive value of pulmonary function tests, Stein and Cassara in 1970 reported that the institution of preventive measures, including cessation of smoking, bronchodilators, antibiotics, postural drainage, inhalation of humidified gases, and chest physiotherapy, could decrease postoperative pulmonary complications.[37] In this study, patients with abnormal pulmonary function tests, according to the criteria in their 1962 paper, were randomized to either the treatment arm in which patients received one or more of the above measures, or the no-treatment arm. Patients in the treatment arm had fewer complications. However, the difference in complications was seen only in those who had thoracotomies. The number of patients who underwent abdominal surgeries was too small to make any statistically meaningful comparisons: Other problems with this study included a lack of strict stratification by type of respiratory maneuvers employed among the treatment group. Even in the no-treatment group, some patients received respiratory treatments based solely on physician preference.

Other better-designed trials have sought to evaluate such interventions as expiratory maneuvers, positive pressure breathing, hyperventilation, and incentive spirometry.[38,39] Incentive spirometry was noted in prospectively randomized trials to be effective in decreasing respiratory complications. Some of the other maneuvers were noted to be of no value and at the same time to be associated with a higher risk of morbidity.[40] None of the respiratory maneuvers noted above were observed to be more efficacious than incentive spirometry in reducing the postoperative pulmonary complication rate (Level I). As a result, the general recommendation is that incentive spirometry should be advocated for all patients undergoing abdominal surgeries, especially upper abdominal surgeries, regardless of whether a patient is at higher risk for complications. This is due to the low cost, efficacy, and absence of associated morbidity attributable to incentive spirometry.[38] In other words, these characteristics of incentive spirometry obviate the need for a screening test to define a subpopulation of patients felt to be at higher risk.

In summary, although preoperative screening spirometry has been demonstrated to be clinically beneficial in the management of lung resection patients, its value in patients undergoing abdominal surgeries has not been clearly proven.[40] Studies have reported value of routine screening spirometry in nonthoracotomy procedures. Nevertheless, all have serious methodological problems that prevent drawing any firm conclusions. It is not clear that screening spirometry contributes any more predictive value beyond a careful history and physical examination alone. In addition, incentive spirometry should be universally utilized in all abdominal surgeries because of its efficacy, low cost, and lack of associated morbidity.

There is currently no support in the literature for the use of screening pulmonary function tests in the routine, general population. There may, however, be some subsets in the general population who may benefit from preoperative spirometry. Although not specifically studied in previously reported research, some pulmonologists have recommended that preoperative spirometry be obtained in patients who have a significant history of cigarette smoking or underlying respiratory conditions. In these cases, spirometry may aid in the assessment of pulmonary impairment, and the information gained may have an impact on surgical and perioperative management.[29,30]

SUMMARY

The value of a careful general history and physical examination that focuses on eliciting signs and symptoms that may alter surgical risk and management cannot be overemphasized. Table 8.3 summarizes the necessity of routine preoperative evaluations and the level of evidence in the literature supporting these recommendations. No laboratory test or radiograph should be used as a substitute for a careful preoperative examination. At the same time, although stud-

TABLE 8.3. **Summary of Recommendations for Preoperative Evaluations and Strength of Evidence Supporting Recommendations**

1. CBC obtained in patients undergoing major surgeries	III, II-3
2. Pregnancy test should be obtained in all female patients with reproductive potential	III
3. PT, PTT should not be routinely obtained without indications	II-2
4. Electrolytes—no evidence to support routine electolytes	II-3
5. BUN/Cr—no evidence to support routine BUN/Cr	II-3
6. Urinalysis—no evidence to support routine urinalysis	II-3
7. Chest X ray—no evidence to support routine chest X ray without underlying cardiovascular/pulmonary disease	II-3
8. Screening spirometry—no evidence to support routine spirometry to be clinically beneficial without underlying pulmonary disease	III, II-3

ies have not proven certain tests to be clinically beneficial, the circumstances surrounding these studies in an individual patient may differ. Thus, the recommendations in this chapter should serve only as guidelines, combining the best published evidence with solid clinical judgment and experience.

REFERENCES

1. Roizen M. Preoperative patient evaluation. *Can J Anesthesiol* 1989;36:S13–17.
2. Kaplan EB, Sheiner LB, Boeckmann AJ, Roizen MF, Beal SL, Cohen SN, Nicoll D. The usefulness of preoperative laboratory screening. *JAMA* 1985;253:3576–3581.
3. Macario A, Roizen MF, Thisted RA, et al. Reassessment of preoperative laboratory testing has changed the test-ordering patterns of physicians. *Surg Gynecol Obstet* 1992;175:539–543.
4. Velanovich V. The value of routine preoperative laboratory testing in predicting postoperative complications: a multivariate analysis. *Surgery* 1991;109:236–243.
5. Thompson JD, Rock JA. *TeLinde's Operative Gynecology*, 8th ed. Philadelphia: Lippincott-Raven, 1996, pp. 70–71.
6. Gershenson DM, DeCherney AH, Curry SL. *Operative Gynecology.* Philadelphia: WB Saunders, 1993, p. 30.
7. Rohrer MJ, Michelotti MC, Nahrwold DL. A prospective evaluation of the efficacy of preoperative coagulation testing. *Ann Surg* 1988;208:554–557.
8. Eisenberg JM, Clarke JR, Sussman SA. Prothrombin and partial thromboplastin times as preoperative screening tests. *Arch Surg* 1982;117:48–51.
9. Robbins JA, Rose SD. Partial thromboplastin time as a screening test. *Ann Intern Med* 1979;90:796–797.
10. Robbins JA, Mushlin AI. Preoperative evaluation of the healthy patient. *Med Clin N Am* 1979;63:1145–1156.
11. Watson-Williams EJ: Hematologic and hemostatic considerations before surgery. *Med Clin N Am* 1979;63:1165–1189.
12. Office of Medical Applications of Research. Summary of NIH Consensus Development Conference on perioperative red cell transfusion 1. *Am J Hematol* 1989;31:144.
13. Heughan C, Grislis G, Hunt TK. The effect of anemia on wound healing. *Ann Surg* 1974;179:163–167.
14. Silberstein LE, Kruskall MS, Stehling LC, et al. Strategies for the review of transfusion practices. *JAMA* 1989;262:1993–1997.
15. Stehling L, Luban NLC, Anderson KC, et al. Guidelines for blood utilization review. *Transfusion* 1994;34:438–448.
16. Wallace EL, Surgenor DM, Hao HS, An J, Chapman RH, Churchill WH. Collection and transfusion of blood and blood components in the United States. *Transfusion* 1993;33:139.
17. National Heart, Lung, and Blood Institute Expert Panel on the Use of Autologous Blood. Transfusion alert: use of autologous blood. *Transfusion* 1995;35:703–711.

18. Etchason L, Potz L, Keeler E, et al. The cost-effectiveness of preoperative autologous blood donations. *N Engl J Med* 1995;332:719–724.

19. McCullough J. *Transfusion Medicine*, 1st ed. New York: McGraw-Hill, 1998.

20. Blery C, Szatan M, Fourgeaux B, Charpak Y, Darne B, Chastang CL, Gaudy JH. Evaluation of a protocol for selective ordering of preoperative tests. *Lancet* 1986;1:139–141.

21. Tape TG, Mushlin AI. The utility of routine chest radiographs. *Ann Intern Med* 1986;104:663–670.

22. Royal College of Radiologists. Preoperative chest radiology. *Lancet* 1979;2:83–86.

23. Mendelson DS, Khilnani N, Wagner LD, Rabinowitz JG. Preoperative chest radiography: value as a baseline examination for comparison. *Radiology* 1987;165:341–343.

24. Sagel SS, Evens RG, Forrest JV, Bramson BE. Efficacy of routine screening and lateral chest radiographs in a hospital-based population. *N Engl J Med* 1974;291:1001–1004.

25. Tornebrandt K, Fletcher R: Pre-operative chest X-rays in elderly patients. *Anaesthesiology* 1982;37:901–902.

26. Rucker L, Frye EB, Staten MA. Usefulness of screening chest roentgenograms in preoperative patients. *JAMA* 1983;250:3209–3211.

27. Harman E, Lillington G. Pulmonary risk factors in surgery. *Med Clin N Am* 1979;63:1289–1298.

28. Zibrak JD, O'Donnell CR, Marton K. Indications for pulmonary function testing. *Ann Intern Med* 1990;112:763–771.

29. Garibaldi RA, Britt MR, Coleman ML, Reading JC, Pace NL. Risk factors for postoperative pneumonia. *Am J Med* 1981;70:677–680.

30. Tisi GM. Preoperative evaluation of pulmonary function. *Am Rev Respir Dis* 1979;119:293–310.

31. Jackson CV. Preoperative pulmonary evaluation. *Arch Intern Med* 1988;148:2120–2127.

32. Wightman JAK. A prospective survey of the incidence of postoperative pulmonary complications. *Br J Surg* 1968;55:85–91.

33. Latimer RG, Dickman M, Day WC, Gunn ML, Schmidt CD. Ventilatory patterns and pulmonary complications after upper abdominal surgery determined by preoperative and postoperative computerized spirometry and blood gas analysis. *Am J Surg* 1971;122:622–632.

34. Stein M, Koota GM, Simon M, Frank HA: Pulmonary evaluation of surgical patients. *JAMA* 1962;181:765–770.

35. Appleberg M, Gordon L, Fatti LP. Preoperative pulmonary evaluation of surgical patients using the vitalograph. *Br J Surg* 1974;61:57–59.

36. Fan ST, Lau WY, Yip WC, Poon GP, Yeung C. et al. Prediction of postoperative pulmonary complications in esophagogastric cancer surgery. 1987;74:408–410.

37. Stein M, Cassara EL. Preoperative pulmonary evaluation and therapy for surgery patients. *JAMA* 1970;211:787–790.

38. Celli BR, Rodriguez KS, Snider GL. A controlled trial of intermittent positive pres-

sure breathing, incentive spirometry, and deep breathing exercises in preventing pulmonary complications after abdominal surgery. *Am Rev Respir Dis* 1984;130:12–15.

39. Bartlett RH, Gazzaniga AB, Geraghty TR. Respiratory maneuvers to prevent postoperative pulmonary complications. *JAMA* 1973;224:1017–1021.

40. Lawrence VA, Page CP, Harris GD. Preoperative spirometry before abdominal operations. *Arch Intern Med* 1989;149:280–285.

CHAPTER 9

POSTOPERATIVE SURVEILLANCE AND PERIOPERATIVE PROPHYLAXIS

HARRIET O. SMITH, M.D., MARK C. GENESEN, M.D.,
and DOROTHY N. KAMMERER-DOAK, M.D.

Excellence in gynecologic surgery depends on experience in a wide variety of operative techniques, and an adequate working knowledge of the effects of anesthesia and surgical trauma on healthy and diseased organ systems. Perioperative morbidity is reduced, costs are minimized, and patient satisfaction is enhanced when the operative procedure selected is tailored to the patient's specific needs and limitations, preoperative and postoperative counseling is supportive and comprehensive, and the intensity of perioperative surveillance is proportionate to previously recognized risk factors.

PHYSIOLOGICAL RESPONSES TO SURGERY (LEVEL II-2)

Changes associated with surgical trauma adversely affect practically every organ system of the human body. Particularly susceptible are the very young, the elderly, or patients with medical conditions that reduce tolerance to anesthetic and surgical stress. The metabolic response to surgery may be divided into (1) an early *ebb phase*, characterized by hypovolemia and associated endocrine and sympathetic responses; (2) a *flow phase*, characterized by oxidation of muscle protein to supply glucose; and (3) the *convalescence phase*, which begins immediately postoperatively and may extend 3 to 12 months.[1] The first 24 hours following surgery are the most hazardous: In one large study of 2,153 consecutive operations, 80% of patients who experienced major morbidity began to deteriorate within 24 hours (Level II-2). With more aggressive management, major morbidity might have been prevented in 12% of these patients.[2] The patho-

Perioperative and Supportive Care in Gynecologic Oncology: Evidence-Based Management,
Edited by Steven A. Vasilev.
ISBN 0-471-24788-X   Copyright © 2000 by Wiley-Liss, Inc.

physiologic effects and management of surgical trauma may be categorized by the specific organ systems involved.

Changes in Fluid and Electrolytes (Level II-1)

Total body water constitutes 50% to 70% of total body weight. It is dependent on lean body mass, or muscle, which decreases with age; body fat contains little water. Consequently, at comparable weights, a young athletic woman will have 20% to 30% more body water per kg than an elderly obese woman. Body water is dispersed into three functional compartments: (1) *intracellular volume*, which represents 40% of body weight, *extracellular fluid*, which comprises 20% of body weight and is disproportionately distributed between the (2) *plasma*, and (3) *interstitial fluid*. Plasma, the intravascular volume compartment, comprises only 5% of body weight, and interstitial fluid (lymph, joint, and *third-spaced fluid*) constitutes the remaining 15%. Body compartment protein and electrolyte composition and hydrostatic pressures vary significantly. Within cells, the major cations are potassium and magnesium; phosphates and proteins are the principal anions. The total *ionic* concentration (mEq/L) within plasma and interstitial fluid is considered for all practical purposes the same. The principal cation in the extracellular compartment is sodium, and chloride and carbonate are the principal anions. The total intracellular particulate concentration is 200 mEq/L, 1.3-fold higher than extracellular compartment particle concentration. Differences in ionic composition between the cellular and extracellular compartment are maintained by semipermeable cell membranes, energy-dependent cell transport mechanisms, and transmembrane differences in electrical potential, particle charge, and oncotic pressure. Oncotic pressure is dependent on the total number of osmotically active particles in each compartment, usually 290–310 mOsm. *Effective oncotic pressure* reflects membrane impermeable particles such as plasma proteins and extracellular sodium. *Colloid oncotic pressure*, the effective osmotic pressure between plasma and interstitial spaces, plays a critical role in maintaining body water distribution between compartments.

Surgery, especially abdominal, is associated with a decline in total body protein, albumin, and total lymphocyte counts that correlates with severity of blood loss, duration of surgery, and weight gain postoperatively. Perioperative hypoalbuminemia of some degree is almost universal and results from crystalloid dilution, increases in capillary permeability and sequestration of albumin in interstitial fluid, and/or intraoperative loss. Postoperative albumin levels do not accurately reflect nutritional status (Level II-2).[3]

Fluid balance disturbances are divided into (1) volume changes: depletion, redistribution, and excess; (2) changes in extracellular sodium; and (3) compositional alterations, including changes in acid-base and departmental concentrations of potassium, magnesium, and calcium.[4] In surgical patients, volume depletion from poor intake, vomiting, nasogastric suction, diarrhea, or fistula drainage is the most common extracellular volume deficit (Table 9.1). A healthy

TABLE 9.1. Average Losses per Day

	Volume (ml/24 hr)	Na (mEq/L)	K (mEq/L)	Cl (mEq/L)	HCO_3 (mEq/L)
Salivary	1500	10	26	10	30
	(500–2,000)	(2–10)	(20–30)	(8–18)	
Stomach	1500	60	10	130	—
	(100–4,000)	(9–116)	(0–32)	(8–154)	
Duodenum	100–2,000				
Ileum	3000	140	5	104	30
	(100–9,000)	(80–150)	(2–8)	(43–137)	
Colon	—	60	30	40	—
Pancreas		140	5	75	115
	(100–800)	(113–185)	(3–7)	(54–95)	
Bile	50–800	145	5	100	35
		(131–164)	(3–12)	(89–180)	

Source: Adapted from Shires GT, Canizaro PC. Fluid and electrolyte management of the surgical patient. In Sabiston DC Jr (Ed), *Textbook of Surgery*, 14th ed. Philadelphia, WB Saunders Co., 1991, pp. 57–76.

70 kg woman requires approximately 2,000–2,500 cc of fluid replacement per day.[4,5] Extra fluid is needed to compensate for increased extracellular fluid losses including perspiration losses, fever, and tachypnea, which increase insensible losses to approximately 1,000–1,500 cc/day. Ascites, pleural effusions, fluid sequestration into the bowel lumen, and extravasation into soft tissues are examples of third-space losses that result from malignancy-associated lymphatic obstruction, colloid oncotic pressure changes (hypoalbuminemia or excessive fluid or crystalloid resuscitation), extensive surgical dissection, or ileus. Bowel preps and poor oral intake aggravate preoperative volume contraction. Volume excess is usually secondary to renal failure or excessive hydration.

Serum levels of sodium generally reflect body fluid tonicity, because sodium is the principal ion responsible for the osmolarity of the extracellular space.[4] *Hypernatremia* is associated with efflux of water from the intracellular to the extracellular compartment, usually in response to acute water loss.[4] To maintain a normal plasma osmolality, renal free-water clearance must equal the free-water intake minus insensible losses. Generation of free water to dilute urine depends on an intact renal collecting system, normal suppression of antidiuretic hormone (ADH), adequate renal profusion, and a normal glomerular filtration rate. *Hypertonic hyponatremia* results in the redistribution of body water from the intracellular space (Fig. 9.1) and is corrected with hydration with normal saline. Insulin therapy increases cellular uptake of glucose, thereby decreasing extracellular osmolality. *Hypotonic hyponatremia* may be associated with expanded, normal, or deficient total body water. Unless the rate of change in sodium concentration is quite rapid, symptoms are typically absent until sodium concentrations are severely abnormal or corrective measures are exces-

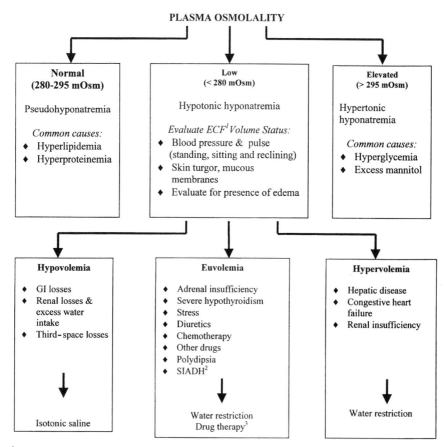

[Extracted from figure]

PLASMA OSMOLALITY

Normal **(280-295 mOsm)**	**Low** **(< 280 mOsm)**	**Elevated** **(> 295 mOsm)**
Pseudohyponatremia *Common causes:* ♦ Hyperlipidemia ♦ Hyperproteinemia	Hypotonic hyponatremia *Evaluate ECF^1 Volume Status:* ♦ Blood pressure & pulse (standing, sitting and reclining) ♦ Skin turgor, mucous membranes ♦ Evaluate for presence of edema	Hypertonic hyponatremia *Common causes:* ♦ Hyperglycemia ♦ Excess mannitol

Hypovolemia	**Euvolemia**	**Hypervolemia**
♦ GI losses ♦ Renal losses & excess water intake ♦ Third-space losses	♦ Adrenal insufficiency ♦ Severe hypothyroidism ♦ Stress ♦ Diuretics ♦ Chemotherapy ♦ Other drugs ♦ Polydipsia ♦ SIADH^2	♦ Hepatic disease ♦ Congestive heart failure ♦ Renal insufficiency
Isotonic saline	Water restriction Drug therapy^3	Water restriction

[1]Extracellular fluid volume.

[2]Syndrome of inappropriate antidiuretic hormone secretion (urine Osm >200 mOsm/kg and elevated urinary sodium [>20 mEq/L] without other etiologies).

[3]Demeclocycline, lasix, increased salt intake.

FIGURE 9.1. Recognition and management of hyponatremia (Level III). (Adapted from O'Shea MH. Fluid and electrolyte management. In Woodley M, Whelan A (Eds), *Manual of Medical Therapeutics*, 27th ed. Boston: Little, Brown, & Company, 1992, pp. 42–61 [Levels II-2, II-3, III].)

sive. Thus, postoperative sodium concentrations should be checked frequently in patients at risk (Level III).[6,7]

Cardiovascular and Thermoregulatory Effects

Effects of inhalation anesthetics upon the endocrine stress response are agent and dose dependent, and include an increase in circulating catecholamines, ADH, ACTH (adrenocorticotrophic hormone), and cortisol (Level III). Systemic blood pressure is maintained by factors that influence cardiac output (CO) as well as systemic vascular resistance (SVR), which reflects afterload. Peripheral vascular tone is regulated by receptors within the arterioles and the central nervous system (CNS). In response to surgical stress, norepinephrine and epinephrine are locally and/or systemically released, resulting in an increase in cardiac output secondary to catecholamine-mediated inotropic and chronotropic effects. Venoconstriction further increases venous return, enhancing stroke volume (SV) and CO. In addition to the hypothalamic-hypophyseal-adrenal mechanisms, systemic blood pressure is regulated by the renin-angiotensin-aldosterone system.

Renin release by the juxtaglomerular cells is mediated by a decrease in wall tension or sodium, as well as by sympathetic activation. Renin coverts angiotensinogen into angiotensin I, which in turn is converted into angiotensin II, a potent vasoconstrictor that stimulates aldosterone secretion from the renal cortex. Aldosterone increases sodium and water retention, resulting in increased venous return and consequently stroke volume, CO, and blood pressure.[8,9] Hypertension may also result from bladder distension, direct laryngoscopy/intubation, pain, and as a rebound effect from hypotension.[9] Inhalation agents alter cerebral blood flow by opposing direct (vasodilatation, which results in increased cerebral blood flow) and indirect (decreased metabolism, which reduces cerebral blood flow) mechanisms. Anesthetics attenuate cerebral autoregulation, which normally assures that cerebral blood flow does not fluctuate with changes in arterial blood pressure (Level III).[10]

All volatile anesthetics depress myocardial contractility. Compared with nitrous oxide or isoflurane, halothane and enflurane decrease CO by 20% to 40%. Intravenous narcotics (e.g., morphine) induce hypotension, especially when given at rates above 10 mg/min (1–4 mg/kg).[11] Fluctuations in the intraoperative mean arterial pressure (MAP) of more than 20 mmHg, congestive heart failure (CHF), myocardial infarction, and renal failure are all significant predictors of major postoperative morbidity (Level II-2).[12] In patients with longstanding or newly diagnosed essential hypertension, blood pressure should be optimally controlled prior to elective surgery, and on the morning of surgery, antihypertensives should be taken orally in the usual doses. Although sedation preoperatively may prevent intraoperative hypotension, since oversedation may result in hypoxia and hypercapnia, and consequently, significant hypertension, sedatives should be used cautiously, in the lowest possible effective doses (Level II-2).[8,9] Optimization of preload and afterload is especially important in patients with ventricular dysfunction; inotropic support guided by pulmonary artery catheterization may be warranted.[13]

Hypothermia, defined as a core temperature of less than 36°C, affects approximately 14 million patients annually and nearly 70% of patients requiring surgery (Level III).[14] Temperature regulation is under the control of the posterior hypothalamus, which receives signals from *core zone receptors* in the preoptic area of the hypothalamus as well as from the spinal cord, major vasculature, and viscera, and *shell zone receptors* within the skin. Hypothalamic response to hypothermia includes (1) activation of motor nerves responsible for shivering; (2) stimulation of catecholamine release, which induces vaso-constriction and consequently an increase in the basal metabolic rate; and (3) increased thyroxine secretion.[15] Hypothermia is an iatrogenic complication of surgery, resulting from prolonged exposure to a cold ambient environment and from the physiological effects of anesthesia. Anesthetic agents lower the basal metabolic rate, inhibit redirection of blood flow from the skin, and prevent shivering.[14] Even without shivering, a decrease in core body temperature of 0.3° to 1.2°C increases oxygen consumption by approximately 92%; shivering may magnify this effect by as much as 500%. Oxygen demand is consequently increased at a time when pulmonary reserve is diminished, increasing the risk for arterial desaturation, which in turn increases heart rate, cardiac output, and oxygen consumption.[14] In addition to patient discomfort, unintentional hypo-thermia is associated with transient hypoxia (a reduction in $Pa_{O_2} < 80$ mmHg), and a higher incidence of angina and myocardial ischemia in the early postop-erative period.[15,16] Coagulopathies secondary to impaired enzymatic reactions of the clotting cascade and/or impaired platelet function with or without throm-bocytopenia often develop; hypothermia also predisposes to hypercoagulability, which increases the risk of pulmonary embolism.[17]

Pulmonary Effects

All inhalation agents are respiratory depressants. Atelectasis has been demon-strated in approximately 50% of patients postoperatively (Level II-2).[18] Dur-ing and following general anesthesia, gas exchange is impaired by paralysis of the chest wall and diaphragm, loss of the normal hypoxic drive to ventila-tion, and inhibition of hypoxic pulmonary vasoconstriction that serves to redi-rect oxygen to underventilated pulmonary segments.[19] Sighing, a physiologi-cal mechanism that reduces alveolar collapse, is also diminished by anesthesia and postoperative sedation (Level II-2).[20] Opioid analgesics slow the respira-tory rate, decrease minute ventilation, and further reduce the functional residual capacity (FRC) to approximately 60% of the preoperative value.[21] Mucociliary action is inhibited, resulting in a reduced capacity to clear mucus secretions. Depressed macrophage, neutrophil and lymphocyte function contribute to the increased risks of bacterial colonization and subsequent infection.[11] Reduced lung compliance and FRC results in microatelectasis and pulmonary shunting, further increasing the alveolar-arterial oxygen gradient. Compared with general anesthesia, epidural anesthesia offers several potential advantages: In the period immediately postoperatively, its blocking effects reduce plasma epinephrine release, thereby reducing oxygen consumption and consequently mixed oxy-gen saturation (Level II-2).[22,23] Although epidural anesthesia appears to provide superior pain relief, in a controlled randomized study of 150 patients, the inci-dence and severity of pulmonary complications following epidural anesthesia compared with parenteral morphine were not improved (Level I).[24]

Effects on Protein Catabolism and Immune Response

Following uncomplicated surgery, weight loss averages about 3 kg, and, in the absence of preexisting deficits, is usually restored within 3 months. Weight loss results from oxidation of fat and protein breakdown.[1] When carbohydrate intake is inadequate, glycogen stores are rapidly depleted and, to supply fuel essential for the brain and healing tissues, gluconeogenesis occurs at the expense of protein catabolism. The rate of metabolism is further accelerated in critically ill patients.[1] High-dose inhalation anesthesia appears to reduce perioperative catabolism and may be an important means of reducing perioperative morbidity in patients with preexisting protein deficits (Level II-2).[25] Protein loss does not account for postoperative fatigue, a syndrome found exclusively in humans, characterized by muscle weakness and fatigue for days or weeks following surgery, although the mechanisms involved are poorly understood and there appears to be both a physiological and psychological basis.[1,25]

Systemically and at the site of tissue injury, mediators including cytokines, vasoactive amines, and arachidonic acid products act to increase protocoagulant activity, vascular permeability, and vasodilatation.[26] Following general surgery, there is an increase in total leukocyte count; function, however, as measured by directed motility (chemotaxis), serum opsonic activity, and ingestive capacity, is depressed for hours to days.[27] Phagocytosis by monocytes and macrophages is also suppressed. Perioperatively, macrophages excrete a variety of factors, including cytokines (IL-1, IL-6, TNF), which are the major mediators of the acute-phase response, as well as proteases, prostaglandin products, and interferon.[11,27] The effect of surgery upon the release and activity of these mediators is under intense investigation. IL-6 is consistently elevated 4–6 hours postoperatively, and has been implicated in the pyrogenic response and in the stimulation of acute-phase protein production by hepatoma cells.[28] Transient increases in serum levels of IL-1β are consistently preceded by elevations in IL-6 levels;[29] however, since TNF, a potent pyrogenic cytokine implicated in septic shock, is not detected, a role for TNF in mediating the acute-phase response is doubtful.[28,29] Complement activity, cell-mediated immunity, and humoral immunity may all be depressed, the severity of which is proportionate to the duration of anesthesia and surgical trauma.[27] The clinical significance of these physiological alterations has yet to be elucidated (Level II-2).[27,28,30]

Gastrointestinal Changes

Entry into the peritoneal cavity and/or the neuroinhibitory effects of general anesthesia result in a transient loss of gastrointestinal peristaltic activity termed *postoperative ileus* (POI; Level III).[31] Symptoms of POI include bloating secondary to air swallowing, abdominal distension, emesis, and pain. Treatment is generally supportive, and includes nasogastric intubation and intravenous hydration. This self-limiting condition generally lasts from 1 to 3 days.[32] In uncomplicated POI, small intestinal transit recovers first with return of phase

III activity of the interdigestive migrating motor reflex (MMC), followed by gastric and then colonic activity.[33] Resolution of POI is assessed clinically by auscultation of normoactive bowel sounds and by the passage of flatus and stool. *Paralytic ileus*, or complicated ileus lasting more than 3 days after surgery, is frequently associated with excessive intestinal manipulation, peritonitis, pancreatitis,[34] opiate administration (Level II-2),[35] and high vasopressin levels,[36] and probably reflects inhibition of small-bowel activity.[34] Inhalation anesthetic agents, especially enflurane and halothane, but not nitrous oxide, suppress motor activity throughout the colon.[37] Although presentation and symptoms are similar, the pathophysiologic mechanisms of paralytic ileus are poorly understood. Paralytic ileus must be distinguished from ileus resulting from intestinal obstruction, and mechanical ileus.

GENERAL PERIOPERATIVE PROPHYLAXIS

Medical History, Physical Examination, and Informed Consent

Preoperative medical history should include thorough investigation of the presenting complaint, past medical history including prescription and over-the-counter medications, and inquiry with respect to prior hospitalizations, exposure to general anesthesia, and all food and drug allergies. A complete review of systems and physical examination provide the basis for indicated laboratory and radiographic investigation, as well as the need for consultation and collaborative management involving other clinical services. Informed consent should include, in layman's terms, a detailed discussion of the planned operative procedure, the potential risks and benefits, the likelihood of success or failure of the anticipated procedure, and treatment alternatives (Table 9.2). A useful way to clarify misconceptions and improve rapport is to have the patient keep a diary of her questions and concerns, and to address these issues preoperatively. Timely charting of relevant history, physical findings, and preoperative discussions cannot be overstressed. The patient's chart is a legal document and can be the physician's best testament to the quality of care rendered.

Laboratory Testing

Preoperative laboratory testing should be performed as indicated by a thorough assessment of the patient, including performance status, medical history, and complexity of the planned operative procedure. Routine laboratory screening (CBC, urinalysis, and ECG) and chest X ray are generally recommended in patients over 40, when extensive surgery is anticipated, and in patients with underlying medical disease or malignancy (Fig. 9.2). However, when performed routinely in healthy young patients undergoing ambulatory surgery, including hysterectomy, elective preoperative screening is costly, unlikely to affect outcome, and increases the probability that additional expensive and potentially

TABLE 9.2. Guidelines for Informed Consent

1. Define the disease process and its severity.
2. Describe the planned operative procedure in understandable language.
    What organs will be removed or altered?
    What is the planned operative incision?
    How will intraoperative findings affect:
        The planned procedure?
        The extent of surgery?
        The need for blood products?
3. Provide a discussion of the risks and potential complications of the proposed
        procedure.
    What is the probability of success or failure?
    What are the anesthetic risks?
    Define risks within the context of the patient's underlying physical condition.
4. Describe the level of care anticipated in the immediate postoperative and
        recovery period.
    Will the patient require intensive care monitoring or ventilatory support?
    What is the anticipated length of hospitalization and convalescence?
    How will fertility and ovarian function be affected?
    Will special devices (e.g., prolonged urinary catheterization or central venous
        access, ostomy products) or medications be necessary, and for how long?
    What, if any, additional therapy will be required?
5. List the treatment alternatives and their risks and benefits
6. Describe the usual course of the patient's disease if the proposed treatment is
        withheld.

harmful tests will be ordered (Level II-2).[38-41] Although intravenous pyelography (IVP) may be occasionally helpful (malignancy, extensive pelvic inflammatory disease, or congenital anomalies of the genitourinary tract), the potential risks—reaction to contrast, nephrotoxicity, and radiation exposure—in addition to costs, prohibit obtaining IVPs routinely (Level II-3).[42-44] Following administration of contrast material, mild, generalized reactions including hives, pruritus, syncope, and gastrointestinal symptoms are common, affecting 5% to 10% of patients, and fatal anaphylactic reactions occur in approximately 1 per 14,000 procedures performed.[42] Prophylactic steroid administration may prevent life-threatening reactions in patients with a history of allergies to contrast material or seafood.[45] Intravenous contrast agents can also induce acute renal insufficiency by reducing renal blood flow, resulting in medullary ischemia.[46] In patients with chronic renal failure, intravenous hydration 12 hours before and after radiocontrast administration reduces this risk; mannitol or furosemide do not improve the protective effects of hydration alone.[47]

Perioperative Cardiac Assessment   The incidence of myocardial infarction (MI) following noncardiac surgery is approximately 0%–0.7%;[48] a nonfatal infarction rate in patients over 40 years of age (with or without coronary artery

**TABLE 9.3. Perioperative Cardiac Morbidity
(Noncardiac Surgery)**

Cardiac Complication	Estimated Incidence (%)
Myocardial Ischemia	
Preoperative	24
Intraoperative	18–74
Postoperative	27–38
Myocardial Infarction (MI)	
General population	0.1–0.7
Prior MI	1.9–7.7
Vascular surgery	1–15
Recent MI (<3 months)	0–37
Unstable angina	—
	—
Congestive Heart Failure	
Intraoperative	4.8
Postoperative	14–40.5
Cardiac Death with Perioperative MI	36–70

Source: Adapted from Mangano DT. Perioperative cardiac morbidity.
Anesthesiology 1990;72:153–184.

disease) is approximately 0.15% (Level II-2).[49] Cardiac morbidity is a leading cause of perioperative death, which is exceeded in frequency only by deaths from anesthetic or surgical complications (Table 9.3).[48] Goldman et al. developed a multifactorial index of independent factors associated with cardiac risk (Table 9.4).[49,50] Based on stratification of these risks factors, the incidence of life-threatening or fatal myocardial morbidity was found to be I (1%), II (7%), III (14%), and IV (78%) (Level II-3).[50] Reinfarction rates are increased following vascular surgery (1–15%) and previous MI (1–7.7%), especially within the antecedent 3 months (0–37%).[48] In recent years, aggressive hemodynamic monitoring has reduced the rate of reinfarction in patients to 1.9% overall, and to 5.7% following a recent (<3 months) MI (Level II-2).[51]

Noninvasive screening tests including preoperative exercise testing, dipyridamole-thallium scintigraphy, stress echocardiography, and ambulatory ischemia monitoring may be useful to identify patients at high risk for postoperative myocardial infarction; in general, however, the cost-benefit ratio of these tests are prohibitive for routine screening.[52] Stratification of perioperative MI risks (Table 9.5) has been modified by Ashton[53] to take into account the three most important risk factors for perioperative myocardial infarction: (1) recent MI (antecedent 3 months), (2) congestive heart failure (CHF), and (3) unstable angina (Level II-2). Cardiac evaluation other than preoperative ECG is not rec-

TABLE 9.4. Goldman Risk Factors for Postoperative Myocardial Infarction (Noncardiac Surgery)

Criteria	Points
S3 gallop or jugular venous distension on preoperative physical examination	11
MI within the previous 6 months	10
Premature ventricular beats (>5 per minutes)	7
Rhythm other than sinus or premature atrial contractions on preoperative ECG	7
Age >70 years	5
Emergency surgery	4
Site of surgery, intrathoracic, intraperitoneal, or aortic	3
Significant valvular stenosis	3
Poor general medical condition[a]	3

[a]Poor respiratory function (PaO2 < 60 mmHg or PaCO2 > 50 mmHg); significant electrolyte disturbances (K < 3.0 or HCO3 < 20 mEq/L); renal insufficiency (BUN > 50 or creatinine > 3.0 mg/dl); liver dysfunction (increased SGOT, SGPT, chronic liver disease); chronically bedridden.

Source: Adapted from Goldman L. Cardiac risks and complications of noncardiac surgery. *Ann Int Med* 1983;98:504–513; Goldman L, Caldera DL, Nussbaum SR, et al. Multifactorial index of cardiac risk in noncardiac surgical procedures. *N Engl J Med* 1977;297:845–850.

ommended for asymptomatic patients lacking a history or physical evidence of cardiovascular disease;[52] however, patients at high or intermediate risk[53] may benefit from aggressive perioperative evaluation including cardiac screening, preoperative cardiac consultation, and aggressive postoperative monitoring.

The Role of Other Perioperative Tests CT contrast studies, ultrasound, barium enema, upper gastrointestinal studies, flexible proctosigmoidoscopy and/or colonoscopy should be performed only in select cases for specific indications, such as symptoms or clinical findings suggestive of involvement of other organs within proximity to the planned operative field (e.g., advanced ovarian cancer or severe endometriosis). When the origin of a pelvic mass is uncertain, such as distinguishing diverticular disease or a gastrointestinal tumor from an ovarian neoplasm, additional clinical or radiographic studies may be helpful (Level III).

Prevention of Surgical Wound Infection

Nosocomial bacteremias in the United States, 25% of which are accounted for by postoperative wound infections,[54] adversely affect approximately 200,000 patients each year, increasing morbidity and mortality, duration of hospital stay, additional antibiotic use, and health care costs by up to $860 million each year (Level II-2).[55] The past 25 years have witnessed a dramatic reduction in the postoperative wound infection rate, mainly due to the use of

TABLE 9.5. Risk for Perioperative Myocardial Infarction[a]

Risk Assessment[b]	Prevalence of CAD	Observed MI Rate	Cardiac Death Rate
Negligible: No evidence of atherosclerosis (AS), low atherogenic risk-factor profile	Almost 0%	Unknown	0 (0/652)
Low risk: >75 years old, high AS risk index, no evidence of AS	5–30%	0 (0/256)	0.4% (1/256)
Intermediate risk: No evidence of CAD; history of CVA, vascular surgery, carotid bruit, TIA, claudication, atypical chest pain	30–70%	0.8% (2/260)	0.4% (1/260)
High risk: CAD, history of MI, abnormal ECG consistent with previous MI, atypical angina pectoris, angiographic evidence of significant CAD or prior coronary bypass surgery	Nearly 100%	4.1% (13/319)	2.3% (7/319)

[a]Risk assessment based on preexisting coronary artery disease (CAD).
[b]Based on age, sex, smoking history, elevated BP, abnormal glucose tolerance, elevated cholesterol, risk of cardiac event within 6 years ≥15%.
Source: Adapted from Ashton CM. Perioperative myocardial infarction with noncardiac surgery. *Am J Med Sci* 1994;308:41–48.

prophylactic antibiotics.[56] For cesarean section alone, judicious use of prophylactic antibiotics may reduce medical costs by $9 million per year.[57] In contrast, indiscriminate use of antibiotics (prolonged use, three or more agent therapy, and timing) increases the risks of toxicity, allergic reactions, and overgrowth of resistant organisms.[58,59] Traditionally, risk for wound infection and need for prophylactic antibiotics was based on stratification by severity of wound contamination—clean, clean contaminated, contaminated, and dirty or infected—which carries an expected risk of infection of 2% or less, 5–15%, 15–30%, and over 30%, respectively.[58,59]

Strictly defined, *prophylactic antibiotics* are given in the absence of contamination and infection to reduce the risks of perioperative infection; antibiotics used for underlying infection are considered *therapeutic antibiotics*.[58] Previously, antibiotic prophylaxis has not been recommended for surgically clean cases except for prosthesis insertion; however, the study on the Efficacy of Nosocomial Infection Control has identified other risk factors associated with increased wound infection, including abdominal surgery, operative time of more than 2 hours, and intrinsic patient risk factors (extremes of age, undernutrition, obesity, and underlying medical diseases), all of which may increase the indications for antibiotic prophylaxis (Level II-1).[58,60] To achieve and main-

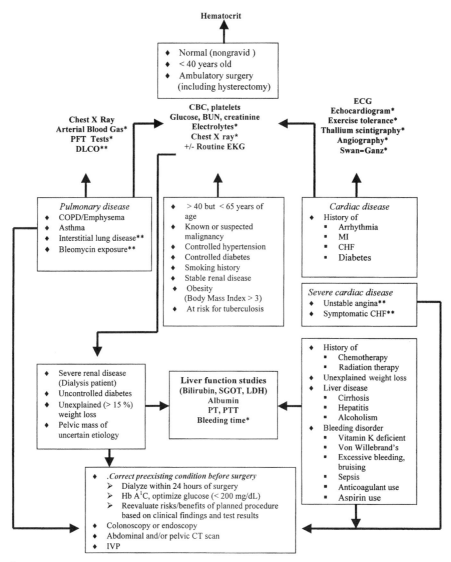

Hematocrit

- Normal (nongravid)
- < 40 years old
- Ambulatory surgery
  (including hysterectomy)

CBC, platelets
Glucose, BUN, creatinine
Electrolytes*
Chest X ray*
+/- Routine EKG

Chest X Ray
Arterial Blood Gas*
PFT Tests*
DLCO**

ECG
Echocardiogram*
Exercise tolerance*
Thallium scintigraphy*
Angiography*
Swan-Ganz*

Pulmonary disease
- COPD/Emphysema
- Asthma
- Interstitial lung disease**
- Bleomycin exposure**

- > 40 but < 65 years of age
- Known or suspected malignancy
- Controlled hypertension
- Controlled diabetes
- Smoking history
- Stable renal disease
- Obesity (Body Mass Index > 3)
- At risk for tuberculosis

Cardiac disease
- History of
  - Arrhythmia
  - MI
  - CHF
  - Diabetes

Severe cardiac disease
- Unstable angina**
- Symptomatic CHF**

- Severe renal disease (Dialysis patient)
- Uncontrolled diabetes
- Unexplained (> 15 %) weight loss
- Pelvic mass of uncertain etiology

Liver function studies (Bilirubin, SGOT, LDH)
Albumin
PT, PTT
Bleeding time*

- History of
  - Chemotherapy
  - Radiation therapy
- Unexplained weight loss
- Liver disease
  - Cirrhosis
  - Hepatitis
  - Alcoholism
- Bleeding disorder
  - Vitamin K deficient
  - Von Willebrand's
  - Excessive bleeding, bruising
  - Sepsis
  - Anticoagulant use
  - Aspirin use

- *.Correct preexisting condition before surgery*
  - ➢ Dialyze within 24 hours of surgery
  - ➢ Hb A^{1}C, optimize glucose (< 200 mg/dL)
  - ➢ Reevaluate risks/benefits of planned procedure based on clinical findings and test results
- Colonoscopy or endoscopy
- Abdominal and/or pelvic CT scan
- IVP

*Depending upon severity of clinical symptoms and/or physical findings.
**Test is indicated for specific indication as highlighted.

FIGURE 9.2. Guidelines for preoperative screening tests (Levels II-2, III).[38-41]

tain effective tissue levels, parenteral antibiotics should be given 30 minutes or more before the skin incision and at maximum (loading) doses; repeated doses should be given every 2 to 4 hours intraoperatively (not to exceed the half-life of the drug) or when blood loss exceeds 1,000 cc.[59] To be effective, perioperative prophylaxis must be administered on schedule.

A 1991 survey found that 83% of patients undergoing abdominal or arterial surgery underwent inappropriate perioperative prophylaxis consisting of missed doses (35%), excessive duration (71%), or questionable agents (25%).[61] Established hospital guidelines with formal instruction of new surgical and anesthesia staff significantly reduces inappropriate antibiotic dosing, particularly with respect to prolonged administration, in up to 40% of cases.[61,62] Prophylactic antibiotics should provide coverage consistent with the antibiotic flora most likely to be involved. In gynecologic surgery, pelvic infection frequently involves aerobic (β-hemolytic streptococci, *Escherichia coli*, *Neisseria gonorrhoeae*, *Chlamydia trachomatis*, and coagulase negative staphylococci) and anaerobic (peptostreptococci, peptococci, *Bacteroides* sp., and *Fusobacterium* sp.) organisms.[63] Prophylactic antibiotics may consist of a single preoperative dose,[64] or may be followed by two postoperative doses; however, except for select indications, prophylactic antibiotics should not be continued beyond the day of surgery.[59] Finally, the agent and dosing schedule should consist of the least expensive regimen that provides adequate protection.

Prophylaxis for Cesarean Section and Abdominal or Vaginal Hysterectomy Prophylactic antibiotics for emergency cesarean section have significantly reduced the incidence of postoperative infection from 27–86% to approximately 15% (Level II-1).[65–67] Risk factors for infection include prolonged labor, ruptured membranes, low socioeconomic status, internal fetal monitoring, obesity, and anemia.[66] Despite prophylaxis, one of two women receiving multiple vaginal examinations (six or more) will develop infectious complications.[68] In *elective* cesarean sections performed in community hospitals, prophylactic antibiotics were responsible for reducing the infectious morbidity rate from 3.7% to 0.9% (Level II-1).[57] The incidence of infectious morbidity, approximately 15%, is high compared to the infection rates, 5% or less, generally associated with clean surgical cases, and has been attributed to the routine practice of withholding antibiotic antibiotic therapy until after clamping the unbilical cord.[66] This practice has been questioned by Fejgin et al. (1993), who demonstrated in a prospective randomized trial that antibiotic administration preoperatively compared with after clamping the unbilical cord significantly reduced the incidence of serious infections, hospital stay, and wound infections (Level-I).[69] Prophylactic preoperative ceftriaxone results in adequate maternal but very low fetal serum or tissue levels.[67] A single perioperative dose of broad-spectrum cephalosporins (cefotetan,[70] cefuroxime,[71] or ceftriaxone[72]) are as effective as a three-dose regimen of cefoxitin. Although the rates of wound infection and endometritis were not significantly different, ceftriaxone significantly reduced the rate of urinary tract infection from 17.8% to 9.7%.[72] Hagar et al. found no differences in the incidence of perioperative infection rates when cefazolin (three doses) or cefoxitin (three doses) were compared with single-dose cefotaxime.[65]

Significant febrile morbidity occurs in 20–30% of abdominal and 30–50% of vaginal hysterectomies. Although serious postoperative infections are uncommon after abdominal or vaginal hysterectomy (0–1% versus 1–4%, respectively), prophylactic antibiotics are associated with a 5–15% reduction in febrile morbidity.[73] Significant risk factors for infection include prolonged operative time, abdominal compared with vaginal surgery, premenopausal versus postmenopausal status, the absence of perioperative prophylactic antibiotics, and low socioeconomic status.[74] A meta-analysis of 25 prospective randomized studies published since 1971 found that patients not receiving antibiotic prophylaxis had significantly higher infection rates (21.2% compared with 9.0%, $p = 0.00001$); at least three drugs—cefazolin, metronidazole, and tinidazole—were found to be effective prophylactic agents. Based on these results, the authors proposed that the practice of withholding prophylactic antibiotics at the time of abdominal hysterectomy was no longer justifiable.[75] The role of third-generation cephalosporins for prophylaxis in gynecologic surgery are yet to be defined. Single-dose cefotaxime was found to be more effective than either multiple doses of cefoxitin or cefazolin in reducing perioperative infectious complications.[76] However, a double-blind comparison of efficacy and cost-effectiveness of single-agent ceftriaxone found no improvement in infection rates and greater costs when compared with multidose cefazolin (Level I).[77]

Patients undergoing radical pelvic surgery for gynecologic malignancy are at increased risk for postoperative infection. Predisposing factors include the presence of pelvic tumor, subclinical infections, prior pelvic radiation therapy, as well as the numerous host factors previously mentioned. Effective antibiotic regimens for radical abdominal hysterectomy include single- and short-term (three doses) cefoxitin or piperacillin therapy.[64,78–80] Broad-spectrum beta-lactam-antibiotic/beta-lactamase-inhibitor combinations such as ticarcillin/clavulanate alone or in combination with aminoglycosides are the agents of choice for ultraradical pelvic surgery (Level III).[81]

Bowel Preparation and Antibiotic Prophylaxis for Intestinal Surgery

Postoperative infections are usually caused by the endogenous microflora present at the operative site rather than by exogenous contamination during surgery (Level II-3).[59,82–84] The high density of bacteria in the large intestine increase the risks for infectious complications in colorectal surgery or appendicitis.[85] Postoperative infections are caused by the endogenous microflora present at the operative site and are significantly reduced by reducing the bacterial concentration below levels necessary to cause infection, usually 10^5 or 10^6 organisms per gram of tissue. The most common pathogens involved in infectious morbidity following colorectal surgery include *E. coli*, *Klebsiella*, *Enterobacter*, *B. fragilis*, *Bacteroides* sp., peptostreptococci, and *Clostridia* sp.[59] By comparison, in the absence of obstruction, the proximal small bowel has no resident flora, and prophylaxis is unnecessary. With obstruction, the small bowel becomes contaminated with colonic flora and antibiotic prophylaxis is recommended.[59]

Bowel Preps

Full mechanical bowel preps are indicated when intestinal injury or bowel resection is anticipated.[86] Exposure for laparoscopic surgery may also be facilitated by cleansing the gastrointestinal tract of feces and air. Traditional methods for bowel cleansing have included clear liquid intake with cathartics (e.g., oral magnesium citrate 240 cc 1–2 days prior to surgery) and enemas (saline or Fleet® [C. B. Fleet Co., Inc., Lynchburg, Virginia]) the evening and morning before surgery until efflux is clear. Golytely® (Braintree Laboratories, Inc., Braintree, Massachusetts) is an isotonic solution of polyethylene glycol, sodium sulfate, NaCl, and KCl that induces diarrhea within 3–4 hours following oral intake. Oral administration is at a rate of 240 cc per hour until 4 liters are consumed. Compared with traditional methods of cleansing, Golytely® is associated with less weight loss, better patient tolerance, and is as effective in colon cleansing.[87,88] Side effects include fullness, cramps, nausea, and vomiting; occasionally NG tube placement and/or antiemetics are necessary to complete an adequate prep. Although the manufacturers do not recommend artificial flavorings or additives, some patients find the salty taste unpleasant, and hard candy or apple juice may improve tolerance (Level III).

Poor oral intake and multiple bowel cleansing for tests, as well as the surgical preparation, predispose the patient to hypovolemia, the extent of which is often underestimated. In patients with little cardiac reserve, hypovolemia may induce clinically significant increases in cardiac work, hypotension, as well as increase operative blood loss. Hydration with 12 or more hours of intravenous fluids (125–150 cc/hr) and/or encouraging additional oral fluid intake (eight or more 8 oz glasses per day) helps to reduce these adverse effects. For patients at increased risk, potassium levels should be checked early the morning of surgery and losses replaced (Level II-3).

Antibiotic Prophylaxis In addition to mechanical bowel cleansing, infectious morbidity following colorectal surgery is significantly reduced by oral, parenteral, or a combination of oral and parenteral antibiotic prophylaxis, especially when the duration of surgery exceeds 3.5–4 hours (Level II-2).[89] By reducing bacterial counts,[90] oral antibiotics reduce the risks of postoperative wound infection from 43% to 9%, compared with mechanical bowel cleansing alone.[90] The gold standard is oral prophylaxis, which consists of neomycin combined with either erythromycin or metronidazole, 1 gram each at 1 P.M., 2 P.M., and 11 P.M. the evening before surgery, after completion of bowel cleansing.[90,91] The role of intravenous agents including cefoxitin, ceftriaxone/metronidazole, or cefotaxime/metronidazole in addition to oral prophylaxis has recently become a more common practice. Although some studies have demonstrated no benefit,[92] others have found that systemic agents significantly reduce infection rates compared with oral agents used alone.[93–96] When oral agents were not given, cefotaxime/metronidazole was found to be superior prophylaxis compared with aztreonam/metronidazole, presumably because aztreonam provides little activity against gram-positive organisms; in this study, *Staphylococcus* was found to be the major organism involved in postoperative surgical sepsis and abscess formation.[97] Intravenous antibiotics should also be given when surgery is delayed beyond 12 hours past the last oral antibiotic

TABLE 9.6. Regimens of Endocarditis Prophylaxis for GI and GU[a] Procedures

Low-risk regimen	Amoxicillin 3.0 g orally 1 hr before procedure followed by 1.5 g every 6 hr after procedure
High-risk[b] regimen	IV or IM ampicillin 2.0 g with gentamicin 1.5 mg/kg (not to exceed 80 mg) 30 min before procedure, followed by two doses every 8 hr[c]
Alternate regimen[d]	Parenteral vancomycin 1.0 g administered over 1 hr prior to procedure with gentamicin

[a]Gastrointestinal and genitourinary.
[b]History of endocarditis or prosthetic valve replacement.
[c]Oral amoxicillin 2 g may be substituted.
[d]Penicillin-allergic patients.
Source: Adapted from Dajani AS, Bisno AL, Chung KJ, et al. Prevention of bacterial endocarditis—recommendations by the American Heart Association. *JAMA* 1990;264:2919–2222.

dose. When there is insufficient time to complete an oral bowel preparation, parenteral prophylaxis should be extended to cover gram-negative bacilli and anaerobic organisms. Options include the addition of clindamycin or metronidazole with an aminoglycoside, or cefoxitin (2 grams) continued for 24 hours postoperatively. Contaminated cases involving fecal spillage should be treated with broad-spectrum antibiotic therapy, which is continued for a full therapeutic course.

Other Indications for Antibiotic Prophylaxis

Endocarditis Prophylaxis Conditions for which endocarditis prophylaxis is recommended include prosthetic valves, most congenital anomalies, rheumatic and other acquired valvular dysfunction, hypertrophic cardiomyopathy, and symptomatic mitral valve prolapse. The genitourinary system is second only to the oral cavity as the major portal of entry for organisms causing endocarditis. *Streptococcal (viridans)* species are the causative organisms associated with oral and dental procedures, whereas *Enterococcus faecalis* usually causes endocarditis associated with urinary and gastrointestinal procedures. Recommended prophylaxis for gynecologic surgery is outlined in Table 9.6 (Level II-3).[98] The duration of antibiotic administration is controversial and depends upon presence of continued foreign materials such as urinary catheters.

Intensive Care Patients and Special Considerations Critically ill patients are especially susceptible to hospital-acquired infections. Predisposing factors include altered resistance of the digestive tract and oropharynx, underlying disease, advanced age, medical and surgical interventions, prolonged ICU admissions, and altered immune response (Level II-2).[99–101] Nosocomial colonization of the oropharyngeal and digestive system in mechanically ventilated patients approaches 70–90%, and over 60% of colonized patients subsequently become infected (Level I).[102] Pathogens involved are predominantly gram-negative microorganisms (*Enterobacteriaceae* or *Pseudomonas* species). Oral tobramycin, amphotericin B, and polymixin E reduce endotracheal and gastrointestinal colonization, and in critically ill patients requiring ICU admission and ventilatory support, they reduce nosocomial infection rates by 60.7 (Level I).[102] The use of nystatin "swish and swallow" (5–10 cc of nystatin [100,000 U/cc]) prophylactically has been found to reduce the incidence of *Candida* wound infection and systemic candidiasis (Level II-1)[103] and should be used routinely in patients with granulocytopenia, on broad-spectrum antibiotics, or following radical pelvic or gastrointestinal procedures.

Neutropenic patients who develop fever are at high risk for infection that, without appropriate therapy, may rapidly develop into sepsis and death. Broad-spectrum beta-lactam-antibiotic/beta-lactamase-inhibitor combinations such as ticarcillin/clavulanate, alone or in combination with aminoglycosides, are the agents of choice for neutropenic fever.[81] Klastersly et al. demonstrated that, in combination with an aminoglycoside, extended-spectrum penicillins (azlocillin, mezlocillin, and pipercillin) compared with extended-spectrum cephalosporins (cefoxtaxime, moxalactam, cefoperazone) are more active against gram-negative bacteremias in febrile granulocytopenic patients (Level 1).[104]

Whenever possible, antibiotics should be directed against the specific organisms(s) involved, and should be given for the shortest possible effective time. Healthy intestinal mucosa functions as a protective barrier to prevent bacteria from invading the host. When the normal endogenous microflora is altered by prolonged antibiotic use, endotoxemia, impaired host defenses, or injury, bacteria within the GI tract can pass through the epithelial mucosa to infect mesenteric lymph nodes, a process known as bacterial translocation (Level II-3).[99,105,106] Translocation of pathogens contributes to the development of sepsis syndrome, septic shock, and multiorgan failure, which carries a mortality rate of 30% to 100%.[107,108] Intravenous antibiotics, especially clindamycin, cephalosporins, and ampicillin (or amoxicillin) are frequently associated with the development of diarrhea and/or pseudomembraneous colitis.[109–116] Alteration in the normal gut flora from antibiotic use or bowel preps permits the overgrowth of a gram-positive anaerobic bacillus, *Clostridium difficile*. Heat-resistant spores produced by the organism are very hearty and may persist in the environment for years. Infection is by oral-fecal contamination. Diarrhea and colitis result from colonization of the colon by toxin-producing strains of *C. difficile*; strains incapable of producing toxins are not pathogenic.

Although fewer than 1% of healthy adults are carriers, approximately 25% of adults recently treated with antibiotics are colonized with *C. difficile*, and most carriers remain asymptomatic.[110,114] Although the treatment of asymptomatic carriers is not recommended, colonized health care providers may be an important source of infection in hospitalized and immunocompromised patients.[116] Other factors that increase susceptibility include chemotherapy, severe debilitation, and hospitalization.[109,110,112,113,116] Reported outbreaks of this organism in intensive care units involving patients not receiving antibiotics emphasize the nosocomial nature of this infection and the importance of vector transmission (bedpans, floors, toilets, and shelves where bedpans are stored).[114] *C. difficile* infection usually presents with mild to moderate diarrhea, occasionally accompanied by lower abdominal cramping.

Most patients lack systemic symptoms including fever or chills, and other than slight tenderness in the lower abdomen, physical examination is normal. Severe colitis with or without pseudomembrane formation may occur, and it is associated with profuse, debilitating diarrhea, abdominal pain, and distention. Rarely, patients present with an acute abdomen and fulminant, life-threatening colitis. These patients are acutely ill, with lethargy, fever, abdominal pain, marked abdominal distension, and toxic megacolon. A history of recent antibiotic use and the presence of *C. difficile* toxins (toxin A or B) in the stool confirm the diagnosis.[116] Although lower abdominal endoscopy (proctosigmoidoscopy/colonoscopy) is the only diagnostic test for pseudomembranous colitis, it is expensive, invasive, insensitive (51–55%), and should be avoided when fulminant colitis is present because of the risk of perforation.[110] Whenever possible, the first step in treatment is discontinuation of antibiotics, and in mild cases this is the only intervention required.[116]

Since life-threatening toxic megacolon[115] or bowel perforation has been associated with antibiotic use, in addition to the potential risks of increased metronidazole systemic absorption, reducing its effectiveness, antiperistaltic agents (e.g., Lomotil, G. D. Searle and Co., Chicago, IL) should be avoided alone or in conjunction with antibiotic therapy.[112] When symptoms are persistent or severe, or when antibiotic therapy must be continued, the treatment of choice is oral metronidazole (250 mg 4 times per day), or vancomycin (125 mg 4 times per day) when symptoms persist or metronidaxole is not tolerated. More severe symptoms require intravenous hydration, and when patients cannot tolerate oral medication because of ileus or recent abdominal surgery, they may be effectively treated with metronidazole (but not vancomycin) intravenously.[111,116] Alternative agents include bacitracin, anion-exchange resins, rifampin, and ciprofloxacin (but not norfloxacin). In most instances, symptomatic colonization in patients with a history of *C. difficile* diarrhea do not require retreatment. For those patients who must receive antibiotic therapy, antimicrobial agents, infrequently or rarely associated with *C. difficile*, such as aminoglycosides, bacitracin, metronidazole, or quinolones, should be considered (Level II-2).[111,116]

Prevention of Deep Venous Thrombosis and Pulmonary Embolus

Major risk factors predisposing to the development of deep venous thrombosis (DVT), as defined by Virchow's triad, include hypercoagulability, venous stasis, and vessel injury. Gynecologic surgery patients are at risk for postoperative DVT because of perioperative venous stasis produced from immobility, activation of clotting factors at the operative site, and vessel damage. Patients with malignancies are at added risk of thrombosis, because some tumors produce thromboplastin, and other tumors produce procoagulants that predispose to hypercoagulability.[117] Other factors associated with an increased risk for thromboembolism (Table 9.7) include age greater than 50 years, preg-

TABLE 9.7. Risk Factors for Deep Venous Thrombosis (Level II-2)[117–119,121]

Risk Factor	Etiology	Comment
Older age	Activation of peripheral vascular system; increased venous stasis	Risk increases exponentially above 50 years of age
Malignancy	Increased thromboplastin and other procoagulants produced by malignant tissues; direct tumor extension or compression of veins	Increases risk three- to fivefold
Immobility; operative time	Venous dilation and stasis; reduced mechanical fibrinolysis	
Obesity	Increased venous stasis; impaired fibrinolytic activity	
Varicose veins	Increased venous stasis; minor varicosities not significant	Increases risk twofold
Pregnancy; oral contraceptives[a]	Increased factor VII and X activity and platelet aggregation; decreased antithrombin III activity	Increases risk four- to sevenfold; dissipates 6–8 weeks after discontinuation of pregnancy or contraceptive use
Previous thromboembolic event		Increases risk two- to threefold
Surgery/trauma	Venous stasis; activation of coagulation system	Risk dependent on length of surgery and type of procedure performed; risk with gynecologic surgery: 7–45%
Hypercoagulable states; inherited risk factors	Deficiencies of protein S, C, antithrombin III; antiphospholipid antibody syndromes	
Smoking	Nicotine-induced reduction in venous stasis; improved fibrinolysis	Increases risk threefold

[a]Postmenopausal hormone replacement therapy does not alter coagulation factors.

Source: Adapted from Weinmann EE, Saltzman EW. Deep-vein thrombosis. *N Engl J Med* 1994;24:1630–1640.

nancy, general anesthesia, obesity, recent radiation therapy, varicose veins, and medical diseases associated with hypercoagulability, such as protein C or S deficiency.[117–120].

Following gynecologic surgery, the majority of pulmonary emboli arise from venous thrombosis of the deep lower extremity leg and pelvic veins. Using I 125–fibrinogen uptake tests, it has been demonstrated that the thrombotic process usually starts in the calf veins (Level II-2). The majority of thrombi within the calf veins remain localized and spontaneously resolve. However, approximately 20% propagate into the proximal thigh and pelvic veins, and about 50% develop into pulmonary emboli, the majority of which are not fatal.[121–123] Thrombosis may originate in the pelvic veins, but it is usually in association with trauma to the veins, such as occurs at the time of a lymphadenectomy.

The incidence of DVT developing after gynecologic surgery overall is approximately 15%; the rate varies from 7% for vaginal hysterectomy to 45% for oncologic procedures.[117,119–121,124] Following gynecologic surgery, the incidence of fatal pulmonary emboli is estimated to be 0.01% to 0.87% and accounts for approximately 40% of all postoperative deaths.[121,124,125] Two-thirds of patients die from pulmonary emboli within one-half hour of the onset of symptoms, and approximately 80% of pulmonary emboli occur in the absence of clinical signs of peripheral venous thrombosis.[126] Since the majority of pulmonary emboli arise from thrombi developing in the deep veins of the pelvis or legs, prevention of thromboembolic events should be aimed at the cause: alterations in coagulability, and venous stasis (Fig. 9.3).

To be effective, preventive measures should be initiated preoperatively and should be continued for the first 7–10 days postoperatively, or until the patient is fully ambulatory (Level II-2). In controlled studies, low-dose heparin is effective in preventing DVT and subsequent fatal and nonfatal pulmonary emboli (Level II-1);[127] low-molecular-weight heparin, dihydroergotamine, dihydroergotamine-heparin, dextran, and warfarin are also effective (Table 9.8, Level II-1).[117–145] Standard heparin contains a mixture of polysaccharide molecules (5–30 kd in weight) that vary widely in their anticoagulant ability.[118] The initial dose is an 80 U/kg bolus, followed by 18 U/kg per hour; APTT is repeated every 6 hours, and dose adjusted to maintain the APTT 46–70 seconds (>1.5–2.3 × control value). Other nomograms recommend maintaining the APTT at 2–2.5 × control value (APTT 55–85 seconds).[118] Nomograms are guidelines; dosing must take into account the severity of the thrombosis, patient characteristics that can alter the clotting profile (advanced age, malignancy, malnutrition), and the risks of bleeding must be weighted against the therapeutic benefit of aggressive anticoagulation, especially immediately postoperatively (Level III). Alternatively, patients may be treated by a 5,000 U bolus followed by 1,280 U per hour (40,000 U/24 hr if patient is at low risk for bleeding (30,000 U if at high risk). Rebolusing (40–80 U/kg) and rate increases (2–4 U/kg/hr (120–240 U/hr) are indicated for subtherapeutic levels; low APTT levels (<35 seconds) require greater incremental changes than higher subtherapeutic levels (APTT 35–55 seconds).[11] When APTT levels exceed therapeutic

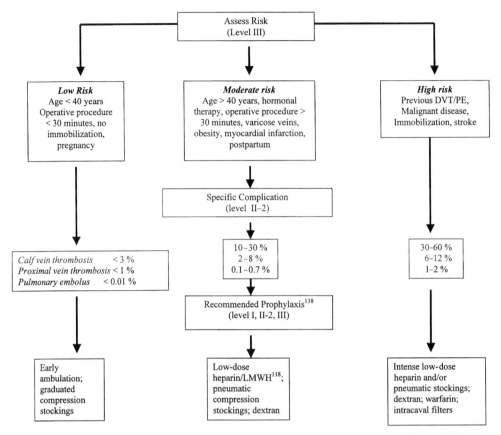

FIGURE 9.3. Deep venous thrombosis risk and prophylaxis (Levels I, II-2, III).[117,118,138]

range, depending on the severity of elevation, therapy should be held 0.5–1 hour, and reinfusion rates reduced 2–3 U/kg/hr (120–240 U/hr).[118]

Animal data suggest that lower-molecular-weight heparins (LMWH), which are less than 7 kd in weight, are associated with less antiplatelet activity and less hemorrhagic complications.[129–131,143,144] Compared with heparin, LMWH have a longer biological half-life, a more predictable dose-response, increased bioavailability, do not require serum level monitoring, and are associated with lower rates of DVT recurrence but are more costly. For treatment of DVT, total cost difference depends upon laboratory monitoring regimens for standard heparin dosing, inpatient versus outpatient therapy, and complication rates. On balance, LMWH have been associated with improved cost effectiveness in treatment at renous thrombosis.[145b,c,d] Cost effectiveness for prophylaxis also appears improved with LMWH versus infractionated heparin.[145e] (34–67% [Level I]).[118,131] For general surgical prophylaxis, an initial dose 1–2 hours before surgery is followed by once daily dosing. Dosing must be based on the specific agent given, since LMWH preparations differ in biological efficacy per unit and half-life.[131] Dihydroergotamine (DHE) is an ergot derivative that has vasoconstrictive effects on capacitance vessels—veins and venules—and minimal effect on arterial resistance vessels.[133,145] DHE reduces venous stasis and accelerates lower extremity venous return. Dextran, a partially hydrolyzed glucose polymer, affects blood flow, platelet activity, coagulation factors V and VIII, and fibrinolysis, and is available in two preparations: Dextran 70 and Dextran 40.[117,118] Aspirin and other oral antiplatelet agents are either less effective than heparin or are ineffective in DVT prevention.[118–120] When administered 24–48 hours preoperatively, oral anticoagulants such as warfarin are among the most effective to prevent both DVT and fatal pulmonary embolism.[120] However, the need for close laboratory control and unacceptable bleeding complications preclude their routine use. Low-dose warfarin therapy appears to be a promising preventive agent. A prospective trial that compared low-dose warfarin (1 mg/day begun 6–42 days preoperatively, continued until discharge from the hospital) with full oral-dose warfarin anticoagulation, demonstrated a significant decrease in thromboembolic sequela without increasing adverse hemorrhagic consequences (Level II-1).[134] Investigational antithrombotic agents include (1) relatives of *hirudin*, a natural anticoagulant component of saliva of the leech; (2) a murine monoclonal antibody fragment that competes with fibrinogen for its platelet receptor; and (3) recombinant human factor Xa, which blocks prothrombinase activity.[118]

Physical measures that decrease venous stasis, such as intermittent pneumatic compression stockings and graduated compression stockings, have also been shown to decrease DVT postoperatively (Level 1).[135–137] Graduated compression stockings, however, are not as effective as other prophylactic means, and should be used only in low-risk patients or in combination with other measures.[118,120,138] Patients at high risk (Fig. 9.3), especially those with malignancy, require more intensive low-dose heparin regimes than those with benign disease.[139] Prolonged use of pneumatic compression stocking are also effective in this group of patients.[137,146] The indications, dosages, risks, and benefits of the various DVT prophylactic measures are listed in Table 9.8.

Postoperative thromboembolic complications do occur after discharge from the hospital. The exact incidence of late venous thromboembolism is unknown, but in a recent review this complication was noted clinically in 1% of patients and in about 10% of patients when screening diagnostics were utilized.[140] Current trials are underway to evaluate the value of long-term DVT prophylaxis in postoperative patients.[140] An alternative to anticoagulation in patients at greatest risk for perioperative pulmonary emboli and hemorrhage, such as the patient with advanced ovarian cancer and a DVT, is fluoroscopic placement of vena cava filters preoperatively. Pulmonary complications are uncommon and are similar in frequency to those of CVP placement (pneumothorax, arrhythmias, vascular injury); however, since clots may propagate above the filter and patients may develop extensive venous thrombosis associated with debilitat-

TABLE 9.8. Perioperative Thromboembolism Prophylaxis

Method	Dose	Indications	Mechanism	Drawbacks	Benefits
Low-dose heparin	5,000 IU SC 2 hr[a] preop and q 12 hr[b] po[127]	Moderate risk	Increased AT-III activity; inactivation of factors Xa, thrombin; possibly coats endothelial walls; decreases thrombogenesis	Bleeding complications;[127] wound hematomas;[141] increases transfusions;[139] increases retroperitoneal drain output; thrombocytopenia[118]	Decreased risk of DVT from 7–45% to 6.2–11.9%;[142] easy to administer and highly effective
LMWH[d]	2,500 IU SC 2 hr preop and daily for 7–10 days[130]	Moderate and high risk	Similar to heparin	High DVT rates;[118] increases bleeding complications, especially with doses >5,000 IU/day[118,143]	Single daily injections as effective as low-dose heparin;[132,143] fewer bleeding complications[142]
DHE[c,f]	0.5 mg po 2 hr preop and twice daily po[b]	Not recommended	Selective venoconstrictor decreases venous stasis	Vasoconstrictive complications; bowel necrosis, vascular spasm, skin/muscle necrosis, many contraindications[145]	Probably not as effective as heparin[143]
DHE and heparin/L[d] MWH	0.5 mg po and 5,000 IU H or 1,500 IU SC LMWH[143] 2 hr preop and daily postop	High risk			No more effective than low-dose heparin, or LMWH[135,143]

Dextran 70[e]	1 L IV/q 6 hr at onset of surgery; effects last 7 days	Moderate and high risk	Increases microcirculation; antiplatelet activity; increases fibrinolysis; alters factors V, VIII[117]	Increases risks for CHF, renal failure, bleeding complications, allergic reactions, anaphylaxis (0.001–0.1%);[142] avoid use with heparin	Volume expander; probably as effective as heparin[117,135]
Pneumatic compression stockings	Placed at induction of anesthesia	Moderate to high risk	Increases venous flow velocity; decreases venous stasis[146]	Patient discomfort rare	As effective as heparin, even in high-risk patients; few or no contraindications[137]

[a]High-risk patients may alternatively be treated with one or two 5,000 IU q 8 hr preop and q 8 hr postop for 7–10 days.[139]
[b]Postoperative administration.
[c]Dihydroergotamine.
[d]Low-molecular-weight heparin.
[e]Alternatively, dextran 70, 500 m IV every 4 hr daily for 2–5 days after surgery.
[f]Contraindicated in pregnancy, hypertension, coronary artery disease, renal failure, or in patients using beta-adrenergic antagonists or dopamine.

ing leg edema, even when coincident anticoagulation is used, filters should be reserved for the high-risk patient.[147]

GI Bleeding Prophylaxis

Bleeding within the upper GI tract secondary to stress ulcers and aggravated by nasogastric intubation is a potentially life-threatening complication in perioperative patients. Histamine type 2 (H2) blockers, such as ranitidine and cimetidine, and/or antacids, are frequently prescribed as prophylaxis against stress-induced bleeding.[148,149] Antacids, which inhibit peptic activity, and H2 blockers, which inhibit gastric acid secretion, reduce bleeding risks by elevating gastric pH.[150,151] Dose efficacy is dependent on elevation of pH in the 3–5 range, which requires serial gastric pH determinations. Unfortunately, gastric acidity is an important physiologic mechanism that prevents upper GI tract colonization with enteric pathogens and may predispose to pneumonia. Hospital-acquired pneumonia, a complication of 0.5% to 1% of all patients undergoing hospitalization, is the leading cause of death secondary to nosocomial infection.[152] Sucralfate is a weak buffer that probably acts through pepsin adsorption, mucosal protein binding, and cytoprotection.[153] In a comparative study of sucralfate and H2 blockers with and without antacids, sucralfate administration resulted in reduced gastric colonization by gram-negative bacteria that was associated with lower rates of hospital-acquired pneumonia and reduced mortality, without increasing the incidence of gastric bleeding (Level I).[154]

Adrenal Insufficiency and Steroid Prophylaxis

The stress of surgery leads to an increase of adrenal corticosteroids. With adrenal insufficiency, circulatory shock may result secondary to inability of the adrenal glands to produce the necessary glucocorticoids. Basal, daily adrenal cortisol production is the equivalent of hydrocortisone, 30 mg, or prednisone, 7.5 mg. Corticosteroids are given for a variety of medical conditions. Exogenous steroids may suppress the hypothalamic-pituitary-adrenal axis; doses equivalent to 20–30 mg of prednisone/day for at least 1 week are probably sufficient to produce adrenal suppression, and recovery of the adrenal glands may take up to 1 year.[155,156] Cosyntropin, a synthetic ACTH, can be utilized in a dose of 25 units, intramuscularly or intravenously, as a stimulation test to assess the integrity of the hypothalamic-pituitary-adrenal axis. Cortisol levels are measured before and 60 minutes after the injection. Normal values, indicating sufficient adrenal reserve for the stresses of surgery, are an absolute rise in cortisol of 7 micrograms, a doubling of the baseline control value, or a stimulated value greater than 18 micrograms.[157] Patients with a history of suppressive dose of exogenous steroids within 1 year prior to surgery or those with an abnormal suppression test need perioperative stress doses of glucocorticoids. Traditionally, these doses have been four times the current steroid dosage.[158]

Studies have demonstrated that the normal adrenal output of cortisol is about 75–150 mg per day in response to major surgery, and 50 mg per day during minor surgery, with cortisol secretion in the first 24 hours after surgery rarely exceeding 200 mg.[158] There are no data to support that administration of doses exceeding these amounts is beneficial. After major surgery, plasma cortisol levels usually return to normal within 24–48 hours. Postoperative complications such as infection require continued administration of stress doses of glucocorticoids. As soon as the patient is able to tolerate oral intake, the preoperative steroid dose is resumed. A tapering of the steroid dose is probably not necessary unless the patient has been on prolonged high doses of glucocorticoids (Level II-3).

High-dose glucocorticoids may increase susceptibility to infection secondary to suppression of the immune response and may have adverse effects on wound healing. Consequently, assessment of the hypothalamic-pituitary-adrenal axis is recommended whenever possible to avoid steroid administration. The current recommendation for major surgical corticosteroid stress dosage is the equivalent of hydrocortisone, 100 mg, given intraoperatively and every 8 hours postoperatively for 24 hours.[159] Although these doses may be excessive, until lower doses of perioperative steroids have been evaluated in a large number of patients, physiological doses cannot be recommended (Level II-3).[158]

Splenectomized Patients

Splenectomy is rarely indicated as part of cytoreductive surgery for ovarian cancer, and is occasionally performed to control bleeding from capsular avulsion, usually resulting from traction in the course of total omentectomy.[160,161] Splenectomized patients are at increased risks for left lower lobe atelectasis, thrombocytosis, and increased infection risks. In these patients, postoperative care should emphasize deep breathing exercises, broad-spectrum prophylactic antibiotics, and administration of 0.5 ml pneumococcal polyvalent vaccine (Pneumovax®, Merck, Sharp & Dome). Thrombocytosis (platelet counts in the range of 625,000–1,221,000 mg/dl) has been reported in up to 66% of these patients and is usually detected 2 to 3 weeks postoperatively. Although it does not affect platelet counts, low-dose heparin therapy is generally advocated in the immediate postoperative period, because of the risks for DVT and pulmonary embolus (Level II-2).[160]

GENERAL PROBLEMS IN POSTOPERATIVE MANAGEMENT

Initial Management in the Postoperative Recovery Room Area

Until the effects of anesthesia are reversed and physiological and mental function returns, adequate oxygenation, airway maintenance, frequent monitoring of vital signs, and correcting hypothermia are primary concerns. Untoward com-

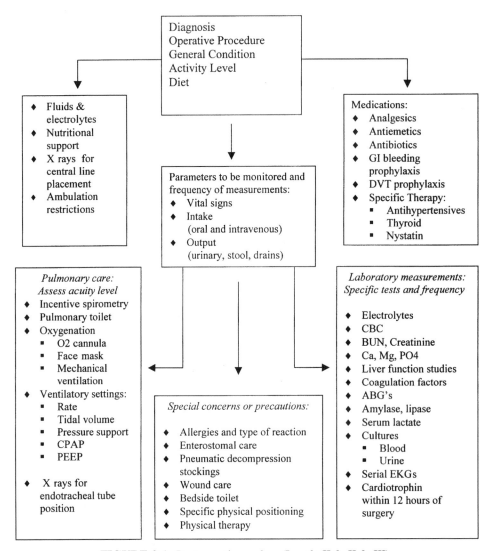

FIGURE 9.4. Postoperative orders (Levels II-2, II-3, III).

plications of anesthesia (neuromuscular blockade, hyperthermia, bronchospasm, or cardiovascular or respiratory insufficiency) should be recognized immediately and therapy instituted. Fluid, electrolyte, and blood product replacement are instigated based on vital signs, urinary output, and preexisting deficits or excesses. In addition to immediate replacement needs, postoperative orders (Fig. 9.4) define activity level, doses and frequency of analgesia and other medications, which physical parameters are to be measured and how often, and other care needs specific for each patient in the recovery area and after transfer to the wards. All hypothermic patients should be actively treated with warming therapy. Shivering can be suppressed by application of heat to the patient's skin, or with sedation (meperidine 15–25 mg intravenously). Traditional methods of warming patients (warmed cotton blankets, warmed intravenous fluids, and use of warm-water mattresses) provide little benefit. Hypothermia may be successfully treated or prevented by using heated and humidified inspired gases, maintaining an ambient operating room temperature over 70°C whenever possible, using radiant heat, and using convective warming therapy consisting of a disposable plastic and tissue paper cover that is inflated with warm air from a heating unit (Level II-2).[14,162]

In uncomplicated patients, recovery care is safely accomplished in 1 to 2 hours in a specifically designed unit. Critically ill patients requiring aggressive hemodynamic monitoring, inotropic agents, or ventilatory support should undergo postoperative recovery in an intensive care unit supervised by a critical care team of doctors, nurses, nutritionalists, and respiratory therapists (Level III). When the postoperative intensive care unit is anticipated, preoperative consultation with the critical care team is recommended.

Fluid and Electrolyte Replacement

Immediately postoperatively, fluid, electrolytes, and/or blood product replacement is guided by clinical, and when indicated, laboratory assessment of the patient's postoperative volume status. The uncomplicated surgical patient who is NPO requires 2,000–3,000 cc/day to compensate for insensible losses and to maintain urinary output at approximately 1,000–1,500 cc/day (minimum 0.5 cc/kg/hr).[6] Solutions (Table 9.9) that also replace physiological and excess losses of sodium, potassium, magnesium, calcium, and glucose are commercially available.[163] Volume replacement should be based on the preoperative volume status, intraoperative losses and replacement, and compartmental shifts in cellular water that occur in response to surgical stress. Additional fluids are required to compensate for increased losses from postoperative fever, gastric suctioning, and third-space losses resulting from sequestration of fluid within the bowel lumen or actual losses, as from abrupt drainage of ascites. Gastrointestinal losses should be replaced based on the electrolyte and acid-base composition of the source of loss (Table 9.1). A solution that is isotonic with plasma with additional potassium and chloride is required to correct for gastric losses, whereas small intestinal losses (ileostomies, fistula, or obstruction) benefit from isotonic saline replacement with added sodium bicarbonate.[4,6] Diarrhea losses typically require replacement with hypotonic buffered solutions.[6] A useful guide for replacement is that approximately one-third of the volume of isotonic fluid given will remain in the intravascular space, and the reminder will redistribute into the interstitium or within cells (Level II-3).

Postoperative *hyponatremia* most frequently results from fluid replacement in excess of water loss.[4] Additional causes include hyperglycemia, physiologic

TABLE 9.9. Composition of Common Parenteral Fluids

Solution	Cation (mEq/L)					Anion (mEq/L)			
	Na+	K+	Ca+	Mg+	NH$_{4+}$	Cl–	HCO$_{4-}$	HPO$_3^4$–	Protein
Plasma	142	4	5	3	0.3	103	27	3	
Intracellular fluid	10	150		40			10	150	40
Ringer's lactate[a]	130	4	2.7			109	28		
0.9% sodium chloride (normal saline)	154					154			
0.45% sodium chloride (half-normal saline)	77					77			
3% sodium chloride	513					513			
5% sodium chloride	855					855			
0.9% ammonium chloride	168					168			

[a]Lactate in solution is converted to bicarbonate.

Source: Modified from Orr JW Jr. Introduction to pelvic surgery: pre- and postoperative care (Level II-3). In Gusberg SB, Shingleton HM, Deppe G (Eds), *Female Genital Cancer*. New York: Churchill Livingstone, 1988.

and pathologic changes in renal water and sodium excretion, and congestive heart failure (Fig. 9.1). Management of hyponatremia usually requires isotonic fluid replacement or restriction, depending on the cause within the context of the extracellular fluid compartment (Level II-3)[5,6] *Hypernatremia* (serum sodium concentration above 150 mEq/L) is usually secondary to insufficient replacement of excess losses. Fever results in excess hypotonic losses through the skin and respiratory system of up to 1–1.5 L/day.[4] Renal losses may be increased in response to increased solute load resulting from high protein intake or hyperglycemia, diuretic therapy, acute and chronic renal insufficiency, a deficiency in ADH, or nephrogenic diabetes insipidis. Treatment depends on recognition of the underlying cause; as with hyponatremia, correction of hypernatremia should proceed slowly to avoid central nervous system dysfunction (Level II-3).

Hypokalemia is a frequent postoperative surgical problem that may be secondary to diuretics, other medications (digitalis, beta-agonists, aminoglycosides, high doses of some penicillins), and gastrointestinal losses. Severe hypokalemia, or moderate in the patient at increased risk (digitalized patients, history of arrhythmias), can result in cardiac arrhythmias, cardiac arrest, muscular paralysis, and respiratory failure (Level II-2).[164] Although oral replacement of 40–60 mEq/day is preferred, intravenous replacement is safely accomplished with 20–40 mEq of potassium per liter of isotonic solution or, when more rapid replacement is advisable, given at a rate of up to 10 mEq per hour. In an ICU setting, severe and life-threatening hypokalemia may be safely replaced by using peripheral or central venous access to infuse KCl at a rate of 20 mEq per hour (Level II-2).[164] When volume restriction is essential, as little as 25–50 cc of compatible solution may be used for dilution.

Manifestations of severe hyperkalemia include weakness, paresthesias, respiratory failure, bradycardia, and cardiac arrhythmias that predispose to complete heart block, ventricular fibrillation, or asystole. EKG changes include ST segment depression, first-degree AV block, and widening of the QRS (principal deflection in an ECG) interval that, without treatment, may progress into a biphasic sinusoidal pattern, predicting impending asystole. Causes include decreased renal potassium excretion from intrinsic renal disease, hypoaldosteronism, medications (potassium-sparing diuretics, neuromuscular blocking agents, heparin, etc.), adrenal insufficiency, excessive potassium administration, tissue destruction (burns, malignant hyperthermia, massive blood transfusion), and acidosis that results in shifts of intracellular potassium into the extracellular fluid compartment.[165] Treatment directed at shifting potassium to the intracellular compartment includes infusion with glucose and insulin (10 U regular insulin after 1 ampule of 50% glucose), sodium bicarbonate,[6] and albuterol.[166] When life-threatening (serum K > 7 mEq/L or associated with ECG changes), calcium gluconate, 10 ml of 10% solution, should be given intravenously over 2–5 minutes, with a second dose if indicated.[6] Calcium exchange resins, such as sodium polystyrene sulfonate, bind potassium in exchange for sodium within the gastrointestinal tract, and are frequently used in patients with chronic renal disease. The usual dose is 15–30 g in 50–100 cc of 20% sorbitol. Oral administration is preferable to enemas; intestinal necrosis has been reported in patients receiving Kayexalate enemas, especially when preexisting diverticular disease or other colorectal pathology is present (Level II-2).[167] Chronic therapy for hyperkalemia includes dietary restriction and loop diuretics (Level II-2).

Nutritional Support

Critically ill and malnourished patients are at an increased risk for prolonged hospitalization and postoperative morbidity and mortality compared with healthy patients.[168–171] Postoperative nutritional support with central hyperalimentation has been found to effectively reverse compromised immunologic function that is frequently present in severely malnourished patients.[168] A standard nutritional assessment begins with dietary history, physical examination, and laboratory evaluation. Physical assessment of nutritional status includes the use of anthropometric measurements to estimate skeletal muscle, changes in body weight over time, and creatinine-height index. Laboratory parameters include measurement of albumin, transferrin, thyroxine-binding prealbumin, and somatomedin-C.[172] Oral feeding, or enteric nutrition via gastroduodenal or jejunal tubes, is preferable to central venous hyperalimentation (TPN), as starvation disrupts indigenous GI tract microflora and allows for overgrowth of pathogenic gram-negative and aerobic bacteria.[104,105,173] Glutamine, a nonessential amino acid that is unstable in aqueous solutions, and thus cannot be provided by standard TPN solutions, has been found to be important in preventing skeletal muscle catabolism,[174] which further supports the practice of intestinal feeding. Nevertheless, enteric feeding is frequently insufficient in critically ill patients because of problems with tube placement or subtle bowel dysfunction. Augmentation of enteric feeding with TPN in critically ill patients improves calorie delivery as well as helps to maintain the integrity of the gastrointestinal mucosa.[175]

Regardless of whether oral or intravenous nutrition is used, caloric, protein, and trace element requirements are the same. Basal metabolic requirements (BMR) for women may be calculated using the Harris–Benedict equation: BMR (kcal/day) = 65.5 + 9.6 (weight in kg) + 1.7 (height in cm) – 4.7 (age). Depending on energy expenditure, caloric needs are usually between 20 and 35 kcal/kg/day; the unstressed elderly female patient typically requires approximately 20 kcal/kg/day.[176] A rule of thumb is that approximately half of calories should be provided by fat (1 gram of fat is equivalent to 9 kcal; 1 cc 10% intralipid provides 1.1 kcal) and the remaining half by carbohydrates (1 gram of CHO supplies 3.4 kcal; 1,000 cc of 10% dextrose provides 340 kcal). Additional calories are indicated in patients who are severely malnourished or stressed patients; however, overzealous supplementation may result in hyperglycemia and hyperosmolar states that predispose the patient to respiratory failure.[177] Protein requirements should be based on nitrogen balance studies, and a positive nitrogen balance is the goal of therapy. Usually, 1.0–1.5 grams of amino acids per kg of body weight is sufficient to maintain a state of positive nitrogen balance. Trace elements (zinc, copper, chromium, and manganese),[178] as well as electrolytes, calcium, magnesium, and phosphorus, should also be provided (Level II-2).

Solutions with high osmotic loads require central venous access. In the past, septicemia was a common complication of central venous catheterization, reported in 6–27% of patients (Level II-2).[179–181] The risk of central venous catheter infection is significantly reduced by adherence to strict aseptic maintenance of the catheter and limiting its use to TPN only,[182] and use of single-lumen compared with double-lumen catheters.[181] Other complications include arterial catheterization, air or catheter embolism, thrombosis, injury of the brachial plexus, pneumothorax, and mediastinal hematoma formation.[183] Very low doses of warfarin (2.5 mg daily) are effective in preventing central venous catheter thrombosis.[184] Although instillation of 5,000 U urokinase with one or two repeat doses is sufficient to relieve thrombosis in the majority of patients with permanent-access catheters, persistent withdrawal occlusion may be effectively managed with high doses of urokinase infusion (250,000 U dissolved in 150 cc D5W infused over 90 min[185]), or a 12-hour infusion of urokinase at 40,000 U/hr.[186]

Pain Management

Despite effective agents and methods of delivery, postoperative pain remains a major source of postoperative morbidity, adversely affecting approximately 30–40% of patients.[187] Analgesics are typically ordered on a prn (as needed) basis, and underdosing frequently occurs because of failure by the nursing staff to adequately assess the patient's requirements for analgesia, and, all too often, because patients are reluctant to ask for pain relief, as a certain amount of pain is expected.[188] Pain increases the risk for pulmonary complications as well as thromboembolic events.[189,190] Patient-controlled anesthesia, which provides intravenous analgesia on demand, has become tremendously popular over the past several years, as it overcomes many of the delivery problems associated with prn orders.[191–194] Regardless of the analgesic agent selected, front loading is necessary to provide adequate serum levels and sufficient analgesia immediately postoperatively.[187] Epidural anesthesia, compared with intramuscular administration of standard agents such as morphine, has also been demonstrated to reduce pulmonary dysfunction and provide superior pain relief;[195–199] however, costs for surveillance are significantly increased (Level I).

Nonsteroidal anti-inflammatory drugs (NSAID) have gained popularity in the postoperative setting. These agents are safe in the majority of patients; pain control comparable to narcotic analgesia is achieved; the frequency and intensity of drowsiness, nausea, and vomiting is reduced; and in some reports, the length of hospital stay is reduced.[200–204] Toradol® (Syntex Laboratories, Inc.), 30–60 mg load (intravenously or intramuscularly), followed by 15–30 mg every 6–8 hours for up to 5 days, is the usual recommended dose; dose reductions or alternative agents are recommended for patients who are elderly, have impaired renal or hepatic function, or who are at significant risk for bleeding complications (Level II-1).[205] A more comprehensive discussion of cancer related pain management is presented in Chapter 20.

Postoperative Nausea and Vomiting

Emesis, the most frequently reported minor complication of surgery, affects approximately 30% of patients and is a major source of patient discomfort (Level II-3).[206] Multiple factors, including age, sex, operative procedure performed and duration, anesthetic agents, preoperative and postoperative opioids, anxiety, a history of motion sickness or previous postoperative nausea, and pain, affect the severity of perioperative nausea and vomiting. Anesthetics, especially nitrous oxide and cyclopropane, compared with isoflurande, enflurane, halothane, and propofol, are associated with higher rates of nausea and vomiting. Perioperative emesis is two- to fourfold more common in women, especially during the luteal phase, and abdominal and gynecologic surgery including laparoscopy is associated with higher rates of perioperative nausea and vomiting than many other surgical procedures.[206,207]

The vomiting reflex results from central or gastrointestinal (GI) stimulation of the chemoreceptor trigger zone (CTZ) in the area postrema. Vagal afferents within the upper GI tract relay stimuli to the CTZ from chemoreceptors and mechanoreceptors that are triggered by intestinal manipulation or luminal distension.[208] Commonly used antiemetics include droperidol, metoclopramide, and hyosine, which effectively alleviate nausea and vomiting but may be associated with distressing extrapyramidal side effects.[206] Serotonin (5 hydroxytryptamine [5-HT]) appears to mediate emesis via activation of receptors, specifically, the 5-HT$_3$ receptor.[208,209] Ondansetron, a 5-HT$_3$ receptor agonist, significantly reduces nausea and vomiting associated with chemotherapy as well as opioid administration. Ondansetron is now licensed for the treatment of postoperative nausea and vomiting.[206,210] Prophylactic ondansetron[210] is superior to both droperidol and metoclopramide in preventing nausea and vomiting following gynecologic surgery, and reduces the emetogenic effects of opioids administered postoperatively.[211]

Tubes and Drains

Open and Closed Suction Tubes and Drains   Surgical drains are commonly used to prevent seroma formation and to drain abscesses, blood, and lymphatic fluid. The Penrose drain, the prototype of an open drain,[212] functions by capillary action to facilitate drainage. However, open drains also permit ingress of bacteria, which increases infection rates.[213] Consequently, closed suction drains are popular in breast and gynecologic surgery. Although closed suction drainage after lumpectomy and axillary node dissection significantly reduces the incidence and severity of seromas,[214] use of drains after radical hysterectomy has recently been challenged.[215] Modern surgical techniques such as use of hemoclips and electrocautery, prophylactic antibiotic therapy, and leaving the retroperitoneum open have reduced the incidence of pelvic lymphocysts following radical hysterectomy from 15–49[215] to 5% or less.[216,217] When pelvic drainage is necessary, complications may be reduced by subfascial operative placement of the perforated portion of the drain to prevent peritubal extravasation, avoidance of irrigation solutions,[218] frequent drain "stripping" to remove clots, and removal within a few days of surgery (Level II-2).[219]

Lymphocysts usually develop within 3 weeks of surgery, but they have been described months or years following radical hysterectomy.[217] Observation is usually adequate therapy for small cysts (4–5 cm). Cysts may be managed by simple needle drainage, insertion of catheters using radiographic guidance,[217] sclerosis with povidone-iodine,[220] and as a final alternative, surgical excision (Level II-2).

Foley Catheter Care and Percutaneous Nephrostomies   Foley catheters are routinely inserted perioperatively in the operating room to facilitate examination under anesthesia, to document urinary output, and to minimize patient discomfort from urinary retention associated with anesthesia or immobility. The most common complication from Foley catheter insertion is urinary tract infection, affecting approximately 3.9% to 40% of patients.[221,222] The incidence and severity of urinary tract infections are dramatically reduced by use of prophylactic antibiotics,[223] leaving the catheter in site for 1 day or less, and by avoiding the use of Foley catheters entirely when clinically unnecessary.[221] Percutaneous nephrostomy tubes require peritubal dressing changes and irrigation with sterile saline once or twice per week. Tubes should be exchanged every 3 months, or preferably, whenever ureteral patency is established, with a universal stent that restores continuity with the bladder.

Nasogastric Decompression   Since its introduction in the 1920s and 1930s, prophylactic nasogastric (NG) decompression has become standard therapy following laparotomy for intestinal procedures and cholecystectomy, despite retrospective and prospective randomized studies condemning this practice (Level I).[224–231] Although NG tube placement reduces the frequency of emesis, postoperative nausea and vomiting is usually self-limited, and several randomized studies have found that NG tubes significantly increase discomfort and duration of hospitalization, costing on average, $1,500 per patient (Level II-2).[34,232] Early enteric feeding reduces the duration of postoperative ileus and helps to restore the normal gastrointestinal barrier mechanism (Level I).[233] There are no data to support the notion of routine NG suction until gastric output is under 1,000–1,500 cc/day. In uncomplicated patients, the routine use of NG tubes following gynecologic surgery is unnecessary and should be discouraged.

On busy gynecologic oncology services, NG tube drainage is often routine and excessively prolonged. "Indications" include ovarian staging and debulking with total omentectomy and/or splenectomy to reduce the risks of postoperative omental pedicle bleeding, extensive retroperitoneal dissection, and/or following intestinal surgery. The care of these patients may also be complicated by a history of prior radiation or chemotherapy, advanced disease, rapid reaccumulation of ascites, and peritonitis, which predispose to paralytic ileus and/or obstruction. Routine NG suction following gynecologic oncology surgery should be reevaluated in light of evidence in the surgical literature, where withholding their use postoperatively did not increase the incidence of anastomotic leaks, abdominal dehiscence, and/or paralytic or mechanical ileus (Level II-2).[224,225,228] These patients are particularly susceptible to gram-negative sepsis that may be precipitated by well-intended but potentially harmful interference with normal, physiologically protective gastrointestinal barriers. In the absence of paralytic ileus or obstruction, NG tubes should be removed in the majority of these patients within 1 to 3 days of surgery (Level II-2).

Wounds, Wound Healing, and Infectious Complications

Wound infections, for the purpose of postoperative surveillance, are divided into incisional surgical site infections (SSI) and organ/space SSIs (Level II-3). Superficial incisional SSIs are infections that occur within 30 days of the operative procedure and involve only skin or subcutaneous tissue. One of the following must also be present: purulent drainage, positive culture from the wound, signs or symptoms of infection (heat, redness, or swelling), or a diagnosis of superficial infection by the attending physician. Stitch abscesses, infection of episiotomy or circumcision incision, and infected burn wounds are not considered superficial infections.[84,234]

Deep incisional SSIs involve the deep soft tissues, including fascial and muscle layers of the incision. Characteristics of deep incisional SSIs include purulent drainage that is not arising from an infected organ/space component of the surgical site, deep incisional dehiscence or surgical separation, or an abscess found on direct examination or using radiographic studies. Criteria for organ/space surgical site infections include infections in any organ or body space with purulent drainage, positive cultures, or those identified by radiographic studies. Wound infections involving both deep and superficial sites are considered deep incisional surgical site infections.[84,234]

Management of a suspected wound infection includes opening and cleaning the wound, debridement of any necrotic tissue, and wet to dry dressing changes with normal saline, until the wound granulates closed. Although these infections are usually self-limiting and resolve over time with sufficient wound care, they must be distinguished from necrotizing fasciitis, a life-threatening condition characterized by infection of the superficial and deep fascia with associated thrombus formation. Mortality rates of 8.7% to 73% have been reported; morbidity and mortality are significantly reduced by early recognition, broad-spectrum antibiotic coverage, and operative debridement within 12 hours of diagnosis.[235] Intra-abdominal abscesses also require drainage, either by reoperation[236] or by CT scan–directed drainage, in addition to broad-spectrum antibiotic therapy (Level II-2).

The most common complication following hysterectomy is febrile morbidity (oral temperature over $38°C$ on two or more occasions at least 6 hours apart during any consecutive 48-hour period, excluding the first 24 hours), often resulting from low-grade infection at the vaginal cuff. Postoperative fever prolongs hospital stay and increases patient anxiety and discomfort; however, in the majority of cases, low-grade fevers resolve spontaneously without antibiotic therapy.[237] Hysterectomy exposes the pelvic peritoneum and soft tissues to bacteria commonly residing in the vaginal vault, which are the most common organisms involved in infection.[63] Risk factors for the development of postoperative infections, such as cuff infections, pelvic cellulitis or abscess, and/or abdominal wound infections following abdominal or vaginal hysterectomy, include the abdominal approach, an indigent population, long duration of surgery, and excessive blood loss. However, menopausal status, obesity, recent antibiotic administration, and pathological diagnosis were not found to be significant risk factors, and, using multivariate analysis, the effect of blood loss was found to be insignificant when corrected for the length of surgery (Level I).[74]

Mild vaginal cuff inflammation is an expected complication of hysterectomy and generally resolves spontaneously. Pelvic cellulitis associated with fever, pelvic pain, and marked vaginal induration with or without a local collection of pus should be treated with broad-spectrum antibiotics aimed at the probable offending organisms. Since the vaginal vault flora is polymicrobial, antibiotic coverage should be sufficient to cover gram-positive, gram-negative, and anaerobic bacteria.[237,238] Ampicillin/sulbactam has been found to be as effective in the management of soft-tissue infections as metronidazole-gentamicin (Level II-2).[239] Although many antibiotic combinations have comparable efficacy, the therapeutic regimen should consist of different antibiotics than those given for surgical prophylaxis. If the cuff is fluctuant or a mass is palpable, the vaginal cuff should also be gently probed and opened with a blunt surgical instrument with or without placement of a drain (Level II-3).

Methods to prevent wound infection include perioperative antibiotic prophylaxis, hexachlorophene showers before surgery, avoiding or minimizing surgical shaving, reducing operative time and length of hospital stay, strict adherence to asepsis, and meticulous surgical technique (Level II-3).[240] Risk factors include advanced age, preexisting illness, diabetes mellitus, obesity, length of preoperative hospitalization, abdominal operations, malignancy, other sites of infection remote from the surgical incision, malnutrition, and cigarette smoking.[241] In one study of high-risk patients, delayed primary closure (postop day 4) using the vertical mattress technique and nonabsorbable sutures reduced the incidence of postoperative surgical wound infections from 23.3% to 2.1%.[242] Finally, the incidence of wound infection from contamination by vectors can be reduced by careful hand-washing techniques and the use of gloves for surgical dressing changes. To reduce the risks of contamination of fresh surgical incisions, we have adopted the practice of morning wound care by individuals other than the operative team of the day.

Decubital Care

Decubitus ulcers are pressure sores that develop as a result of tissue ischemia due to continual pressure on the skin. The soft tissues are compressed between two hard surfaces: an underlying bony structure inside the body, and a bed or chair outside the body. This causes occlusion of tissue capillary perfusion, leading to ischemia and necrosis.[243,244] With the body in the reclining position, the greatest pressures are exerted over the sacrum and the heels.[245,246] In the sitting position, pressure is concentrated over the ischial tuberosities; when lying on the side, pressure is greatest over the trochanter of the femur. Elevation of the head above 30° increases pressure to the sacrum. Normally, capillary perfusion pressure is approximately 30 mmHg.[246] Prolonged pressure greater than the vascular perfusion pressure may lead to pressure sores. There is an inverse relationship between amount of pressure and time needed to cause damage. Pressures on soft tissues above 45–50 mmHg are likely to cause reversible damage, whereas pressure on soft tissues greater than 70 mmHg applied for 2 or more hours leads to irreversible tissue damage (Level II-2).[247]

Patients at risk for the development of decubitus ulcers are those with decreased mobility, most commonly spinal injury and orthopedic patients.[243,244] Individuals with impaired microvascular circulation, such as those with diabetes and peripheral vascular disease, are more susceptible to the development of pressures sores.[248] Gynecologic surgery patients are also at risk, and careful positioning of patients during surgery to avoid pressure points is important to reduce the risks, which are further aggravated postoperatively by altered levels of consciousness and prolonged immobility. Tissue integrity and wound healing may also be enhanced by optimum nutrition, especially protein, ascorbic acid, and zinc replacement, maximizing tissue perfusion and avoidance of anemia.[249,250] Hypotension reduces tissue perfusion and lowers the pressure necessary to occlude capillary blood flow.

Prevention is aimed at the four etiologic factors involved in the development of pressure sores: (1) *shear forces*, (2) *friction*, (3) *moisture*, and (4) *compressive forces*.[248] Various pressure-reduction devices such as foam, cushions, and special beds allow diffusion of pressure to surrounding tissue areas, rather than concentrating force over small, susceptible areas. Sheep skin and egg-crate mattresses are not very effective. Control of exposure time to pressure forces is achieved by turning patients in bed at least every 2 hours on a regular mattress.[245] Repositioning without sliding or rubbing, and keeping the patient dry, helps to reduce friction and shear forces, which can predispose to tissue breakdown.[251] Despite these preventive measures, approximately 9.2% of hospitalized patients and up to 35% of critical care patients develop pressure sores.[252,253] Pressure sores are staged or graded according to the depth of tissue destruction (Level II-3):

Stage I: Nonblanchable erythema of intact epidermis. Erythema of skin that does not resolve within 30 minutes of relief of skin pressure.

Stage II: Partial-thickness skin loss involving the epidermis with or without partial dermis involvement. The wound base is painful and free of necrotic tissue.

Stage III: Full-thickness skin loss penetrating through to the full-thickness dermis and involving subcutaneous tissues, but not underlying fascia, muscle layers, joints, or bone. The wound base is a shallow and nonpainful ulcer, and necrosis, exudates, sinus tract formation, and infection may be present.

Stage IV: Full-thickness skin loss with extension into underlying fascia, muscles, joints, or bone. The wound base has a nonpainful, deep crater, necrosis, tissue undermining, sinus tract formation, infection, and exudate may be present.[254]

Pressure sores may be treated by conservative and surgical methods. Stages I and II can usually be managed nonoperatively with pressure relief and cleansing of the ulcerated area. Pressure relief may be best managed by pressure-redistributing/decreasing mattresses such as the Comfortex DeCube®

mattress.[247,255] Localized treatment is aimed at debridement of necrotic areas and relief of infection. As necrotic tissue is usually colonized by skin flora only, debridement with application of a topical antibiotic, such as bacitracin or silver sulfadiazine, is generally adequate to clear local infection. Systemic antibiotics are not recommended unless cellulitis or osteomyelitis is present, as they may slow wound healing and promote resistant bacterial growth. Prompt treatment of these infectious processes is imperative, however, because bacteremia in association with pressure sores carries a 50% mortality rate.[256]

Debridement can be accomplished surgically, mechanically, or chemically with enzymatic preparations. Whirlpools are helpful with large ulcers. The healing process may be accelerated once the ulcer is cleaned with the use of tissue growth factors such as platelet-derived growth factor.[257] In the absence of necrosis and infection, occlusive, semiocclusive, and hydrocolloid wound dressings, including DuoDerm®, Op-Site®, and IntraSite®, may be applied to create a physiologic wound-healing environment. Most ischial ulcers have a deep underlying cavity and small outlet and are best managed with saline gauze packing to allow healing from the bottom up; an abscess cavity may form if the outlet closes first. Surgery is the preferred treatment for Stages III and IV pressure sores over 2 cm in size (Level II-2).[248,257] After the ulcer bed is clean and free of infection or necrosis, simple excision of devitalized tissue followed by closure, with or without the use of skin grafts, muscle flaps, or myocutaneous grafts, may be used.

Stomal Care

The surgical management of gynecologic malignancies frequently requires intestinal surgery. Rubin et al., in a retrospective review, found that 10.4% of all laparotomies on a busy gynecologic oncology service were complicated by intestinal surgery.[258] In a 1992 summary of complications of colostomy performed on patients with gynecologic cancer, Hoffman et al. found a 6.3% incidence of early complications and a 15.3% incidence of delayed complications that compared favorably with the 8–27% complication rate reported in the surgical literature (Level II-2).[259] Common stomal complications are summarized in Table 9.10. Peristomal skin irritation, the most common early stomal complication, affects approximately 42.1% of all ostomies,[260] occurs three times more frequently in ostomies created at unmarked sites, and is usually the result of improper site selection, suboptimum stomal construction, or inadequate peristomal skin protection.[260,261] Management directed to the specific etiology includes avoidance of irritants and adhesive products, topical treatment of yeast and other infections, steroidal creams, control of diarrhea, and avoidance of trauma.[261] Stomas that are flushed or retracted, on soft abdomens, or have deep peristomal creasing are particularly difficult management problems and may cause significant emotional distress and social incapacitation. Treatment options include the creation of convexity using belts, inserts, or faceplates, and custom-made abdominal supports.

Surgical revision is sometimes accomplished by stomal mobilization and

TABLE 9.10. Peristomal and Stomal Complications (Level II-3)[258-262]

Early Complications	Late Complications	Dermatologic Complications
Bleeding	Prolapse/parastomal	Caput Medusae
Necrosis	herniation	Allergic dermatitis
Mucocutaneous separation	Stenosis	Irritant dermatitis
Ostomy wound infection	Retraction	Folliculitis
Melanosis coli	Tumor involvement	Hyperplastic (pseudo-
Partial stomal obstruction	Site choice problems	verrucos) lesions
Peritonitis/sepsis		Infectious
		Candida
		Bacterial
		Mucosal transplantation
		Preexisting dermatoses
		Dermatomyositis
		Psoriasis
		Pemphigus
		Mycosis fungoides

advancing the loop of bowel so that a stoma can be created without tension.[262] More frequently, laparotomy with additional intestinal resection is required. In a series of 123 patients undergoing 156 colostomy revisions, Allen-Mersh and colleagues[262] achieved a 63% success rate after one or more attempts. However, because a high failure rate was anticipated, morbidly obese and "frail" patients were excluded (Level II-2). Ileostomies and ileal and jejunal conduits have higher complication rates than colostomies or transverse colon conduits; ostomies constructed in the course of resection of gynecologic pelvic malignancies have also been associated with higher complication rates.[260]

Our patients frequently have comorbid conditions that increase the risks for peristomal complications; therefore, the gynecologic surgeon must be especially attuned to the construction and management of intestinal stomas, as prevention is clearly preferable to repair (Table 9.11). Prior to surgery, ostomy site selection and patient education should be performed by a trained enterostomal nurse. Within the context of the individual's psychosocial needs, dietary restrictions, and physical limitations, thorough perioperative counseling regarding stomal care improves adjustment to enterostomal lifestyle changes. Skin site problems are reduced by careful preoperative site selection, delineating skin folds and pannus creases with the patient in various positions. Other surgical options include use of turmbull ostomies for additional mesenteric length, transverse colon conduits in heavily radiated patients, and placement of the colostomy and mucous fistula at separate skin sites. Seromuscular to fascial tacking sutures may increase local infection rates and fistula formation (II-3).[260]

TABLE 9.11. Guidelines for Stomal Construction (Level II-3)[258–262]

Preoperative counseling by a trained enterostomal nurse
Assess the abdominal wall in supine, sitting, and standing positions
Avoid skin folds, scars, belt lines, bony protuberances, and incisions
Place all stomas through the rectus muscle
Avoid fecal spillage into the peristomal space
Stomas should be placed without tension
Adequately mobilize intestinal segment with mesenteric blood supply
Avoid trimming peristomal fat and epiploic appendages
Mature stomas primarily using mucosubcutaneous closures
Apply peristomal protection

SPECIAL MANAGEMENT CONSIDERATIONS IN THE HIGH-RISK SURGICAL PATIENT

Early recognition of potentially life-threatening complications such as hemorrhage, intestinal perforation, or sepsis reduces morbidity and mortality. In physiologically compromised patients, critical care units capable of intensive hemodynamic monitoring and cardiorespiratory support have dramatically improved survival.

Surgical Complications

Perioperative Bleeding and Blood Component Therapy Perioperative bleeding requiring transfusion complicates approximately 8% of vaginal hysterectomies and 15% of abdominal hysterectomies for benign disease. When radical abdominal hysterectomy and pelvic exenterative procedures are performed, the average blood loss is 1,500 and 3,000 cc, respectively.[263] It has been estimated that about 60% of all blood transfused in the United States is given to surgical patients.[264] Because oxygen-carrying capacity is met in most healthy women by a hemoglobin of 7 g/dl, the concept of empiric transfusion at hemoglobin levels of 8, 9, or 10 mg/dl is no longer justifiable.[265] Loss of approximately 20% of blood volume is equivalent to a 1,500 cc blood loss in a 70 kg individual and is not associated with a significant reduction in oxygen-carrying capacity or ventricular filling pressures when appropriate crystalloid resuscitation is provided. In the absence of preexisting coagulation defects, duration of surgery (>3 hours), pelvic malignancy with associated extensive dissection, and surgical expertise are the most important factors that affect blood loss. Most healthy gynecologic patients require a preoperative type and screen only, as crossmatching in the absence of antibodies can be completed in less than an hour in most hospitals. Preoperative crossmatch is routine, however, for patients with significant cardiopulmonary disease, preexisting anemia, or when extensive abdominal or pelvic dissection is anticipated (Level III).

Blood component therapy specific for the component needed has replaced transfusion with whole blood as the standard of care. Adverse effects of the transfusion of blood products include infection, alloimmunization, and transfusion reaction.[265] An acute hemolytic reaction occurs in 1 per 6,000 units transfused and is associated with a 1 : 17 mortality rate, or 1 in 100,000 units.[266] Prior to blood product transfusion, correct identification of each unit of blood and the patient receiving the product should be checked by two trained personnel. All blood products should be administered through filtered lines with normal (9.0%) saline without electrolyte or drug additives. Other crystalloid solutions should be avoided because of the risks of hemolysis, agglutination, and/or clotting.[265]

Warming is indicated when the volume infused exceeds 50 ml/kg/hr to prevent cardiac-induced hypothermia, and in the presence of cold agglutinin disease, using an in-line blood warmer. Packed RBCs have a volume of 200–250 ml, a hematocrit of 70%, and combined with crystalloid therapy for volume expansion, are the component of choice for hemorrhagic shock. Whole blood or packed RBCs with fresh frozen plasma (FFP) in a 4 : 1 ratio are appropriate when blood loss exceeds 25% of the blood volume. Platelet transfusions are indicated in the presence of severe thrombocytopenia, platelet dysfunction, and may be indicated after massive transfusion (10 U/24 hr in a 70 kg individual). One unit of platelet concentrate will usually increase the count of a 70 kg patient by 5,000–10,000/mm.[267] Fresh frozen plasma is indicated for patients with disseminated intravascular coagulation, severe liver disease, massive transfusion, coumadin therapy reversal, and specific clotting disturbances when the specific factor concentrate is not available. FFP transfusion should be based on coagulation studies that generally should be repeated and checked after every 5–10 units of blood transfused. FFP is never indicated for volume expansion, nutritional support, or prophylactically with massive blood transfusion (Level III).[268]

Cryoprecipitate is concentrated FFP in a small volume of 10–15 ml (1 bag per 5 kg in a 70 kg individual). Because cryoprecipitate represents pooled factor components from multiple donors, risk of infection is significantly increased. Cryoprecipitate is reserved for deficiencies in factor VIII, von Willebrand factor, fibrinogen factor XIII, and fibronectin. If disseminated intravascular coagulation is suspected based on massive transfusion and persistence of significant bleeding and oozing, FFP rather than cryoprecipitate is the component of choice.[269]

Gastrointestinal Injury, Paralytic Ileus, and Intestinal Obstruction
Because serosal injuries are rarely documented, it is difficult to document the incidence of laceration injuries encountered in gynecologic surgery. Obese patients have a 2.5-fold greater risk of injury.[270] Other factors that increase risk for injury and for which preoperative bowel preparation is strongly recommended include previous abdominal surgery, pelvic inflammatory disease, endometriosis, and pelvic malignancies.[271] Thermal injuries complicate 1% to 2% of all laparoscopic surgical procedures and are often not recognized until the patient presents with peritonitis 4 to 7 days postoperatively. Management

consists of prompt surgical exploration, wide resection (3–5 cm) of the thermal burn, and reanastomosis whenever feasible (Level II-2).[271]

Intestinal obstruction complicates only about 0.2% of surgical procedures for benign gynecologic conditions. In contrast, nearly half of patients with ovarian malignancies and 3% of patients with other gynecologic cancers experience this complication. Obstruction usually involves the small bowel (77% of cases).[270,272] In the Western world, adhesions following general surgical and gynecological procedures are the most common cause, and precede the obstructive event by an average of 6 to 10 years.[273–276]

Differentiating between paralytic ileus and complete obstruction is critical, as ileus and partial small-bowel obstruction will resolve in approximately 80% of postoperative patients with medical management.[261] However, unrecognized ischemia and strangulation increase risks of peritonitis, perforation, sepsis, and death. Complete history and physical examination are crucial for appropriate decision making (Fig. 9.5). Both conditions are characterized by volume contraction resulting from third spacing into the intestinal lumen. Metabolic alkalosis may result from NG losses and is often associated with respiratory acidosis; metabolic acidosis is an ominous finding indicative of cellular ischemia. Initial management consists of volume resuscitation with isotonic crystalloid solutions, electrolyte and blood product replacement based on laboratory findings, and nutritional support. Radiographic findings consistent with partial or complete obstruction include "bird's peak" luminal narrowing, air-fluid levels, and absence of air in the distal colon. In the absence of recent celiotomy, intraperitoneal free air on upright abdominal films or chest X ray signifies perforation. Broad-spectrum antibiotics should be administered for associated abscess and perioperatively.

Proximal small-bowel obstruction frequently presents with bilious vomiting, upper abdominal and/or generalized abdominal pain, and high-pitched hyperactive bowel sounds. Patients with partial obstruction who are likely to respond to conservative management usually do so within 24 hours of presentation (Level II-2). In one large series, 75% of patients managed conservatively with clinical improvement within 24 hours ultimately avoided surgery, compared with only 5% of patients with no improvement after 48 hours.[276] Laparotomy is indicated in patients who fail to respond after 48 hours of conservative management to prevent ischemia or perforation. As obstruction progresses, NG drainage may become feculent, reminiscent of distal obstruction; a suddenly "quiet" abdomen with fever, leukocytosis, or leukopenia is an omnious finding associated with strangulation or ischemia from mesenteric arterial or venous thrombosis. Surgical management should be conducted in consultation with a general surgical specialist or gynecologic oncologist, and consists of lysis of adhesions, adequate mobilization, isolation of the involved intestinal segment, and resection with primary anastomosis or bypass. Surgical stapling devices shorten operative time and improve blood supply and may reduce risks of anastomotic leaks or strictures.

Large-bowel obstruction is common in the elderly and often results from

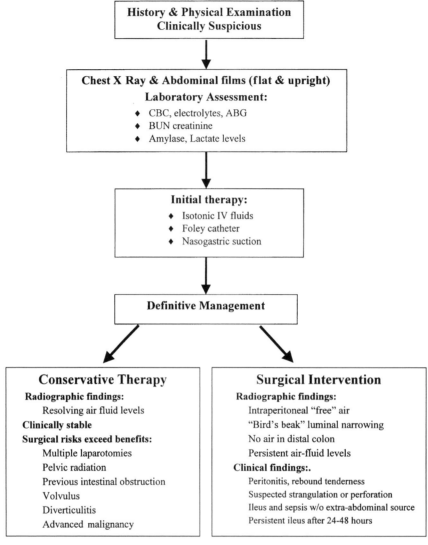

FIGURE 9.5. Intestinal obstruction—diagnosis and management (Level II-2).[271–276]

fecal impaction, diverticular disease, and benign or malignant luminal tumors. Pseudo-obstruction and volvulus can often be managed conservatively with colonoscopy. Clinical findings include generalized abdominal distension, feculent vomiting, and fever with leukocytosis and left shift. Surgical management with resection and primary reanastomosis frequently is impossible because of fecal contamination. Operative management may require extirpation of both intestinal loops and protective colostomy.

Risks for intestinal obstruction, primary or repetitive, are reduced by meticulous operative management. Adhesion formation can be minimized by gentle handling of bowel and peritoneal surfaces, sharp dissection, meticulous hemostasis, careful repositioning of the bowel in an anatomical position, use of the omentum or peritoneum to cover denuded surfaces or to fill pelvic defects, use of delayed absorbable sutures, gentle and limited intestinal packing with moist laparotomy pads, and avoidance of foreign-body contamination, including cotton fibers from sponges and talc from surgical gloves.[271–274]

Medical Conditions Requiring Special Surveillance

Diabetes Mellitus Diabetes mellitus, a group of closely related disorders characterized by insulin insufficiency that results in hyperglycemia, is the most common endocrine disease that the gynecologist is likely to encounter. Over 11 million Americans are affected; of these, approximately half will undergo one or more operations in their lifetime, usually after the age of 50.[277] Clinical manifestations are variable and depend on disease duration and severity. Symptoms at onset include polyuria, polydipsia, and weight loss that, without appropriate intervention, progress to ketoacidosis or nonketotic hyperosmolar syndrome.[278] Longstanding diabetes adversely affects multiple-organ systems, and is characterized by microvascular insufficiency, resulting in the development of cardiovascular disease, diabetic retinopathy, neurological deficits, gastrointestinal disturbances, and peripheral neurovascular impairment that predisposes to lower extremity skin ulcerations, infection, tissue necrosis, and fracture (Level III).[278]

Vascular disease related to diabetes is the single most important risk factor for perioperative morbidity and mortality. Over half of diabetics ultimately succumb to complications of cardiovascular disease.[279] Cardiovascular complications are the leading cause of mortality in diabetic patients, accounting for approximately 30% of perioperative deaths.[280] The rates of postoperative morbidity are highest among patients undergoing coronary artery bypass surgery and patients with severe renal insufficiency, with an increase in average hospitalization stay by 30% to 50%.[281] Although the extent of ischemia and infarction is comparable in patients with and without angina, diabetics have a significantly higher incidence of painless myocardial ischemia perioperatively, increasing the probability of progression to irreversible injury.[282] Hyperglycemia in patients undergoing coronary artery bypass surgery has been reported to significantly reduce the ratio of the arterial partial pressure of oxygen to the inspired oxygen gradient, as well as elevate the alveolar-arterial oxygen gradient to levels consistent with significant pulmonary dysfunction.[283] Nevertheless, with optimal preoperative assessment and perioperative control, patients with diabetes mellitus have similar rates of surgical complications as patients without diabetes.[284] Thus, the surgeon's responsibility prior to elective surgery is to adequately access the patient to determine the extent of organic manifestations, correct existing hyperglycemia, and stabilize any related electrolyte disturbances. This evaluation includes a complete history, physical examination, and laboratory testing including electrolytes, glucose, BUN, creatinine, preoperative cardio-vascular screening proportionate to cardiovascular involvement, and endocrine consultation where appropriate.

The stress response is characterized by metabolic alterations that affect the rate of hepatic glucose production and peripheral glucose disposal. Cortisol and glucagon accelerate hepatic gluconeogenesis, whereas adrenaline stimulates glycogenolysis; increased glucose production coupled with relative insulin resistance results in hyperglycemia.[285] Postoperative hyperglycemia is not indicative of diabetes; surgical stress and its associated glucose load reduces both the number and the affinity of insulin receptors, a possible mechanism for physiologic insulin resistance that accompanies surgical stress.[286] In uncompli-cated cases, insulin resistance is reversible by administration of insulin that, coupled with nutritional supply sufficient to meet metabolic demands, effec-tively preserves body protein and energy stores.[287] Hyperglycemia also lowers serum insulin levels, an effect counterbalanced and exceeded by the glycogenic effects of adrenaline, glucagon, growth hormone, and cortisol.[288] In the absence of insulin, the metabolic effects of these hormones includes glycogenolysis; once glycogen stores are depleted, protein catabolism and lipolysis ensue.[285,289] The consequences of this hyperosmotic load include diuresis, potentially result-ing in hypotension and decreased cellular perfusion, ketoacidosis, and redistri-bution of potassium from within cells to the extracellular space. Insulin ther-apy reverses hyperkalemia by stimulating sodium and potassium exchange via the adenosine triphosphate Na^+–K^+ pump mechanism.[285] Both hyperglycemia and hypoglycemia may induce significant neurological damage, especially in patients at greatest risk.[285,289] Altered mental consciousness, often the most sen-sitive indicator of brain functions, cannot be assessed intraoperatively, when the patient is at greatest risk of hypoxia.[279] Thus, operative management includes adjusting insulin infusion based on the results of frequency blood glucose sam-pling every 2 or 3 hours to keep the serum glucose in the range of 120–250 mg/dl.[285]

Hyperglycemia (>240–250 mg/dl) impairs wound healing by altered leuko-cyte function including impaired phagocytosis, chemotaxis, and ability to kill bacteria, and inhibition of collagen synthesis, fibroblast formation, and neovascularization.[289] Risks of wound infection, gram-negative and staphy-lococcal pneumonia, and gram-negative and beta-hemolytic streptococcal septicemia are increased, probably in association with impaired neutrophil function.[289,290] Thromboembolic complications are common in diabetic patients secondary to increased levels of thromboxane-mediated platelet activation, which are partially reversible with metabolic control as well as with the admin-istration of low-dose aspirin therapy (Level II-2).[291]

When surgery is elective, diabetes should be optimally controlled prior to the operative procedure. Elevated glycosylated hemoglobin levels have been found to accurately reflect the level of diabetic control within the antecedent 2 or 3 months (Level II-2).[292] Long-acting oral glycosemic agents should be discon-tinued at least 36 hours prior to surgery; shorter-acting agents such as glyburide

(Micronase®, Diabeta®) and glipizide (Glucotrol®) should be withheld the day prior to surgery to reduce the risks of hypoglycemia (Level II-3).[285]

Although it is generally agreed that perioperative hyperglycemia should be prevented, the ideal method to accomplish this is controversial. Traditionally, on the morning prior to surgery, approximately one-half to two-thirds of the usual insulin dose is administered in combination with low-dose carbohydrate infusion such as D5W at 100–125 cc/hr to prevent hypoglycemia and ketosis.[293] Alternatively, the patient may be maintained by a low-dose dextrose infusion along with an insulin drip at 1–2 U/hr to maintain a serum glucose level in the 120–180 mg/dl range,[281,293,294] followed postoperatively by subcutaneous insulin titrated to severity. As serum glucose determinations are only reflective of glucose levels at the time they are drawn, it is important that levels be checked frequently and acted upon promptly. Severe hyperglycemia with associated ketosis, metabolic acidosis, and hyperkalemia is managed by aggressive volume replacement, intravenous insulin infusion, and laboratory-directed replacement of potassium and phosphate. In complicated patients requiring prolonged nutritional support, continuous insulin infusion may be administered in parenteral nutrition. In insulin-dependent diabetes, as soon as oral nutritional replacement is tolerated, enteric feeding should be supplemented by the combination of regular and intermediately acting insulin, which peak in activity 3 and 10 hours, respectively, after administration.[288]

Cardiac Insufficiency   While the reported incidence of perioperative myocardial infarction (MI) varies widely, ranging from <1% following minor low-risk procedures to >10% with vascular procedures,[53] the risk of fatality, 36–70%, emphasizes the seriousness of this complication.[295] Although it is recommended that patients over 70 years of age or with a history of cardiovascular disease be followed postoperatively with serial electrocardiograms (ECG), the ECG is an insensitive and nonspecific tool for the diagnosis of perioperative MI. Over half of perioperative MIs are diagnosed on or before the third postoperative day. Measurement of MB creatine kinase has been the marker of choice for the detection of cardiac ischemia, although false positives may result from skeletal muscle injury. Serum CK-MB bands in excess of 5% of the serum CK, or greater than 50 IU per liter, are considered diagnostic of perioperative myocardial infarction.[296] An elevated CK-MB, 6–9 hours postoperatively, which remains elevated, with one or more confirmatory studies (new Q waves on ECG and/or a positive myocardial pyrophosphate scan), enhances the predictive value of serum CK-MB.[297] The serum level of cardiac troponin I, a regulatory protein produced only within the myocardium, is a highly sensitive (100%) and specific (99%) marker for myocardial infarction that avoids the high false positives (19%) associated with CK-MB measurement (Level I).[295]

The ACC/AHA task force in 1990 published guidelines of recommended indications for diagnostic procedures and therapeutic interventions, including triage and transport, ECG monitoring, invasive hemodynamic monitoring, antiarrhythmic therapy, and thrombolytic therapy, which are based on classification of risk.[298] In uncomplicated myocardial infarction, basic support includes oxygen therapy to alleviate hypoxemia; nitroglycerin to reduce preload and improve epicardial blood flow; morphine sulfate to alleviate pain, reduce preload and afterload, and decrease myocardial oxygen demand; and recognition and management of arrhythmias. Invasive hemodynamic monitoring including balloon flotation right heart catheters and/or arterial pressure catheters are indicated for patients with hemodynamic instability manifested by hypotension (systolic <80 mmHg) requiring presser agents, cardiogenic shock, pulmonary edema, and severe or progressive congestive heart failure (Level II-2).[298] The case fatality rate for acute MI in patients receiving thrombolytic therapy is 10–15%, significantly reduced from the 30–50% mortality rate from perioperative MI.[53] However, because surgery or trauma within 2 weeks are relative contraindications to thromboembolytic therapy,[298] coronary angioplasty, which has been associated with success rates comparable to thrombolysis, may be a viable alternative in the high-risk postoperative patient.[53]

Congestive heart failure (CHF) following surgery is a particularly ominous finding. In a series of 15 patients developing postoperative CHF, 5 patients (33%) developed pulmonary edema, including 4 patients (26.7%) with concomitant myocardial ischemia; 7 patients (46.7%) had evidence of postoperative myocardial ischemia. Risk factors associated with postoperative CHF included diabetes mellitus, age over 70 years, less than 500 ml intake or urine output in the 24 hours preceding surgery, and preexisting cardiac disease (Level II-2).[299]

Pulmonary Complications The most common respiratory complications following hospitalization or surgery are nosocomial infections of the respiratory tract, affecting 0.5–5.0% of all hospitalized patients (Level II-2).[300] There appears to be no significant difference in the incidence of nosocomial pneumonia on surgical compared with medical services, approximately 75 to 80 cases per 10,000 patient discharges. Approximately half of hospital-acquired pneumonias are caused by gram-negative organisms.[301] The most common organisms involved in nosocomial pneumonia (12–22%) include *Pseudomonas* sp., *Staphylococcus* sp., *Klebsiella* sp., and *Enterobacter* sp., while the frequencies of other organisms less commonly isolated, including *Serratia* sp., *Candida* sp., *Haemophilus* sp., and *Acinetobacter* sp., are in the order of 4–9% of cases.[301-303] In normal individuals, death associated with gram-negative bacteremia is only 10%, compared with high mortality rates (45–70%) from nosocomial infection.[304]

Hypoventilation in the immediate postoperative period predisposes to the development of atelectasis, which is characterized by collapse of the small airways, resulting in intrapulmonary venous shunting as well as entrapment of bacteria (Level II-2). Atelectasis is the most common cause of postoperative fever within the first 24 hours of surgery. There is no evidence that antibiotic therapy reduces the probability of pneumonia in high-risk patients; rather, empiric antibiotic use predisposes to the development of resistant organisms.[300,305] Uncomplicated atelectasis should be treated with early ambulation and incentive spirometry. Persistent fever and leukocytosis associated with rales and/or rhonchi on clinical examination and with purulent sputum production signify the development of pneumonia, which is confirmed by pulmonary infiltrates on chest X ray.[305]

In hospitalized patients, antibiotic therapy should cover both gram-positive and gram-negative organisms until cultures are available. Choice of antibiotic coverage should depend on a number of high-risk factors including whether the patient is or has recently been intubated, whether aspiration is suspected, whether systemic manifestations of sepsis are present, and whether recent antibiotic therapy has been prescribed.[300,305] In uncomplicated patients, single-agent therapy aimed at pneumococcal or *Haemophilus* sp. is usually sufficient, with therapy continued for approximately a week, and until after clinical and chest X-ray findings have abated. For patients in the ICU, vancomycin in doses of 2–4 g/day is frequently used.[300] When aspiration is suspected, and in patients on mechanical ventilation, coverage is often extended to include anaerobic flora. Aminoglycoside dosing in high-risk patients (patients with significant metabolic derangement, sepsis, or renal failure) should be based on pharmacokinetics as well as peak and trough levels, to prevent either overdosing and associated ototoxicity and nephrotoxicity, or underdosing, resulting in inadequate tissue levels. For patients with normal renal function, doses of gentamicin or tobramicin should be in the 3–5 mg/kg/day range, whereas elderly patients and patients with renal dysfunction require major dose reductions and/or interval spacing between doses. Third-generation penicillins and cephalosporins are preferred in patients with renal insufficiency; however, when *Pseudomonas* is suspected, single-agent therapy with these agents is inadequate because of the rapid development of resistance to these agents when they are used alone.

Risks for all forms of respiratory dysfunction including nosocomial pneumonia are dramatically increased by the presence of pulmonary compromise, as measured by alterations in ventilation, lung water content, perfusion, and resistance to infection.[20] Ventilation may be impaired by structural defects (scoliosis, kyphosis), mechanical uncoupling (effusions, hemorrhage, pneumothorax), muscular weakness (severe malnutrition, ventilatory paralysis, chronic muscular diseases), conditions that increase the work of breathing (abdominal distention from ascites or pregnancy, obesity), imbalance in nutritional supply and demand (thyroid disease, hypoperfusion states), and conditions that restrict lung movement (pulmonary edema, pulmonary fibrosis, adult respiratory distress syndrome [ARDS]).[20] Increased lung water, which may result from alterations in permeability (ARDS, aspiration, sepsis) or hemodynamic alterations (CHF, valvular heart disease), increases the risk of hypoxia resulting from ventilation-perfusion mismatch. Any condition that reduces immune function, such as use of steroids, smoking, or COPD, increases the risk of postoperative infection. Although controversy exists as to the potential risk of H-2 blockers and the development of pneumonia,[154] use of these agents to prevent gastrointestinal hemorrhage continues to be advocated in some intensive care units.[305]

Patients with COPD and hypoxemia/hypercapnia are particularly susceptible to postoperative complications and/or requirements for postoperative ventilatory support (Level II-2).[306,307] Preoperative interventions that reduce infection risks include cessation of smoking, use of bronchodilators, antibiotic coverage when a purulent cough is present, chest physical therapy with postural drainage, use of nebulizers, and control of congestive heart failure.[20] Postoperatively, meticulous attention to pulmonary toilet and incentive spirometry are imperative in these patients.

For many years, ventilation has been routinely quantified using pulmonary function tests and arterial blood gas determinations. Predictors of postoperative atelectasis include a reduction in the maximal breathing capacity to 50% or less of that predicted, FEV_1 of less than 1 liter, forced vital capacity (FVC) of less than 70% of that predicted, and FEV_1/FVC of less than 65% of the predicted value. Low serum oxygenation ($PaO_2 < 60$ mmHg) and carbon dioxide retention ($PaCO_2 > 45$ mmHg) are also predictive of postoperative complications.[308] Despite their routine use, there is little evidence that preoperative spirometry and pulmonary exercise testing improve the sensitivity of history and physical examination in identifying patients at risk for postoperative pneumonia, prolonged hospitalization, or death, with the exception of patients undergoing lung resection.[309,310]

Asthma is a common condition in the Western world, affecting approximately 5% of the population; the incidence appears to be increasing. Asthma is an inflammatory disease characterized by infiltration of the airways with inflammatory cells (Level III). Chronic asthma is also associated with bronchial hyperresponsiveness that is induced by inflammatory cell mediators. The treatment of choice includes the use of inhalant steroids (up to 2 mg/day) and β_2-adrenergic agents. Anticholinergic agents are as effective as β_2-adrenergic agents; there appears to be no therapeutic advantage to combining these agents (Level II-2).[311] In adults, chronic use of inhalant steroids in recommended doses (up to 2 mg/day) does not appear to be associated with adrenal insufficiency. When severe refractory asthma and acute asthmatic exacerbations are encountered, the immediate treatment of choice includes inhalant and intravenous steroids rather than intravenous theophylline, which, although it is a useful adjunctive agent in asthmatics, appears to have no effect on inflammatory cell-mediated hyperresponsiveness.[312]

Renal Disease Acute renal failure is a complication affecting only approximately 2% to 5% of all hospitalized patients. Surgery, however, with its associated hemodynamic and neuroendocrine changes, is second only to decreased renal perfusion as the cause of acute renal failure, and accounts for 18% to 47% of all cases.[313–315] Development of acute renal failure in one case-controlled study was associated with a 6.2 relative odds of death.[316] Although isolated acute renal failure carries a mortality rate of only approximately 10%, multiorgan-system failure is more common; renal failure in association with multisystem-organ failure (three or more organ systems) carries a mortality rate of over 90%.[314] Significant risk factors for the development of postoperative renal failure include hypertension, diabetes mellitus, volume depletion, aminoglycoside use, congestive heart failure, radiocontrast exposure, and septic shock (Level II-3).[316–320]

Acute renal failure may be divided into three main categories: (1) *prerenal azotemia*, which is reversible renal failure caused by decreased effective arterial blood flow to the kidneys; (2) *intrinsic renal disease*, which accounts for approximately 30% of cases of acute renal failure in hospitalized patients; and (3) *obstructive uropathy*, which accounts for approximately 10% of all cases arising on inpatient services. Prerenal azotemia may be caused by induction anesthesia, severe volume overload resulting in CHF and shunting of blood flow away from the kidneys, or sepsis. A serum BUN to creatinine ratio of 40 : 1 is considered indicative of prerenal azotemia, although other conditions such as sepsis, urea absorption from gastrointestinal bleeding, and steroid use may also elevate serum urea nitrogen levels.[315]

The most common cause of intrinsic renal disease, accounting for more than 90% of cases, is *acute tubular necrosis* that usually develops in association with ischemia or nephrotoxin use, and is frequently aggravated by perioperative hypotension.[308] In patients with preexisting hypertension or diabetes, Charlson et al. found that continuous infusion of 300 cc or more per hour of isotonic solutions significantly reduced the risk of postoperative renal insufficiency. Because decompensated CHF was found to be associated with a 36% rate of postoperative renal dysfunction, the authors strongly advised against elective surgery in these patients until cardiac function improved.[317] Renal dysfunction associated with aminoglycoside therapy is related to dose, dosing intervals, duration of therapy, previous use of aminoglycoside therapy, use of other nephrotoxic agents such as intravenous contrast materials, volume status, and host factors. In the adult population, the incidence of nephrotoxicity from a single therapeutic cycle of aminoglycosides is approximately 5–10%, and is the fourth leading cause of renal failure, after hypoperfusion, surgery, and administration of radiographic contrast.[303,309] Another uncommon but life-threatening cause of operative renal failure is malignant hyperthermia and associated disorders. Malignant hyperthermia, an autosomal-dominant pharmacogenetic disorder of the musculoskeletal system instigated by exposure to certain anesthetic agents including isoflurane and succinylcholine, is characterized by rhabdomyolysis, hyperthermia, generalized muscle rigidity, and renal failure. Prior to the use of dantrolene, which has reduced mortality rates to approximately 10%, the mortality from this condition approached 80%.[320]

Causes for obstructive uropathy in the postanesthetic period include the anticholinergic effects of certain anesthetics and antihistamines, which result in acute urinary retention, especially in patients with diabetes mellitus. Ureteral obstruction may result from retroperitoneal hematoma formation and iatrogenic ureteral injury in the course of pelvic surgery. Patients with advanced cervical cancer or a pelvic mass with hydronephrosis and partial ureteral obstruction may have renal dysfunction disproportionate to the serum creatinine; postoperative obstructive diuresis may induce profound hypotension that further predisposes to acute tubular necrosis.

Factors that reduce the risk of acute renal failure in surgical patients include maintaining an adequate volume status preoperatively, intraoperatively, and postoperatively, avoidance of nephrotoxic agents whenever possible, and documenting the existing level of renal function prior to surgery. When contrast studies are essential, hydration with isotonic saline solution before and after the procedure reduces the risk of renal dysfunction in patients at increased risk (Level II-3).[47]

Chronic renal failure is characterized by fluid retention, disturbances in electrolyte function, hematologic and coagulation abnormalities including normocytic, normochromic anemia, and increased bleeding time probably in association with reduced factor VIII in the serum of uremic patients. In a study of over 300 chronic dialysis patients, the overall operative mortality was 3 in 312 procedures (0.96%), with an operative mortality following major surgery of 2%, although a high complication rate, 68%, was also reported.[321] Management consists of performing renal dialysis within 24 hours of surgery and correcting any existing problems of volume overload and/or electrolyte disturbances. Postoperatively, patients are at high risk for fluid overload, arrhythmias, respiratory decompensation, and shunt thrombosis. Analgesic and sedative doses must be decreased to reduce deterioration in respiratory and mental function.

The most common electrolyte disturbance is hyperkalemia, which, in the report by Pinson et al., developed in 19% of all renal failure patients postoperatively. Contributing factors included massive blood transfusion and elevations in preoperative serum potassium levels.[321] Insulin in glucose is more effective than epinephrine or bicarbonate solutions in reducing hyperkalemia;[322] in postoperative patients, however, the most effective management of hyperkalemia is dialysis.[321] When surgery is elective, recombinant human erythropoietin, 500 U/kg, may elevate the hematocrit by as much as 10% within 3 weeks, and may significantly reduce transfusion requirements.[323] Conjugated estrogen therapy results in a prolonged (14-day) improvement in the bleeding time in patients with chronic renal failure, compared with the short-term effects of more commonly used agents including cryoprecipitate or desmopression.[324] Postoperatively, patients on chronic dialysis therapy are also at increased risk for infection, most commonly *Staphylococcus aureus*, followed by *S. epidermidis* and *E. coli*, which partly results from alterations in neutrophil and monocyte function.[325]

Liver Disease   Although there is no evidence that currently used anesthetic agents are direct hepatotoxins, all agents reduce hepatic blood flow, resulting in decreased oxygen uptake by the liver and splanchnic organs.[326] Additionally, other factors associated with surgery including hypotension, blood loss, use of vasoactive drugs, surgical manipulation of abdominal viscera, and hypoxemia reduce hepatic blood flow and contribute to the morbidity associated with preexisting significant hepatobiliary disease.[327] Sedatives, narcotics, and neuromuscular blocking agents must be used with caution in these patients because of reduced metabolic clearance that may result in severe respiratory depression and/or result in requirements for prolonged postoperative ventilation. In addition to increased risk for morbidity and mortality from exacerbated hepatic dysfunction, patients with significant liver failure are at increased risk for bleeding complications resulting from coagulopathies, renal failure, and pulmonary compromise from ascites or coexisting derangement in hemodynamic function. In managing the patient with liver disease, it is imperative that the risks of morbidity be weighed against the potential operative risks; thus, a thorough preoperative assessment, including history, physical examination, and laboratory investigation, including PT, PPT, albumin, total and direct bilirubin, and transaminases, be obtained prior to surgery.

Acute and chronic viral hepatitis, alcoholic liver disease, and cirrhosis are among the most common conditions associated with liver dysfunction. Active viral hepatitis is felt to be a contraindication to elective surgery.[327] However, surgery is well tolerated in chronic persistent hepatitis, which is characterized by mild persistent elevations in serum aminotransferases and does not progress to cirrhosis. In contrast, chronic active hepatitis associated with portal inflammation and marked elevations in serum aminotransferase and bilirubin levels may develop into cirrhosis. Preoperative liver biopsy is usually necessary to determine the level of hepatic injury.[326] Mild elevations in hypothrombinemia can be corrected with one or serial (3-day) injections of vitamin K, 10 mg, intramuscularly.[328,329]

Cirrhosis is an irreversible condition of the liver characterized by parenchymal necrosis, nodular regeneration, and fibrosis. Severe metabolic derangement (hyponatremia, hypoalbuminemia, glucose intolerance, prolonged protime/partial thromboplastin times) may be present. Clinical findings may include weight loss, nausea and vomiting, gynecomastia, and ascites. Although more data are available regarding operative risks for cirrhosis compared with liver disease from other causes, most of the available literature is retrospective, consisting of anecdotal reports or studies with small patient numbers.[326] The best predictor of tolerance to surgery is the Child's Classification (Level II-2).[330–332] In patients with Child's Class A (no evidence of encephalopathy or ascites, a normal serum albumin, and elevations in bilirubin or prothrombin time less than two times the normal values), surgery is usually well tolerated. In patients with Child's Class B or C (ascites, encephalopathy, marked elevations in bilirubin levels and prothrombin time, and hypoalbuminemia), the substantial risks of operative morbidity and mortality must be carefully weighted against the expected benefits of surgery.

Thyroid Disease

Hyperthyroidism   Hyperthyroidism, most commonly secondary to Grave's disease, is a state of increased metabolic rate secondary to increased levels of thyroid hormone. Increased thyroid function can also occur in association with gestational trophoblastic disease as a result of circulating thyroid stimulator secreted by trophoblastic tissue. The effects of surgery and anesthesia on thyroid function are very complex; laboratory evaluation may not completely reflect the thyroid status, as chronic illness or surgery can inhibit the conversion of T4 to T3, with a shift to conversion to reverse T3. Recognition of the hyperthyroid state is imperative and relies on careful clinical assessment as well as laboratory data. Thyroid storm, defined as extreme hyperthyroidism with cardiovascular collapse, can be precipitated by an operative procedure in 10% to 32% of insufficiently treated patients.[159,333,334] Elective surgery should be postponed, awaiting return to the euthyroid state (Level II-3).

Treatment of hyperthyroidism includes medications and/or ablative therapy with radioactive iodine or surgery. Propylthiouracil and methimazole interfere with thyroid hormone production (Level II-3). The starting dose of propylthiouracil is 100 mg po (by mouth) 3 times daily; in severely symptomatic patients, 150–200 mg is recommended.[334] Methimazole is administered in a starting dose of 30 mg/day; up to 90 mg/day may be required. Methimazole is contraindicated in pregnancy. Clinical response to these antithyroid medications takes weeks to months, as their mode of action is on the production of hormone, whereas release of stored hormone is minimally affected. Consequently, thyrotoxic symptoms are managed with beta-blockers, such as propranolol, 10–20 mg/6 hr, increased to up to 320 mg/6 hr, to decrease the heart rate to less than 90 beats/min.[159,333,334] Propranolol can also be given slowly intravenously, 2–10 mg/6 hr.[159] An alternative is diltiazem, a calcium channel blocker, initiated at 30 mg/6 hr, with a gradual increase to up to 360 mg/day, to control symptoms.[334] Iodide is used to treat patients in thyroid storm, patients undergoing emergency surgery, and patients with significant underlying cardiovascular disease; iodide interferes with treatment with radioactive iodine. It is given as SSKI, 1–2 drops BID (twice daily).[51] Finally, dexamethasone, 2 mg IV or po every 6 hours, or hydrocortisone, 100 mg IV or po every 8 hours, which inhibits the release of thyroid hormones and peripheral conversion of T4 to T3, can be used in the management of thyroid storm.[159,333,334] In the postoperative period, antithyroid medications can be withheld for several days until oral intake is possible. If this period is prolonged, these medications may be administered via nasogastric tube.[159]

Hypothyroidism   Decreased thyroid function is associated with decreased metabolic rate, decreased serum T4, and elevated TSH. The diagnosis may be subtle but should be suspected in patients with symptoms of weight gain, cold intolerance, constipation, bradycardia, edema, especially of the hands and the face, and delayed deep tendon reflexes. Underlying cardiac disease may be masked by hypothyroidism (Level II-3).[159,333,334]

Elective surgery should be postponed several months until thyroid medication, levothyroxine, 1.6 mcg/kg/day (usual dose 0.10–0.125 mg/day) renders the patient euthyroid. To avoid the complications of angina and cardiac arrhythmias in elderly patients and patients at greatest risk, therapy should begin at a lower dose, with gradual dose escalation as clinical evidence of myxedema resolves and thyroid function improves (Level II-3).[334,335] The final dose is determined by TSH and T4 levels. Serious illness, including surgery, can precipitate myxedema coma, an illness characterized by hypotension, hypothermia, hyponatremia, hypoglycemia, and respiratory difficulties. Cardiomegaly and pericardial effusion can also develop.[159,333,334] This disease is treated with IV levothyroxine, 200–500 mcg, followed by IV levothyroxine, 100 mcg/day.[334] Following most gynecologic procedures, thyroid medication can be safely withheld until the patient is tolerating oral intake. However, if the recovery interval becomes unduly prolonged, levothyroxine may be given intravenously or via the nasogastric tube.[159]

Pituitary Insufficiency and Hypoparathyroidism Hypopituitarism is a rare disorder that may develop secondary to profound systemic hypotension and infarction of portions of the pituitary gland (Level II-3).[335] Particularly susceptible are lactotropes and gonadotropes, which account for lack of milk production that characterizes Sheehan's syndrome, and subsequent alterations in reproductive function.

The parathyroid gland mediates calcium balance between the intravascular and extravascular spaces and the bone via parathyroid hormone (PTH) and calcitonin. PTH increases serum calcium, mainly by increasing bone resorption and renal reabsorption.[336] Hypercalcemia most commonly is caused by primary hyperparathyroidism secondary to adenoma, hyperplasia, or carcinoma. Malignancies, such as breast cancer that has metastasized to the bone, and ovarian cancer (e.g., small cell carcinoma and clear cell adenocarcinoma), with malignant production of PTH-like peptides, are causes of increased serum calcium that are likely to be encountered on a gynecologic service. Although hypercalcemia is asymptomatic in approximately half of affected patients, preoperative chemistry screening should identify the patient with asymptomatic elevated serum calcium, and appropriate evaluation should establish the diagnosis. When primary hyperparathyroidism is diagnosed, elective surgery should be delayed until treatment is initiated to avoid the risks of hypercalcemic parathyroid crisis, which is characterized by marked dehydration and coma. Unfortunately, the only effective therapy is parathyroidectomy. After correcting calcium, phosphate, magnesium, and electrolyte disturbances in collaboration with endocrine and surgical consultants, the preferred surgical management may involve a multidisciplinary approach, combining parathyroidectomy with the gynecologic procedure under the same anesthetic.

Hypercalcemic patients undergoing nonelective surgery or those with malignant hypercalcemia are managed with measures that increase calcium excretion and decrease bone calcium resorption.[336] Acute management is initiated when serum calcium levels are greater than 12 mg/dl; lower serum levels can usually be managed expectantly. Simple hydration with 1–3 L of isotonic solution will generally effectively lower serum calcium levels. After sufficient hydration, lasix diuresis may also be beneficial; however, urine electrolytes should be obtained prior to diuretic administration if kidney disease is the suspected etiology.

Hypocalcemia can occur as a consequence of renal failure, hypoparathyroidism, abnormal serum magnesium levels, pancreatitis, tumor lysis syndrome, or multiple citrated blood transfusions.[336] Calcium replacement is administered as calcium gluconate 10% in ampules containing 90 mg elemental calcium per 10 mg. Magnesium levels must be evaluated and replaced if indicated in order to correct hypocalcemia. The most common cause of decreased serum calcium is hypoalbuminemia; for every 1 g/dl decrease in albumin, serum calcium will decrease by 0.8 mg/dl.[336] An ionized serum calcium level, or correction for low albumin, should be performed before initiation of calcium repletion.

Surgery in Pregnant Patients   During pregnancy, 0.75% to 2.2% of women undergo surgery for nonobstetrical indications.[337,338] Morbidity and mortality, both maternal and fetal, are dictated by severity of preexisting disease and are not adversely affected by pregnancy. Surgery during the first and second trimesters has been associated with a slight but significant increase in spontaneous abortion.[337] In the largest study published to date, an increase in preterm delivery, low- and very low–birth–weight infants, as well as intrauterine growth retardation, was reported, with no increase in the rate of stillbirths (Level II-2).[337] Fortunately, multiple studies have demonstrated no increase in congenital anomalies associated with operative procedures during pregnancy, even when surgery is performed in the first trimester, which is considered the period of greatest risk because of ongoing organogenesis.[338–340]

Beginning at about 16 weeks estimated gestational age (EGA), perioperative fetal heart rate (FHR) monitoring is indicated, with continuous monitoring of FHR and uterine activity once fetal viability (24 weeks) is reached so that tocolytics may be given where appropriate.[340] Beta-mimetics use is not recommended in patients with cardiovascular disease. Magnesium sulfate, another commonly used tocolytic, has been associated with pulmonary edema as well as with decreasing respiratory effort. In preterm pregnancies (EGA less than 32 weeks), the antiprostaglandin indomethacin can be safely used with little toxicity, but should be avoided in later gestations because of risks of premature closure of the ductus. The loading dose is 60 mg given orally or per rectum, followed by 25–50 mg every 6–8 hours for a total of 24 hours.[341] Prophylactic perioperative hydroxyprogesterone has not been demonstrated to be of any benefit in prevention of fetal wastage.[342] If the adnexa containing the corpus luteum is removed prior to the 10th week of pregnancy, however, hormonal support becomes essential. Progesterone in oil, 100 mg intramuscularly per day, should be given until hormonal production by the corpus luteum is superceded by placental hormonal production, which predominates at approximately 10 weeks gestation.[343] Continuous fetal assessment with heart rate monitoring after 24 weeks is important, as maternal blood pressure, pulse, and oxygen status as determined by pulse oximetry may not reflect uterine perfusion and fetal status.[344] Because fetal physiology is exquisitely sensitive to changes in maternal ventilation and hemodynamic status, changes in fetal heart rate may indicate maternal compromise long before changes in maternal vital signs become apparent.

Surgery in the Elderly Our society is continuing to age. It is estimated that 21% of the U.S. population, approximately 53 million people, are over 55 years of age, and 31.5 million are over 65. By 2050, approximately 21.7% are expected to be over 65 years of age, and women will constitute the majority of this group. Today, there are 19 million women over 65 years of age.[345] About 50% of all cancers are detected in patients within this age group (Level II-2).[346]

Until recently, few reports existed in the literature that provided data regarding the perioperative care or morbidity of surgery in the elderly. Genitourinary cancers, including cancer of the bladder, breast, ovary, cervix, and uterus, are significantly more likely to be diagnosed at advanced stages in older patients.[347] There is an inverse relationship between frequency in gynecologic examinations and Pap smears and advancing age, which supports the premise that inadequate screening among the elderly is a major factor in failure to diagnose gynecological cancers at early, potentially treatable stages.[348,349] The increased side effects of cytotoxic chemotherapy and/or radiation therapy in elderly patients often requires major reductions in dose, which partly accounts for the higher incidence of treatment failures in elderly patients, including those with local disease only.[350,352] Several studies have confirmed that surgery can safely be accomplished, even in the very elderly, although the rate of perioperative morbidity is increased proportionate to age and preexisting health problems.[353–356] With the advent of critical care surveillance, even ultraradical surgery including ovarian debulking, radical hysterectomy, and pelvic exenteration may be safely accomplished with acceptable morbidity in older patients who are in otherwise good health.[357–359]

Nevertheless, blood loss, morbidity, length of hospital stay, and multiorgan failure are complications that are significantly increased with surgery in the elderly. Coronary artery disease, congestive heart failure, and malignancy with its associated immunological suppression and malnutrition, and other preexisting diseases predispose the elderly to more perioperative complications by virtue of organ system dysfunction. Wound complications and skin breakdown are increased in older patients.[360] Recovery in muscle strength including handgrip and respiratory muscle strength is significantly reduced in the elderly and may contribute to the development of atelectasis, pneumonia, and DVTs, which are major contributors to morbidity and mortality in these patients.[361,362] Reduced morbidity and mortality require a thorough preoperative assessment of preexisting medical diseases with appropriate perioperative medical and intensive care consultation.[356]

REFERENCES

1. Hill GL, Douglas, RG, Schroeder D. Metabolic basis for the management of patients undergoing major surgery. *World J Surg* 1993;17:146–153.
2. Gamil M, Fanning A. The first 24 hours after surgery. *Anaesthesia* 1991;46:712–715.

3. Sun H, Iles M, Weissman C. Physiologic variables and fluid resuscitation in the postoperative intensive care unit patient. *Crit Care Med* 1993;21:555–561.

4. Shires GT, Canizaro PC, Lowry SF. Fluid, electrolyte, and nutritional management of the surgical patient. In Schwartz SI, Shires GT, Spencer FC, Storer EH (Eds), *Principles of Surgery*, 4th ed. New York: McGraw-Hill, 1984, pp. 45–80.

5. Shires GT, Canizaro PC. Fluid and electrolyte management of the surgical patient. In Sebastian DC Jr, *Textbook of Surgery*, 14th ed. Philadelphia: WB Saunders Company, 1991, pp. 57–76.

6. O'Shea MH. Fluid and electrolyte management. In Woodley M, Whelan A (Eds), *Manual of Medical Therapeutics*, 27th ed. Boston: Little, Brown, & Company, 1992, pp. 42–61.

7. DeFronzo RA, Thier SO. Pathophysiologic approach to hyponatremia. *Arch Intern Med* 1980;140:897–902.

8. Levi R. Therapies for perioperative hypertension: pharmacodynamic considerations. *Acta Anaesthesiol Scand* 1993;37(S99):16–19.

9. Heuser D, Guggenberger H, Fretschner R. Acute blood pressure increase during the perioperative period. *Am J Cardiol* 1989;63:26C–31C.

10. Aken HV, Hemelrijck JV. The influence of anesthesia on cerebral blood flow and cerebral metabolism: an overview. *Agressologie* 1991;32:303–306.

11. Layon JA. Physiologic effects of anesthesia in the critically ill. In Civetta JM, Taylor RW, Kirby RR (Eds), *Critical Care*. Philadelphia: JB Lippincott, 1988, pp. 145–156.

12. Charlson ME, MacKenzie CR, Gold JP, Ales KL, Topkins M, Shires GT. Intraoperative blood pressure: What patterns identify patients at risk for postoperative complications? *Ann Surg* 1990;212:567–580.

13. Kolansky DM, Cohen LS. Immediate postoperative management. In Frankl WS, Brest AN (Eds), *Valvular Heart Disease: Comprehensive Evaluation and Treatment*. Cardiovascular Clinics, vol. 23, 1992, pp. 277–291.

14. Augustine SD. Hypothermia therapy in the postanesthesia care unit: a review. *J Post Anesth Nurs* 1990;5(4):254–263.

15. Osguthorpe SG. Hypothermia and rewarming alter cardiac surgery. *AACN Clin Issues Crit Care Nurs* 1993;4(2):276–292.

16. Frank SM, Beattle C, Christopherson R, et al. Unintentional hypothermia is associated with postoperative myocardial ischemia. *Anesthesiology* 1993;78:468–476.

17. Danzl DF, Pozos RS. Current concepts: accidental hypothermia. *N Engl J Med* 1994;331:1756–1760.

18. Strandberg AA, Tokics L, Brismar B, Lundquist H, Hedenstierna G. Atelectasis during anaesthesia and in the postoperative period. *Acta Anaesthesiol Scand* 1986;30:154–158.

19. Jones JG, Sapsford DJ, Wheatley RG. Postoperative hypoxaemia: mechanisms and time course. *Anesthesia* 1990;45:566–573.

20. Pett Jr SB, Wernly JA. Respiratory function in surgical patients: perioperative evaluation and management. *Surg Ann* 1988;20:311–329.

21. Meyers JR, Lembeck L, O'Kane, Baue AE. Changes in functional residual capacity of the lung after operation. *Arch Surg* 1975;110:576–583.

22. Hosoda R, Hattori M, Shimada Y. Favorable effects of epidural analgesia on hemodynamics, oxygenation and metabolic variables in the immediate post-anesthetic period. *Acta Anaesthesiol Scand* 1993;37:469–474.

23. Licker M, Suter PM, Krauer F, Rifat NK. Metabolic response to lower abdominal surgery: analgesia by epidural blockade compared with intravenous opiate infusion. *J Anaesthesiol* 1994;11:193–199.

24. Jayr C, Mollie A, Bourgain JL, et al. Postoperative pulmonary complications: general anesthesia with postoperative morphine compared with epidural anesthesia. *Surgery* 1988;104:57–63.

25. Giesecke K, Klingstedt C, Ljungovist O, Hagenfeldt L. The modifying influence of anaesthesia on postoperative protein catabolism. *Br J Anaesthesiol* 1994;72:697–699.

26. Schulze S. Humoral and neural mediators of the systemic response to surgery. *Dan Med Bull* 1993;40:365–377.

27. Salo M. Effects of anaesthesia and surgery on the immune response. *Acta Anaesthiol Scand* 1992;36:201–220.

28. Pullicino EA, Carli F, Poole S, et al. The relationship between the circulating concentrations of interleukin 6 (IL-6), tumor necrosis factor (TNF) and the acute phase response to elective surgery and accidental injury. *Lymphokine Res* 1990;9:231–238.

29. Baigrie RJ, Lamont PM, Kwaitkowski D, Dallman MJ, Morris PJ. Systemic cytokine response after major surgery. *Br J Surg* 1992;79:757–760.

30. Lennard TWJ, Shenton BJ, Borzotta A, et al. The influence of surgical operations on components of the human immune system. *Br J Surg* 1985;72:771–776.

31. Bowling TE. Does disorder of gastrointestinal motility affect food intake in the post-surgical patient? *Proc Nutr Soc* 1994;53:151–157.

32. Clevers GJ, Smout AJ. The natural course of postoperative ileus following abdominal surgery. *Neth J Surg* 1989;41:97–99.

33. Waldhausen JHT, Shaffrey ME, Skenderis II BS, Jones RS, Schirmer BD. Gastrointestinal myoelectric and clinical patterns of recovery after laparotomy. *Ann Surg* 1990;211(6):777–785.

34. Livingston EH, Passaro EP. Review article. Postoperative ileus. *Dig Dis Sci* 1990;35:121–132.

35. Ingram DM, Catchpole BN. Effect of opiates on gastroduodenal motility following surgical operation. *Dig Dis Sci* 1981;26:989–992.

36. Mitchell A, Collin J. Vasopressin effects on the small intestine: a possible factor in paralytic ileus? *Br J Surg* 1985;72:642–465.

37. Condon RE, Cowles V, Ekbom GA, Schulte WJ, Hess G. Effects of halothane, enflurane, and nitrous oxide on colon motility. *Surgery* 1987;101:81–132.

38. Johnson Jr H, Knee-Ioli S, Butler TA, Munoz E, Wise L. Are routine preoperative laboratory screening tests necessary to evaluate ambulatory surgical patients? *Surgery* 1988;104:639–645.

39. Velanovich V. The value of routine laboratory testing in predicting postoperative complications: a multivariate analysis. *Surgery* 1991;109:236–243.

40. Rohrer JM, Michelotti MC, Nahrwold DL. A prospective evaluation of the efficiency of preoperative coagulation testing. *Ann Surg* 1988;208:554–557.

41. Roizen MI. Preoperative evaluation. In Miller RD (Ed), *Anesthesia*, vol. 1, 4th ed. New York: Churchill Livingstone, 1994, pp. 827–882.

42. Mushlin AI, Thornbury JR. Intravenous pyelography: the case against its routine use. *Ann Intern Med* 1989;111:58–70.

43. Simel DL, Matchar DB, Piscitelli JT. Routine intravenous pyelograms before hysterectomy in cases of benign disease: possibly effective, definitely expensive. *Am J Obstet Gynecol* 1988;159:1049–1053.

44. Piscitelli JT, Simel DL, Addison WA. Who should have intravenous pyelograms before hysterectomy for benign disease? *Obstet Gynecol* 1987;69:541–545.

45. Lasser EC, Berry CC, Talner LB, et al. Pretreatment with corticosteroids to alleviate reactions to intravenous contrast material. *N Engl J Med* 1987;317:845–849.

46. Heyman SN, Brezis M, Epstein FH, Spokes K, Silva P, Rosen S. Early renal medullary hypoxic injury from radiocontrast and indomethacin. *Kidney Int* 1991:40:632–642.

47. Solomon R, Werner C, Mann D, D'Elia J, Silva P. Effects of saline, mannitol, and furosemide on acute decreases in renal function induced by radiocontrast agents. *N Engl J Med* 1994;331;1416–1420.

48. Mangano DT. Perioperative cardiac morbidity. *Anesthesiology* 1990;72:153–184.

49. Goldman L, et al. Cardiac risk factors and complications in non-cardiac surgery. *Medicine* 1978;57:357–370.

50. Goldman L, Caldera DL, Nussbaum SR, et al. Multifactorial index of cardiac risk in noncardiac surgical procedures. *N Engl J Med* 1977;297:845–850.

51. Rao TLK, Jacobs KH, El-Etr AA. Reinfarction following anesthesia in patients with myocardial infarction. *Anesthesiology* 1983;59:499–505.

52. Goldman L. Assessment of perioperative cardiac risk (editorials). *N Engl J Med* 1994;330:707–709.

53. Ashton CM. Perioperative myocardial infarction with noncardiac surgery. *Am J Med Sci* 1994;308(1):41–48.

54. Nichols RE. Surgical wound infection. *Am J Med* 1991;91(suppl 3B):54–64.

55. Maki DG. Nosocomial bacteremia: an epidemiologic overview. *Am J Med* 1981;70:719–732.

56. Leaper DJ. Prophylactic and therapeutic role of antibiotics in wound care. *Am J Surg* 1994;167:15–20S.

57. Ehrenkranz NJ, Blackwelder WC, Pfaff SJ, Poppe D, Yerg DE, Kaslow RA. Infections complicating low-risk cesarean sections in community hospitals: efficacy of antimicrobial prophylaxis. *Am J Obstet Gynecol* 1990;162:337–343.

58. Page CP, Bohnen JMA, Fletcher JR, McManus AT, Solomkin JS, Wittmann DH. Antimicrobial prophylaxis for surgical wounds. *Arch Surg* 1993;128:79–88.

59. Ludwig KA, Carlson MA, Condon RE. Prophylactic antibiotics in surgery. *Ann Rev Med* 1993;44:385–393.

60. Culver DH, Horan CT, Gaynes RP, et al. Surgical wound infection rates by wound class, operative procedure, and patient risk index. *Am J Med* 1991;91:152–157S.

61. Drobrzanski S, Lawley DI, McDermott I, Selby M, Ausobsky JR. Research and reports: the impact of guidelines on perioperative antibiotic administration. *J Clin Pharm Therapist* 1991;16:19–24.

62. Dellinger EP, Gross PA, Barrett TL, et al. Quality standard for antimicrobial prophylaxis in surgical patients. *Clin Infect Dis* 1994;18:422–427.

63. Stein GE. Patient costs for prophylaxis and treatment of obstetric and gynecologic surgical infections. *Am J Obstet Gynecol* 1991;164:1377–1380.

64. Orr JW, Sisson PF, Patsner B, et al. Single-dose antibiotic prophylaxis for patients undergoing extended pelvic surgery for gynecologic malignancy. *Am J Obstet Gynecol* 1990;162:718–721.

65. Hagar WD, Rapp RP, Billeter M, Bradley BB. Choice of antibiotic in nonelective cesarean section. *Antimicrob Agents Chemother* 1991;35:1782–1784.

66. Galask RP. The challenge of prophylaxis in cesarean section in the 1990s. *J Reprod Med* 1990;35:1078–1081.

67. Lang R, Shalit I, Segal J, et al. Maternal and fetal serum and tissue levels of ceftriaxone following preoperative prophylaxis in emergency cesarean section. *Chemotherapy* 1993;39:77–81.

68. Chang PL, Newton ER. Predictors of antibiotic prophylactic failure in post-cesarean endometritis. *Obstet Gynecol* 1992;80:117–122.

69. Fejgin MD, Markov S, Goshen S, Segal J, Arbel Y, Lang R. Antibiotic for cesarean section: the case for "true" prophylaxis. *Int J. Gynecol Obstet* 1993;43:257–261.

70. McGregor JA, French JI, Makowski E. Single-dose cefotetan versus multidose cefoxitin for prophylaxis in cesarean section in high-risk patients. *Am J Obstet Gynecol* 1986;154:955–960.

71. Kristensen GB, Beiter E-C, Mather O. Single-dose cefuroxime prophylaxis in non-elective cesarean section. *Acta Obstet Scand* 1990;69:497–500.

72. Von Mandach U, Huch R, Malinverni R, Huch A. Ceftriaxone (single dose) versus cefoxitin (multiple doses): success and failure of antibiotic prophylaxis in 1052 cesarean sections. *J Perinat Med* 1993;21:385–397.

73. Swartz WH. Prophylaxis of minor febrile and major infectious morbidity following hysterectomy. *Obstet Gynecol* 1979;54:284–288.

74. Shapiro M, Munoz A, Takger IB, Schoenbaum SC, Polk BF. Risk factors for infection at the operative site after abdominal or vaginal hysterectomy. *N Engl J Med* 1982;307:1661–1666.

75. Mittendorf R, Aronson MP, Berry RE, et al. Avoiding serious infections associated with abdominal hysterectomy: a meta-analysis of antibiotic prophylaxis. *Am J Obstet Gynecol* 1993;169:1119–1124.

76. Campillo F, Rubio JM, Comparative study of single-dose cefotaxime and multiple doses of cefoxitin and cefazolin as prophylaxis in gynecologic surgery. *Am J Surg* 1992;164:12S–15S.

77. Stiver HG, Binns BO, Brunham RC, et al. Randomized doubleblind comparison of the efficacies, costs and vaginal flora alterations with single dose ceftriaxone and multidose cefazolin prophylaxis in vaginal hysterectomy. *Antimicrob Agents Chemother* 1990;34:1194–1197.

78. Sevin BU, Ramos R, Lichtiger M, Girtanner RE, Averette HE. Antibiotic prevention of infections complicating radical hysterectomy. *Obstet Gynecol* 1984;64:539–545.

79. Cartana J, Cortes J, Yarnoz MC, Rossello JJ. Antibiotic prophylaxis in Wertheim–Meigs surgery. A single dose vs. three doses. *Eur J Gynaecol Oncol* 1994;XV:14–18.

80. Kobamatsu Y, Makinoda S, Yamada T, et al. Evaluation of the improvement of cephems on the prophylaxis of pelvic infection after radical hysterectomy. *Gynecol Obstet Invest* 1991;32:102–106.

81. Graham JE Jr. Infectious morbidity in gynecologic oncology. *J Reprod Med* 1990;35:348–352.

82. Morris WT. Prophylaxis against sepsis in patients undergoing major surgery. *World J Surg* 1993;17:178–183.

83. McDonald PJ, O'Loughlin JA. Prophylactic antibiotics and prevention of surgical sepsis. *Bailliere's Clin Obstet Gynecol* 1993;7:219–236.

84. Sheridan RL, Tompkins RG, Burke JF. Prophylactic antibiotics and their role in the prevention of surgical wound infection. *Adv Surg* 1994;27:43–65.

85. Gorbach SL. Session II: Clinical uses of prophylaxis. Antimicrobial prophylaxis for appendectomy and colorectal surgery. *Rev Infect Dis* 1991;13:S815–820.

86. Menaker GJ. The use of antibiotics in surgical treatment of the colon. *Surg Gynecol Obstet* 1987;164:581–586.

87. Beck DE, Harford FJ, DiPalma JA. Comparison of cleansing methods in preparation for colonic surgery. *Dis Colon Rectum* 1985;28:491–495.

88. Wolff BG, Beart RW Jr, Doxois RR, et al. A new bowel preparation for elective colon and rectal surgery: a prospective, randomized clinical trial. *Arch Surg* 1988;123:895–900.

89. Kaiser AB, Herrington JL Jr, Herrington JL Jr, Mulherin JL Jr, Roach AC, Sawyers JL. Cefoxitin versus erythromycin, neomycin and cefazolin in colorectal operations: importance of the duration of the surgical procedure. *Ann Surg* 1983;198:525–530.

90. Nichols RL. Effects of preoperative neomycin erythromycin intestinal preparation on the incidence of infectious complications following colon surgery. *Ann Surg* 1973:178:453–462.

91. Clarke JS, Condon RE. Bartlett JG, et al. Preoperative oral antibiotics reduce septic complications of colon operations: results of prospective randomized, double-blind clinical study. *Ann Surg* 1977;186:251–259.

92. Stellato TA, Danziger LH, Gordon N, et al. Antibiotics in elective colon surgery. A randomized trial of oral, systemic, and oral/systemic antibiotics for prophylaxis. *Am Surg* 1990;56:251–254.

93. Weaver M, Burdon DW, Youngs DJ, Keighley MRB. Oral neomycin and erythromycin compared with single-dose systemic metronidazole and ceftriaxone prophylaxis in elective colorectal surgery. *Am J Surg* 1986;151:437–442.

94. Coppa GF, Eng K. Factors involved in antibiotic selection in elective colon and rectal surgery. *Surgery* 104;1990:383–386.

95. Schoetz DJ Jr, Roberts PL, Murray JJ, Coller JA, Veidenheimer MC. Addition

of parenteral cefoxitin to regimen of oral antibiotics for elective colorectal operations. A randomized prospective surgery. *Ann Surg* 1990;212:209–212.

96. Portnoy J, Kagan E, Gordon P, Mendelson J. Prophylactic antibiotics in elective colorectal surgery. *Dis Colon Rectum* 1983;26:310–313.

97. Morris DL, Wilson SR, Pain J, et al. A comparison of aztreonam/metronidazole and cefotaxime/metronidazole in elective colorectal surgery: antimicrobial prophylaxis must include gram-positive cover. *J Antimicrob Chemother* 1990;25: 673–678.

98. Dajani AS, Bisno AL, Chung KJ, et al. Prevention of bacterial endocarditis: recommendations by the American Heart Association. *JAMA* 1990;264:2919–2922.

99. Offenbartl K, Bengmark S. Intraabdominal infections and gut origin sepsis. *World J Surg* 1990;14:191–195.

100. Stoutenbeek CHP, van Sacne HKF, Miranda DR, et al. The effect of selective decontamination of the digestive tract on colonization and infection rate in multiple trauma patients. *Intensive Care Med* 1984;10:185–192.

101. Kerver AJH, Rommes JH, Mevissen-Verhage EAE, et al. Colonization and infection in surgical intensive care patients—a prospective study. *Intensive Care Med* 1987;13:347–351.

102. Kerver AJH, Rommes JH, Mevissen-Virhage EAE, et al. Prevention of colonization and infection in critically ill patients: a prospective randomized study. *Crit Care Med* 1988;16:1087–1093.

103. Desai MH, Rutan RL, Heggers, JP, Herndon DN. *Candida* infection with and without nystatin prophylaxis: an 11-year experience with patients with burn injury. *Arch Surg* 1992;127:159–162.

104. Klastersky J, Glauser MP, Schimpff C, Zinner SH, Gaya H, EORTC Antimicrobial Therapy Project Group. Prospective randomized comparison of three antibiotic regimens for empirical therapy for suspected bacteremic infection in febrile granulocytopenic patients. *Antimicrob Agents Chemother* 1986;29:263–270.

105. Deitch EA, Winterton J, Berg R. The gut as a portal of entry for bacteremia: role of protein malnutrition. *Ann Surg* 1987;205:681–691.

106. Deitch EA, Winterton J, Berg R. Effect of starvation, malnutrition, and trauma on the gastrointestinal tract flora and bacterial translocation. *Arch Surg* 1987;122:1019–1024.

107. Cerra FB. Hypermetabolism, organ failure, and metabolic support. *Surgery* 1987;101:1–13.

108. Gallup DG, Nolan TE. The gynecologist and multiple organ failure syndrome (MOFS). *Gynecol Oncol* 1993;48:293–300.

109. Cirisano FD, Greenspoon JS, Stenson R, Farias-Eisner R, Karlan BY, Lagasse JD. The etiology and management of diarrhea in the gynecologic oncology patient. *Gynecol Oncol* 1993;50:45–48.

110. Reinke CM, Messick CR. Update on *Clostridium difficile*–induced colitis, part 1. *Am J Hosp Pharm* 1994;51:1771–1781.

111. Reinke CM, Messick CR. Update on *Clostridium difficile*–induced colitis, part 2. *Am J Hosp Pharm* 1994;51:1892–1901.

112. Gerding DN, Johnson S, Peterson LR, Mulligan ME, Silva Jr J. *Clostrid-*

ium difficile–associated diarrhea and colitis. *Infect Control Hosp Epidemiol* 1995;16:459–477.

113. Anand A, Glatt AE. *Clostridium difficile* infection associated with antineoplastic chemotherapy: a review. *Clin Infect Dis* 1993;17:109–113.

114. Walters BAJ, Roberts RK, Seneviratne E. Contamination and cross infection with *Clostridium difficle* in an intensive care unit. *Aust N Z J Med* 1982;12:255–258.

115. Trudel JL, Deschenes M, Mayrand S, Barkun AN. Toxic megacolon complicating pseudomembranous enterocolitis. *Dis Colon Rectum* 1995;38:1033–1038.

116. Kelly CP, Pothoulakis C, LaMont JT. *Clostridium difficile* colitis (review article). *N Engl J Med* 1994;330:257–262.

117. Bonnar J. Venous thromboembolism and gynecologic surgery. *Clin Obstet Gynecol* 1985;28(2):432–446.

118. Weinmann EE, Salzman EW. Deep-vein thrombosis. *N Engl J Med* 1994;24:1630–1640.

119. Clarke-Pearson DL, DeLong ER, Synan IS, Coleman RE, Creasman WT. Variables associated with postoperative deep venous thrombosis: a prospective study of 411 gynecology patients and creation of a prognostic model. *Obstet Gynecol* 1987;69:146–150.

120. Genton E, Turpie AGG. Venous thromboembolism associated with gynecologic surgery. *Clin Obstet Gynecol* 1980;23(1):209–241.

121. Walsh JJ, Bonnar J, Wright FW. A study of pulmonary embolism and deep vein thrombosis after major gynecological surgery using labeled fibrinogen, phlebography and lung scanning. *J Obstet Gynaecol Br Commonw* 1974;81:311–316.

122. Nicolaides A, Kakkar V, Field ES, Renney J. The origin of deep vein thrombosis: a venographic study. *Br J Radiol* 1971;44:653–663.

123. Kakkar VV, Howe CT, Flang C, Clarke MB. Natural history of postoperative deep-venous thrombosis. *Lancet* 1969;2:230–232.

124. Ballard RM, Bradley-Watson PJ, Johnston FD, Kenney A, et al. Low doses of subcutaneous heparin in the prevention of deep vein thrombosis after gynaecological surgery. *J Obstet Gynaecol Br Commonw* 1973;80:469–663.

125. Clayton JK, Anderson JA, McNicol GP. Effect of cigarette smoking on subsequent postoperative thromboembolic disease in gynaecological patients. *Br Med J* 1978;2:402.

126. Kakkar VV. Prevention of fatal pulmonary embolism. *Haemostasis* 1993;23S:42–50.

127. Kakkar VV. An International Multicenter Trial: Prevention of fatal postoperative pulmonary embolism by low doses of heparin. *Lancet* 1975;2:45–51.

128. Ginsberg JS. Management of venous thromboembolism (review). *N Engl J Med* 1996;335:1816–1828.

129. Carter CJ, Kelton JG, Jirsh J, Cerskus A, Santos AV, Gent M. The relationship between the hemorrhagic and antithrombotic properties of low molecular weight heparin in rabbits. *Blood* 1982;59:1239–1245.

130. Salzman EW, Rosenberg RD, Smith MH, Lindon JN, Favreau L. Effect of heparin and heparin fractions on platelet aggregation. *J Clin Invest* 1980;65:64–73.

131. Kakkar VV, Cohen AT, Edmonson RA, Phillips MJ, et al. Low molecular weight

versus standard heparin for prevention of venous thromboembolism after major abdominal surgery. *Lancet* 1993;341:259–265.

132. Weitz JI. Low-molecular-weight heparins (review). *N Engl J Med* 1997;37(10): 688–698.

133. Multicenter Trial Committee. Dihydroergotamine-heparin prophylaxis of postoperative deep vein thrombosis: a multicenter trial. *JAMA* 1984;251:2960–2966.

134. Poller L, McKernan A, Thomson JM, Elstein M, Hirsch PJ, Jones JB. Fixed minidose warfarin: a new approach to prophylaxis against venous thrombosis after major surgery. *Br Med J* 1987;295:1309–1312.

135. Turner GM, Cole SE, Brooks JH. The efficacy of graduated compression stockings in the prevention of deep vein thrombosis after major gynaecological surgery. *Br J Obstet Gynaecol* 1984;91:588–591.

136. Clarke-Pearson DL, Synan IS, Hinshaw WM, Coleman RE, Creasman WT. Prevention of postoperative venous thromboembolism by external pneumatic calf compression in patients with gynecologic malignancy. *Obstet Gynecol* 1984;63:92–98.

137. Clarke-Pearson DL, Synan IS, Dodge R, Soper JT, Berchuck A, Coleman RE. A randomized trial of low-dose heparin and intermittent pneumatic calf compression for the prevention of deep venous thrombosis after gynecologic oncology surgery. *Am J Obstet Gynecol* 1993;168:1146–1154.

138. Consensus Conference. Prevention of venous thrombosis and pulmonary embolism. *JAMA* 1986;256(6):744–749.

139. Clarke-Pearson DL, DeLong E, Synan IS, Soper JT, Creasman WT, Coleman RE. A controlled trial of two low-dose heparin regimens for the prevention of postoperative deep vein thrombosis. *Obstet Gynecol* 1990;75:684–689.

140. Wille-Jorgensen, Lausen I, Jorgensen LN. Is there a need for long-term thromboprophylaxis following general surgery? *Haemostasis* 1993;23(S1):10–14.

141. vanOoijen B. Subcutaneous heparin and postoperative wound hematomas. *Arch Surg* 1986;121:937–940.

142. Oster G, Tuden RL, Colditz GA. Prevention of venous thromboembolism after general surgery: cost-effectiveness analysis of alternative approaches to prophylaxis. *Am J Med* 1987;82:889–899.

143. Samama M, Bernard P, Bonnardot JP, Combe-Tamzali S, Lanson Y, Tissot E. Low molecular weight heparin compared with unfractionated heparin in prevention of postoperative thrombosis. *Br J Surg* 1988;75:128–131.

144. Sasahara AA, Koppenhagen, Haring R, Welzel D, Wolf H. Low molecular weight heparin plus dihydroergotamine for prophylaxis of postoperative deep vein thrombosis. *Br J Surg* 1986;73(9):697–700.

145. Abramowicz M, et al. Dihydroergotamine-heparin to prevent postoperative deep vein thrombosis. *The Medical Letter on Drugs and Therapeutics* 1985;27(688): 45–46.

145b. Gould MK, Dembitzer AD, Sanders GD, Garber AM. Low molecular weight heparins compared with unfractionated heparin for treatment of acute deep venus thrombosis: A cost-effectiveness analysis *Ann Int Med* 1999;130:789–799.

145c. Rodger M, Bredeson C, Wells PS, Beck J, Kearns B, Haebsch LB. Cost effectiveness of low molecular weight heparin and unfractionated heparin in treatment at deep venous thrombosis. *CMAJ* 1998;159:931–938.

145d. Fishman A, Altaras M, Klein Z, Aviram R, Byeth Y. Low molecular weight heparin (Enoxaparin) as an alternative treatment of acute deep venous thrombosis in gynecologic oncology patients. *Eur J Gynaecol Oncol* 1996;17:365–367.

145e. Bergqvist D, Lindgren B, Matzseh T. Comparison at cost in preventing postoperative deep venous thrombosis with either unfractionated or low molecular weight heparin. *Br J Surg* 1996;83:1548–1552.

146. Salvian AJ, Baker JD. Effects of intermittent pneumatic calf compression in normal and postphlebitic legs. *J Cardiovasc Surg* 1988;29:37–41.

147. Schwarz RE, Marrero AM, Conlon KC, Burt M. Inferior vena cava filters in cancer patients: Introduction and outcome. *J Clin Oncol* 1996;14(2):652–657.

148. Zinner MJ, Zuidema GD, Smith PL, Mignosa M. The prevention of upper gastrointestinal tract bleeding in patients in an intensive care unit. *Surg Gynecol Obstet* 1981;153:214–220.

149. Priebe HJ, Skillman JJ, Bushness LS, Long PC, Silen W. Antacid versus cimetidine in preventing acute gastrointestinal bleeding: a randomized trial in 75 critically ill patients. *N Engl J Med* 1980;302:426–430.

150. Ruddell WSJ, Axon ATR, Findaly JM, Bartholomew BA, Hill MJ. Effect of cimetidine on the gastric bacterial flora. *Lancet* 1980;1:672–674.

151. Donowitz LG, Page MC, Mileut BL, Guenthner SH. Alteration of normal gastric flora in critical care patients receiving antacid and cimetidine therapy. *Infect Control* 1986;7:23–26.

152. Horan TC, White JW, Jarvis WR, et al. Nosocomial infection surveillance, 1984. *MMWR CDC Surveill Summ* 1986;35(1):17SS–29SS.

153. Samloff IM, O'Dell C. Inhibition of peptic activity by sucralfate. *Am J Med* 1985;79S–2C:15–18.

154. Drisk MR, Craven DE, Celli BR, et al. Nosocomial pneumonia in intubated patients given sucralfate as compared with antacids or histamine type 2 blockers. *N Engl J Med* 1987;317:1376–1382.

155. Axelrod L. Glucocorticoid therapy. *Medicine* 1976;55:39–65.

156. Graber AL, et al. Natural history of pituitary-adrenal recovery following long-term suppression with corticosteroids. *J Clin Endocrinol Metab* 1965;25:11–16.

157. Kehlet H, Binder C. Value of ACTH test in assessing HPA function in glucocorticoid-treated patients. *Br Med J* 1973;1:147–149.

158. Salem M, Tainsh RE, Bromberg J, Loriaux DL, Chernow B. Perioperative glucocorticoid coverage: a reassessment 42 years after emergence of a problem. *Ann Surg* 1994;219(4):416–425.

159. Goldmann DR. Perioperative endocrinologic problems. In Merli GJ, Weitz HH (Eds), *Medical Management of the Surgical Patient*. Philadelphia: WB Saunders Company, 1992, pp. 227–245.

160. Sonnendecker EWW, Guidossi F, Margolius KA. Splenectomy during primary maximal cytoreductive surgery for epithelial ovarian cancer. *Gynecol Oncol* 1989;35:301–306.

161. Morris M, Gershenson DM, Burke TW, Wharton JT, Copeland LJ, Rutledge FN.

Splenectomy in gynecologic oncology: indications, complications, and technique. *Gynecol Oncol* 1991;43:118–122.

162. Feroe DD, Augustine SD. Hypothermia in the PACU. *Crit Care Nurs Clin N Am* 1991;3(1):135–144.

163. Orr JW Jr, Holloway RW, Orr PF. Postoperative care of the gynecologic patient. In Copeland LJ, Jarrell JF, McGregor JA (Eds), *Textbook of Gynecology*. Philadelphia: WB Saunders Company, 1992, pp. 670–694.

164. Kruse JA, Carlson RW. Rapid correction of hypokalemia using concentrated intravenous potassium chloride infusions. *Arch Intern Med* 1990;150:613–617.

165. Kunis CL, Lowenstein J. The emergency treatment of hyperkalemia. *Med Clin N Am* 1981;65:165–175.

166. Allon M, Copkney C. Albuterol and insulin for treatment of hyperkalemia in hemodialysis patients. *Kidney Int* 1990;38:869–872.

167. Lillemoe KD, Romolo JL, Hamilton SR, Pennington LR, Burdick JF, Williams GM. Intestinal necrosis due to sodium polystyrene (Kayexalate) in sorbitol enemas: clinical and experimental support for the hypothesis. *Surgery* 1987;101:267–272.

168. Mullen JL, Buzby GP, Matthews DC, Smale BF, Rosato EF. Reduction of operative morbidity and mortality by combined preoperative and postoperative nutritional support. *Ann Surg* 1980;192:604–613.

169. Massad LS, Vogler G, Herzog TJ, Mutch DG. Correlates of length of stay in gynecologic oncology patients undergoing inpatient surgery. *Gynecol Oncol* 1993;51:214–218.

170. Campos ACL, Meguid MM. A critical appraisal of the usefulness of perioperative nutritional support. *Am J Clin Nutr* 1992;55:117–130.

171. Veterans Affairs Total Parenteral Nutrition Cooperative Study Group. Perioperative total parenteral nutrition in surgical patients. *N Engl J Med* 1991;325: 525–532.

172. Grant JP (Ed). *Handbook of Total Parenteral Nutrition*, 2nd ed. Philadelphia, WB Saunders Company, 1992, pp. 15–47.

173. Baue AE. Nutrition and metabolism in sepsis and multisystem organ failure. *Surg Clin N Am* 1991;71:549–565.

174. Vinnars E, Hammarqvist F, von der Decken A, Wernerman J. Role of glutamine and its analogs in posttraumatic muscle protein and amino acid metabolism. *J Parent Enteral Nutrition* 1990;14:125S–129S.

175. Kemper M, Weissman C, Hyman AI. Caloric requirements and supply in critically ill surgical patients. *Crit Care Med* 1992;20:344–348.

176. Schlichtig R, Ayres SM. Nutritional assessment of the critically ill. In *Nutritional Support of the Critically Ill*. Chicago: Year Book Medical Publishers, 1988, pp. 75–95.

177. Willatts SM. *Br J Anaesthesiol* 1986;58:201–222.

178. AMA Department of Foods and Nutrition. Guidelines for essential trace element preparations for parenteral use. *JAMA* 1979;241:2051–2054.

179. Bozzetti F, Terno G, Camerini E, Baticci F, Scarpa D, Pupa A. Pathogenesis and predictability of central venous catheter sepsis. *Surgery* 1982;91:383–389.

180. Bjornson HS, Colley R, Bower RH, Duty VP, Schwartz-Fulton JT, Fischer JE. Association between microorganism growth at the catheter insertion site and colonization of the catheter in patients receiving total parenteral nutrition. *Surgery* 1982;92:720–727.

181. Pemberton B, Lyman B, Lander V, Covinsky J. Sepsis from triple- vs. single-lumen catheters during total parenteral nutrition in surgical or critically ill patients. *Arch Surg* 1986;121:591–594.

182. Padberg FT, Ruggiero J, Blackburn GL, Bistrain BR. Central venous catheterization for parenteral nutrition. *Ann Surg* 1981;193:264–270.

183. Haire WD, Lieberman RP. Defining the risks of subclavian-vein catheterization. *N Engl J Med* 1994;331:1769–1770.

184. Bern MM, Lokich JJ, Wallach SR, et al. Very low doses of warfarin can prevent thrombosis in central venous catheters. *Ann Intern Med* 1990;112:423–428.

185. Tschirhart JM, Rao MK. Mechanism and management of persistent withdrawal occlusion. *Am Surg* 1988;54:326–328.

186. Haire WD, Lieberman RP, Lund GB, Edney J, Wieczorek BM. Obstructed central venous catheters: restoring function with a 12-hour infusion with low-dose urokinase. *Cancer* 1990;66:2279–2285.

187. Edwards TW. Optimizing opioid treatment of postoperative pain. *J Pain Symptom Manage* 1990;5:S24.

188. Donovan M, Dillon P, McGuire L. Incidence and characteristics of pain in a sample of medical-surgical inpatients. *Pain* 1987;30:69–78.

189. Hopf HW, Weitz S. Postoperative pain management. *Arch Surg* 1994;129:128–132.

190. Lutz LJ, Lamer TJ. Management of postoperative pain: review of current techniques and methods. *Mayo Clin Proc* 65;1990;584–596.

191. Rose PG, Piver MS, Batista E, Lau T. Patient-controlled analgesia in gynecologic oncology. *J Reprod Med* 1989;34:651–654.

192. Lange MP, Dahn MS, Jacobs LA. Patient-controlled analgesia versus intermittent analgesia dosing. *Heart Lung* 1988;17:495–498.

193. Moss G, Regal ME, Lichtig L. Reducing postoperative pain, narcotis, and length of hospitalization. *Surgery* 1986;99:206–210.

194. Dahl JB, Daugaard JJ, Larsen HV, Mouridsen P, Nielsen TH, Kristofferson E. Patient-controlled analgesia: a controlled trial. *Acta Anaesthesiol Scand* 1987;31:744–747.

195. Rybro L, Schurizek BA, Petersen TK, Wernberg M. Postoperative analgesia and lung function: a comparison of intramuscular with epidural morphine. *Acta Anaesthesiol Scand* 1982;26:514–518.

196. Hjortso NC, Neumann P, Frosig F, et al. A controlled study on the effect of epidural analgesia with local anaesthetics and morphine on morbidity after abdominal surgery. *Acta Anaesthesiol Scand* 1985;29:790–796.

197. Drummond GB, Littlewood DG. Respiratory effects of extradural analgesia after lower abdominal surgery. *Br J Anaesthesiol* 1977;49:999–1004.

198. Cuschieri RJ, Morran CG, Howie JC, McArdle CS. Postoperative pain and

pulmonary complications: comparison of three analgesic regimens. *Br J Surg* 1985;72:495–498.

199. Cullen ML, Staren ED, El-Ganzouri A, et al. Continuous epidural infusion for analgesia after major abdominal operations: a randomized, prospective, double-blind study. *Surgery* 1985;98:718–728.

200. Lysak SZ, Anderson PT, Carithers RA, DeVane GG, Smith ML, Bates GW. Post-operative effects of fentanyl, ketorolac, and piroxicam as analgesics for outpatient laparoscopic procedures. *Obstet Gynecol* 1994;83:270–275.

201. Stouten EM, Armbruster S, Houmes RJ, Prakash O, Erdmann W, Lachmann B. Comparison of ketorolac and morphine for postoperative pain after major surgery. *Acta Anaesthesiol Scand* 1992;36:716–721.

202. Parker RK, Holtmann BH, Smith I, White PF. Use of ketorolac after lower abdominal surgery. *Anesthesiology* 1994;80:6–12.

203. Bradford TH, Robertson K, Norman PF, Meeks GR. Reduction of pain and nausea after laparoscopic sterilization with bupivacaine, metoclopramide, scopolamine, ketorolac, and gastric suctioning. *Obset Gynecol* 1995;85:687–691.

204. Wong HY, Carpenter RL, Kopacz DJ, Fragen RJ, Thompson G, Maneatis TJ, Bynum LJ. A randomized, double-blind evaluation of ketorolac tromethamine for postoperative analgesia in ambulatory surgery patients. *Anesthesiology* 1993;78:6–14.

205. Rogers JEG, Fleming BG, Magintosh KC, Johnston B, Morgan-Hughes JO. Effect of timing of ketorolac administration of patient-controlled opioid use. *Br J Anaesthesiol* 1995;75:15–18.

206. Joslyn AF. Ondansetron, clinical development for postoperative nausea and vomiting: current studies and future directions. *Anaesthesia* 1994;49S:34–37.

207. Kenny GNC. Risk factors for postoperative nausea and vomiting. *Anaesthesia* 1994;49S:6–10.

208. Naylor RJ, Inall FC. The physiology and pharmacology of postoperative nausea and vomiting. *Anaesthesia* 1994;49S:2–5.

209. Watcha MF, White PF. Postoperative nausea and vomiting: its etiology, treatment, and prevention. *Anesthesiology* 1992;77:162–164.

210. Alon E, Himmelseher S. Ondansetron in the treatment of postoperative vomiting: a randomized double-blind comparison with droperidol and metoclopramide. *Anesth Analg* 1992;75:561–565.

211. Anderson R, Krohg K. Pain as a major cause of postoperative nausea. *Can Anaesth Soc J* 1976;23:366–369.

212. Abramson DJ. Charles Penrose and the Penrose drain. *Surg Gynecol Obstet* 1973;136:285–286.

213. Sarr MG, Parikh KJ, Minken SL, et al. Closed-suction versus Penrose drainage after cholecystectomy. *Am J Surg* 1987;153:394–398.

214. Somers RG, Jablon LK, Kaplan MJ, Sandler GL, Rosenblatt NK. The use of closed suction drainage after lumpectomy and axillary node dissection for breast cancer: a prospective randomized trial. *Ann Surg* 1992;215:146–149.

215. Jensen JK, Lucci III JA, DiSaia PJ, Manetta A, Berman M. To drain or not to

drain: a retrospective study of closed-suction drainage following radical hysterectomy with pelvic lymphadenectomy. *Gynecol Oncol* 1993;51:46–49.

216. Petru E, Tamussino K, Lahousen M, Winter R, Pickel H, Haas J. Pelvic and paraaortic lymphocysts after radical surgery because of cervical and ovarian cancer. *Am J Obstet Gynecol* 1989;161:937–941.

217. Choo YC, Wong LC, Wong KP, Ma HK. The management of intractable lymphocyst following radical hysterectomy. *Gynecol Oncol* 1986;24:309–316.

218. Galanduik S, Fazio VW. Postoperative irrigation-suction drainage after pelvic colonic surgery. *Dis Colon Rectum* 1991;34:223–228.

219. Orr JW Jr, Barter JF, Kilgore LC, Soong SJ, Shingleton HM, Hatch KD. Closed suction pelvic drainage after radical pelvic surgical procedures. *Am J Obstet Gynecol* 1986;155:867–871.

220. Cohen RH, Saeed M, Schwab SJ, Perlmutt LM, Dunnick NR. Povidone-iodine sclerosis of pelvic lymphoceles: a prospective study. *Urol Radiol* 1988;10:203–206.

221. Bartzen PJ, Hafferty FW. Pelvic laparotomy without an indwelling catheter: a retrospective review of 949 cases. *Am J Obstet Gynecol* 1987;156:1426–1432.

222. Kingdom JCP, Kitchener HC, MacLean AB. Postoperative urinary tract infection in gynecology: implications for an antibiotic prophylaxis policy. *Obstet Gynecol* 1990;76:636–638.

223. Ireland D, Tacchi D, Bint AJ. Effect of single-dose prophylactic co-trimoxazole on the incidence of gynaecological postoperative urinary tract infection. *Br J Obstet Gynecol* 1982;89:578–580.

224. Burg R, Geigle CF, Faso JM, Theuerkauf Jr FJ. Omission of routine gastric decompression. *Dis Colon Rectum* 1978;21:98–100.

225. Colvin DB, Lee W, Eisenstat TE, Rubin RJ, Salvati EP. The role of nasointestinal intubation in elective colonic surgery. *Dis Colon Rectum* 1986;29(5):295–313.

226. Cheadle WG, Vitale GC, Mackie CR, Cushieri A. Prophylactic postoperative nasogastric decompression: a prospective study of its requirement and the influence of cimetidine in 200 patients. *Ann Surg* 1985;202:361–366.

227. Moss G. Discharge within 24 hours of elective cholecystectomy. *Arch Surg* 1986;121:1159–1161.

228. MacRae HM, Fischer JD, Yakimets WW. Routine omission of nasogastric intubation after gastrointestinal surgery. *Can J Surg* 1992;35:625–628.

229. Bauer JJ, Gelernt IM, Salky BA, Kreel I. Is routine postoperative nasogastric decompression really necessary? *Ann Surg* 1985;202:233–236.

230. Schippers E, Holscher AH, Bollschweiler E, Siewert JR. Return of interdigestive motor complex after abdominal surgery: End of postoperative ileus? *Dig Dis Sci* 1991;36:621–626.

231. Frankel AM, Horowitz GD. Nasoduodenal tubes in short-stay cholecystectomy. *Surg Obstet Gynecol* 1989;168:433–436.

232. Moss G, Regal ME, Lichtig LK. Reducing postoperative pain narcotics and length of hospitalization. *Surgery* 1986;90:206–210.

233. Bickel A, Shtamler B, Mizrahi S. Early oral feeding following removal of naso-

gastric tube in gastrointestinal operations: a randomized prospective study. *Arch Surg* 1992;127:287–289.

234. Horan TC, Gaynes RP, Martone WJ, et al. CDC definitions of nosocomial surgical site infections, 1992: a modification of CDC definitions of surgical wound infections. *Am J Infect Control* 1992;20:271–274.

235. Sudarsky LA, Laschinger JC, Coppa GF, Spencer FC. Improved results from a standardized approach in threatening patients with necrotizing fascitis. *Ann Surg* 1987;206:661–665.

236. Fry DE, Clevenger FW. Reoperation for intra-abdominal abscess. *Surg Clin N Am* 1991;71:159–174.

237. Boyd ME. Postoperative gynecologic infections. *Can J Surg* 1987;30:7–9.

238. Houang ET. Antibiotic prophylaxis in hysterectomy and induced abortion: a review of the evidence. *Drugs* 1991;41:19–37.

239. Crombleholme WR, Ohm-Smith M, Robbie MO, DeKay V, Sweet RL. Ampicillin/sulbactam versus metronidazole-gentamicin in the treatment of soft tissue pelvic infections. *Am J Obstet Gynecol* 1987;156:507–512.

240. Cruse PJE. The epidemiology of surgical infection: a 10-year prospective study of 62,939 wounds. *Surg Clin N Am* 1980;60:27–40.

241. Sawyer RG, Pruett TL. Wound infections. *Surg Clin N Am* 1994;74:519–536.

242. Brown SE, Allen HH, Robins RN. *Am J Obstet Gynecol* 1977;127:713–717.

243. Woolsey RM, McGarry JD. The cause, prevention and treatment of pressure sores. *Neuro Clin* 1991;9(3):797–808.

244. Alvarez OM, Jarczynski E. Pressure ulcers: physical, supportive, and local aspects of management. *Clin Pod Med Surg* 1991;8(4):869–890.

245. Jester J, Weaver V. A report of clinical investigation of various tissue support surfaces used for the prevention, early intervention and management of pressure ulcers. *Ostomy Wound Manage* 1990;19:39.

246. Lindan O, Girbenway RM, Piazza JM. Pressure distribution on the human body. I. Evaluation of lying and sitting positions using a "bed of springs and nails." *Arch Phys Med Rehab* 1965;45:378–385.

247. Landis EM. Microinjection studies of capillary blood pressure in human skin. *Heart* 1930;15:209–228.

248. Kosiak M. Etiology and pathology of ischemic ulcers. *Archiv Phys Med Rehab* 1959;40:62–69.

249. Taylor TV, Rimmer S, Day B, Butcher J, Dymock IW. Ascorbic acid supplementation in the treatment of pressure sores. *Lancet* 11974;2(7880):544–546.

250. Hallbook T, Lanner E. Serum zinc and healing of venous leg ulcers. *Lancet* 1972;2(7881):780–782.

251. FaLyons J. Monitoring practice. *Nurs Times* 1994;90(16):69–78.

252. Meechan M. Multisite pressure ulcer prevalence survey. *Decubitus* 1990;3:14.

253. Robnett MK. The incidence of skin breakdown in a surgical intensive care unit. *J Nurs Qual Assur* 1986;1:77–81.

254. National Pressure Ulcer Advisory Panel. Pressure ulcers prevalence, cost and risk assessment: Consensus Development Conference Statement. *Decubitus* 1989;2:24.

255. Hofman A, Geelkerken RH, Wille J, Hamming JJ, Hermans J, Breslau PJ. Pressure sores and pressure-decreasing mattresses: controlled clinical trial. *Lancet* 1994;343:568–571.

256. Bryan CS, Dew CE, Reynolds KL. Bacteremia associated with decubitus ulcers. *Arch Intern Med* 1983;143:2093–2095.

257. Mustoe TA, Cutler NR, Allmand RM, et al. A Phase II study to evaluate recombinant platelet-derived growth factor-BB in the treatment of Stage 3 and 4 pressure ulcers. *Arch Surg* 1994;129:213–219.

258. Rubin SC, Benjamin I, Hoskins WJ, Pierce VK, Lewis JR JL. Intestinal surgery in gynecologic oncology. *Gynecol Oncol* 1989;34:30–33.

259. Hoffman MS, Barton DP, Gates J, et al. Complications of colostomy performed on gynecologic cancer patients. *Gynecol Oncol* 1992;44:231–234.

260. Pearl RK, Prasad L, Orsay CP, Abcarian H, Tan AB, Melzl MT. Early local complications from intestinal stomas. *Arch Surg* 1985;120:1145–1147.

261. Hampton BG. Peristomal and stomal complications. In Hampton BG, Bryant RA (Eds), *Ostomies and Continent Diversions: Nursing Management*. St. Louis, Mosby-Year Book Inc, 1992, pp. 105–128.

262. Allen-Mersh TG, Thomson JPS. Surgical treatment of colostomy complications. *Br J Surg* 1988;75:416–418.

263. Orr JW Jr. Introduction to pelvic surgery—pre- and post-operative care. In Gusberg SB, Shingleton HM, Deppe G (Eds), *Female Genital Cancer.* New York: Churchill Livingstone, 1988, pp. 497–534.

264. Stgehling L. Preoperative blood ordering. *Int Anesth Clin* 1982;20:45–57.

265. Blood Component Therapy. *ACOG Technical Bulletin, Number 199*, November 1994.

266. Sazama K. Reports of 355 transfusion-associated deaths: 1976 through 1985. *Transfusion* 1990;30:583–590.

267. Goldberg GL, Gibbon DG, Smith HO, DeVictoria C, Runowicz CD, Burns ER. Clinical impact of chemotherapy-induced thrombocytopenia in patients with gynecologic cancer. *J Clin Oncol* 1994;12:2317–2320.

268. National Institutes of Health Consensus Conference. Fresh-frozen plasma: indications and risks. *JAMA* 1985;253:551–557.

269. Ness PM, Perkins HA. Cryoprecipitate as a reliable source of fibrinogen replacement. *JAMA* 1979;241:1690–1691.

270. Krebs HB. Intestinal injury in gynecologic surgery: a ten year experience. *Am J Obstet Gynecol* 1986;155:509–514.

271. Alvarez RD. Gastrointestinal complications in gynecologic surgery: a review for the general gynecologist. *Obstet Gynecol* 1988;72:533–540.

272. Krebs HB, Goperud DR. Mechanical intestinal obstruction in patients with gynecologic disease: a review of 368 patients. *Am J Obstet Gynecol* 1987;157:467–471.

273. Holder WD Jr. Intestinal obstruction. *Gastroenterol Emer* 1988;17(2):317–340.

274. Fabri PJ, Rosemurgy A. Reoperation for small intestinal obstruction. *Surg Clin N Am* 1991;71:131–146.

275. Monk BJ, Berman ML, Montz FJ. Adhesions after extensive gynecologic surgery: clinical significance, etiology, and prevention. *Am J Obstet Gynecol* 1994;170:1396–1403.

276. Brolin R, Crasna M, Mast B. Use of tubes and radiographs in the management of small bowel obstruction. *Ann Surg* 1987;206:26–133.

277. Butts DE. Perioperative care of the patient with diabetes mellitus. *Plastic Surg Nurs* 1990;10:7–31.

278. Orland MJ. Diabetes mellitus. In Woodly M, Whelan A (Eds), *Manual of Medical Therapeutics*, 27th ed. Boston: Little, Brown, & Company, 1992, pp. 375–399.

279. Unger RH, Foster DW. Diabetes mellitus. In Wilson JD, Fostor DW, (Eds), *Williams Textbook of Endocrinology*, 8th ed. Philadelphia: WB Saunders Company, 1992, pp. 1255–1333.

280. Vinico F. Atherosclerosis and diabetes mellitus. *Diabetes Spect* 1988;1:319.

281. Gavin LA. Perioperative management of the diabetic patient. *Endocrinol Metabol Clin N Am* 1992;21:457–473.

282. Nesto RW, Phillips RT, Kett KG, Hill T, Perper E, Young E, Leland S Jr. Angina and exertional myocardial ischemia in diabetic and nondiabetic patients: assessment by exercise thallium scintigraphy. *Ann Intern Med* 1988;108:170–175.

283. Seki S, Yoshida H, Monoki y, Ooba O, Termato S, Komoto Y. Impaired pulmonary oxygenation of diabetic origin in patients undergoing coronary artery bypass grafting. *Cardiovasc Surg* 1993;1:72–78.

284. Hjortrup A, Sorensen C, Dyremose E, Hjortso NC, Kehlet H. Influence of diabetes mellitus on operative risk. *Br J Surg* 1985;72:783–785.

285. Schumann D. Postoperative hypoglycemia: clinical benefits of insulin therapy. *Heart Lung* 1990;19:165–173.

286. Kaukinen S, Salmi J, Marttinen A, Koivula T. Postoperative hyperglycaemia—Are the patients diabetic? *Exp Clin Endocrinol* 1992;100:85–89.

287. Brandi LS, Frediani M, Oleggini M, et al. Insulin resistance after surgery: normalization by insulin treatment. *Clin Sci* 1990;79:443–450.

288. Hoogwerf BJ. Perioperative management of diabetes mellitus: striving for metabolic balance. Cleveland J Med 1992;59(5):447–449.

289. McMurray JF Jr. Wound healing with diabetes mellitus: better glucose control for better wound healing in diabetes. *Surg Clin N Am* 1984;64:769–778.

290. Wheat LJ. Infection and diabetes mellitus. *Diabetes Care* 1980;3:187.

291. Davi G, Catalano I, Averna M, et al. Thromboxane biosynthesis and platelet function in Type II diabetes mellitus. *N Engl J Med* 1990;322:1769–1774.

292. Goldstein DE, Parker KM, England JD, et al. Clinical application of glycosylated hemoglobin measurements. *Diabetes* 1982;31(suppl 3):70–78.

293. Walts LF, Miller J, Davidson MB, Brown J. Perioperative management of diabetes mellitus. *Anaesthesiology* 1981;55:104–109.

294. Ljungvist O, Thorell A, Gutniak M, Haggmark T, Efendic S. Glucose infusion instead of preoperative fasting reduces postoperative insulin resistance. *J Am Coll Surg* 1994;178:329–336.

295. Adams III JE, Sigard GA, Allen BT, et al. Diagnosis of perioperative myocardial infarction with measurement of cardiac troponin I. *N Engl J Med* 1994;330:670–674.

296. Graeber GM. Creatine kinase (CK): its use in the evaluation of perioperative myocardial infarction. *Surg Clin N Am* 1985;65:539–551.

297. Val PG, Pelletier LC, Hernandez MG, et al. Diagnostic criteria and prognosis of preoperative myocardial infarction following coronary bypass. *J Thorac Cardiovasc Surg* 1983;86:878–886.

298. ACC/AHA Task Force Report. Guidelines for the early management of patients with acute myocardial infarction. *JACC* 1990;16(2):249–292.

299. Charlson ME, MacKenzie CR, Gold JP, et al. Risk for post-operative congestive heart failure. *Surg Gynecol Obstet* 1991;172(2):95–104.

300. Eickhoff TC. Pulmonary infections in surgical patients. *Surg Clin N Am* 1980;60:175–183.

301. Rodriguez JL, Giboons KJ, Bitzer LG, et al. Pneumonia: incidence, risk factors, and outcome in injured patients. *J Trauma* 1991;31:907–912.

302. Martin LF, Asher EF, Casey JM, et al. Postoperative pneumonia: determinants of mortality. *Arch Surg* 1984;119:379–383.

303. Centers for Disease Control. Nosocomial infection surveillance, 1984. *CDC Surveill Summ* 1986;35:17S–29S.

304. Dunn DL. Gram-negative bacterial sepsis and sepsis syndrome. *Surg Clin N Am* 1994;74:621–635.

305. Fry DE. Postoperative pneumonia in the intensive care unit. *Surg Obstet Gynecol* 1993;177:41S–49S.

306. Milledge JS, Nunn JF. Criteria of fitness for anaesthesia in patients with chronic obstructive lung disease. *Br Med J* 1975;3:670–673.

307. Flenley DC. Chronic obstructive pulmonary disease. *Dis Mon* 1988;34:543–599.

308. Bosser SA, Rock P: Asthma and chronic obstructive lung disease. In Breslow MJ, Miller CJ, Rogers MC (Eds), *Perioperative management*. St. Louis: CV Mosby Company, 1990, pp. 259–280.

309. Zibrak JD, O'Donnell CR, Marton K. Indications for pulmonary function testing. *Ann Int Med* 1990;112:763–771.

310. Meyers JR, Lembeck L, O'Kane H, Baue AE. Changes in functional residual capacity of the lung after operation. *Arch Surg* 1975;110:576–583.

311. Easton PA, Jadue C, Dhingra S, Anthonisen NR. A comparison of the bronchodilating effects of a beta-2 adrenergic agent (albuterol) and an anticholinergic agent (ipratropium bromide) given by aerosol alone or in sequence. *N Engl J Med* 1986;315:735–739.

312. Barnes PJ. A new approach to the treatment of asthma. *N Engl J Med* 1989;321:1517–1527.

313. Hou SH, Bushinsky DA, Wish JB, Cohen JJ, Harrington JT. Hospital-acquired renal insufficiency: a prospective study. *Am J Med* 1983;74:243–248.

314. Smithies NM, Cameron JS. Can we predict outcome in acute renal failure? *Nephron* 1989;51:297–300.

315. Kellerman PS. Perioperative care of the renal patient. *Arch Intern Med* 1994;154: 1674–1688.

316. Schusterman N, Strom BL, Murray TG, Morrison G, West SW, Maislin G. Risk factors and outcome of hospital-acquired acute renal failure. *Am J Med* 1987;83:75–71.

317. Charlson ME, MacKenzie R, Gold JP, Ailes KL, Shires TG. Postoperative renal dysfunction can be predicted. *Surg Gynecol Obstet* 1989;169:303–309.

318. Wilkes BM, Mailloux LU. Acute renal failure: pathogenesis and prevention. *Am J Med* 1986;80:1129–1136.

319. Meyer RD. Risk factors and comparisons of clinical nephrotoxicity of aminoglycosides. *Am J Med* 1986;80:119S–125S.

320. Allen GC. Malignant hyperthermia and associated disorders. *Curr Opin Rheumatol* 1993;5:719–724.

321. Pinson CW, Schuman ES, Gross GF, Schuman GA, Hayes JF. Surgery in long-term dialysis patients: experience with more than 300 cases. *Am J Surg* 1986;151: 567–571.

322. Blumberg A, Wiedmann P, Shaw S, Gnadinger M. Effect of various therapeutic approaches on plasma potassium and major regulating factors in terminal renal failure. *Am J Med* 1988;85:507–512.

323. Eschback JW, Egrie JC, Downing MR, Browne JK, Adamson JW. Correction of the anemia of end-stage renal disease with recombinant human erythropoietin: results of a combined phase I and II clinical trial. *N Engl J Med* 1987;316:73–78.

324. Livio M, Mannucci PM, Vigano G, et al. Conjugated estrogens for the management of bleeding associated with renal failure. *N Engl J Med* 1986;315:731–735.

325. Lewis SL, van Epps DE. Neutrophil and monocyte alterations in chronic dialysis patients. *Am J Kid Dis* 1987;9:381–395.

326. Friedman LS, Maddrey WC. Surgery in the patient with liver disease. *Med Clin North Am* 1987;71:453–476.

327. Harville DD, Summerskill WHJ. Surgery in acute hepatitis. *JAMA* 1963;184:257–261.

328. Martinez J, Palescak JE. Hemostatic alterations in liver disease. In Zakim D, Boyer TD (Eds), *Hepatology: A Textbook of Liver Disease.* Philadelphia: WB Saunders Company, 1992, pp. 546–580.

329. Roberts HR, Cederbaum AI. The liver and blood coagulation: physiology and pathology. *Gastroenterology* 1979;63:297–320.

330. Child CG, Turcotte JC. Surgery and portal hypertension. In Child CG (Ed), *The Liver and Portal Hypertension.* Philadelphia: WB Saunders Company, 1994, pp. 1–85.

331. Pugh RNH, Murray-Lyon IM, Dawson JL, et al. Transection of the oesophagus for bleeding oesophageal varices. *Br J Surg* 1973;60:646–649.

332. Stone HH. Preoperative and postoperative care. *Surg Clin N Am* 1977;57:409–419.

333. Goldmann DR. Surgery in patients with endocrine dysfunction. *Med Clin North Am* 1987;71(3):499–509.

334. Semenkovich CF. Endocrine diseases. In Woodley M, Whelan A (Eds), *Man-*

ual of Medical Therapeutics. Boston: Little, Brown and Company, 1993, pp. 400–405.

335. Daniels GH, Martin JB. Neuroendocrine regulation and diseases of the anterior pituitary and hypothalamus. In Isselbacher KJ, Braunwald E, Wilson JD, Martin JB, Fauci AS, Kasper DL (Eds), *Harrison's Principles of Internal Medicine.* New York: McGraw-Hill, 1994, pp. 1911–1913.

336. Clutter WE. Mineral and metabolic bone disease. In Woodley M, Whelan A (Eds), *Manual of Medical Therapeutics.* Boston: Little, Brown and Company, 1993, pp. 427–433.

337. Mazze RI, Kallen B. Reproductive outcome after anesthesia and operation during pregnancy: a registry study of 5405 cases. *Am J Obstet Gynecol* 1989;161: 1178–1185.

338. Brodsky JB, Cohen EN, Brown BW, Wu ML, Whitcher C. Surgery during pregnancy and fetal outcome. *Am J Obstet Gynecol* 1980;138:1165–1167.

339. Levinson G, Shnider SM. Anesthesia for surgery during pregnancy. In Shnider SM, Levinson G (Eds), *Anesthesia for Obstetrics.* Baltimore: Williams and Wilkins, 1994, pp. 188–277.

340. Vincent RD. Anesthesia for the pregnant patient. *Clin Obstet Gynecol* 1994;37(2):256–273.

341. Moise KJ. Effect of advancing gestational age on the frequency of fetal ductal constriction in association with maternal indomethacin use. *Am J Obstet Gynecol* 1993;168:1350–1353.

342. Hill LM, Johnson CE, Lee RA. Cholecystectomy in pregnancy. *Obstet Gynecol* 1975;46:291–293.

343. Speroff L, Glass RH, Kase NG. The endocrinology of pregnancy. In *Clinical Gynecologic Endocrinology and Infertility.* Baltimore: Williams and Wilkins, 1989, p. 251.

344. Dilts PV, Brinkman CR, Kirschbaum TH, Assali NS. Uterine and systemic hemodynamic relationships and their response to hypoxia. *Am J Obstet Gynecol* 1965;103:138–157.

345. U.S. Bureau of the Census. *Statistical Abstract of the United States,* 113th ed. Washington, DC, 1993.

346. Yancik R. Frame of reference: old age as the context for prevention and treatment of cancer. In Yanci, R (Ed), *Perspectives on Prevention and Treatment of Cancer in the Elderly.* New York: Raven Press, 1993, p. 5.

347. Goodwin JS, Samet JM, Key CR, Humble C, Kutvirt D, Hunt C. Stage at diagnosis of cancer varies with the age of the patient. *J Am Geriatr Soc* 1986;34:20–26.

348. Grover SA, Cook EF, Adam J, Coupal L, Goldman L. *Am J Med* 1989;86: 151–157.

349. Wheat ME, Mandelblatt JS, Kunitz G. Pap smear screening in women 65 and older. *J. Am Geriatr Soc* 1988;36:827–830.

350. Samet J, Hunt WC, Key C, Humble CG, Goodwin JS. Choice of cancer therapy varies with age of patient. *JAMA* 1986;255:3385–3390.

351. Kennedy AW, Flagg JS, Webster KD. Gynecologic cancer in the very elderly. *Gynecol Oncol* 1989;32:49–54.

352. Grant PT, Keffrey JF, Fraser RC, Tompkins G, Filbee JF, Wong OS. Pelvic radiation therapy for gynecologic malignancy in geriatric patients. *Gynecol Oncol* 1989;33:185–188.

353. Kirshner CV, DeSerto TM, Isaacs JH. Surgical treatment of the elderly patient with gynecologic cancer. *Surg Gynecol Obstet* 1990;170:379–384.

354. Lawton FG, Hacker NF. Surgery for invasive gynecologic cancer in the elderly female population. *Obstet Gynecol* 1990;76:287–289.

355. Warner MA, Hosking MP, Lobdell CM, Offord KP, Melton LJ III. Effectsof referral bias on surgical outcomes: a population-based study of surgical patients 90 years of age or older. *Mayo Clin Proc* 1990;65:1185–1191.

356. Lichtinger M, Averette H, Penalvaer M, Sevin B-U. Major surgical procedures for gynecologic malignancy in elderly women. *South Med J* 1986;79:1506–1510.

357. Fuchtner C, Manetta A, Walker JL, et al. Radical hysterectomy in the elderly patient: analysis of morbidity. *Am J Obstet Gynecol* 1992;166:593–597.

358. Matthews CM, Morris M, Burke TW, Gershenson DM, Wharton JT, Rutledge FN. Pelvic exenteration in the elderly patient. *Obstet Gynecol* 1992;79:773–777.

359. Altaras MM, Ben-Baruch G, Aviram R, et al. Treatment results for ovarian cancer in women older than 70 years (abstract). *Gynecol Oncol* 1993;50:270.

360. Lau HC, Granick MS, Aisner AM, Solomon MP. Wound care in the elderly patient. *Surg Clin N Am* 1994;74:441–463.

361. Watters JM, Clancey SM, Moulton SB, Briere KM, Zhu J-M. Impaired recovery of strength in older patients after major abdominal surgery. *Ann Surg* 1993;218:380–393.

362. Harper CM, Lyles YM. Physiology and complications of bedrest. *J Am Geriatr Soc* 1988;36:1047–1054.

CHAPTER 10

PERIOPERATIVE ANESTHETIC EMERGENCIES

JOAN CHRISTIE, M.D. and ROY D. CANE, M.D., B.Ch.

Cardiopulmonary and neurologic function are unstable during and after anesthesia and surgery. This chapter reviews some common but potentially serious conditions that present in the perioperative period. Some of these problems may be preexisting, such as hypertension, whereas others are unique to anesthesia, such as emergence delirium or malignant hyperthermia.

If preexisting illness is delineated prior to surgery, patient risk can be defined or reduced. An example is a patient with a recent myocardial infarction. Appreciation of cohort data and evaluation of the patient allow for development of an individualized perioperative management plan. The timing of surgery, type of anesthetic, and extent of perioperative monitoring may play a role in the outcome for such a patient. This chapter addresses preoperative strategies to reduce perioperative emergencies.

RESPIRATORY DISEASE

Preoparative Evaluation

Anesthesia and surgery may have deleterious effects on pulmonary function. Lung volumes are decreased secondary to supine position and induction of general anesthesia. Gas exchange is altered due to changes in hypoxic pulmonary vasoreactivity and mucociliary clearance.[1] In addition to anesthesia, surgery can impose profound effects on pulmonary oxygenation and pulmonary mechanics. Vital capacity is often less than 50% of normal immediately after abdominal surgery and is still 17% below normal at 4 months postoperatively. Lung disease affects up to 5% to 15% of the general population and respiratory complications are common in the perioperative period.

Perioperative and Supportive Care in Gynecologic Oncology: Evidence-Based Management, Edited by Steven A. Vasilev.
ISBN 0-471-24788-X   Copyright © 2000 by Wiley-Liss, Inc.

TABLE 10.1. Risk Factors for Postoperative Pulmonary Failure

Definite Risk Factors

Site of surgery (upper abdominal, thoracic)
General medical condition
Symptomatic pulmonary disease
Chronic obstructive pulmonary disease

Probable Risk Factors

Obesity
Age >60 years
Smoker
Hypercapnia
Patients taking amiodarone
Severe chest-wall or spinal deformities

Possible Risk Factors

Male gender
Length of surgery
Hypoalbuminemia
Chest X-ray abnormality

The object of preoperative evaluation with respect to pulmonary complications is to identify persons at risk, to determine the degree of risks, and to remediate factors associate with increased risk. Studies of postoperative pulmonary dysfunction establish definite, probable, and possible risk factors (Table 10.1). Respiratory failure is more commonly associated with smoking, obesity, neuromuscular disease, chest-wall or spine deformities, preexisting pulmonary disease, the elderly, and occurring after thoracic or upper abdominal surgery (Level II-2).[1,4]

The degree of risk for a given individual may relate to the extent of disease. Preoperative evaluation to identify disease should include inquiry regarding medications taken and patient's functional status. The presence of intercurrent acute illness suggested by sputum, cough, stridor, dyspnea, or wheezing should prompt further evaluation and treatment prior to elective surgery. Functional limitations secondary to respiratory disease or a history of severe exacerbations warrant more exhaustive information.

While no universal guidelines are available to suggest who should have pulmonary function testing, the history and physical findings should predict which patients are more likely to have postoperative complications and therefore benefit from preoperative therapy. Pulmonary function studies, chest X ray, and arterial blood gases may provide invaluable information on the extent and reversibility of pulmonary disease.[2] Such information may suggest the desirability for a specific anesthetic or surgical technique, or the application of more intensive respiratory monitoring postoperatively.

The efficacy of various perioperative maneuvers to reduce postoperative pulmonary complications (PPC) has been the subject of many studies (Level 1).[3,6,8,10] The results suggest that lung expansion techniques lessen PPC, especially after upper abdominal incision. Beginning treatment prior to surgery confers added benefits for 48 to 72 hours postoperatively. Incentive spirometry, mask continuous positive pressure, and chest physical therapy all decrease the risk of PPC.

Early studies advocating regional anesthesia to prevent PPC have been challenged by recent studies demonstrating no differences (Level II-2).[4,5] Postoperative pain control using epidural analgesia may, however, provide superior pain relief and earlier intensive care unit (ICU) discharge.

The available literature suggests that PPC are more common in patients with chronic obstructive pulmonary disease and that the preoperative treatment of airflow obstruction and infection may lessen this risk.[6,7] Smoking cessation does not confer clinically significant physiologic benefits for at least 2 months prior to surgery.[8]

Postoperative Ventilatory Failure

Postoperative pulmonary dysfunction may result in inadequate ventilation or oxygenation. Inadequate ventilation with resultant carbon dioxide retention occurs when the neuromuscular apparatus of breathing (the pump) fails or when inspiratory work demands exceed functional reserves (Table 10.2). Respiratory drive can be blunted due to the residual effects of anesthetic agents. The type and time of administration of anesthetic agents are important, since certain techniques can cause delayed or biphasic respiratory depression (e.g., epidural morphine or high-dose IV [intravenous] fentanyl). Administration of excessive postoperative analgesics may cause hypoventilation. Patients with extraordinary sensitivity to respiratory depressants include those with morbid obesity, sleep apnea, or chronic airway obstruction. Such patients may best be managed with regional analgesia or IV nonsteroidal analgesics.

Respiratory muscle function may be inadequate postoperatively if residual neuromuscular relaxants still exert an influence. Overt paralysis is easily recognized in the anxious patient who has airway obstruction. Subtle hypoventilation or aspiration may not be easily detected. Patients with preexisting neuromuscular problems—for example, myasthenia gravis or muscular dystrophy—can hypoventilate even when muscle relaxants are not used. Severe hypermagnesemia, hypophosphatemia, or hypokalemia may impair ventilatory muscle function.[9] Sensitivity to succinylcholine occurs in patients with atypical pseudocholinesterase. Ventilation should be supported and the underlying process treated in patients with neuromuscular dysfunction in the postanesthesia care unit (PACU).

Increased dead space—that is, more ventilation to areas of lung that are not perfused—mandates a higher total minute ventilation and can result in impaired carbon dioxide elimination. Dead space is increased with connectors and tubes,

TABLE 10.2. Postoperative Ventilatory Failure

Pump Failure

Depressed ventilatory drive
  residual anesthetics, opiates
  decrease in noxious stimuli
  abnormal CO_2 responses
  COPD, sleep apnea, obesity
  increased intracranial pressure
Depressed Neuromuscular Function
  residual neuromuscular blockade
  preoperative neuromuscular dysfunction
  myasthenia gravis, muscular dystrophy
  neuromuscular blockade enhancement
  aminoglycosides, furosemide, hypermagnesemia
  high spinal or epidural
  phrenic nerve damage
  severe scoliosis

Inspiratory Work Demand Exceeds Reserves

Increased Dead Space
  excessive tubing, connectors in breathing apparatus
  positive end-expiratory pressure
  high ventilator rates, short expiratory time
  pulmonary embolus
  pulmonary hypotension
Increased Airway Resistance or Airway Obstruction
  laryngospasm, edema, tongue, foreign body
  extrinsic airway compression
  hematoma, abscess
  small airway resistance
  bronchospasm, secretions, edema
  too small endotracheal tube
  ventilator flows low
Decreased Compliance
  obesity
  increased intra-abdominal pressure
  ascites, tumor, pregnancy, bowel obstruction
  pulmonary edema, fibrosis, pneumothorax, adult
    respiratory distress syndrome

and excessive application of positive end-expiratory pressure (PEEP) or continuous positive airway pressure (CPAP). Auto PEEP can occur if the patient is not given an adequate period of exhalation as when excessive ventilatory rates are used on mechanical ventilators. Less common causes of increased dead space include pulmonary emboli or hypotension secondary to hemorrhage or sepsis.

Increased airway resistance and all forms of acute lung disease may increase work of breathing excessively. Increased airway resistance may occur because of laryngospasm, bronchospasm, or extrinsic airway compression. Upper airway obstruction can usually be relieved by clearing secretions and elevating the jaw. Nasopharyngeal or oropharyngeal airway insertion may be necessary until the patient is more alert.

Laryngospasm or airway closure occurs in emerging patients who are still partially anesthetized or partially obstructed. Stimulation of the larynx by secretions can also cause laryngospasm. Clearing and opening the airway and applying positive pressure with a face mask usually resolves the problem. Occasionally, upper airway edema occurs secondary to a difficult intubation, and reintubation may be necessary. Bronchospasm may be subtle in the immediate postoperative period manifest by excessive peak airway pressures in ventilated patients or tachypnea in those who are extubated. Increased small airway inspiratory resistance may be secondary to loss of lung volume with secretions or pulmonary edema and is not responsive to $beta_2$ sympathomimetic or parasympatholytic agents.

Decreased lung compliance can result in increased work of breathing and ventilatory failure. Obesity and increased intra-abdominal pressure decrease total respiratory system compliance. Atelectasis, pneumonia, and heart failure may all lead to decreased lung compliance, which would most likely be noted in the ICU or on the floor some time after surgery and discharge from the PACU.

The etiology of low lung compliance should be discovered and treatment instituted to reexpand collapsed airways and thus restore functional residual capacity. CPAP is useful in preventing and treating lung volume loss after general anesthesia.[3]

Postoperative hypoxemia can occur secondary to hypoventilation, and ventilation perfusion (VQ) mismatch. Hypoventilation can usually be identified because it is often associated with carbon dioxide retention as described above. VQ mismatch is common postoperatively, often secondary to reduction in functional residual capacity (FRC). Some patients are at increased risk for VQ mismatch, including the elderly and those with obesity, chronic lung disease, and upper abdominal surgery patients. Prone, Trendelenburg, and lithotomy positions and abdominal insufflation for laparoscopic surgery reduce FRC. Efforts to reduce VQ mismatch in the PACU should include the semisitting position, analgesia, clear airway maintenance, use of CPAP or PEEP, and maintenance of adequate cardiac output. Pulse oximetry should be utilized in all PACU patients and oxygen saturation should be at least 90%.

Asthma

Asthma is characterized by a reversible component of airway obstruction. The majority of the obstruction occurs secondary to mucosal edema and inflammation and is commonly treated with steroids and adrenergic agents. Hyperplasia of goblet cells and hypertrophy of mucous glands is common, and a number of

TABLE 10.3. Pharmacologic Management of Acute

β_2-agonists	Stimulate β_2 receptor, activate adenylate cyclase, increase cyclic adenosine monophophate, inhibit phosphorylation of myosin. Increase ciliary activity, decrease mediator release from mast cells.
Anticholinergics	Ablate vagal tone, synergistic effects with β_2 agonists.
Corticosteroids	Anti-inflammatory, prevent arachidonic acid release, inhibit neutrophil-endothelial interaction, decrease mast cell mediators, modulate calcium entry into cells, synergism with β_2 agonists.
Methylxanthines	Inhibit phosphodiesterase only at supra-therapeutic concentrations. Modulate β_2 receptor function.

mediators, both inhaled and systemic, may trigger constriction of bronchi and edema.[10]

Medications used to treat asthma usually include anticholinergics, beta-agonists, and steroids (Table 10.3). Theophylline is used less frequently as the risk-to-benefit ratio with this agent is high. Minor side effects include gastrointestinal upset and atrial arrhythmias. However, the more serious ventricular arrhythmias or seizures may occur even at low therapeutic serum levels. Beta-agonists are useful for acute asthmatic exacerbation by increasing synthesis of cyclic adenosine monophosphate (AMP), which results in bronchial smooth muscle relaxation. Most of the side effects of beta-agonists lie in their lack of specificity, and a number of disturbing studies indicate higher mortality in patients who use them chronically even when adjustments are made for assessments of severity of disease. Beta$_2$-selective adrenergics are preferable to less specific agents, which may cause undesirable side effects such as tachycardia, angina, and tremors. Ipratropium bromide, a congener of atropine, is also useful in asthma treatment. By blocking muscarinic receptors, anticholinergics decrease vagal tone. Ipratropium is less selective than beta$_2$ agonists and has a later peak bronchodilator effect of 15 to 30 minutes. Steroids are used, and beclomethasone and triamcinolone are available in metered-dose inhalers. If patients are taking systemic steroids, they should receive replacement with hydrocortisone 100 mg prior to, during, and after surgery. If inhaled steroids are used, no systemic replacement is necessary.

Bronchodilator drugs should be continued prior to surgery. Supplementation with IV corticosteroids is recommended as above if patients are taking systemic steroids for asthma. Intercurrent infections should be treated and drugs known to exacerbate symptoms, for example, aspirin, should be avoided. Anesthetic choice will depend on the severity of the asthma and the type of surgery proposed. Regional anesthesia is often appropriate and may be an attractive alternative to general endotracheal anesthesia. All anesthetic induction agents have been successfully used for intubation in asthmatics including barbiturates, benzodiazepines, propofol, and etomidate. Ketamine (1–2 mg/kg IV) may be useful as it prevents increases in airway resistance. However, increased secretions associated with its use somewhat limit its effectiveness.

Inhalational anesthetics are used for maintenance but must be given in sufficient concentrations to depress airway hyperactivity. All inhaled anesthetics are effective bronchodilators and all have been used to treat life-threatening bronchoconstriction. IV lidocaine (1.5 mg/kg) may be given 3 minutes prior to intubation or on extubation to decrease bronchospasm. Although some authorities suggest that histamine-releasing muscle relaxants (e.g., atracurium curare) be avoided, others have found no clinically relevant deleterious effects.

Ventilator management should allow sufficient time in exhalation to promote adequate alveolar emptying without gas trapping. A slow inspiratory flow rate provides optimal ventilation relative to perfusion. PEEP is not usually recommended in asthmatics. Humidification of the airways by particulate droplets may induce bronchospasm. The endotracheal tube should be removed while the patient still has a depth of anesthesia sufficient to suppress bronchospasm. Bronchospasm occurring intraoperatively must be distinguished from mechanical obstruction of the tracheal tube, active expiration, one-lung intubation, aspiration, pulmonary edema, retained secretions, pulmonary embolus, and pneumothorax. All of these disorders produce wheezing noise and altered end-tidal CO_2 trace and thus mimic bronchial constriction. Treatment of true bronchospasm consists first of increasing the depth of anesthesia and instituting beta$_2$-agonist therapy by metered inhaler or by IV.

NEUROLOGIC COMPLICATIONS

Emergence from General Anesthesia

Emergence from general anesthesia is associated with a fluctuating state of consciousness. Patient response may range from lethargy to restless combative confusion. If the patient does not become increasingly more alert, the situation should be investigated. Residual anesthesia is most frequently the cause of lethargy in the PACU. Other factors include prolonged surgical procedure, the elderly patient, long-acting or excessive sedation, or neuromuscular blockers that are not reversed (Table 10.4). In general, most patients should be responsive to tactile stimulus 1 hour after discontinuation of all anesthetics. Reversal of opiates with 0.04 mg increments of naloxone, and benzodiazepines with 0.2–1 mg of flumazenil, will predict eventual recovery from the drug effect. Hypothermia potentiates residual sedative effects; hypoglycemia is uncommon. Electrical status epilepticus, cerebral thromboembolism (usually from air), and severe metabolic disturbances may also impair mentation. Postoperative stroke

TABLE 10.4. Postoperative Lethargy

Cause	Treatment
Preoperative lethargy secondary to drugs or alcohol	Await drug elimination
Intraoperative anesthetic drugs, e.g., opiates, benzodiazepines	Reverse specific drug, i.e., naloxone for opiates, flumazenil for barbiturates
Hypothermia	Warm
Metabolic effect, hypoglycemia, hyperosmolar state, ketosis	Glucose, fluids, insulin
Hypoxemia, hypercarbia	Increase ventilation
Status epilepticus	Antiepileptics
Cerebral anoxic injury	Supportive care
Thromboembolism: blood, air, amniotic fluid	Anticoagulate, extract air, PEEP to support ventilation

in gynecology patients is rare and usually occurs later in the postoperative period.

Combativeness or delirium that persists may suggest serious abnormalities such as hypoxemia (Table 10.5). Transient exaggerated emergence responses are more prevalent in the very old or young and those with preexisting personality disorders. Patients with organic mental dysfunction, psychiatric disorders, or merely a language barrier may have a difficult emergence. Drugs given in the perioperative period including scopalamine, ketamine, and opiates may produce emergence delirium.

Hypoxemia, lactic acidemia, and hypoglycemia can present with restlessness and agitation. Identification of common metabolic, respiratory, and drug effects will suggest appropriate treatment. Patients are at risk during periods of agitation and may dislodge drains, tubes, lines, grafts, and so forth. Corneal abrasions and sprains are not uncommon. Patients should receive verbal reassurance in addition to specific treatment for pain, anxiety, hypoxemia, etc. Physical restraint and IV sedation are warranted when safety is jeopardized.

Recovery from Regional Anesthesia

Patients may emerge from regional anesthesia alone or in combination with general anesthesia. Epidural and spinal techniques are commonly employed for surgery of the pelvis and abdomen. Sequelae from regional anesthetics are related to the type of medication used in the block. Local anesthetics, such as lidocaine and bupivacaine, disturb autonomic, sensory, and motor spinal cord function. The final height of the achieved block occurs as a result of the spinal segment where the local is placed; the volume, concentration, and speed of injection of the local; and the position of the patient. Excessively high levels

**TABLE 10.5. Factors Associated with
Postoperative Delirium During Emergence from
Anesthesia**

- Young children
- Mental impairment
- Breast or testicular biopsy
- Tracheal intubation
- Scopolamine, atropine premedicant
- Ketamine
- Alcohol, cocaine withdrawal
- Corneal abrasion, tight dressings
- Constraints
- Partial muscle paralysis
- Hypoxemia
- Pulmonary edema
- Acidosis
- Seizure
- Cerebral hemorrhage, infarct

of anesthesia may occur, resulting in hypotension, respiratory embarrassment, and cardiovascular collapse.

If surgery is very brief, under 1 hour, a subarachnoid block may not have achieved its final height and the patient may be hypotensive in the PACU. Usually, epidural or spinal local block progressively recede and patients are discharged from the PACU when they can move both legs. Persistent or prolonged neurologic deficit in the PACU warrants investigation. The addition of epinephrine to the local anesthetic or the use of a long-acting agent such as tetracaine may result in prolonged block (up to 5 hours).

Early postoperative central nervous system damage may occur secondary to peripheral nerve injury from retraction, positioning, hematoma, or surgical disruption of nerves (Table 10.6). The lithotomy position may injure the peroneal or sciatic nerve and the lumbosacral plexus may be disrupted after oncologic surgery of the pelvis. Persistent central nervous system (CNS) disturbances that can be solely attributed to regional anesthesia are extremely rare, occurring in more than 1 in 100,000 cases (Level II-2).[11] Such injuries fall into three main categories: (1) exacerbation of preexisting deficits, (2) bacterial or chemical meningitis, and (3) myelitis (Table 10.6). The causes of neural injury solely secondary to regional anesthesia include spinal cord ischemia, trauma, compression, contamination of injectate, and the neurotoxic effects of local anesthetics themselves or the preservatives used in their preparation.

A common recovery problem of regional anesthesia is urinary retention. Urinary retention occurs after epidural or spinal anesthesia, particularly when an opiate is added to the injectate (Table 10.7). Peridural opiates may also cause nausea, vomiting, and trigeminal distribution pruritis. Hypotension may occur even in patients who have been stable for some time after epidural or spinal

TABLE 10.6. Neural Impairment in the PACU

Injury Types	Cause or Associated Factor
Prolonged block	Long-acting local, additional of epinephrine
Ulnar nerve	Males, sternal retraction or compression
Brachial plexus	Nerve stretch
Lumbosacral root	Nerve compression
Transverse myelitis	Spinal cord ischemia, compression, or injectate contamination
Cauda equina syndrome	Neurotoxic effects of local anesthetic
Exacerbation of previous neural deficit	Residual anesthetics, retractors, hematoma, stirrups, lithotomy position

analgesia, particularly if the patients have been moved. This problem occurs because autonomic responses to modulate blood pressure with changes in position may be attenuated by the block, especially with high levels of regional anesthesia.

Nausea and vomiting after spinal opiates should be treated with antiemetics plus metaclopramide. Itching is first treated with hydroxyzine and if refractory with naloxone (Table 10.7). Care must be taken not to use large doses of naloxone, which would reverse the opiate-induced analgesia. Bladder distension should be relieved with intermittent or indwelling catheter drainage as untoward reflex responses may ensue (e.g., hypertension).

MALIGNANT HYPERTHERMIA

Malignant hyperthermia (MH) is an inherited disease of muscle that is frequently asymptomatic until triggered by the administration of anesthetic agents.[12] The disorder was described in the 1950s, and dantrolene, and first

TABLE 10.7. Complications of Peridural Opiates

Complication	Treatment
Respiratory depression	Ventilate, stimulate, naloxone
Urinary retention	Catheterize bladder
Nausea and emesis	Antiemetics, transdermal scopolamine
Pruritis	Hydroxyzine, naloxone

effective drug treatment for MH, was introduced in 1974. Untreated or unrecognized, MH is associated with a high mortality rate.

MH is associated with a number of disorders including King–Denborough syndrome (dwarfism, mental retardation, facial deformities), central core disease (a myopathy), and Duchenne muscular dystrophy. Some other disorders have been sporadically linked to MH, including myotonia, sudden infant death syndrome (SIDS), and heat stroke.

Laboratory and clinical evidence suggest genetically susceptible individuals exposed to specific anesthetic agents develop abnormalities in intracellular calcium. Studies demonstrate abnormal release of calcium into sarcoplasm during acute MH and reversal of calcium gradients between sarcoplasmic reticulum, mitochondria, and extracellular fluid.

A number of clinical signs may be exhibited by patients with acute MH. Tachycardia, rigidity, increased temperature, hypertension, and arrhythmias are frequently seen. Hypercarbia, rhabdomyolysis, and profound metabolic acidosis ensue. Anesthetic triggering agents include succinylcholine and potent volatile inhalation agents such as halothane, enflurane, and isoflurane. Total body metabolism increases, and mixed venous oxygen saturation and pH fall while $PaCO_2$ rises. If the clinical syndromes of rigidity, tachycardia, and hyperthermia occurs, MH should be diagnosed and treated. Rising end expired CO_2 may be the most sensitive method of detecting MH.

Treatment begins by discontinuing all anesthetics and providing 100% oxygen. Dantrolene 2–3 mg/kg (up to 10 mg/kg) every 5 minutes is given. Cooling and correction of metabolic acidosis with fluids and bicarbonate is necessary. Rhythm disturbances usually respond to correction of hypermetabolism and acidosis, but lidocaine or procainamide may be administered. Calcium channel blockers are not effective and may lead to cardiovascular collapse when combined with dantrolene.

MH susceptibility testing is offered in several North American centers and a registry of families is available.[13] If results of the halothane-caffeine contracture test are normal, then patients may be given by anesthetic. If the test is positive or if a known MH patient requires surgery, then anesthesia can still be provided. Contraindicated agents are excluded. An anesthesia machine that has been cleared of gases is used. Nontriggering anesthetics that may be given include opiates, barbiturates, propofol, N_2O, and nondepolarizing muscle relaxants. Dantrolene is available, but prophylaxis is unnecessary.

CIRCULATORY PROBLEMS

Systemic hypotension is not uncommon in the postoperative period and can result in inadequate oxygen and substrate delivery. Hypotension is less well tolerated in those with preexisting hypertension, valvular heart disease, renal disease, or atherosclerotic heart disease. The most common causes of hypoten-

TABLE 10.8. Postoperative Hypotension

Hypovolemia

Hemorrhage
Third space
Sweating
Insensible losses
Ascites

Decreased Peripheral Vascular Resistance

Regional anesthesia
α-adrenergic blockers
Opiates
Phenothiazines
Warming
Blood products
Histamine
Acidemia
Hypoxemia

Ventricular dysfunction

Fluid overload
Anesthetics
Pulmonary or systemic hypertension
Myocardial ischemia
Tachycardia
Bradycardia
Hypertension
Infarction

Miscellaneous

Spurious BP value
Adrenal cortical insufficiency
Hypocalcemia

sion are hypovolemia, decreased systemic vascular resistance, drug effects, left ventricular failure, and myocardial ischemia (Table 10.8).

Hypovolemia does not cause hypertension until compensatory mechanisms such as tachycardia and vasoconstriction fail. In healthy patients, loss of 15% to 20% of circulating blood volume is well tolerated. Intravascular volume depletion may occur long before surgery when patients undergo radiographic dye studies and bowel preparations that result in urinary and colonic loss of fluid and electrolytes.

Fluid overload, hypoxemia, drugs that impair contractility, hypothermia, ischemia, and excessive ventilation may all contribute to hypotension in the

PACU. Blood loss may also be occult and third-space losses can be very profound in the first 48 hours after surgery. Rewarming increases venous capacity as do many drugs given postoperatively, including opiates for pain and phenothiazines for nausea. Monitoring urine output and systemic blood pressure may be sufficient in healthy young patients, but invasive monitoring is preferable for the elderly or those with cardiac or renal disease.

Decreased systemic vascular resistance (SVR) frequently occurs postoperatively secondary to inhaled and IV anesthetics, warming, and other factors. Fluid challenge or administration of alpha-agonists may be necessary if hypotension occurs due to decreased SVR. Systolic hypotension with positive pressure ventilation may suggest intravascular volume depletion.

Hypotension due to ventricular systolic dysfunction is usually seen in patients with preexisting poor myocardial contractility. Preoperative determination of exercise intolerance or a history of ischemic heart disease may suggest the possibility of perioperative ventricular hypofunction. Systolic failure is usually treated by mobilizing fluid, providing afterload reduction if systemic vascular resistance is elevated, and augmenting myocardial contractility with an inotropic agent. Support of the myocardium is important, since pure alpha-agonists such as norepinephrine may potentiate failure by increasing peripheral resistance. Hypoxemia and pulmonary hypertension should be treated, as well as myocardial ischemia, if present.

Myocardial ischemia resulting in hypotension may become evident if the patient has tachycardia, bradycardia, or high sympathetic tone. Pain, anxiety, shivering, and hypoxemia can all precipitate increased myocardial oxygen demands. Signs and symptoms of ischemia are not typical in the perioperative period when analgesics may mask chest pain and cerebral hypoperfusion can be unnoticed as the patient recovers from anesthesia. Aggressive intraoperative monitoring including invasive techniques continued into the postop period are warranted in high-risk patients or those who develop ischemia by EKG. Treatment of the underlying precipitants and support of the blood pressure until ischemia is resolved are important.

ARRHYTHMIAS

Mechanisms Responsible for Arrhythmias

Rhythm disturbances that arise in the perioperative period occur as a result of abnormal impulse formation (automaticity) or conduction (reentry). Automaticity refers to the tendency of a focus in the heart to undergo spontaneous depolarization. Increasing the slope of phase 4 depolarization of the action potential leads to enhanced automaticity and increased heart rate or myocardial irritability. Reentry rhythm disturbances require two pathways that conduct cardiac impulses of different velocities. One pathway conducts the impulse forward (antegrade). The second pathway conducts the impulse backward (retrograde) to restimulate the forward pathway. There is a tenuous balance between the conduction velocities and refractory periods of these dual pathways that may be influenced by physiological or pharmacological manipulations. The importance of preexisting or perioperative rhythm disturbances relates to the effects of the rhythm on cardiac output and hence myocardial and systemic perfusion.

Arrhythmias may be a manifestation of heart disease and thus are indicators of perioperative cardiac complications. The presence of a rhythm other than sinus or frequent premature ventricular contraction (PVC) is included in the Goldman multifactorial index of cardiac risk in surgical procedures. This index refers to the risk of cardiac event in patients with cardiac disease undergoing noncardiac surgery (Level 1).[14,18] Others authors have not found risk association independent of that attributable to the underlying heart disease. For example, frequent PVCs in patients with no heart disease have a benign perioperative prognosis, whereas PVCs in patients with coronary artery disease are associated with increased cardiac morbidity. Atrial rhythm disturbances other than sinus tachycardia suggest atrial enlargement, which is often associated with pulmonic or systemic hypertension, or stenotic valvular disease.

In general, the risk of preoperative rhythm disturbance is related to the underlying disease process. Therefore, in asymptomatic patients it is not necessary to control every rhythm disturbance preoperatively. For example, in the patient with well-controlled atrial fibrillation secondary to known chronic disease, cardioversion should not be performed unless it is otherwise indicated. Asymptomatic PVCs require no treatment.

Rhythm Disturbances Requiring Treatment

Symptomatic dysrhythmia or hemodynamically significant rhythm disturbances should be treated preoperatively. Patients with complete heart block (third-degree AV dissociation) require treatment with a pacemaker (Table 10.9). Bifascicular block preoperatively can be intimidating, since a significant number of patients who develop this abnormality during myocardial infarction progress to complete heart block. However, in several prospective perioperative studies, progression to bifascicular block did not occur in patients without previous third-degree heart block (Level II-3).[15] Thus, first-degree and second-degree type I (Wenckebach) atrioventricular block do not require preoperative pacing. Patients with bifascicular block and second-degree AV type 2 or transient third-degree AV block should have temporary pacemakers inserted prior to surgery.

Patients with permanent pacemakers should be evaluated preoperatively to ensure that the pacemaker functions properly. Electrocautery can interfere with demand pacemakers. The cautery ground pad should be as far away from the pacemaker unit as possible. Continuous cautery produces more interference than brief bursts. Bipolar cautery is less likely to interfere with implanted pacemakers. The pacemaker programmer or a magnet should be available in the operating room to convert the pacemaker to a fixed rate if necessary. Pulmonary artery catheters may be used in patients who have permanent pacemakers but

TABLE 10.9. Indications for Perioperative Pacemaker

Third-Degree Atrioventricular Block

Second-Degree Atrioventricular Block

Symptomatic type I
Symptomatic type II

Acute Myocardial Infarction

New bifascicular block
New bundle branch with transient third degree
Type II second-degree atrioventricular block
Complete heart block

Sinus Node Dysfunction

Symptomatic bradyarrhythmias

Tachycardia

Bradycardia-dependent arrhythmia
Medically unresponsive reentrant arrhythmia

---

should be placed under fluoroscopy if the pacemaker has been inserted within the past 6 weeks to avoid dislodging the pacemaker wire.

Intraoperative and Postoperative Rhythm Disturbance

Rhythm disturbances are extremely common during and after surgery. Arrhythmias in this setting do not usually represent a primary cardiac event but rather reflect extracardiac factors such as hypovolemia, hypoxemia, hypercarbia, metabolic disturbances, catecholamine excess, or acid-base imbalance. Sinus tachycardia is the most common perioperative dysrhythmia and is related to a host of noncardiac factors (Table 10.10). These noncardiac factors are far more likely to cause sinus tachycardia than ischemia, infarction, or congestive heart failure. Primary cardiac causes must be sought when other etiologies have been ruled out.

Nonsinus supraventricular tachycardias (SVT) develop in about 4% of patients after major noncardiac surgery.[16] Of those who developed SVT in one study, 46% had acute cardiac conditions such as ischemia or systolic failure; the remainder had metabolic derangements or hypoxemia. SVT alone was not associated with morbidity, but several patients died from other conditions. Thus, new postoperative SVT often suggests a concurrent, perhaps severe, medical problem or cardiac dysfunction.

Atrial fibrillation is a common postoperative rhythm disturbance and usu-

TABLE 10.10. Perioperative Sinus Tachycardia

Pain anxiety
Shivering
Visceral distension (bladder, gastric)
Endotracheal tube stimulation
Fever, including malignant hyperthermia
Anemia
Hypervolemia, hypovolemia
Drug withdrawal (alcohol, opiates, β-blockers, clonidine)
Drug effects (cocaine, ketamine, atropine, β-agonists, epinephrine)
Catecholamine excess
Hypercarbia, hypoxemia
Light anesthesia
Surgical stimulation
Pulmonary emboli
Hypotension
Hypomagnesemia, hypokalemia

ally occurs because of atrial distension. Causes of perioperative atrial distension include ventricular failure, hypervolemia, pulmonary hypertension, and emboli. The perioperative patient with new-onset atrial fibrillation should have the ventricular rate controlled with one of the several classes of drug that slows AV node conduction. Such drugs include digitalis, calcium channel blockers, and beta blockers. The choice of agent will depend on the patient's status. Cardioversion is usually unsuccessful and can wait until the underlying process is reversed (e.g., the pneumonia is treated). With resolution of the precipitant there is often spontaneous conversion to sinus rhythm.

Atrial flutter is not well tolerated and resultant ventricular rates can become very rapid. AV node blockade, electrical cardioversion, and administration of a type 1A or type III antiarrhythmic are the treatments of choice.

Ventricular rhythm disturbances including PVCs may occur because of mechanical stimulation from central venous lines, electrolyte disturbance, or excessive sympathetic or parasympathetic input. A significant percentage of wide, complex EKG changes postoperatively represents aberrantly conducted atrial complexes or reentry rhythms. PVCs should not be treated unless they cause hemodynamic compromise. Rather, the underlying cause should be sought and reversed. Ventricular tachycardia (VT) usually indicates profound myocardial ischemia, hypoxemia, or severe electrolyte abnormality. VT must be aggressively treated or fibrillation will ensue.

Sinus bradycardia occurs when parasympathetic tone is increased and is usually asymptomatic unless the heart rate declines below 45 beats per minute. Hypoxemia is commonly the cause, although reflexes such as bladder distention, drugs such as fentanyl, or anesthetic technique may induce bradycardia (Table 10.11). Treatment of the underlying stimulus is indicated. Occasionally, when sinus bradycardia is symptomatic, atropine is necessary.

TABLE 10.11. Bradycardia in the PACU

Reflex

Valsalva
Bladder distention
Raised intraocular or intracranial pressure
Emesis

Medications

β-blockers
Opiates
Local anesthetics
Acetylcholinesterase inhibitors
α-agonists
Digitalis

Myocardial

Ischemia
Failure
Infarction
Conductance failure
Heart block
Hypoxemia
Hypomagnesemia

A patient who develops a perioperative rhythm disturbance should not necessarily receive long-term antiarrhythmic therapy, particularly since most of these rhythms are caused by noncardiac stimuli. Medications can frequently be discontinued before discharge and the patient can be observed as an outpatient to assess the need for long-term therapy.

MYOCARDIAL INFARCTION

Ischemic heart disease is common in the United States. However, there are striking differences in the clinical presentation and prognosis of coronary heart disease in men and women.[17] The onset of heart disease consistently occurs later in women, with angina as the predominant presentation. Women with angina have a more favorable prognosis than men and may be treated less often with invasive techniques. Myocardial infarction (MI) is less often the initial manifestation of coronary artery disease in women than men (Table 10.12). However, initial episodes of infarction are more often fatal in women. Unrecognized myocardial infarction and non-Q-wave (subendocardial) infarct are more frequent in women. Once coronary artery disease is manifest in women, mortality equals

TABLE 10.12. Epidemiology of Ischemic Cardiac Disease in Women

Positives	Negatives
Overall lower age-adjusted rates	Leading cause of death
Older age of onset	IF MI is presentation, higher death rate
Usually present with angina	MI more often unrecognized
MI more often subendocardial	Fewer invasive cardiac procedures performed
Less multivessel disease	
Less restenosis postbypass or PTCA	Early postbypass mortality higher
Prevalence of hypertension less overall	More severe hypertension in black women

that of men. Following bypass surgery, the mortality for women is twice that for men despite their lesser incidence of multivessel disease, failure, and previous infarction (Table 10.12). Later survival after bypass and percutaneous transluminal coronary angioplasty (PTCA) is similar in men and women and women may have less restenosis.

Perioperative Risk

During the 1970s, several reports suggested increased risk of perioperative reinfarction when noncardiac surgery was performed in persons who had previously suffered from an MI. Operations within 3, 6, and more than 6 months after MI were associated with reinfarction or cardiac death rates of 30%, 15%, and 5%, respectively. In the 20 years since these data were collected, the application of invasive hemodynamic monitoring and changes in anesthetic techniques produced a reduction in complication rates. Rao described a 6% incidence and Wells and Kaplan reported no reinfarction in 48 patients operated on within 3 months of MI.[23,24]

When can patients with a history of MI have surgery? Clearly, life-threatening procedures can be performed on patients with previous MI, with little expected mortality. Purely elective procedures should be delayed for 6 months postinfarction when stable, long-term risk values are achieved.

The less clear-cut situation involves a patient with a potentially curable cancer with very recent MI. One approach to such a patient is to obtain cardiac studies between 4 weeks and 3 months postinfarction. Absolute risk may depend on the severity of the insult as reflected by the development of Q-waves, systolic failure, rhythm disturbance, or angina. Evaluation of ventricular function and exercise tolerance is important in deciding the timing of the proposed operation. Stress thallium testing and echocardiographic determination of ejection fraction may help provide the information necessary to establish the risk of reinfarction.

Preoperative Evaluation

Patients with ischemic heart disease should be evaluated by history, physical exam, EKG, chest X ray, and possibly specialized tests prior to undergoing surgery. Useful elements of the history include exercise tolerance, description of chest pain, dyspnea, or fatigue.

EKG may demonstrate rhythm disturbance, MI, ischemia, or evidence of conduction disturbance. Chest X ray may suggest heart failure or concomitant lung disease. Invasive and noninvasive testing may be especially useful if the history is unreliable or if the patient is unable to exercise because of noncardiac disability. The exercise treadmill has been used, but has limited sensitivity and specificity for diagnosing coronary artery disease. Ambulatory ischemia monitoring has been used in vascular surgery patients with normal EKGs and has identified more than 90% of patients who subsequently had postoperative ischemic events. In several reports, preoperative ischemia predicted major postoperative cardiac events, but asymptomatic postoperative ischemia appeared to be a better predictor of morbidity in one recent study.[18]

Dipyridamole thallium imaging successfully identified high-risk patients undergoing vascular surgery. The specificity of both Holter monitoring and dipyridamole thallium scanning increases when appropriate subsets of patients are tested. If a patient's history suggests Class I or Class II activities can be performed, further testing is not necessary. If the history is not reliable or if the patient cannot exericse, then dipyridamole thallium screening may demonstrate transient defects reflective of myocardium at risk for infarction. Patients who cannot perform Class I or Class II activities, or who have positive ambulatory ischemia monitoring or dipyridamole thallium scans, should be optimized medically and then undergo repeat testing. If physical status or tests remain positive, coronary arteriography is advisable to determine if PTCA or invasive revascularization is indicated.

Patients undergoing noncardiac operations who have been revascularized have a low mortality rate except in the first 10 days postbypass. One study showed that the operative mortality was 2.4% in 548 patients with significant coronary artery disease who had noncardiac surgery without bypass grafting. Operative mortality was 0.9% in a similar cohort who first had bypass grafting performed.[19] The combined mortality for bypass surgery plus noncardiac surgery (2.3%) was similar to noncardiac surgery in the nonbypass group (2.4%). Thus, preoperative bypass for patients whose symptoms would not independently warrant bypass is not recommended.

Intraoperative and Postoperative Monitoring

Patients with underlying heart disease undergoing noncardiac surgery may benefit from invasive hemodynamic monitoring including a pulmonary artery catheter, arterial line, and transesophageal echocardiography. Such monitoring allows for optimization of reload and other cardiac parameters. From 1973 to

1976, little invasive monitoring was used and the risk of new infarction in patients with previous MI was 7.7%. From 1977 to 1982, such patients were aggressively monitored, with reinfarction reduced to 1.9%. Patients considered good candidates for invasive monitoring include those with MI within 3 months, those with Canadian Class II or greater angina, those in heart failure, or those at high risk on a multifactorial cardiac risk index such as the Goldman scale. Invasive monitoring is usually extended into the postoperative period. In view of Mangano's data suggesting that postoperative ischemia has the closest association with major postoperative cardiac morbidity, continuing hemodynamic monitoring postoperatively in the ICU seems warranted.[18]

HYPERTENSION

Preoperative Assessment

Hypertension is a common illness and the largest contributor to death from cardiovascular, cerebral, and renal disease. Despite its prevalence in aging women, all epidemiologic studies have shown that woman live longer and experience fewer complications than do men for similar levels of hypertension.[20] After menopause, the incidence of cardiac complications in women approaches that in males.

Blood pressure (BP) is distributed along a Gaussian curve; thus, there is no unequivocal division between "normal" and "abnormal," merely gradations of risk. Values above the 95th percentile are frequently used to distinguish high- from low-risk populations. The Fourth Joint National Committee on the Detection, Evaluation and Treatment of High Blood Pressure (JNC IV) recommended that diastolic BP > 90 mmHg be considered mild hypertension (Table 10.13).[25] Systolic BP of 140–159 mmHg is borderline isolated systolic hypertension. Hypertension is most common in blacks and men. However, white women >60 years of age and black women >45 years of age have rates equivalent to their male counterparts.

TABLE 10.13. Definition of Hypertension[a]

	Value mmHg	Classification
Systolic	<140	Normal
(when diastolic	140–159	Borderline
<90 mmHg)	≤160	Isolated systolic hypertension
Diastolic	<85	Normal
	85–89	High normal
	90–104	Mild hypertension
	105–114	Moderate hypertension
	≤115	Severe hypertension

[a]Fourth Joint National Committee Classification.

TABLE 10.14. Causes of Secondary Hypertension

Coartation of the Aorta

Renal Disease

Glomerulonephritis
Pyelonephritis
Autoimmune nephritis
Fibromuscular dysplasia
Atherosclerosis

Endocrine Disease

Diabetes
Thyrotoxicosis
11β- or 17α-hydroxylase deficiency
Cushing's disease
Catecholamine excess

Drugs

Cocaine
Steroids
Oral contraceptives
Amphetamines
Nicotine
Antidepressants, MAO inhibitors, β-blockers

Drug Withdrawal

Catecholamine administration

Miscellaneous

Pregnancy-induced hypertension
Autonomic hyperreflexia
Alcohol withdrawal

Primary hypertension is a complex phenomenon. Several factors, including genetics, weight, race, sodium intake, environment, use of alcohol or tobacco, renin levels, and hormone status, influence the expression of essential hypertension. Secondary hypertension occurs in less than 5% of all hypertensive women, often beginning in childhood or after age 50 in women with negative family history. The secondary causes of hypertension may be classified as congenital, renal, endocrine, and miscellaneous (Table 10.14). The most common congenital cause of hypertension in females is coarctation of the aorta, which is relatively frequent in women with Turner's karyotype. Renal disease constitutes the most prevalent cause of secondary hypertension in women. Endocrine disorders such as mineralocorticoid, glucocorticoid, or aldosterone excess may cause hypertension in women as do pheochromocytomas. Multiple endocrine neoplasia types 2A and 2B occur more frequently in women than in men. Drugs may induce hypertension, including amphetamines, oral contraceptives, antidepressants, steroids, alcohol, nicotine, beta-adrenergics, and narcotics.

Hypertension influences morbidity and mortality in the perioperative period. Studies have documented increased incidence of major cardiac complications after noncardiac surgery in hypertensive versus normotensive patients, especially in type 2 diabetic patients.[26–28] Most of the apparent excess risk occurs in patients with hypertension that has resulted in end organ damage, such as ischemic heart disease, left ventricular dysfunction, or renal failure. Thus, in patients with mild hypertension, diastolic BP < 104 mmHg, and no serious end organ dysfunction, general anesthesia and major surgery are well tolerated. Halothane anesthesia may engender more intraoperative hypotension in hypertensive patients than other inhaled anesthetics. Hypertensive patients are at higher risk for labile blood pressures in the perioperative period, although it is not clear whether such episodes are associated with adverse outcomes.

Medications taken for the treatment of hypertension may be important in the perioperative period. Diuretics may cause some degree of volume or electrolyte depletion; beta-adrenergic blockers may decrease cardiovascular stress responses. Nitrates and afterload reducers may exaggerate hypotension. Several agents, such as clonidine and propranolol, if withdrawn abruptly, precipitate untoward cardiac responses.

Although medications for control of H may interact with anesthetic agents and uncontrolled earlier studies suggested hypotension was more common if they were continued, substantial recent data suggest that patients do better if blood pressure medicine is continued peri-operatively. Patients should be given their usual BP medications up until surgery. It is not necessary to delay or avoid surgery to achieve ideal blood pressure in the stable patient with mild to moderate hypertension who has no evidence of end organ effects. If the patient has symptomatic hypertension (for example headache or angina) the surgery should be delayed.

Intraoperative Management

Laryngoscopy with or without endotracheal intubation may be associated with excessive hemodynamic responses including hypertension and tachycardia. The sequence and choice of drugs for anesthetic induction and maintenance depend on patient condition and the anesthesiologist's preference. A smooth transition from the awake state to the anesthetized state without exaggerated responses is desirable in hypertensive patients. Numerous pharmacologic regimens have been espoused to attenuate or eliminate hyperdynamic responses to laryngoscopy. All carry some risk and none is 100% successful. Fentanyl, intravenous or aerosolized lidocaine, esmolol, captopril, and nitroprusside have all been demonstrated to diminish the hemodynamic response to laryngoscopy. Clearly, the overall clinical picture, including the assessment of the airway, the extent of coexisting cardiac disease, and other factors, will suggest specific techniques appropriate for a given patient.

TABLE 10.15. Causes of Intraoperative Hypertension

Preexisting hypertension
Operative stimulation
Manipulation of tubes (endotracheal, urinary)
Light anesthesia
Reflex—oculocardic, carotid baroresponse
Fluid overload
Excessive catecholamine release
Drugs—ketamine, epinephrine
Hypercarbia, hypoxemia
Acidosis

Hypertension may occur intraoperatively in patients with known preexisting hypertension or may be seen in those who are normotensive (Table 10.15). Light levels of anesthesia, fluid overload, reflex responses, hypoxemia, drugs, and hypercarbia are a few of the many causes of intraoperative hypertension. The etiology of blood pressure elevation must be identified and treated appropriately. It is important perioperatively to maintain hypertensive patients close to their normal pressures, since cerebral perfusion autoregulation is shifted to higher levels in longstanding hypertension.

Postoperative Management

Mild to moderate elevations in systemic blood pressure are common postoperatively; however, significant hypertension increases morbidity and should be treated. Hypertension increases postoperative bleeding, third-space losses, and intracranial pressure, and can cause heart failure, ischemia, and rhythm disturbances. Systolic or diastolic elevations of 20% to 30% above baseline or end organ complication such as headache or angina should prompt evaluation and treatment.

Postoperative care of the hypertensive patients involves reinstitution of preoperative BP medications and attention to factors that stimulate pressure responses. Hypertension in the recovery room may occur secondary to pain or stimulation from urinary catheters, endotracheal tubes, medications, fluid overload, hypoglycemia, and so forth.

After correction of easily identified causes of hypertension, antihypertension medications may be given. The choice of medication will depend on the clinical circumstances. Nifedipine, in 10 mg increments, is well tolerated and may be given sublingually. IV labetolol, in 5 mg increments, is helpful if the patient is also tachycardiac, but must be used with caution in brochospastic patients. Nitroglycerin is indicated if the patient has ischemic myocardial disease or hypertension associated with ST segment depression. IV nitroprusside may be administered when hypertension is refractory or profound, but requires concomitant use of invasive BP monitoring.

AIRWAY DIFFICULTIES

The presence of a patent airway is a fundamental prerequisite to the provision of operative anesthesia or cardiovascular resuscitation. Airway loss constitutes a true perioperative emergency. Brain damage or death results after a few minutes of hypoxemia. Failure to successfully manage the difficult airway is responsible for about 30% of the deaths entirely attributable to anesthesia. Recognition of the difficult airway prior to attempts at intubation provides an opportunity to decrease morbidity through provision of the safest setting for the intubation.[21]

Identification of the Difficult Airway

Identification of the difficult airway may be quite easy or very subtle. Careful history and physical examination of every patient who requires an airway is mandatory to consistently recognize patients who may be difficult to intubate. The history should include previous problems with anesthetics, neck or airway surgery, trauma, and the presence of specific disease states such as rheumatoid arthritis, ankylosing spondylitis, and amyloidosis. At physical examination the airway may be grossly abnormal, such as in patients with head and neck trauma, abscess, or mandibular deformities. Three elements can be used to identify the difficult airway: atlanto-occipital joint mobility, thyromental distance, and Mallampati's tongue/pharyngeal classification.

When the neck is somewhat flexed and the atlanto-occipital joint is extended, the oral, pharyngeal, and laryngeal axes form a straight line. It has been described as the sniffing position and produces the optimal laryngoscopic view. The normal atlanto-occipital joint can achieve 35° of extension. Evaluation of extension is made by observing the range of motion achieved when the patient voluntarily extends her head. Certain diseases reduce neck mobility, including cervical spine fracture and ankylosing spondylitis. The space anterior to the larynx is called the thyromental or hyomental distance. This area can be expressed as the number of finger breadths that can be inserted horizontally between the hyoid and the tip of the mandible. If the distance is short (less than three finger breadths), the laryngeal and pharyngeal axis will be acute and alignment may be difficult. The size of the tongue in relation to the oral cavity can be estimated using Mallampati's classification. The patient sits upright with the mouth opened and the tongue protruded maximally. The observer assigns a classification based on the visualized pharyngeal structures.

Class I: soft palate, fauces, uvula, tonsilla or pillars

Class II: soft palate, fauces, uvula

Class III: soft palate, base of uvula

Class IV: no soft palate

The significance of Mallampati's classification lies in its correlation with laryngoscopic view. Laryngoscopic views affect intubation difficulty and are assigned four grades. A grade I view includes the entire laryngeal opening, grade II just the posterior elements, grade III only the epiglottis, and grade IV just the hard palate. The degree of difficulty in placing an endotracheal tube roughly corresponds to the laryngoscopic grade. Most brain damage and death secondary to problems with intubation occur with grades III and IV. A class I airway produces a grade I laryngoscopic view 99% of the time. A class IV airway is associated with a grade III or IV laryngoscopy view 100% of the time. Class II and III airways are distributed among all four laryngoscopic grades. Thus, it is predictable that persons with class I airways will be easily intubated and that those with class IV will be relatively difficult. Taken together, these three anatomic assessments of the airway are extremely useful in predicting difficulty with intubating. When airway difficulty is predicted, intubation should be performed with the patient awake.

Management of the Difficult Airway

The American Society of Anesthesiology Study Group formulated a practice algorithm for the management of recognized and unrecognized difficult airways (Fig. 10.1) (Level III).[21] Awake intubation preserves the patients' ability to breathe and protect their lungs from aspiration of stomach contents. Awake intubation is more unpleasant for the patient and it is more time-consuming and difficult for the anesthesiologist. However, it is safe and preserves airway anatomy, whereas paralysis causes the larynx to move to an anterior position and the tongue to become more posterior. If the patient has eaten or is otherwise considered to have a full stomach for another reason, then sodium citrate ranitidine, metoclopramide, and nasogastric tube decompression may be considered prior to airway manipulation.

Supplemental oxygen, an airway-drying agent, IV sedation, topical anesthetics, and nerve blocks are usef to prepare the airway. If nasal intubation is planned, vasoconstrictor and local anesthetics are given. After patient and airway preparation, several techniques are available for awake intubation. Blind nasal or oral intubation may be associated with less overall success than other techniques. Direct visualization may be aided with a lighted stylet or special laryngoscope. Fiberoptic bronchoscopy (FOB) may be performed orally or nasally and is easier to tolerate than direct laryngoscopy. Retrograde intubation techniques have been successfully employed for decades. Patients with maxillofacial trauma, trismus, cervical ankylosis, and airway masses have all been intubated using retrograde technology. The cricothyroid membrane is pierced and the trachea is entered with a cannula or large needle. A thin guide wire is passed into the trachea until it emerges out of the oral cavity or nares. The endotracheal tube is directly inserted over the guide wire and blindly advanced to the point where the retrograde enters the trachea from the neck. The guide wire is then removed.

Unanticipated difficulties with intubation also occur, necessitating a thought-

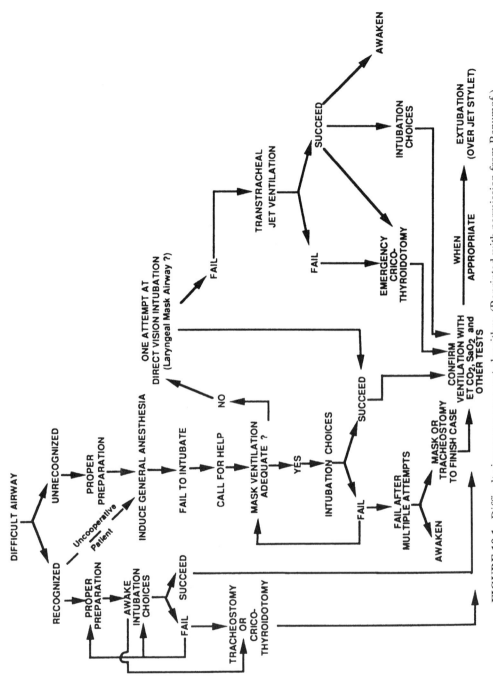

FIGURE 10.1. Difficult airway management algorithm. (Reprinted with permission from Benumof.)

ful and coordinated sequence of responses to ensure ventilation and oxygenation. If ventilation cannot be performed, transtracheal jet ventilation, cricothyroidotomy, or tracheostomy can be performed. A laryngeal mask airway (LMA) might be inserted to provide ventilation and can be successfully placed over 90% of the time. The LMA is positioned blindly and does provide an airway; however, it will not prevent aspiration of gastric content unless an endotracheal tube is placed through it into the trachea. Percutaneous transtracheal jet ventilation (TTJV) is easy, very effective, and will permit excellent oxygenation until a surgical tracheostomy or cricothyroidotomy can be performed. All that is required is a high-pressure (50 psi) oxygen source and some simple equipment found on the anesthesia cart.

Obesity

Morbidity obesity poses special challenges for both intubation and intraoperative ventilation. Difficulty with intubation occurs in about 20% of morbidly obese patients. There is a particular increased risk for gastric aspiration that occurs more often during difficult intubation and in obese patients. Premedications frequently do not end up in muscle in obese patients, so they should be given IV or by mouth. A suggested preop might include metoclopramide 10 mg and ranitidine 50 mg IV with nasogastric decompression 1 hour before the operation.

A focused history should assess for respiratory disease and sleep apnea, and chest X ray and room air arterial blood gases should be obtained. Detailed pulmonary evaluation may be warranted if history, physical findings, or lab work suggests severe abnormalities. Intubation must avoid hypoxia and aspiration, and awake intubation is often the best choice. If IV induction is planned, cricothyroid pressure (the Sellick maneuver) should be employed to protect the airway from gastric contents.

Preoxygenation is important, since functional residual capacity is reduced in the obese patient, particularly in the supine position. Auscultation of the lungs after endotracheal tube placement may be difficult and end tidal CO_2 monitoring is necessary. Ventilation and oxygenation must be provided after intubation. Problems achieving adequate CO_2 and O_2 exchange include suboptimal positioning (Trendelenburg or lithotomy), high peak airway pressures needed to overcome chest-wall resistance, decreased lung volumes, and hypoventilation with spontaneous ventilation. Adequate pain relief without respiratory depression is very important in the obese patient and epidural analgesia continued into the postoperative period may be the technique of choice.

Postoperative Monitoring

Extubation of patients with difficult airways should occur in a controlled, reversible manner. If extubation is performed and respiratory distress ensues, reintubation becomes emergent and may be impossible. The patient should be wide awake with good analgesia (epidural) and no evidence of acute respiratory distress such as wheezing or hypoxia. A special instrument called a jet stylet can be inserted into the endotracheal tube, which is withdrawn over the stylet. The stylet can be left in situ long enough to ensure that the patient does not require reintubation. If reintubation is necessary, it can be accomplished by threading an endotracheal tube over the jet stylet.

Important advances for management of the difficult airway have occurred in the 1990s. Recognition of the potential problem airway, proper patient and anesthetic preparation, and controlled extubation are the keys to a successful outcome. The American Society of Anesthesiology Clinical Practice Guidelines summarize most of these advances and provide a rational basis for caring for difficult airway patients. As we become increasingly able to manage these challenging patients, respiratory-related morbidity should decrease.

AIR EMBOLISM

Air embolism may occur whenever a pressure gradient can develop between a vein open to air and the right atrium. When the operative field is elevated 5 cm or more above the atrium, air entrainment may occur. Certain surgical positions, such as the sitting position, increase the risk of air embolus. Although air embolus is more common (20–35%) with the sitting position, it has also been reported in supine, lateral, or Trendelenburg positions and during gynecologic surgery. Air returning to the right side of the heart may be distributed into the pulmonary circulation or to the left side of the heart. The conditions favorable for air emboli to enter the coronary or cerebral circulation occur when right atrial pressure exceeds left atrial pressure and when a communication (patent foramen ovale) exists between the right and left heart. The specific pathology in venous air embolism is local vasoconstriction of the pulmonary vasculature and pulmonary hypertension resulting in profound ventilation-perfusion mismatch in the lung, pulmonary edema, and reduced cardiac output.

Monitoring for venous air entrainment consists of a precordial Doppler or 2D echo plus end tidal capnography. Pulmonary artery catheterization has been advocated as changes in pulmonary artery pressure correlate with volume of air entrained. If air is detected by the monitoring devices, aspiration of the atrial catheter should be attempted. Retrieval of air from a pulmonary artery catheter is not as great as that from a right atrial catheter. Maximal retrieval of air is achieved using a polyorifice catheter tip, with the patient positioned left lateral decubitus and head down. In more emergent circumstances, a percutaneous needle can be placed through the chest wall directly into the right ventricle.

Unfortunately, despite best efforts, mortality may be high with a large embolus. Hyperbaric therapy may be useful in theory as it is in diving accidents, but it is not used routinely in critical care patients. Animal data suggest that corticosteroids may reduce lung injury, although no clear role has been demonstrated.[29–30]

The following statement sums up the need for great care in prevention of this potentially lethal complication in line placement: A pressure gradient of 4 mmHg along a 14-gauge catheter can entrain air at a rate of 90 ml/sec and can produce a fatal air embolus within 1 second.

REFERENCES

1. Williams-Russo P, Charlson ME, MacKenzie RC, Gold JP, Shires TG. Predicting postoperative pulmonary complications. *Arch Intern Med* 1992;152:1209.
2. Crapo RO. Pulmonary function testing. *N Engl J Med* 1994;331:25.
3. Lindner KH, Lotz P, Ahnefeld FW. Continuous positive airway pressure effect on functional residual capacity, vital capacity and its subdivisions. *Chest* 1987;91:66.
4. Ah J, Weisel RD, Layaug AB, et al. Consequences of postoperative alterations in respiratory mechanics. *Am J Surg* 1974;128:376.
5. Ravin Me. Comparison of spinal and general anesthesia for lower abdominal surgery in patients with chronic obstructive pulmonary disease. *Anesthesiology* 1971;35:319.
6. Dohi S, Gold MI. Comparison of two methods of postoperative respiratory care. *Chest* 1978;73:592.
7. Stein M, Cassara EL. Preoperative pulmonary evaluation and therapy for surgery patients. *JAMA* 1970;211:787.
8. Buist AS, Sexton GH, Magy JM, et al. The effect of smoking cessation and modification on lung function. *Am Rev Respir Dis* 1976;114:115.
9. Aldrich TK. Respiratory muscle fatigue. *Clin Chest Med* 1988;9:225.
10. Pien LC, Grammer LC, Patterson R. Minimal complications in a surgical population with severe asthma receiving prophylactic corticosteroids. *J Allergy Clin Immunol* 1988;82:696.
11. Horlocker TT, McGregor DG, Matsushige DK, et al. A retrospective review of 4767 consecutive spinal anesthetics: central nervous system complications. *Anesth Analg* 1997;84:578–584.
12. Kaplan R. *Hypothermia/Hyperthermia: Manual of Complications During Anesthesia*, Gravenstein N (Ed). Philadelphia: JB Lippincott, 1991.
13. Grovert GA, Schulman SR, Mott J. Malignant hyperthermia. In Miller RD (Ed), *Anesthesia.* New York: Churchill Livingston, 1991, p. 935.
14. Goldman L, Caldera DL, Southwick FS, et al. Cardiac risk factors and complications in noncardiac surgery. *Medicine* 1978;57:357.
15. Pastore JO, Yurchak PM, Janis KM, et al. The risk of advanced heart blocks in surgical patients with right bundle branch block and left axis deviation. *Circulation* 1978;57:677.
16. Goldman L. Supraventricular tachyarrhythmias in hospitalized adults after surgery. *Chest* 1978;73:450.
17. Eaker ED, Packard B, Thom TJ. Coronary heart disease. In Douglas PS (Ed), *Heart Disease in Women.* Philadelphia: FA Davis Co., 1989, p. 127.
18. Mangano DT, Browner WS, Hollenberg M, et al. Association of perioperative myo-

cardial ischemia with cardiac morbidity and mortality in men undergoing noncardiac surgery. *N Engl J Med* 1990;323:1781.

19. Foster ED, Davis KB, Carpenter JA, et al. Risk of noncardiac operation in patients with defined coronary disease: The Coronary Artery Surgery Study (CASS) registry experience. *Ann Thorac Surg* 1986;41:42.

20. Perloff DP. Hypertension in women In Douglas PS (Ed), *Heart Disease in Women.* Philadelphia: FA Davis Co., 1989, p. 207.

21. Benumof, JL. Management of the difficult adult airway. *Anesthesiology* 1991;75: 1087.

22. Sladen A. Complications of invasive hemodynamic monitoring in the intensive care unit. *Curr Probl Surg* 1988;25:69–145.

23. Rao TL, Jacobs, KH, El-Etr AA. Reinfarction following anesthesia in patients with myocardial infarction. *Anesthesiology* 1983;59:499–505.

24. Wells PM, Kaplan JA. Optimal management of patients with ischemic heart disease for noncardiac surgery by complementary anesthesiologist and cardiologist interaction. *Am Heart J* 1981;102:1029–1937.

25. Joint National Committee on Detection, Evaluation and Treatment of High Blood Pressure: The 1988 Report. *Arch Intern Med* 1988;148:1023–1038.

26. Shackelford DP, Hoffman MK, Kramer PR Jr, Davies MF, Kaminski PF. Evaluation of preoperative cardiac risk index valves in patients undergoing vaginal surgery. *Am J Obstet Gynecol* 1995;173(1):80–84.

27. Hypertension in Diabetes Study (HDS): II. Increased risk of cardiovascular complications in hypertensive type 2 diabetic patients. *J Hypertens* 1993;11(3):319–325.

28. Maggio C, Bonzano A, Conte E, Libertucci D, Panarelli M, Bobbio M, Pinton P. Preoperative evaluation in non-cardiac: cardiac risk assessment. *Qual Assur Health Care* 1992;4(3):217–224.

29. Goldstein G, Luce JM. Pharmacologic treatment of the adult respiratory distress syndrome. *Clin Chest Med* 1990;11(4):773–787.

30. Luce JM. Acute lung injury and acute respiratory distress syndrome. *Crit Care Med* 1998;26(2):369–376.

CHAPTER 11

PERIOPERATIVE INFECTIONS: PREVENTION AND THERAPEUTIC OPTIONS

SUBIR ROY, M.D., and STEVEN A. VASILEV, M.D., M.B.A.

POSTOPERATIVE FEVER

Postoperative fever is common, but not usually indicative of an infectious process, which may be present in as few as 2% of febrile surgical patients (Level II-3).[1–3] Of course, the true risk depends on many perioperative factors, including the type of surgery performed. Other high-risk factors include surgery of greater than 2 hours duration, preexisting infection, and administration of prophylactic antibiotics. Differential diagnosis should be established by physical examination and history, not by an immediate and expensive battery of laboratory and radiologic tests. Testing should then follow, based on findings.

Infectious processes usually produce fever later (2.7 vs. 1.6 days) than inflammatory changes and last longer (5.4 versus 3.4 days).[1] Conversely, a septic process could be underway in the absence of fever in up to 50% of postoperative patients.[1] Also, patients with prophylactic drains in place are at higher risk for postoperative fever, but in most cases this is due to inflammation rather than infectious etiology, (Levels I and II-1).[2,4]

Most often, postoperative fever is due to operative site inflammation and/or atelectasis. Rare and nonfectious etiologies may include delayed posttransfusion reaction, anesthetic hepatotoxicity, and underlying inflammatory conditions such as systemic lupus and rheumatoid arthritis.[3,5]

Perioperative and Supportive Care in Gynecologic Oncology: Evidence-Based Management, Edited by Steven A. Vasilev.
ISBN 0-471-24788-X   Copyright © 2000 by Wiley-Liss, Inc.

SURGICAL INFECTION GENESIS

Contamination by endogenous bacteria may occur at the time of gynecologic operations despite vigorous preoperative skin and vaginal cleansing. The combination of hemostatic sutures around crushed tissue, blood products, and bacterial contaminants from the vagina may lead to postoperative abdominal wound infections, pelvic cellulitis, or pelvic abscesses. Prolonged hospitalization with therapeutic antibiotic administration and a second operation may be necessary if prophylaxis fails, rapidly escalating costs and morbidity.

The vagina contains both aerobic and anaerobic organisms (anaerobes > aerobes).[6] Pelvic infections may occur as a consequence of the introduction of pathogenic exogenous organisms and/or by the presence of normal vaginal flora in an abnormal location (e.g., in the endometrium, oviducts, peritoneal cavity) in sufficient numbers to overwhelm the host defense system.

When an inoculation of mixed (aerobic and anaerobic) organisms derived from bowel flora is introduced into an abnormal location (e.g., peritoneal cavity), a biphasic infection pattern may ensue.[7] Initially, peritonitis secondary to the effects of aerobic gram-negative organisms such as *Escherichia coli* precedes abscess formation, composed largely of anaerobic organisms, predominantly of the *Bacteroides* group. Approximately 40% of laboratory animals infected in this manner but not treated with antibiotics die of peritonitis while nearly 100% of surviving animals develop abscesses.[7]

Kelly demonstrated that a small number of *E. coli* or *B. fragilis* colony-forming units introduced into a wound do not produce a wound infection whereas large numbers ($>10^8$) of the former can induce a wound infection. Even greater numbers of the latter by itself can be harmless.[8] However, once a threshold is exceeded for either, a wound infection develops. Thus, an innoculum of single or multiple organisms, which can overwhelm the host-defense mechanism, appears to be necessary to cause disease.[8]

CATHETERS AND DRAINS

Foley Catheters and Ureteral Stents

Foreign objects, whether catheters or other prosthetics, are rapidly enveloped by a biofilm, consisting of thrombin, fibrin, fibronectin, and microbial production of an organic polymer matrix.[9,10] If human cells attach to the artificial material ahead of bacteria, the likelihood of an infection is less likely.[11] Microbial adherence depends on the material of the prosthetic, with Teflon or silicon being more resistant to adherence than polyvinylchloride. The microbes may not initially derive sufficient nutrients to replicate and to produce disease. However, when the devices are exposed to the outside environment (e.g., Foley catheter into the bladder through a highly colonized distal urethra), the replicating bacteria can serve as a nidus of infection and continue seeding, requiring antibiotic therapy with removal and/or replacement.[12]

Bacteriuria develops in up to 30% of patients with cathethers in place for less than 1 month and in almost all patients with prolonged catheterization.[12–15] Urine cultures may not identify this bacteriuria due to adherence of pathogens to biofil.[16] Patients with diabetes mellitus are at higher risk of catheter-associated infection.[17] Pyelonephritis and systemic sepsis can complicate both short- and long-term catheterization.[14,15]

Although suggested by some, prophylactic antibiotics do not have a clear role for prevention of urinary tract infections in patients with indwelling catheters.[14,15] In the absence of clear data, such a strategy should be individualized relative to the risk factors.

Drains

The use of Penrose drains is associated with an increased rate of infection when compared with closed suction systems (Level I).[2,4] In general, therapeutic use of drains in gynecologic oncology patients with localized infectious processes should be for specific proven indications and favorable risk/benefit. Routine prophylactic use after radical pelvic surgery has not been substantiated (Level I).[18–20] Even in the presence of prepared colonic surgery, in the absence of pus, the routine use of drains has not been validated and can increase morbidity (Level I).[21]

Central Venous Catheters

Short-term catheters are associated with a higher rate of bacteremia and infection than long-term insertions, with a rate as high as 15%.[10] The most common organisms involved are coagulase-negative staph: *Staphylococcus aureus* and *Candida* species.

Skin site contamination, at the time of insertion or subsequent care, is the most common cause of infection and reflects skin flora migrating up along the external surface of the catheter from the skin exit site.[9] The second most common cause is hub infection, whereby breaks in aseptic technique allow microbes to migrate up the internal aspect of the catheter.[9] Seeding from distant infections represents the least frequent mechanism, although *Candida* species infections are likely related to hematogenous seeding from the gastrointestinal tract.

Subcutaneous reservoir port catheters are associated with low infectious complication rates.[9] As already noted, infection depends on minimal contamination at insertion and formation of a synthetic material to human cell adherence before microbial adherence occurs.[11] On the other hand, silver impregnated cuffs have not reduced infection rates (Level I).[22,23]

The definition of catheter infection is not clearly outlined in many reports and includes exit site infections as well as catheter-related bacteremia. Signs of localized exit site infection, in the absence of positive blood cultures, can be treated with local care and intravenous antibiotics. Removal of the catheter should be considered if there is no response to these measures or if tunnel infection/cellulitis is present.[10]

Catheter-related bacteremia due to coagulase-negative staphylococci needs to be confirmed by more than one blood culture because of the high prevalence of contamination by this organism.[10] If confirmed, it should be noted that more than half of these organisms are resistant to antistaphylococcal penicillins and cephalosporins. Vancomycin therapy for 5 to 7 days is indicated. If no rapid response is evident, removal of the catheter should be considered.[10] Bacteremia due to *S. aureus* is more serious, precipitating severe complications in up to 30% of infectious episodes.[24,25] This may be due to the known specific *S. aureus* binding sites to fibronectin and fibrinogen, causing intense biofilm nidation. Some form of interaction with the biofilm markedly increases minimum bactericidal concentration (MBC), even after the organisms are extricated from the biofilm. Catheter removal should be strongly considered and antibiotic therapy administered for 7 to 10 days if uncomplicated. In the event of sepsis despite removal, a prolonged 4-week course is required.

Uncomplicated systemic catheter-related infection can be cured with antibiotics administered through the catheter 85% of the time. An absolute indication for removal is persistence of fevers and positive blood cultures despite antibiotic therapy.[26] If signs of infection persist despite antibiotic therapy and catheter removal, endocarditis or septic thrombophlebitis should be ruled out.[10]

Candidemia induced by a central venous catheter should be treated with a short course of amphotericin (2 weeks at 0.5 mg/kg) and evaluation for systemic candidiasis. If infection persists beyond 48 hours, a longer treatment course is required and the catheter should be removed.[10,25]

Unusual pathogen infections with *Pseudomonas* species, gram-positive bacilli, and atypical mycobacteria should be treated with appropriate antibiotics and removal of the catheter.[10,24,25]

PREVENTION OF SURGICAL INFECTIONS

Both patient and operative environment factors influence infection rates. Many studies are relatively old and address issues that are considered resolved or are perceived to be minor and not likely to be actively researched due to funding limitations.

Patient Factors

It is best not to alter the normal flora of the vagina or abdominal skin prior to surgery. For vaginal hysterectomy patients, a preoperative vaginal douche with an iodophor solution the night before surgery only reduces the total number of organisms from about 10^8 to 10^6–10^7.[27] Instead, a very thorough preoperative cleansing of the vagina in the operating room with either providone-iodine or saline in conjunction with intravenous antibiotics is effective in preventing infection (Level II-1).[27,28] Therefore, vaginal douching the night before surgery is not recommended.

Patients undergoing exploratory laparotomy or abdominal hysterectomy should simply bathe or shower normally the night prior to surgery, removing debris from the skin surface. Using an antiseptic agent such as chlorohexidine or iodophor for 1–2 days prior to surgery could theoretically lead to an altered skin flora, resulting in increased wound infections. Most studies show that skin bacterial counts may be reduced. However, neither clinical nor cost-effectiveness advantage has been demonstrated for antiseptic showering the days prior to surgery (Levels I and II-1).[29–32]

Skin preparation immediately prior to surgery will reduce the bacterial count sufficiently during the operative period. Results have generally been very comparable regardless of the agent used, although many favor the currently unavailable chlorhexidine or alcohol preparations. Similarly, no discernible differences have been appreciated whether the agent is applied by scrubbing, spraying, or painting.[33] The most effective available agent appears to be aqueous povidone-iodine.[34–36]

Hair removal by shaving increases infection rates and depilatories have been associated with dermatitis. Given that hair is usually sterile, it does not need to be removed. If it is in the way of the surgical incision, hair clippers appear to be the most effective method for removal (Level II).[37–43]

Operative Environment

There is no substitute for good operative technique with attention to hemostasis in reducing postoperative infections. No antibiotic or other aids will overcome poor operative technique in reducing postoperative infections.

Use of a Jackson–Pratt drain subcutaneously, brought out through a separate incision, may enhance successful primary closure of incisions associated with clean-contaminated procedures in obese patients or in patients with chronic immune-modulating diseases such as diabetes mellitus.[44] This technique may be more effective in contaminated cases, although further study is required.[45] While closure of dead space via suction drains or percutaneous mattress/stay sutures is a goal, it has been appreciated for a long time that placement of sutures in the subcutaneous tissues only increases necrosis and infection rates.[46]

Alternatively, in contaminated cases, following irrigation of the abdomen and subcutaneous tissues, sutures can be placed in the incision but not tied, and the incision may be packed with gauze with a covering bandage. After 4 days, the packing can be removed, and if the tissues appear uninfected, the sutures may be tied.[47,48] This timing coincides with quantitative bacteriology findings of $< 10^5$ bacteria/gram of tissue.[49,50] This approach results in more rapid wound healing and less morbidity, and appears to be cost-effective (Level I).[51]

Irrigation of the contaminated wound with pressure exerted by syringe (i.e., 35 cc syringe with 19-gauge needle = 8 psi) appears to be superior to volume irrigation in decreasing bacterial counts and infection rates (Level II).[52–54] In contrast, volume irrigation may decrease infection one-third of the time, but does nothing or increases the infection rate two-thirds of the time.

Wounds form a coagulum rapidly and are virtually impermeable to bacterial ingress within 24 to 48 hours, assuming the skin edges are well apposed. Thus, the primarily closed wound may be observed on the first postoperative day with removal of dressings, but the risk of horizontal nosocomial transmission must be guarded against. An alternative is to leave the dressings undisturbed until the second postoperative day. Additionally, some have proposed as long as three decades ago that tape closure minimizes avenues for bacterial ingress, resulting in lower infection rates than seen with suture or clip closure.[55,56] Some continue to champion this technique and the use of fibrin sealant, but randomized trials are needed to determine optimal mix of materials and techniques.[57–62]

Surgeon's Scrub   The surgeon's hands are colonized primarily by coagulase-negative staphylococci and coryneform bacteria, as well as pathogens picked up by patient contact.[63,64] Gloving causes the wet, sweaty skin environment to selectively proliferate gram-negative organisms.

There is strong Level II evidence that a 10-minute scrub should be abandoned as a routine. At the end of 2-hour operations, 5- versus 10-minute surgical scrubs with povidone-iodine or hexachlorophene showed no difference in bacterial counts on surgeons' hands (Level II-3).[65] Cruse has reported no increase in wound infection rates if brush scrub with detergent antiseptics are used for only 3 to 5 minutes for the first operation and for 2 to 3 minutes with a sponge between cases (Level III).[37,38] In fact, a 98.2% reduction in bacterial counts occurs after a 2-minute scrub (Level II-3).[66,67] Chlorhexidine gluconate has been reported effective in less than 1 minute, reducing bacterial colonization from 10^4 to 2.4 colony-forming units.[64,68] It appears that a 2- to 3-minute scrub is more than adequate (Level II-1).[69,70]

The ideal scrub agent should reduce bacterial counts for as long as possible without causing dermatitis, which increases bacterial counts. Alcohol preparations are recognized to be the most effective agents, but due to flammability and skin-drying effects, they are not available. The most commonly used agent today is povidone-iodine, usually in a 7.5% concentration, which also often elicits skin reactions. A little-known study documented that a 5-minute scrub with povidone-iodine results in absorption of four times the daily recommended intake of iodine.[71] When compared to chlorhexidine gluconate, povidone-iodine is substantially less effective in reducing and maintaining low bacterial counts.[66,67,70,72] Although ototoxicity has been reported with chlorhexidine, it was noted in cases of contact through open eardrums during myringotomy.[73]

Masks   Use of face masks prevents large droplets of bacterial contaminant from contacting the surgical wound. However, infection rates are not decreased by their use (Level I).[74–76] Protection of the surgeon from patient secretions and blood appears to be the main reason for this traditional ritual.

Gloves   Studies have shown that glove failure occurs in up to 58% of surgical procedures. Additionally, surface glove contamination occurs often at the time of draping.[77] Yet infection rates do not seem to correlate with glove failure rates.[37,38,77,78] It appears that, although not prospectively and specifically tested, gloves may not reduce infection rates and are mostly useful to protect the surgeon. To that end, double gloving reduces glove failure from 51% to 7%.[79]

Footwear and Covers Shoe covers and tacky mats are not effective in reducing infection rates, since floor contamination does not result in airborne redistribution of bacteria (Level I).[80–82] However, the former may still be useful for protection from blood and other products.

Operating Room Cleansing and Surveillance Although stringent cleansing protocols are abundant, there is no proof of clinical efficacy or cost-effectiveness.[82,83] In dirty cases, debris cleanup is recommended, but the environment bacterial counts after such cases are equivalent to those seen after clean cases.[84] No evidence exists to support extensive cleanup procedures between clean and clean/contaminated cases (see "Wound Classes"). Routine microbiological surveillance of operating theaters is not cost-effective.[83]

In contradistinction, dedicated infection surveillance programs have demonstrated cost-effectiveness.[85] Close monitoring allows evaluation of trends and rapid initiation of required changes based on statistical process control as discussed in Chapter 2.

WOUND CLASSES

The National Research Council has categorized surgical procedures as being clean, clean/contaminated, contaminated, or dirty.[19] The likelihood of operative site infection without and with antibiotic prophylaxis, respectively, is as follows: clean: 1–2% versus 0%; clean/contaminated: 10–20% versus 7%; contaminated: 20–35% versus 10–15%. Within the realm of gynecologic surgery, clean cases are non-traumatic and do not enter the gastrointestinal or genitourinary (GU) tract. In a clean-contaminated case, the vagina or non-infected. GU tract is entered, or the GI tract is entered without significant spillage. A contaminated case involved trauma, major break in technique, gross GI tract spillage or entry into an infected GU tract.

Thus, the only category of surgery for which prophylactic antibiotic use is of benefit is the clean contaminated case (i.e., one that requires operation into or through the vagina). There is insufficient data to warrant use of prophylactic antibiotics for clean procedures. For contaminated or dirty cases, therapeutic antibiotics should be used.

Prophylactic antibiotics administration is generally defined to be perioperative administration not to exceed 24 hours. However, in more recent years, it has been redefined by some to involve a preoperative administration only (Level III),[27,86] unless the surgery extends beyond 4 hours or blood loss has exceeded

1,500 cc (Level I),[87] and if a short half-life antibiotic is used for prophylaxis (e.g., cefoxitin). At least one prospective study specifically addressing patients undergoing radical pelvic surgery suggests improved efficacy of multiple perioperative dosing (Level I).[88]

INTRA-ABDOMINAL AND PELVIC INFECTIONS

Risk factors for intraperitoneal infections include both conditions related to the patient and those related to the operation. Among the former conditions are medical conditions such as obesity, medical conditions such as diabetes mellitus, hypertension, renal or liver disease, and immunosuppressive therapy. Among the latter conditions are duration of surgery, tissue damage (especially injury to the genitourinary [GU] or gastrointestinal [GI] tract), blood loss, and vaginal flora (Level II-3).[89,90]

Gynecologic Ascending Infections

As noted, the vagina normally harbors bacteria, and bacterial vaginosis has been linked to the development of upper genital tract infections, especially at midcycle when the cervical mucus is thin and penetrable or at menses when it is absent. Sexually transmitted disease pathogens such as *Gonococci GC* and *Chlamydia* are thought to damage surface epithelium in an ascending fashion from the endocervix, endometrium, and fallopian tube. The female genital tract is susceptible to infection by other organisms whenever there is instrumentation or surgery performed with contact with the endometrium or endocervix. These areas are impossible to sterilize prophylactically with topical agents.

If peritonitis, without evidence of intra-abdominal gas but with elevated WBC and temperature, is observed, then expectant management with aggressive antibiotic therapy should be continued. However, if peritonitis with evidence of a perforated viscus is noted, surgical intervention is mandatory, since the underlying diagnosis may be in error. Chapter 4 should be consulted for appropriate radiologic testing for developing a differential diagnosis, as well as the Centers for Disease Control Guidelines for Treatment Options.[91]

Bowel-Related Infections

Recognized injury of the unprepared large bowel is associated with both aerobic and anaerobic organism contamination. As already described, a biphasic infection pattern may develop. Peritonitis leading to mortality may occur unless appropriate operative management (i.e., repair of injury with or without colostomy) and prophylactic or therapeutic antibiotic therapy is promptly instituted, depending on the degree of contamination.

Small-bowel contents have a very low concentration of potentially pathogenic organisms, depending on the site and presence or absence of obstruction. In general, recognized injury is treated surgically without antibiotic therapy/prophylaxis. In the presence of bowel obstruction, feculent overgrowth can occur, particularly of anaerobes, and production of endo- and exotoxins can lead to septic shock and death.[92] Details of diagnosis and management of bowel obstruction are addressed in Chapters 4 and 17.

Although newer techniques have dramatically improved diagnostic accuracy, there is absolutely no reliable way to distinguish simple from strangulated obstruction, especially in the presence of carcinomatosis (Level II-2).[93–98] Most would suggest that in the presence of any one of the following classical findings, surgery is indicated: (1) fever, (2) tachycardia, (3) localized tenderness, or (4) leukocytosis.[99] Also, in cases of carcinomatosis-induced obstruction, conservative management is usually futile and the obstruction is often amenable to surgical relief.[98] However, morbidity and cost data suggest that conservative management should be considered when possible.[100,101] Decisions have to be individualized depending on localization of the malignant process, probability of successful bypass/resection, and life expectancy. Although limited by degree of carcinomatosis and adhesive disease, and lack of prospective controlled data, laparoscopy may be useful in diagnosis and management.[102,103]

The use of perioperative antibiotics in simple adhesive small-bowel obstruction has not been proven efficaceous, but studies are ongoing.[104] If employed, coverage should include those species which translocate with any frequency. Specifically, they include *Escherichia coli*, *Proteus* sp., *Klebsiella pneumoniae*, other *Enterobacteriaceae*, *Pseudomonas aeruginosa*, enterococci, lactobacilli, and staphylococci. Usually, clinically significant translocation occurs only under conditions of mucosal injury, which may include mesenteric ischemia and strangulation, but may also be due to radiation or other therapeutic insults.[105] In the presence of ischemia or longer-standing obstruction, feculent environment predisposes to anaerobic predominance.[92,106,107]

Abscesses

The second phase of the biphasic infection pattern, especially if the antibiotic choice was insufficient in its spectrum or activity, is abscess formation. Though there is evidence that abscesses may respond to antibiotic therapy alone, there is a variety of intervention strategies available. It is possible to adequately drain some abscesses with sonographic or radiologic assistance, as reviewed in Chapter 4.

Ultrasound or CT-assisted aspiration (with or without irrigation with Ringer's lactate) may be performed in patients failing antibiotic therapy, especially in postoperative patients in whom reoperative surgery may be hazardous. This therapeutic option should be restricted to individuals in whom there is no evidence of perforation. If there is evidence of perforation, such as with ruptured appendicitis or bowel anastomosis leakage, surgical intervention and correction of the defect is necessary. Exploratory laparotomy may be necessary and is often associated with extirpation of genital tract structures if they are involved, if the patient is unresponsive to antibiotic therapy, and if the patient's clinical condition warrants it.

Lymphocyst Infections

Lymph collections can become infected as a result of direct inoculation from the gut flora or from hematogenous spread. Thus, they are apt to represent mixed infections and should be treated as already discussed with antibiotics and drainage. Prophylactic drains have been proven ineffective in preventing lymphocyst occurrence after radical pelvic surgery.[18–20]

Intravenous Antibiotic Choices

In order to provide antibiotic coverage for aerobes and anaerobes, a variety of therapeutic options can be considered. It has been customary to use combination agents such as penicillin or ampicillin with gentamicin and clindamycin or metronidazole; a monobactam such as aztreonam with clindamycin or metronidazole; a cephamycin such as cefoxitin or cefotetan; a third-generation cephalosporin such as cefotaxime or ceftizoxime alone or with metronidazole; urideopenicillins such as unasyn, timentin, or piperacillin; simple agents with a beta-lactamase inhibitor such as ampicillin with clavulanic acid or piperacillin with tazobactam.[108–111] All of these agents require multiple daily doses and none have an oral therapy equivalent in spectrum and activity alone or in combination.

The newest antibiotic available with spectrum and activity that could be used to treat mixed infections is IV alatrovafloxacin, which is converted to trovafloxacin in the bloodstream, identical to the oral form. This fluoroquinolone antibiotic can be administered once daily with equivalent serum and tissue concentrations, whether administered intravenously or orally (Level I).[112]

Oral Antibiotics: Primary or Completion

The oral antibiotic that follows parenteral antibiotic therapy often does not provide the same spectrum or activity. Exceptions include ciprofloxacin/metronidazole and the newer agent alatrovaloxacin/trovafloxacin. Upon resolution of the peritonitis or upon ability to tolerate enteral medications, oral therapy can be instituted with identical circulating and tissue concentrations as with the IV therapy. Completion therapy for intra-abdominal infection with oral antibiotics has been shown to be effective (Level I).[113] Also, in selected cases, the oral form may be administered primarily. There is insufficient data to provide guidelines for duration of total therapy. Convention has dictated that for infections without abscesses, a 5- to 7-day course of therapy should be administered, while for those with abscesses, a 10- to 14-day course should be administered (Level III).[91] Randomized controlled trials are lacking and are indicated.[110]

EXTRA-ABDOMINAL INFECTIONS

Pneumonia

Nosocomial pneumonia is defined as occurring more than 48 hours after hospital admission and is the most common cause of nosocomial infection–induced mortality.[114] The average addition to length of stay is 9 days, which has a significant economic impact.[115] The most common isolates are aerobic gram-negative rods and *S. aureus*, aspirated from the oropharynx. Mortality rates have been higher with the former, especially when the organism is *P. aeruginosa.*

Mechanical ventilation is often complicated by nosocomial pneumonia, with a relative risk of 7 to 10 times that seen in nonventilated patients. Each hospital and intensive care facility monitors that pathogens associated with these infections. Selective pressures from antibiotic usage leading to resistant organisms responsible for these infections have been routinely reported and may explain the high death rate despite the availability of poten antibiotics. Additionally, breakdowns in standard protocols for ventilator management may lead to infections. Contamination of the condensate forming in the tubing is frequent. If this condensate is not drained frequently and the tubing is not changed every 24 to 48 hours (CDC recommendation is 24 hours), it may be inoculated into the tracheobronchial tree during patient positioning. As few as 10 gram-negative bacilli introduced into the lower airways can produce pneumonia.[116–118]

Personnel may also be responsible for horizontal infection spread (e.g., lack of hand washing or gloving). Although ventilator-associated pneumonia may be due to aspiration of refluxed pathogens colonizing the stomach and duodenum, studies involving selective enteral antibiotic decontamination of the digestive tract as prophylaxis have produced conflicting results. Additionally, although the risk of respiratory infection seems to be decreased in most series, there has been no substantial reduction in overall mortality.[119,120]

Empiric treatment should be based on clinical findings and Gram's stain results from an uncontaminated sputum specimen or tracheal aspirate. Although broncho-alveolar lavage or protected specimen brushing may be more sensitive or specific, the cost-effectiveness is not clear. Radiographic assessment and implications are addressed in Chapter 5.

Treatment modifications are based on clinical response and sensitivity patterns. Consideration should be given to hospital surveillance–based resistance trends. Following are general guidelines:[121–123]

1. Patients with *P. aeruginosa* pneumonia should receive combination therapy with a beta-lactam and an aminoglycoside.

2. In critically ill patients with nosocomial pneumonia due to other gram-negative rods, combination regimens should also be considered. If clinical response is readily apparent, the aminoglycoside may be discontinued. Monotherapy with a beta-lactam may be considerd in less critically ill patients.

3. If monotherapy is selected, the possibility of superinfection and drug resistance should be kept in mind, especially if clinical response is suboptimal.

4. Vancomycin should be initiated for *S. aureus* pneumonia if methicillin resistance (MRSA) is demonstrated.

Lower Urinary Tract Infections

Diagnosis is established based on symptomatology and Gram's stain of uncentrifuged urine showing >1 organism/high-powered field, especially in the presence of pyuria. This amount correlates with a bacteriuria of >100,000 CFU/ml.

Empiric therapy for uncomplicated lower-tract infections should be based on local hospital infection surveillance susceptibility patterns, Gram stain, and patient issues such as allergies, age, and renal function. Multiple recommendations include trimethoprim/sulfamethoxazole, nitrofurantoin, and fluoroquinolone.

Pyelonephritis

Empiric initial therapy is based on the findings associated with UTI along with costovertebral angle (CVA) tenderness, often associated with a higher fever. Ampicillin and gentamicin are often used, as they provide coverage for the often encountered gram-negative bacilli and enterococci. Alternatives include the quinolones, ciprofloxacin, and trovafloxacin. Monotherapy with ceftazidime or aztreonam provides good gram-negative coverage, including for *P. aeruginosa*, but lacks enterococcal coverage. In the event of progressive systemic sepsis, multiagent regimens targeting gram-negative rods and enterococci should be selected. Modifications should be based on clinical response and culture and sensitivity profiles.

CLOSTRIDIUM DIFFICILE COLITIS

Pseudomembranous antibiotic-induced colitis is now a common complication of prolonged broad-spectrum antibiotic therapy.[124] Flexible sigmoidoscopy can quickly identify pseudomembranes in most cases. However, testing for stool cytotoxin presence is more sensitive and is highly specific.[125] Treatment is oral metronidazole for mild to moderate cases, based on equal efficacy, less cost, and less morbidity than vancomycin (Level I).[126] For severe cases, vancomycin continues to be the agent of choice. Patients in whom *C. difficile* is not found, but who have symptoms of enteric infection, can be treated with oral quinolones. In the presence of associated bacteremia, a third-generation cephalosporin is effective against the most common offending pathogens: *Campylobacter*, *Salmonella*, *Shigella*, and *E. coli*.

INCISIONAL WOUND INFECTION

Seromas or infected surgical wounds generally respond to opening, irrigation, debridement, packing with fine mesh gauze with daily irrigation, debridement, and redressing as necessary. Normal saline should be used, not Dakin's solution or iodophor, as these agents lead to decreased wound macrophage and fibroblast function, retarding the healing process. After 3 or 4 days, if the wound looks healthy, it can be reapproximated. Closure by secondary intention generally takes many weeks to months and frequently leads to a less satisfactory cosmetic result.

If the wound is associated with cellulitis, antibiotic therapy may be necessary. Early wound infection with red striae may suggest group A or B hemolytic streptococci and may require therapy with penicillin and clindamycin or cephalosporins. Should the wound not bleed, or if the patient cannot feel the surgical manipulations, the diagnosis of necrotizing fasciitis should be considered, which may be associated with aerobic and anaerobic organisms, especially *Streptococcus*, group A, C, or G, and *Clostridia* species. Findings may include rapidly spreading erythema and subcutaneous crepitus. Treatment should consist of penicillin and clindamycin, and possibly gentamicin, with aggressive surgical resection of diseased tissue to margins that bleed. This surgical course may be required multiple times daily because this disease may pursue a fulminant course with development of multiple-organ dysfunction.[127]

SYSTEMIC SEPSIS

The definitions of systemic inflammatory response syndrome and sepsis are presented in Chapter 6. Empiric antibiotic selection guidelines for sepsis are as follows (Level III):[128-130]

1. Initial treatment: aminoglycoside (gentamicin, tobramycin, or amikacin) plus one of the following:

   Third-generation cephalosporin (cefotaxime, ceftizoxime, or ceftriaxone)

   Ticarcillin-clavulanic acid

   Imipenem

2. Suspected methicillin-resistant *S. aureus:*

   Add vancomycin with or without rifampin

3. Intra-abdominal or pelvic infection:

   Metronidazole or clindamycin plus aminoglycocide

   Any of the following with or without an aminoglycoside: ticarcillin-clavulanic acid, piperacillin-tazobactam, ampicillin-sulbactam, imipenem, cefoxitin, or cefotetan

4. Urinary tract infection origin:

   Third-generation cephalosporin with or without an aminoglycoside

      Ticarcillin-clavulanate or piperacillin-tazobactam

      Imipenem with or without an aminoglycoside

5. Neutropenia (Level II-3):[131–133]

      Ceftazidime with or without an aminoglycoside

      Imipenem with or without an aminoglycoside

      Ceftriaxone and amikacin (both in single daily dose)[134]

      Piperacillin-tazobactam plus amikacin in single daily dose[135]

      Modifications for item 5 may include:

      Infections of oral cavity, or GI tract, or perianal region: add clindamycin or metronidazole

      IV catheter–associated infections: add vancomycin

      Documented infection by GNB (especially *P. aeruginosa*, *Enterobacter*, or *Serratia*): add aminoglycoside

      Prolonged neutropenia or persistent fever: antifungal therapy

      Outpatient completion: ciprofloxacin or trovafloxacin

      Combination therapy:

      Antipseudomonal pericillin (piperacillin, mezlocillin, or ticarcillin) plus an aminoglycoside

      Once daily amikacin plus ceftriaxone[136]

      Tricarcillin-clavulanate with or without an aminoglycoside

      Piperacillin-tazobactam with or without an aminoglycoside[137]

      Aztreonam plus an aminoglycoside

6. Endocarditis: penicillin G (or ampicillin), vancomycin, and gentamicin

7. Fungal infection: *Candida* species accounts for approximately 78% of all nosocomial fungal infections while *Candida albicans* accounts for 76% of all *Candida* infections, which increased from 52% in 1980 to 63% as of 1990.[138–140] This increase in fungemia is thought to reflect the use of total parenteral nutrition, central venous catheterization, and broad-spectrum antibiotics. Mortality, partly because of the fungemia, was 29%—a significant increase from the 17% mortality caused by other pathogens ($P < 0.001$; Level III).[138,139] Risk factors for candidemia include presence of a central venous catheter, urinary catheter, and use of systemic antibiotics and steroids.[141,142] Meticulous aseptic technique when inserting and managing indwelling catheters and shortening inpatient systemic antibiotic usage, if possible, should reduce the risk of fungemia (Level II-1).[143–145]

     In a small comparative study of surgical patients with systemic mycosis, those receiving the combination therapy with amphotericin B/5-flucytosine showed an earlier elimination than patients on monotherapy with fluconazole; however, there were no significantly different cure rates between these therapies (Level I).[146]

G-CSF or GM-CSF increases WBC, but most studies show marginal improvement in rate of response, no change in duration of hospitalization, and no improvement in survival (Level II-3).[147] Monoclonal therapies and specific cytokine-based interventions do not presently have a role in most perioperative infection scenarios, although exciting research is ongoing.

PHARMACOECONOMICS

Description of the various forms of economic analysis is provided in Chapter 2. Use of pharmacoeconomics in formulary decision making provides a better alternative to purchasing the "cheapest" agent as measured by unit cost. Incorporating outcomes analysis and proper attention to total, relevant cost data gathering allows equitable comparison of agents and results in optimized care rather than simple cost cutting.

Economic assessment of antibiotic use should generally be based on comparison of marginal or incremental benefits with marginal costs of administration. This holds true for prophylaxis as well as therapeutic use. As noted in Chapter 2, the actual definition of *costs*, and accurate assigning thereof, significantly influences the outcome analysis. Opportunity costs and human suffering/morbidity cost should not be lost in favor of pure economics. Wasteful infection control measures, such as use of prophylactic antibiotics for greater than 24 hours, compromises patient care and is a reflection of poor scarce resources utilization.

With respect to direct costs, evaluating excess costs of infection per operation takes into account: (1) the costs of infection care, (2) the infection rate, and (3) the number of surgical procedures performed per year.[32] On an excess cost per case basis, clean operations may not rank very highly due to the low expected rate of infection. However, due to the volume of cases, excess cost per year may total more than the clean/contaminated to dirty cases on a sheer volume basis. These factors should be considered in determining the effectiveness of infection-control measures, including use of prophylactic antibiotics and duration of administration.[148]

Formulary decisions and antibiotic usage may be made based on the following types of analyses, depending on the question being posed:

Cost minimization: Do the products have the same patient outcomes but differing vendor prices?

Cost-effectiveness: What is the total cost of therapy versus the outcomes gained if the agents are dissimilar in patient outcomes?

Cost utility: Which antibiotic treatment results in optimal patient outcomes when adjusted for patient preferences (e.g., side effects, duration, and route of therapy, inpatient/outpatient)?

Cost-benefit: Which program area (e.g., antibiotics) of the formulary requires greatest attention and more benefit per dollar due to higher ascribed value of outcomes than another program (e.g., antihypertensives)?

Prior to economic evaluation, clinical effectiveness must be clearly demonstrated. If antibiotic therapy fails, surgery with extirpation of organs or prolonged intensive care is very costly, no matter how costs are defined, and suffering may be extreme. Unfortunately, in many areas there are insufficient definitive studies suggesting that one antibiotic or one combination of antibiotics is superior to another. We are left with having to examine the outcomes of various therapies for the treatment of specific conditions. In the case of treatment of presumed tubo-ovarian abscesses, therapy with a cephamycin with doxycycline or gentamicin, or tobramycin with clindamycin, may fail 15% to 22% of the time (Level I).[149,150]

In earlier reports, antibiotic therapy with similar agents was associated with the need for operative intervention approximately one-third of the time during the primary hospitalization. Additionally, approximately one-third of those who initially responded required surgery with extirpation of some pelvic structures before being cured of their infection (Level I).[151] With such a high failure rate when employing standard therapies, alternate therapies such as alatrovafloxacin/trovafloxacin should be considered and further researched encouraged.

Each intravenous administration is costly, averaging $58 per administration at LA County USC Medical Center. Thus, multiple drug and dosing daily may be far more costly than the direct unit cost of the drug alone, sometimes overshadowing the inflated costs of new agents. Even if the efficacy of a new single daily dose agent is not superior to conventional therapies, there may be a favorable cost-effectiveness ratio to the use of single daily dosing. While clinical and economic evaluation of antibiotic usage is very complex and currently imprecise, treatment patterns should not be based on the best drug detailer pitch or personal anecdotal experience alone. Audit programs, incorporating infection-control surveillance and outcomes analysis, have been proposed as effective means of eliminating wasteful practices while optimizing care.[152]

REFERENCES

1. Galicier C, Richet H. A prospective study of postoperative fever in a general surgery department. *Infect Control* 1985;6:487.
2. Locker D, Norwood SH, Torma MJ, et al. A prospective randomized study of drained and undrained cholecystectomies. *Am Surg* 1983;49:528.
3. Lewis JH, Zimmerman HJ, Ishak KG, et al. Enflurane hepatotoxicity: a clinicopathologic study of 24 cases. *Ann Intern Med* 1983;98:984.
4. Lewis RT, Allan CM, Godall RG, et al. The conduct of cholecystectomy: incision, drainage, bacteriology, and postoperative complications. *Can J Surg* 1982;25:304.

5. Soper DE. Delayed hemolytic transfusion reaction: a cause of late postoperative fever. *Am J Abstet Gynecol* 1985;153:227.

6. Bidwell DE, Bartlett A, Voller A. Enzyme immunoassays for viral diseases. *J Infect Dis* 1977;136:271–277.

7. Weinstein WM, Onderdonk AB, Bartlett JG, Gorbach SL. Experimental intra-abdominal abscesses in rats: development of an experimental model. *Infect Immunol* 1974;10:1250–1255.

8. Kelly MJ. The quantitative and histological demonstration of pathogenic synergy between *Escherichia coli* and *Bacteroides fragilis* in guinea-pig wounds. *J Microbiol* 1976;11:513–523.

9. Goldmann DA, Pier GB. Pathogenesis of infections related to intravascular catheterization. *Clin Microbiol Rev* 1993;6:176–192.

10. Raad II, Bodey GP. Infectious complications of indwelling vascular catheters. *Clin Infect Dis* 1992;15:197–210.

11. Gristina AG. Biomaterial-centered infection: microbial adherence versus tissue integration. *Science* 1987;237:1588–1595.

12. Garibaldi RA, Burke JP, Dickman ML, et al. Factors predisposing to bacteriuria during indwelling urethral catheterization. *N Engl J Med* 1974;291:215–219.

13. Kunin CM, McCormack RC. Prevention of catheter-induced urinary tract infections by sterile closed drainage. *N Engl J Med* 1966;274:1155–1161.

14. Warren JW. Catheter-associated urinary tract infections. *Infect Dis Clin N Am* 1987;1:823–854.

15. Warren JW, Damron D, Tenney JH, et al. Fever, bacteremia and death as complications of bacteriuria in women with long term urethral catheters. *J Infect Dis* 1987;155:1551–1158.

16. Reid G, Densedt JD, Yang YS, et al. Microbial adhesion and biofilm formation on ureteral stents in vitro and in vivo. *J Urol* 1992;148:1592–1594.

17. Platt R, Polk BF, Murdock B, et al. Risk factors for nosocomial urinary tract infection. *Am J Epidemiol* 1986;124:977–985.

18. Lopes AD, Hall JR, Monaghan JM. Drainage following radical hysterectomy and pelvic lymphadenectomy: dogma or need? *Obstet Gynecol* 1995;86(6):960–963.

19. Jensen JK, Lucci JA, DiSaia PJ, Manetta A, Berman ML. To drain or not to drain: a retrospective study of closed-suction drainage following radical hysterectomy with pelvic lymphadenectomy. *Gynecol Oncol* 1993;51:46–49.

20. Franchi M, Ghezzi F, Zanaboni F, Scarabelli C, Beretta P, Donadello N. Nonclosure of peritoneum at radical abdominal hysterectomy and pelvic node dissection: a randomized study. *Obstet Gynecol* 1997;90(4, Pt 1):622–627.

21. Hoffman J, Shokouh-Amiri M, Damm, Jensen R. A prospective controlled study of prophylactic drainage after colonic anastamosis. *Dis Colon Rectum* 1987;30;449–452.

22. Groeger JS, Lucas AB, Coit D, et al. A prospective randomized evaluation of silver-impregnated subcutaneous cuffs for preventing tunneled chronic venous access catheter infections in cancer patients. *Ann Surg* 1993;218:206–210.

23. Babycos CR, Barracas A, Webb WR. A prospective randomized trial comparing

silver impregnated collagen cuff with the bedside tunneled subclavian catheter. *J Parenter Enteral Nutr* 1993;17:61–63.

24. Arnow PM, Quimosing EM, Beach M. Consequences of intravascular catheter sepsis. *Clin Infect Dis* 1993;16:778–784.

25. Maki DG. Pathogenesis, prevention, and management of infections due to intravascular devices used for infusion therapy. In *Infections Associated with Indwelling Medical Devices*. Washington, DC: American Association for Microbiology, 1989, pp. 161–177.

26. Verghese A, Widrich WC, Arbeit RD. Central venous septic thrombophlebitis: the role of medical therapy. *Medicine* 1985;64:394.

27. Roy S, Wilkins J. Comparison of cefotaxime to cefazolin for prophylaxis of vaginal or abdominal hysterectomy. *Clin Ther* 1982;5(suppl A):74.

28. Amstey MS, Jones AP. Preparation of the vagina for surgery: a comparison of povidone-iodine and saline solution. *JAMA* 1992;245:839–842.

29. Garibaldi RA, Skolnick D, Lerer T, et al. The impact of preoperative skin disinfection or preventing intraoperative wound contamination. *Infect Control Hosp Epidemiol* 1988;9:109.

30. Garibaldi RA. Prevention of intraoperative wound contamination with chlorhexidine shower adn scrub. *J Hosp Infect.* 1988;11(suppl B):5.

31. Lynch W, Davey PG, Malek M, et al. Cost effectiveness analysis of the use of chlorhexidine detergent in preoperative whole-body disinfection in wound prophylaxis. *J Hosp Infect* 1992;21:179.

32. Lynch W, Malek M, Davey PG, et al. Costing wound infection in a Scottish hospital. *PharmacoEconomics* 1992;2:163–170.

33. Ritter MA, French MLV, Eitzen HE, et al. The antimicrobial effectiveness of operative site preparative agents: a microbiological and clinical study. *J Bone Joint Surg* 1980;62A:826.

34. Davies J, Babb JR, Ayliffe GAJ, et al. Disinfection of the skin of the abdomen. *Br J Surg* 1978;65:855.

35. Sebben JE, Surgical antiseptics. *J Am Acad Dermatol* 1983;9:759.

36. Brown TR, Ehrlich CE, Stehman FB, et al. A clinical evaluation of chlorhexidine gluconate spray as compared with iodophor scrub for preoperative skin preparation. *Surg Gynecol Obstet* 1984;158:363–366.

37. Cruse PJE. Wound infections: epidemiology and clinical characteristics. In Simmons R, Howard R (Eds), *Surgical Infectious Diseases*. New York: Appleton-Century-Crofts, 1982, p. 429–441.

38. Cruse PJE. Some factors determining wound infection: a prospective study of 30,000 wounds. In Polle HC Jr, Stone HH (Eds), *Hospital-Acquired Infections in Surgery*. Baltimore: University Park Press, 1977, pp. 77–85.

39. Polk HC, Simpson CJ, Simmons BP, Alexander JW. Guidelines for prevention of surgical wound infection. *Arch Surg* 1983;118:1213–1217.

40. Alexander JW, Fischer JE, Boyajian M, et al. The influence of hair removal methods on wound infections. *Arch Surg* 1983;118:347.

41. Seropian R, Reynolds BM. Wound infections after preoperative dipilatory versus razor preparation. *Am J Surg* 1971;121:251.

42. Bird BJ, Chrisp DB, Scrimgeour G. Extensive preoperative shaving: a costly experience. *NZ Med J* 1984;97;727.

43. Price PB. The bacteriology of normal skin: a new quantitative test applied to a study of bacterial flora and the disinfectant action of mechanical cleansing. *J Infect Dis* 1988;63:301.

44. Kozol RA, Fromm D, Ackerman NB, Chung R. Wound closure in obese patients. *Surg Gynecol Obstet* 1986;162:442–444.

45. Farnell MB, Worthington-Self S, Mucha P Jr, Ilstrup DM, McIlrath DC. Closure of abdominal incisions with subcutaneous catheters. A prospective randomized trial. *Arch Surg* 1986;121:641–648.

46. DeHoll D, et al. Potentiation of infection by suture closure of dead space. *Am J Surg* 1974;127:716–720.

47. Edlich RF, et al. Technique of closure: contaminated wounds. *J Am Coll Emerg Phys* 1974;3:375–381.

48. Edlich RF, Rogers W, Kasper G, Kaufman D, Tsung MS, Wangensteen OH. Studies in the management of the contaminated wound. I. Optimal time for closure of contaminated open wounds. II. Comparison of resistance to infection of open and closed wounds during healing. *Am J Surg* 1969;117:323–329.

49. Robson MC, et al. Quantitative bacteriology and delayed wound closure. *S Forum* 1968;19:510–502.

50. Robson MC, Krizek TJ. Predicting skin graft survival. *J Trauma* 1973;13:213–217.

51. Dodson MK, Magann EF, Meeks RF. A randomized comparison of secondary closure and secondary intention in patients with superficial wound dehiscence. *Obstet Gynecol* 1992;80;321–324.

52. Madden JC, et al. Application of principles of fluid dynamics to surgical wound irrigation. *Curr Topics Surg Res* 1971;3:85–93.

53. Stevenson TR, et al. Cleansing the traumatic wound by high pressure syringe irrigation. *J Am Coll Emerg Phys* 1976;5:17–21.

54. Wheeler CB, et al. Side effects of high pressure irrigation. *Surg Gynecol Obstet* 1976;143:775–778.

55. Conolly WB, et al. Clinical comparison of surgical wounds by suture and adhesive tapes. *Am J Surg* 1969;117;318–322.

56. Carpendale MTF, Sereda W. The role of percutaneous suture in surgical wound infection. *Surgery* 1965;58:672–677.

57. Spotnitz WD, Falstrom JK, Rodeheaver GT. The role of sutures and fibrin sealant in wound healing. *Surg Clin N Am* 1997;77(3):651–669.

58. Edlich RF, Becker DG, Thacker JG, Rodeheaver GT. Scientific basis for selecting staple and tape skin closures. *Clin Plast Surg* 1990;17:571–578.

59. Rodeheaver GT, McLance M, West L, Edlich RF. Evaluation of surgical tapes for wound closure. *J Surg Res* 1985;39:251–257.

60. Pickford IR, Brennan SS, Evans M, Pollock AV. Two methods of skin closure in abdominal operations: a controlled clinical trial. *Br J Surg* 1983;70:226–228.

61. Pepicello J, Yavorek H. Five year experience with tape closure of abdominal wounds. *Surg Gynecol Obstet* 1989;4:310–314.

62. Webster DJ, Davis PW. Closure of abdominal wounds by adhesive strips: a clinical trial. *Br Med J* 1975;20:696–698.

63. Casewell M, Phillips I. Hands as a route of transmission for *Klebsiella* species. *Br J Med* 1977;2:1315–1317.

64. Casewell MW, Law MM, Desai N. A laboratory model for testing agents for hygienic hand disinfection: handwashing and chlorhexidine for the removal of *Klebsiella. J Hosp Infect* 1988;12:163–165.

65. Dineen P. An evaluation of the duration of the surgical scrub. *Surg Gynecol Obstet* 1969;129:1181.

66. Lowbury EJL, Lilly HA, Bull JP. Methods for disinfection of hands and operation sites. *Br Med J* 1964;2:531–532.

67. Lowbury EJL, Lilly HA. Use of 4% chlorhexidine detergent solution and other methods of skin disinfection. *Br Med J* 1973;1:510–512.

68. Larson E. Guideline for use of topical antimicrobial agents. *Am J Infect Control* 1988;16:253–256.

69. Hingst V, Juditzki I, Heeg P, et al. Evaluation of the efficacy of surgical hand disinfection following a reduced application time of 3 instead of 5 minutes. *J Hosp Infect* 1992;20:79–82.

70. Ayliffe GAJ. Surgical scrub and skin disinfection. *Infect Control Hosp Epidemiol* 1984;5:23–25.

71. Knolle P, Globel B, Globel H, et al. Release of iodide from povidone-iodine in PVP-1 preparations: a review of iodide tolerances and a comparative clinical pharmacology study. *Proceedings of the International Symposium of Povidone.* University of Kentucky College of Pharmacy, Lexington, 1983, p. 342.

72. Aly R, Maibach HI. Comparative antibacterial efficacy of a 2-minute scrub with chlorhexidine gluconate, povidone iodine and chloroxylenol sponge brushes. *Am J Infect Control* 1988;16:173–176.

73. Bicknell PG. Sensoneural deafness following myringoplasty operations. *J Laryngol Otol* 1971;85:957.

74. Ha'eri GB, Wiley AM. The efficacy of standard surgical face masks: an investigation using tracer particles. *Clin Orthop* 1980;148:160.

75. Orr MWM. Is a mask necessary in the operating theatre? *Ann R Coll Surg Engl* 1981;63:390.

76. Tunevall TG. Postoperative wound infections and surgical face masks: a controlled study. *World J Surg* 1991;15:383.

77. McCue SF, Berg EW, Sanders EA. Efficacy of double gloving as a barrier to microbial contamination during total joint arthroplasty. *J Bone Joint Surg* 1981;63:811.

78. Albin MS, Bunegin L, Duke ES, et al. Anatomy of a defective barrier: sequential glove leak detection in a surgical and dental environment. *Crit Care Med* 1992;20:170.

79. Quebbeman EJ, Telford GL, Wadsworth K, et al. Double gloving: protecting surgeons from blood contamination in the operating room. *Arch Surg* 1992;127:213.

80. Ritter MA, Sieber JM, Carlson SR. Street shoes versus surgical footwear in the operating room. *Infect Surg* 1984;3:81.

81. Garner JS, Emori TG, Haley RW. Operating room practices for the control of

infection in U.S. hospitals, October 1976 to July 1977. *Surg Gynecol Obstet* 1982;155:873.

82. Weber DO, Gooch JJ, Wood WR, et al. Influence of operating room surface contamination on surgical wounds—a prospective study. *Arch Surg* 1976;111:484.

83. Maki DG, Alvarado CJ, Hassemer CA, et al. Relation of inanimate hospital environment to endemic nosocomial infection. *N Engl J Med* 1982;307:1562.

84. Hambraeus A, Bengtsson S, Laurell G. Bacterial contamination in a modern operating suite: III. Importance of floor contamination as a source of airborne bacteria. *J Hygiene* 1978;80:169.

85. Olson M, O'Connor M, Schwartz ML. Surgical wound infections: a 5-year prospective study of 20,193 wounds in the Minneapolis VA Medical Center. *Ann Surg* 1984;199:253.

86. Roy S, Wilkins J. Single dose cefotaxime versus 3 to 5 doses cefoxitin for prophylaxis of vaginal or abdominal hysterectomy. *J Antimicrobial Chemother* 1984;14(suppl B):217–221.

87. Roy S, Hemsell D, Gordon S, Godwin D, Pearlman M, Luke D. Oral trovafloxacin compared with intravenous cefoxitin in the prevention of bacterial infection after elective vaginal or abdominal hysterectomy for nonmalignant disease. *Am J Surg* 1998;176(6A suppl):625–665.

88. Cartana J, Cortes J, Yarnoz MC, Rossello JJ. Antibiotic prophylaxis in Wertheim–Meigs surgery. A single dose vs. three doses. *Eur J Gynaecol Oncol* 1994;15:14–18.

89. Soper DE, Bump RC, Hurt WG. Bacterial vaginosis and trichomoniasis vaginitis are risk factors for cuff cellulitis after abdominal hysterectomy. *AJOG* 1990;163:1016–1023.

90. Larsson PG, Platz-Christensen JJ, Forsum U, Pahlson C. Clue cells in predicting infections after abdominal hysterectomy. *Obstet Gynecol* 1991;77:450–452.

91. Centers for Disease Control and Prevention. *Morbidity and Mortality Weekly Report, 1998 Guidelines for Treatment of Sexually Transmitted Diseases*, p. 47.

92. Sykes PA, Boulter KH, Schofield PF. The microflora of the obstructed bowel. *Br J Surg* 1976;63:721–724.

93. Silen W, Hein MF, Goldman L. Strangulation obstruction of the intestine. *Arch Surg* 1962;85:137–141.

94. Sarr MG, Bulkley GB, Zuidema GA. Pre-operative recognition of intestinal strangulation obstruction. *Am J Surg* 1983;145:176–180.

95. Osteen RT, Guyton S, Steele G Jr, et al. Malignant intestinal obstruction. *Surgery* 1980;87:611–614.

96. Donckier V, Closset J, Van Gansbeke D, Zalcman M, Sy M, Houben JJ, Lambilliotte JP. Contribution of computed tomography to decision making in the management of adhesive small bowel obstruction. *Br J Surg* 1998;85(8);1071–1074.

97. Taourel PG, Fabre JM, Pradel JA, Seneterre EJ, Megibow AJ, Bruel JM. Value of CT in the diagnosis and management of patients with suspected acute small-bowel obstruction. *AJR* 1995;165(5):1187–1192.

98. Tang E, Davis J, Silberman H. Bowel obstruction in cancer patients. *Arch Surg* 1995;130(8):832–836.

99. Stewardson RH, Bombeck CT, Nyhus LM. Critical operative management of small bowel obstruction. *Ann Surg* 1978;187:189–192.

100. Krebs HB, Helmkamp BF. Management of intestinal obstruction in ovarian cancer. *Oncology* 1989;3(5):25–31.

101. Asbun HJ, Pempinello C, Halasz NA. Small bowel obstruction and its management. *Int Surg* 1989;74(1):23–27.

102. Franklin ME Jr, Dorman JP, Pharand D. Laparoscopic surgery in acute small bowel obstruction. *Surg Laparoscopy Endoscopy* 1994;4(4):289–296.

103. Memon MA, Fitzgibbons RJ Jr. The role of minimal access surgery in the acute abdomen. *Surg Clin. N Am* 1997;77(6):1333–1353.

104. Fabian TC, Mangiante EC, Boldreghini SJ. Prophylactic antibiotics for elective colorectal surgery or operation for obstruction of the samll bowel: a comparison of cefonicid and cefoxitin. *Rev Infect Dis* 1984;6:S896–900.

105. Morehouse JL, Specian RD, Stewart JJ, et al. Translocation of indigenous bacteria from the gastrointestinal tract of mice after oral ricinoleic acid treatment. *Gastroenterology* 1986;91:673–675.

106. Bennion RS, Wilson SE, Serota AI, et al. The role of gastrointestinal microflora in the pathogenesis of complications of mesenteric ischemia. *J Infect Dis* 1984;6:S132–S135.

107. Bennion RS, Wilson SE, Williams RA. Early portal anaerobic bacteremia in mesenteric ischemia. *Arch Surg* 1984;119:151–154.

108. Gonzenbach HR, Simmen HP, Amgwerd R. Imipenem (N-F-thienamycin) versus netilmicin plus clindamycin. A controlled and randomized comparison in intra-abdominal infections. *Ann Surg* 1987;205(3):271–275.

109. Solomkin JS, Fant WK, Rivera JO, et al. Randomized clinical trial of imipenam-cilastin to gentamicin-clindamycin in mixed flora infections. *Am J Med* 1985;78:85–89.

110. Solomkin JS. Duration of antibiotic treatment in surgical infections of the abdomen. The future: randomised prospective studies. *Eur J Surg* 1996;S576:33–35.

111. Barie PS, Vogel SB, Dellinger EP, Rotstein OD, Solomkin JS, Yang JY, Baumgartner TF. A randomized, double-blind clinical trial comparing cefepime plus metronidazole with imipenem-cilastatin in the treatment of complicated intra-abdominal infections. Cefepime Intra-abdominal Infection Study Group. *Arch Surg* 1997;132(12):1294–1302.

112. Roy S, Koltun W, Chatwani A, Martens M, Dittrich R, Luke D. Treatment of acute gynecologic infections with trovafloxacin. *Am J Surg* 1998;176(6A suppl):675–735.

113. Solomkin JS, Dellinger EP, Bohnen JM, Rostein OD. The role of oral antimicrobials for the management of intra-abdominal infections. *New Horizons* 1998;6(suppl 2):S46–52.

114. Craven DE, Steger KA, Barber TW. Preventing nosocomial pneumonia. State of the art and perspectives for the 1990's. *Am J Med* 1991;3B:44S–53S.

115. Leu HS, Kaiser DL, Mori M, et al. Hospital-acquired pneumonia. Attributable mortality and morbidity. *Am J Epidemiol* 1989;129:1258–1266.

116. Craven DE, Steger KA. Nosocomial pneumonia in the intubated patient. New concepts on pathogenesis and prevention. *Infect Dis Clin N Am* 1989;3:843–866.

117. Simmons BP, Wong ES. Guidelines for prevention of nosocomial pneumonia. *Infect Control Hosp Epidemiol* 1982;3:327–333.

118. Torres A, Aznar R, Gatell JM, et al. Incidence risk and prognosis factors of nosocomial pneumonia in mechanically ventilated patients. *Am Rev Respir Dis* 1990;152:523–528.

119. Ferrer M, Torres A, Gonzalez J, de la Bellacasa JP, El-Ebiary M, Roca M, Gatell JM, Rodriguez-Roisin R. Utility of selective digestive decontamination in mechanically ventilated patients. *Ann Intern Med* 1994;120:389–395.

120. Kollef MH. The role of selective digestive tract decontamination on mortality and respiratory tract infections. *Chest* 1994;105:1101–1108.

121. Lerner AM. The gram-negative bacillary pneumonias. *Dis Mon* 1980;26:10–11.

122. LaForce FM. Systemic antimicrobial therapy of nosocomial pneumonia. Monotherapy versus combination therapy. *Eur J Clin Microbiol* 1989;8:61–68.

123. Clone LA, Woodward DR, Stoltzman DS, et al. Ceftazidime versus tobramycin-ticarcillin in the treatment of pneumonia and bacteremia. *Antimicrob Agents Chemother* 1985;28:33–36.

124. Kelly CP, Pothoulakis C, LaMont JT. *Clostridium difficile* colitis. *N Engl J Med* 1994;330:257–262.

125. Doern GV, Coughlin RT, Wu L. Laboratory diagnosis of *Clostridium difficile* associated gastrointestinal disease: comparison of a monoclonal antibody enzyme immunoassay for toxins A and B with a monoclonal antibody enzyme immunoassay for toxin A only and two cytotoxicity assays. *J Clin Microbiol* 1992;30:2042–2046.

126. Teasley DG, Gerding DN, Olson MM, et al. Prospective randomized study of metronidazole versus vancomycin for *Clostridium difficile* associated diarrhoea and colitis. *Lancet* 1983;2:1043–1046.

127. Nolan TE, King LA, Smith RP, Gallup DC. Necrotizing surgical infection and necrotizing fascitis in obstetric and gynecologic patients. *South Med J* 1993;86:1363–1367; *Obstet Gynecol* 1995;86(6):960–963.

128. Gibson J, Johnson L, Snowdon L, Joshua D, Young G, MacLeod C, Iland H, Vincent P, Kronenberg H. A randomized dosage study of ceftazidime with single daily tobramycin for the empirical management of febrile neutropenia in patients with hematological diseases. *Int J Hematol* 1994;60:119.

129. Anonymous. Efficacy and toxicity of single daily doses of amikacin and ceftriaxone versus multiple daily doses of amikacin and ceftazidime for infection in patients with cancer and granulocytopenia. The International Antimicrobial Therapy Cooperative Group of the European Organization for Research and Treatment of Cancer. *Ann Inter Med* 1993;119:584.

130. *Medical Letter* 1996;38:25–30.

131. Pizzo PA, Hathorn JW, Hiemenz J, Browne M, Commers J, Cotton D, Gress J, Longo D, Marshall D, McKnight J, et al. A randomized trial comparing ceftazidime alone with combination antibiotic therapy in cancer patients with fever and neutropenia. *New Engl J Med* 1986;315:552.

132. DePauw BE, Deresinkski SC, Feld R, Lane-Allman EF, Donnelly JP. Ceftazidime

compared with piperacillin and tobramycin for the empiric treatment of fever in neutropenic patients with cancer. A multicenter randomized trial. The Intercontinental Antimicrobial Study Group. *Ann Intern Med* 1994;120:834.

133. Winston DJ, Ho WG, Bruckner DA, Champlin RE. Beta-lactam antibiotic therapy in febrile granulocytopenic patients. A randomized trial comparing cefoperazone plus piperacillin, ceftazidime plus piperacillin, and imipenem alone. *Ann Intern Med* 1991;115:849.

134. Freifeld AG, Walsh T, Marshall D, Gress J, Steinberg SM, Hathorn J, Rubin M, Jarosinski P, Gill V, Young RC, et al. Monotherapy for fever and neutropenia in cancer patients: a randomized comparison of ceftazidime versus imipenem. *J Clin Oncol* 1995;13:165.

135. Cometta A, Calandra T, Gaya H, Zinner SH, deBock R, Del Favero A, Bucaneve G, Crokaert F, Kern WV, Klastersky J, Langenaeken I, Micozzi A, Padmos A, Paesmans M, Viscoli C, Glauser MP. Monotherapy with meropenem versus combination therapy with ceftazidime plus amikacin as empiric therapy for fever in granulocytopenic patients with cancer. The International Antimicrobial Therapy Cooperative Group of the European Organization for Research and Treatment of Cancer and the Gruppo Italiano Malattie Ematologiche Maligne dell'Adulto Infection Program. *Antimicrob Agents Chemother* 1996;40:1108.

136. Eggimann P, Glauser MP, Aoun M, Meunier F, Calandra T. Cefepime monotherapy for the empirical treatment of fever in granulocytopenic cancer patients. *J Antimicrob Chemother* 1993;32(suppl B);151–63.

137. Johnson PR, Liu Yin JA, Tooth JA. A randomized trial of high-dose ciprofloxacin versus azlocillin and netilmicin in the empirical therapy of febrile neutropenic patients. *J Antimicrob Chemother* 1992;30:203.

138. Edwards JE, Filler SG. Current strategies for treating invasive candidiasis: emphasis on infections in nonneutropenic patients. *Clin Infect Dis* 1992;14(suppl 1):106–113.

139. Beck-Sagué CM, et al. Secular trends in the epidemiology of nosocomial fungal infections in the United States, 1980–1990. *J Infect Dis* 1993;167:1247–1251.

140. Fraser VJ, Jones M, Dunkel J, et al. Candidemia in a tertiary care hospital: epidemiology, risk factors, and predictors of mortality. *Clin Infect Dis* 1992;15:414–421.

141. Bross J, Talbot GH, Maislin G, et al. Risk factors for nosocomial candidemia: a case-control study in adults without leukemia. *Am J Med* 1989;87:614–620.

142. Komshian SV, Uwaydah AK, Sobel JD, et al. Fungemia caused by *Candida* species and *Torulopsis glabrata* in the hospitalized patient: frequency, characteristics, and evaluation of factors influencing outcome. *Rev Infect Dis* 1989;11:379–390.

143. Wey S, Mori M, Pfaller, M, Woolson R, Wenzel R. Risk factors for hospital-acquired candidemia: a matched case-control study. *Arch Intern Med* 1989;149:2349–2353.

144. Burchard KW, Minor LB, Slotman GJ, et al. Fungal sepsis in surgical patients. *Arch Surg* 1983;118:217–221.

145. Marsh PK, Tally FP, Kellum J, et al. *Candida* infections in surgical patients. *Ann Surg* 1983;198:42–47.

146. Lerch P, Kochendörfer P, Boos C. Comparative study of the efficacy of flucona-

zole versus amphotericin B/flucytosine in surgical patients with systemic mycoses. *Infection* 1993;21(6);376–382.

147. Anaissie EJ, Vartivarian S, Bodey GP, Legrand C, Kantarjian H, Abi-Said D, Karl C, Vadhan-Raj S. Randomized comparison between antibiotics alone and antibiotics plus granulocyte-macrophage colony-stimulating factor (*Escherichia coli*–derived in cancer patients with fever and neutropenia). *Am J Med* 1996;100(1):17–23.

148. Kaiser AB, Roach AC, Mulherin JL, et al. The cost effectiveness of antimicrobial prophylaxis in clean vascular surgery. *J Infect Dis* 1983;147:1103–1107.

149. Walters MD, Gibbs RS. A randomized comparison of gentamicin-clindamycin and cefoxitin-doxycycline in the treatment of acute pelvic inflammatory disease. *Obstet Gynecol* 1990;75:867–872.

150. Landers DV, Wolner-Hanssen P, Paavonen J, Thorpe E, Kiviat N, Ohm-Smith M, Green JR, Schachter J, Holmes KK, Eschenbach DA, et al. Combination antimicrobial therapy in the treatment of acute pelvic inflammatory disease. *Am J Obstet Gynecol* 1991;164–849–858.

151. Landers DV, Sweet RL. Current trends in the diagnosis and treatment of tubo-ovarian abscess. *Am J Obstet Gynecol* 1985;151:1098–1110.

152. Davey PG, Nathwani D. What is the value of preventing postoperative infections? *New Horizons* 1998;6(suppl 2):S64–S69.

CHAPTER 12

INTRAOPERATIVE AND PERIOPERATIVE CONSIDERATIONS IN LAPAROSCOPY

STEVEN A. VASILEV, M.D., M.B.A.

Ott and Kelling developed laparoscopy at the turn of the century.[1,2] Jacobaeus soon thereafter reported his extensive experience.[3a] However, it was not until the 1990s that operative laparoscopy finally came of age, largely due to vastly improved technology. Now an estimated two million laparoscopic procedures are performed in the United States yearly. Although these procedures have decreased morbidity and cost under some circumstances, they are associated with specific perioperative complications and considerations. This chapter reviews fundamental intra- and perioperative physiology related to pneumoperitoneum, medical management, and morbidity associated with advanced laparoscopic surgical procedures, including prevention and care of complications. Most evidence is Level II-3 to III. Areas achieving Level I support are especially noted.

PHYSIOLOGY OF PNEUMOPERITONEUM

Until the 1900s, laparoscopy was largely used in short diagnostic or minimal therapeutic interventions, such as tubal ligation in younger women. When first introduced, these short procedures were well tolerated despite as high as 40 mmHg intra-abdominal pressures commonly used at that time. Therefore, little attention was paid to understanding the physiology of prolonged pneumoperitoneum. Although the physiologic alterations discussed below and summarized in Table 12.1 are generally well tolerated, they may cause significant challenges in elderly or obese patients with cardiopulmonary compromise. There

Perioperative and Supportive Care in Gynecologic Oncology: Evidence-Based Management,
Edited by Steven A. Vasilev.
ISBN 0-471-24788-X   Copyright © 2000 by Wiley-Liss, Inc.

TABLE 12.1. Physiologic Changes/Complications During Laparoscopy

Pneumoperitoneum

Circulatory changes: venous return and filling pressures, cardiac contractility, afterload

Respiration/ventilation changes: minute ventilation, airway pressure, lung volumes, gas exchange

Trendelenburg and Reverse Position

Circulatory changes: heart rate, stroke volume, systemic vascular resistance

Respiration/ventilation changes: minute ventilation, work of breathing, lung volumes, gas exchange

Carbon Dioxide Insufflation

Circulatory changes: arrhythmias, cardiac contractility, venous gas embolization

Respiration/ventilation changes; dead-space ventilation, hypercarbia-acidemia

is an urgent need for further research pertaining to pneumoperitoneum in the critically ill or compromised patient.[3b] In these cases, gasless laparoscopy may be a viable alternative to laparotomy for some of the more limited procedures that these patients could tolerate (Level I).[3c–e]

Carbon Dioxide

Normal cellular oxidative metabolism produces CO_2.[4a] Blood flow to tissues, local tissue perfusion, ventilatory capacity, and buffering systems all contribute to homeostasis and determine plasma CO_2 concentrations, which is discussed further in Chapter 6. During laparoscopy, exogenous CO_2 contributes an additional volume and exposure-length related stress on intracellular and plasma homeostatic mechanisms, acting as an irritant and potential local cellular immune depressant within the peritoneum. With copious intraoperative irrigation, the former effect may be lessened (Level I).[4b,c]

Carbon dioxide is the preferred laparoscopic insufflation gas due to its non-combustion properties and high diffusion coefficient that reduces, but does not eliminate, the potential for gas embolism. However, the latter property also leads to rapid systemic absorption, causing an increase in arterial pCO_2 and decreased pH, which may be arrhythmogenic.[5–7a] Particular care is theoretically warranted in patients with sickle cell disease who may be in danger of crisis precipitated by alterations in pH and pCO_2, although small series have documented laparoscopy to be safe in this setting.[7b]

Controlling mechanical ventilation minute volume (V_T = rate × tidal volume) allows maintenance of a normal pCO_2 and pH in most otherwise healthy patients. A twofold increase in minute ventilation results in a pCO_2 adjustment of 5 mmHg. Thus, ventilation is a highly effective method of clearing volatile acid. However, diaphragmatic elevation due to pneumoperitoneum decreases lung volumes. In order to compensate, peak airway pressures increase to deliver constant tidal volumes for CO_2 homeostasis.[8] The consequences are discussed below. By and large, homeostatic disturbances lead to clinically significant findings only in patients with abnormal cardiopulmonary function and resulting limited homeostatic reserves.[9] These reserves may be limited by increased ventilatory dead space as seen in chronic obstructive pulmonary disease (COPD), impaired tissue perfusion, or poor cardiac output due to cardiovascular disease.

While it is imperative that all patients be closely monitored with end tidal CO_2 readings, it is especially critical in patients with chronic lung or cardiac disease in whom radial artery cannulation may be indicated.[9] End tidal Co_2 ($EtCO_2$) is the most common intraoperative noninvasive method for assessing adequacy of ventilation, and it accurately reflects changes in pCO_2 in normal patients. However, it may differ significantly from $PaCO_2$ in the presence of significant ventilation perfusion (VQ) mismatch.[10–12a] Thus blood gas monitoring should be considered in patients with known cardiorespiratory disease or those who develop intraoperative hypoxemia or high airway pressures.[9]

Alternate Gases

Argon   Argon is an inert gas with a poor solubility index relative to CO_2. Although not ordinarily used as a substitute gas for creation of a pneumoperitoneum, through use of the argon beam coagulator (ABC), argon gas can contribute significantly to the gas mixed achieved intraoperatively. Animal studies suggest lesser effects than CO_2 on most hemodynamic indices and pulmonary gas exchange. However, systemic vascular resistance index (SVRI) and stroke volume (SV) depression by 30% has been reported.[12b] Additionally, due to the solubility characteristics, deleterious effects of an accidental embolism may be more severe.[13a] At the very least, argon gas is more likely to be retained in the abdomen and is associated with greater pain at 72 hours due to decreased solubility and absorption (Level I).[13b] Therefore, when using the ABC, the abdomen should be continuously vented and the argon flow rate limited to 4–6 LPM. One, or preferably two, high-flow CO_2 insufflators will maintain adequate pneumoperitoneum with continuous venting.

Nitrous Oxide   The relatively low blood solubility of nitrous oxide (N_2O) increases risk for gas embolism, and its potential support of combustion generally limits intraperitoneal use to diagnostic procedures. Additionally, the much lower solubility than nitrogen and methane results in nitrous oxide diffusing into the intestinal lumen faster than the latter gases diffuse out. With inspired nitrous oxide anesthesia, the intestine may expand, obstructing the view or the ability to retract intestine, especially during laparoscopic procedures exceeding 4 hours.[14,15a] If intestinal perforation is sustained intraoperatively, an explosion hazard exists due to the nitrogen-methane mix.[15b] On balance, there is little to support use of N_2O for insufflation in operative laparoscopy. However, for shorter diagnostic procedures it may cause less pain than CO_2, possibly due to lack of hydrogen ion–mediated peritoneal irritation.[16,17] Inhalational N_2O use should be limited to shorter cases to prevent bowel distention.[15,18]

Lung Volumes, Compliance, and Ventilation

Changes in lung volumes may accompany laparoscopy due to increased pressures displacing the diaphragm cephalad and deep Trendelenburg position. Total lung compliance and functional residual capacity may be reduced, producing areas of ventilation-perfusion (VQ) mismatch.[19] Although mechanical ventilation may overcome some of these problems, increased peak airway pressures may become prohibitive, risking barotrauma even in patients with normal lungs. A special challenge occurs in the obese patient in whom high peak airway pressures are already required just to overcome chest-wall resistance and decreased lung volumes.[6,8]

Another risk of deep Trendelenburg is inadvertent intraoperative right main stem bronchial intubation with resulting hypoxemia. The proposed mechanism involves a tethered endotracheal tube at the mandible while the diaphragm displaces the lung and carina cephalad.[20,21a] Keeping intra-abdominal pressures in the 10–15 mmHg range and Trendelenburg position at a minimum will help minimize these problems.

Postoperative spirometry demonstrates a significant difference between lower abdominal and upper abdominal surgery effect on lung volumes. Minor pelvic surgery produces no significant changes beyond the day of surgery. In contradistinction, forced vital capacity (FVC), forced expiratory volume at one second (FEV-1), and peak expiratory flow rate are significantly reduced beyond the day of surgery following laparoscopic cholecystectomy.[21b]

Oxygenation

The effect of pneumoperitoneum on oxygenation is minimal in healthy patients—American Society of Anesthesiologists (ASA) Class 1—who are mechanically ventilated during laparoscopy.[6a] The possible causes of hypoxemia are listed in Table 12.2. ASA Class 2 and 3 patients are at higher risk on several parameters as listed.[6a]

As discussed in Chapter 6, intraoperative monitoring via pulse oximetry is usually adequate, correlating well with arterial blood gas measurements. However, if laser-, argon beam coagulation-, or cautery-induced smoke is allowed to accumulate, carboxyhemoglobin levels can become significantly elevated, producing inaccurate pulse oximetry readings (Level II-2).[6b]

Cardiovascular Changes

Changes in central venous return, and, hence, cardiac output, depend on the degree of intra-abdominal pressure and position of the patient.[22,23] While both

TABLE 12.2. Hypoxemia Risk Factors and Etiologies

Preexisting Conditions
Cardiopulmonary dysfunction
Morbid obesity
Hypoventilation
Patient position
Pneumoperitoneum
Endotracheal tube obstruction
Inadequate/dead-space ventilation
VQ Mismatch
Atelectasis and reduced FRC
Endobronchial intubation
Pneumothorax
Reduced Cardiac Output
Pneumomediastinum, pneumopericardium
Arrhythmias
Myocardial depression: anesthesia, sepsis, acidosis
Gas embolism
Reduced filling pressures, vena cava compression
Technical Failure
Hypoxic gas mixture delivery
Ventilator dysfunction

may decrease if pressures exceed 20 mmHg, return and output may increase if pressures are kept between 10 and 15 mmHg due to a shift of circulating blood volume from the abdominal mesentery and vena cava into the chest. Trendelenburg position *may* increase return, while a reverse Trendelenburg position decreases return in euvolemic patients. However, in the hypovolemic patient, Trendelenburg position can decrease filling pressures and increase systemic vascular resistance, resulting in a decreased cardiac output.[24,25] Additionally, higher mean airway pressures during mechanical ventilation may contribute to decreased cardiac output.

Elderly patients with limited cardiovascular reserves do not readily compensate for the above changes and thus more commonly evidence significant hemodynamic alterations with increased abdominal pressures and steep positions. For this reason, right heart catheterization and close monitoring may be indicated for prolonged procedures in the compromised or elderly patient.

Neuroendocrine Hormonal Response

Primarily incited by afferent neural input, levels of stress hormones are typically increased during and after laparotomy, and mediate widespread physiologic effects in proportion to the degree of insult. Cardiovascular changes in heart rate, blood pressure, and myocardial performance are mediated primarily by the catecholamines. Additionally, accelerated fat and protein metabolism combined with impaired glucose utilization contribute to a catabolic state. Overall, these major alterations can be poorly tolerated by compromised patients and can be persistent. After a laparotomy, plasma vasopressin (antidiuretic hormone [ADH]) can remain elevated for 5 to 7 days, reducing the ability to excrete free water, whereas during laparoscopy available data suggests a more rapid ADH normalization despite higher intraoperative levels, ostensibly due to greater peritoneal stretch/pressure receptor activation (Level I).[26]

A key question surrounds whether laparoscopy favorably blunts some of these stress response effects at clinically significant levels. Table 12.3 summarizes the relative alterations found in laparotomy versus laparoscopy. The physiologic effects tend to be complex, variable, time dependent, and synergistic, such that this summary by no means reflects all situations at any given point in time. Although preliminary animal data seems promising, limited clinical data, primarily comparing open versus laparoscopic cholecystecomy, fails to substantiate a major difference in any stress response parameters, with most differences in response being of short duration (Level I).[27–29a,b,c] In addition, there are significant questions regarding the overall impact of immunomodulation/inflammatory response seen with laparoscopy. Even though the beneficial effects are apparent, reflected by reduced pain and fevers, the immunosuppression may alter infection response cascades in a negative fashion.[29d]

Renal Perfusion

Pneumoperitoneum reduces urine output by several mechanisms, similar to that which occurs in other abdominal compartment syndromes such as malignant tense ascites. First, a 15 mmHg intra-abdominal pressure translates into a 15 mmHg decrease in blood perfusion and a 60% reduction in renal cortical perfusion.[30] This in turn leads to a 50% reduction in urine output. If only one kidney is compressed, as may occur in a laparoscopic retroperitoneal para-aortic node dissection with unilateral retroperitoneal insufflation, a 25% reduction in urine output may be evident.[30,31] Second, antidiuretic hormone (ADH) and aldosterone elevation due to increased intraperitoneal pressures further mediates decreased urine output, which may persist into the immediate postoperative period.[32] Maintaining the intra-abdominal pressures between 10 and 15 mmHg may improve renal perfusion and lessens the probability of decreased urine output, thereby lessening the hazard of inadvertent iatrogenic fluid overload.[30,32,33a]

TABLE 12.3. Perioperative Neuroendocrine Response to Surgery and Stress Effects

System/Organ	Effect	Alteration	Lap	LSC
Pituitary	Increased ACTH	Impaired free-water	++	+
	Increased TSH	excretion	+	+
	Increased growth hormone	Hyponatremia	+	+
	Increased vasopressin (ADH)		+	+++
Autonomic nervous system	Increased plasma norepinephrine	Sodium retention Hypokalemia Glucose intolerance Lipolysis Protein catabolism	+	+
Adrenal	Increased catecholamines	Arrhythmogenic tachycardia	+	++
			+	+
	Increased cortisol	Tachypnea	+	+
	Increased aldosterone	Widened pulse pressure Glucose intolerance Lipolysis Protein catabolism		
Pancreas	Increased glucagon	Hyperglycemia	+	+
	Decreased/increased insulin	Lipolysis Protein catabolism	+	+
Thyroid	Variable T4 and T3 effect		+	+

Note: + = minor effect, ++ = moderate effect, +++ = major effect.

Splanchnic and Hepatic Perfusion

Animal data suggests intraperitoneal pressure increase results in mechanical compression of the splanchnic capillary beds, increasing systemic vascular resistance. To limit this effect and its role in reduced cardiac output, maintaining pressures at 10–15 mmHg is recommended.[33b,c] Hepatic blood flow is also affected, but to a much lesser extent.[33b,c]

Gastrointestinal Distention

Spinal and epidural blockade above T5 interrupts sympathetic nervous system innervation to the gastrointestinal tract, with the epidural approach achieving a more controlled and slower onset of blockade. The resulting unopposed parasympathetic activity leads to relaxed sphincters and contracted intestines, facilitating positioning and retraction of bowel for upper retroperitoneal dissection.

Inhalational anesthesia with nitrous oxide increases sympathetic tone and possibly directly influences gaseous intestinal dilatation, making it a less desirable agent when optimal intestinal contraction is desired in longer complicated cases.[15,18,34]

LAPAROSCOPY COMPLICATIONS

In a 1991 survey by the American Association of Gynecologic Laparoscopists (AAGL), a mortality rate of 1.8 per 100,000 procedures was reported.[35a] Although possible underreporting limits interpretation of available data, it appears that operative laparoscopy is still associated with low mortality, although an increase in more complex surgeries has led to higher complication rates.[35b] A large prospective clinical series (25,764 cases) reported an operative laparoscopy complication rate of 17.9 per 1,000, as opposed to 2.7 per 1,000 for diagnostic laparoscopy and 4.5 per 1,000 for sterilization procedures.[35c] This correlation of complexity and morbidity was confirmed by a large French study comprising 29,966 operations. The same series reported a statistically significant correlation between a surgeon's current experience and the rate of complications.[35d]

Cardiovascular Collapse and Cardiac Arrest

Acute cardiovascular collapse during or immediately following laparoscopy is a rare but life-threatening complication, occurring at a rate of less than 0.5%. Causes for cardiovascular collapse are given below.

Metabolic Abnormalities Clinically significant metabolic abnormalities leading to significant cardiac dysfunction occur at a rate of less than 5 per 10,000 laparoscopic cases.[35a] The most frequently occurring changes of hypercarbia, hypoxemia, and acidemia can cause hypertension and cardiac bradyarrythmias or tachyarrhythmias in compromised patients.

These metabolic abnormalities can be minimized by limiting peritoneal CO_2 exposure as much as possible (i.e., by expeditiously completing the operative procedure) and keeping intraperitoneal pressures between 10 and 15 mmHg.[36] Pulse oximetry evaluation should be continuous, and adequate ventilation of the patient must be maintained as reflected by end tidal CO_2 or arterial measurements. Volume cycled mechanical ventilation must be adjusted to compensate for the excess CO_2 absorbed via the peritoneal surface, and Trendelenburg position must be limited in order to minimize pressure against the intra-abdominal diaphragmatic surface. If significant changes in oxygenation are noted or cardiac arrhythmias occur, the pneumoperitoneum must be immediately evacuated, Trendelenburg position reversed, and efforts focused on acutely decreasing pCO_2 while increasing pO_2 and pH. Appropriate medical management of persistent arrhythmias is further discussed in Chapter 10.

Gas Embolism This complication is extremely rare but potentially fatal, occurring in about 15 per 100,000 laparoscopies.[37] CO_2 is used preferentially during laparoscopy partly because of its solubility relative to air and N_2O, minimizing the chances of fatal embolization. Since CO_2 is rapidly absorbed, small amounts can be injected into the venous circulation without clinical consequence.[38] Etiology of clinically significant embolism may be multifactorial, including direct vessel insufflation via the Verres needle or through a significant rent in a low-pressure venous vessel. However, with high intraperitoneal pressures, gas embolism can theoretically occur following extensive tissue dissection without a major vessel injury.

If a large gas embolus lodges in a significant venous channel or right atrium or ventricle, an obstruction to blood flow can result. Clinical sequelae may include cardiovascular collapse, acute pulmonary hypertension and right heart failure, or cerebrovascular accident.

Embolism risk can be minimized by limiting intraperitoneal pressures, especially when alternative gases such as argon are used (argon beam coagulator), closing of open vessels, and using the Trendelenburg position conservatively. Intraoperative findings may include sudden-onset hypoxemia, hypotension, asystole or ventricular fibrillation associated with basilar rales, and a pathognomonic but often fleeting "mill wheel" murmur. One of the earliest signs may be a transient and sudden increase in $EtCO_2$.[39] Postoperatively, there may be associated signs such as seizures, motor/sensory deficits, or bronchoconstriction and noncardiogenic pulmonary edema.[40,41]

Intraoperative therapy includes immediate termination of the procedure with decompression of the pneumoperitoneum, adequate ventilation with 100% O_2, and aggressive cardiovascular support. Cardiac arrest may occur if large-volume air/gas is acutely infused (>100 cc). The patient should be placed in Trendelenburg and a left lateral decubitus position to minimize embolized gas entering the pulmonary circulation, although this traditional maneuver has limited effect on outcome. An attempt may be made to extract larger gas volumes via a right heart catheter. Once the patient is stable, hyperbaric oxygen unit therapy has been suggested for treatment of clinically significant emboli. Proposed therapy is 30 minutes of hyperbaric oxygen at 3 atmospheres.[42] Finally, use of corticosteroids in order to reduce lung injury remains controversial.[43]

Pneumothorax Clinically recognized pneumothorax occurs at a rate of less than 0.08%. CO_2 can either enter the pleural space across congenital defects in the diaphragm, at the time of alveolar bleb rupture, via the transdiaphragmatic lymphatics, or pneumoretroperitoneal dissection of gas through the aortic and esophageal diaphragmatic hiatus.[44] Some of these mechanisms are potentiated by excessive intraperitoneal pressures and the length of time that these pressures are maintained. Alveolar blebs in particular are more likely to rupture at the higher peak inspiratory pressures and volumes that are necessary to counteract the effects of increased intra-abdominal pressure on the diaphragm.

N_2O has a blood : gas partition coefficient (0.47) that is 34 times that of nitrogen (0.014). This differential solubility allows N_2O to enter an air-filled cavity from blood 34 times faster than nitrogen can leave the cavity. Therefore, in the presence of an intraoperatively diagnosed closed pneumothorax, N_2O is contraindicated because it can cause the volume of the pneumothorax to double rapidly. In fact, the presence of subcutaneous emphysema appearing during laparoscopy associated with decreasing pulmonary compliance should raise the possibility of unrecognized pneumothorax, and N_2O use should be discontinued.

Therapy of pneumothorax includes early recognition initially based on a significant decrease or loss of breath sounds on the affected side. Subcutaneous emphysema of the chest wall and neck should alert the anesthesiologist to the possibility of associated pneumothorax and a chest film should be ordered. If pneumothorax is the result of congenital defects in the diaphragm, decompression of the pneumoperitoneum and hyperexpansion of the lungs may suffice. Should the postoperative chest radiograph(s) demonstrate a persistent large (greater than 30%) or expanding pneumothorax, a small-bore tube thoracostomy with the tip placed at the apex is mandated. The chest tube should be connected to water seal, not to wall suction, as the latter may prolong bronchopleural leak. Simple pneumothorax usually requires the chest tube to be in place for 24 hours following resolution of an air leak. If there is clinical perioperative evidence of a tension pneumothorax, emergency chest tube thoracostomy is indicated and should not be delayed by a radiographic work-up.

Pneumomediastinum Occurring at a rate of less than 0.01%, this complication is most likely due to dissection of CO_2 along the aortic or esophageal hiatus or passage of CO_2 through congenital defects in the mediastinum.[44] It may also follow inappropriate placement of the Verres needle into the falciform ligament or dorsal retroperitoneum with the CO_2 dissecting cephalad.

Prevention focuses on appropriate Verres needle placement, minimization of retroperitoneal dissection, and maintenance of low intraperitoneal pressures and degree of Trendelenburg. Diagnosis is usually based on loss, or distancing, of heart sounds with associated hypotension. Pneumomediastinal decompression may be performed using a transcutaneous large-bore spinal needle and the pneumoperitoneum evacuated.

Pneumopericardium There are only a few reported cases of pneumopericardium, which is usually associated with pneumomediastinum.[45,46] Causation, prevention, and management are the same as for pneumomediastinum. Surgical decompression is imperative if a significant decrease in cardiac output occurs.

Myocardial Ischemia Patients predisposed to myocardial ischemia tolerate increased afterload poorly. In ASA III or IV patients, an intraperitoneal pressure of 15 mmHg leads to elevation in mean arterial pressure, peripheral vascular resistance, and central venous pressure, with a significant reduction in cardiac output. Additionally, mixed venous oxygen saturation (sVO_2) drops in half of these patients. The fall in cardiac output is likely due to inadequate ventricular reserve, emphasizing the need for very close monitoring in the presence of cardiac compromise history.[47]

Hemorrhage Hemorrhage may occur as a result of either arterial or venous injury. Whereas arterial or venous injury is readily evidenced by brisk bleeding, pressure equalization between the venous and intraperitoneal compartments may hide or minimize a significant venous injury. Intraoperative surgical management of vascular injury is discussed below. To avoid postoperative cardiovascular collapse from an unrecognized major venous injury, hemostasis should be ascertained at the end of the procedure as the intraperitoneal pressures are slowly decreased during pneumoperitoneum evacuation. If ongoing hemorrhage is suspected in the postoperative period, laparotomy is indicated to arrest the bleeding and evacuate any hematomas that may compromise organ functioning by direct pressure via a compartment syndrome in an enclosed retroperitoneal space.

Cardiac Arrhythmia Acidemia, hypoxemia, and hypercarbia contribute to various arrhythmias, which commonly occur intraoperatively.[7] Most are ventricular in origin. Tachyarrhythmias can be precipitated by surgical stress response increases in catecholamine levels and may be further potentiated by halothane anesthesia.[7,48] In addition to the metabolic etiologies, vagal stimulation via peritoneal distention may result in bradyarrhythmias or asystole.[48–52] Increasing intraperitoneal pressure quickly can lead to a sudden decrease in venous return and bradycardia via the Bainbridge reflex. Additionally, Mobitz type I block has been reported with propofol, fentanyl, and vecuronium, possibly preventable with an anticholinergic premedication.[53] In general, bradycardia may occur more frequently when anticholinergic and nonvagolytic neuromuscular blockers are not used.

Other Causes of Cardiovascular Collapse Excessive compression of the vena cava and vasovagal response have both been proposed as causes of cardiovascular collapse.[51] The former can be minimized by keeping intraperitoneal pressures between 10 and 15 mmHg and limiting the degree of Trendelenburg position. The latter may be prevented by atropine sulfate premedication. Additionally, the possibility of an adverse drug reaction should be entertained in the absence of any of the above.

Subcutaneous Emphysema

Subcutaneous emphysema occurs in up to 50% of patients undergoing laparoscopic lymph node dissections.[54] In the absence of a retroperitoneal dissection, rates are much lower, approximating 2%. The majority of the subcutaneous emphysema cases are due to improper Verres needle placement and insufflation superficial to the rectus fascia or to prolonged cases with improperly sealed sleeves. Genital emphysema is probably due to CO_2 dissection through the inguinal ring and a patent canal of Nuck. Emphysema of the neck and face may be associated with anterior thoracoabdominal-wall emphysema and may accompany a pneumomediastinum/pneumothorax.

Management of subcutaneous emphysema includes adequate analgesics to control the pain associated with cutaneous distension. Pressure dressings can be applied in an attempt to facilitate CO_2 absorption. In rare cases of extensive emphysema, a patient's ability to clear the absorbed CO_2 may be overcome, requiring extended mechanical ventilation.

Extraperitoneal Insufflation

Extraperitoneal insufflation follows either improper placement of a Verres needle or the insertion of an operative sleeve superficial to the peritoneum. Prevention includes open laparoscopy or direct placement of the first sleeve into the peritoneal cavity prior to establishing a pneumoperitoneum. These techniques are described later in the section on gastrointestinal injuries.

Extraperitoneal insufflation at the time of Verres or sleeve placement can be minimized by using a continuous motion through an adequate skin incision. The sleeve should be placed at a 45–60° angle to the peritoneum, which is usually tightly adherent to the anterior abdominal wall fascia. Unfortunately, preperitoneal insufflation is usually not recognized until the laparoscope is placed and it is noted that the peritoneum has been displaced by the insufflating gas. At this time the gas tubing should be disconnected from the sleeve, the stop cock left open, the laparoscope removed, and the diaphragm of the sleeve held open.

The anesthesiologist should be asked to valsalva the patient in an attempt to increase the intraperitoneal pressure and expel the extraperitoneal CO_2 through the open trocar. An attempt should not be made to blindly penetrate the distended peritoneum with a trocar in the sleeve, as such a maneuver has a significant risk of injuring an intraperitoneal structure. After the extraperitoneal insufflation has been maximally decompressed, the Verres needle should be reintroduced via an alternative site such as the left upper quadrant. A low intercostal, subcostal, or cul-de-sac approach can also be used.

Anesthetic Complications

Anesthesia complications independent of laparoscopy are rare, occurring at most in 1.4 of every 1,000 cases.[55] The majority of anesthesia-related deaths are due to hypoventilation. This can be caused by failed or esophageal intubation, but may also follow inadvertent endobronchial intubation. The former can be prevented in the difficult case by use of newer techniques of intubation such as flexible endoscopic direction. Appropriate monitoring via pulse oximetry allows early recognition of hypoxemia. Initial endobronchial intubation can be avoided by using appropriate-length (i.e., shorter) endotracheal tubes. However, the possibility of intraoperative migration of the endotracheal (ET) tube with steep Trendelenburg must be kept in mind.[20,21]

Laryngeal mask airway (LMA) may be a safe alternative for shorter cases. During a 2-year survey study period, a subset of 2,222 patients underwent an abdominal procedure under general anesthesia via LMA, of whom 44% were subjected to positive pressure ventilation. On 579 occasions, the procedures lasted for 2 hours. There were 18 critical incidents involving the airway, none of which involved intensive care management.[56]

Higher intra-abdominal pressures and steep Trendelenburg position increase the risk of regurgitation of gastric contents and subsequent aspiration pneumonitis. This risk can be minimized by assuring that the patient has been NPO (nothing by mouth) for 8 hours prior to surgery and by the use of cuffed endotracheal tubes, the pressure of which requires monitoring in longer cases. Although intraoperative oral-gastric tube suction may not decrease an already low aspiration pneumonitis rate (<0.1%), it may improve surgical field exposure and may decrease the risk of instrument injury.[57]

Hypothermia

Decrease in core body temperature may be minimized in laparoscopic procedures due to less extensive visceral exposure to ambient temperatures and irrigation fluid. However, at least one randomized controlled trial demonstrates that core body temperature can still be lowered during laparoscopy and is a function of the length of anesthesia rather than the irrigant temperature. Use of ambient-temperature, or lower, irrigant poses the greatest risk and can lower the core temperature by $1.7°$ (±0.2) (Level I).[58a] Depending on starting temperatures, this decrease may approach clinical significance and may intraoperatively affect platelet function among other variables. Use of preconditioned CO_2 (heated and hydrated) reduces hypothermia, shortens recovery room stay, and reduces postoperative pain due to the favorable effect of humidification on reducing peritoneal irritation (Level I).[58b]

Deep Venous Thrombosis

Pneumoperitoneum causes pelvic venous compression, which leads to venous stasis in the lower extremities. For gynecologic procedures utilizing Trendelenburg position, this venous stasis is lessened, thus potentially lowering the incidence of deep venous thrombosis (DVT). The incidence of DVT and pulmonary embolism during laparoscopy appears to be low, but may be underreported. The bulk of reported cases/series is found in the general surgery literature, and no randomized trial data is available (Level II-2).[59–62] In the absence of strong evidence, but given the potentially disastrous outcomes due to associated high risk factors, gynecologic oncology patients in whom lengthy operative procedures are planned should receive prophylactic measures. Further study is required in this area.

Vascular Injury

Vascular injury is one of the most frequent laparoscopic-surgery-related complications. Unfortunately, not all injuries are recognized intraoperatively.

Minor Vascular Injury   The superficial and deep inferior epigastric vessels are frequently injured with an incidence approaching 2.5%.[63a,b] If not appreciated intraoperatively, a hemoperitoneum may develop or an anterior abdominal wall extraperitoneal hematoma may form. This occurrence may be heralded by a progressively decreasing hemoglobin/hematocrit, changes in vital signs, a palpable lateral abdominal wall mass, or simply by pain and bleeding from the incision(s).

Management of a significant or expanding hematoma may include wound exploration, hematoma evacuation, and vessel ligation under general anesthesia. In the unstable patient, selective and rapid angiographic embolization may be an option. However, inferior to superior deep epigastric artery arborization and anastamosis is variable, such that embolization may not provide enough decrease in pulse pressure to ensure hemostasis.[64]

Major Vascular Injury   Major vessel injury occurs with a frequency of approximately 0.1%, most often at the aortic bifurcation,[65a,b] usually during Verres needle or umbilical sleeve placement. Mortality rates of 10–40% have been reported with major vessel injury, as well as significant morbidity and high transfusion rates.[65b–d] Injury risk can be minimized by angling the Verres needle or trocar towards the pelvis below the bifurcation of the aorta, which is usually deep to the umbilicus in the nonobese patient.

Injury to major pelvic vessels after the laparoscope has been placed is less common due to the ability to visualize accessory trocar placement. Such injuries can still occur unless the surgeon is very familiar with the retroperitoneal course of the common and external iliac vessels. Injury can also occur due to the misuse or inappropriate settings of a given instrument such as the argon beam coagulator with power set too high and/or directed at one area for too long. Large veins can appear flat and blend into the adjacent anatomy in the presence of pneumoperitoneum and Trendelenburg position. Thus, injury may go undetected until the Venturi effect of CO_2 suction into the vessel is appreciated.

Arterial injury due to placement of a Verres needle will be appreciated immediately, while an injury to a major venous vessel may initially go unrecognized. If bleeding is encountered through the Verres needle, the stopcock should be closed and the needle left in place. This arrangement functionally tamponades the bleeding and leads the surgeon to the site of injury. When the site of injury is identified via laparotomy, a 4-O vascular Prolene® figure-eight suture can be placed around the defect and secured while the Verres needle is removed.

Major vascular injuries due to initial trocar insertion are usually appreciated after the laparoscope is introduced. In the presence of brisk intraperitoneal bleeding or expanding hematoma, it may be prudent to perform a midline laparotomy. A posterior parietal peritoneal incision should be made lateral to the injury and a complete and thorough retroperitoneal exploration performed, including evaluation for concomitant ureteral injury.

Many vascular injuries can be repaired using endoscopic techniques. Laparoscopic vascular clips can be used as the first-line effort to obtain hemostasis. Additionally, as a preemptive measure, placement of a surgical mini-laparotomy sponge in the peritoneal cavity for immediate availability may help stem hemorrhage should an injury occur. It is important to not excessively delay an exploratory laparotomy if laparoscopic repair is not immediately successful. If the patient is in steep Trendelenburg position, blood can drain into the upper abdomen, where it can pool and remain hidden from view despite extensive hemorrhage. If an extensive major vessel laceration has occurred, especially of an artery, intraoperative vascular surgery consultation should be obtained. Perioperative sequelae can be minimized by employing vascular techniques that ensure that the vessel lumen is not narrowed and that a thrombus has not formed.

Mesenteric Vascular Injury The incidence of mesenteric vessel injury is unknown. These injuries may occur at the time of Verres needle or initial trocar placement and often are not appreciated until the laparoscope is placed. Due to extensive anastamoses, most small-vessel injuries can be repaired via laparoscopy using clips and electrocautery. If multiple ligations are required, care must be taken to ensure that blood supply to the nearby bowel segment has not been interrupted to the point of causing ischemia. In addition to visual inspection, options include laparoscopic Doppler examination at the mesenteric border, intravenous fluorescein-facilitated bowel segment evaluation, or a planned second-look laparoscopy within 24 to 48 hours.[66a] A technique that may facilitate these procedures involves leaving a flexible drain in one or two sleeve sites, through which a 5 mm scope and accessory sleeve can be re-placed in 24–48 hours with minimal risk of trocar reinsertion bowel injury.[66b] Injuries to the superior mesenteric artery require revascularization. However, if the injury involves the inferior mesenteric artery, ligation may be safely accomplished in the majority of patients due to excellent collateral blood supply.[66a]

Gastrointestinal Tract Injury and Dysfunction

The incidence of intestinal injury during laparoscopy is apparently 0.002% to 0.2%.[67a–c] The majority of these injuries occur at the time of Verres needle or primary trocar placement. Prior abdominal surgery increases the risk and at one time was considered a strong relative contraindication to laparoscopy.

Open laparoscopy techniques carry the advantage of peritoneal cavity entry under direct visualization. Unfortunately, this does not completely avoid bowel injury, maintenance of pneumoperitoneum may be difficult, and risk of subcutaneous emphysema may be increased if the Hasson sleeve sutures do not provide a tight seal.

An alternative is to place the initial trocar at another site, away from the umbilicus or prior abdominal incisions. Some have described a low intercostal or subcostal Verres needle placement, while others have demonstrated the efficacy of direct 2 mm or 5 mm trocar introduction in the left upper quadrant, just lateral to the midclavicular line (Level II-1).[68a,b,69] If the left upper quadrant entry is chosen, a nasogastric tube should be preemptively placed to ensure stomach decompression. Once the anatomy and adhesion location is appreciated, additional ports can be safely introduced under direct visualization.

Electrosurgical bowel injury usually occurs with the use of unipolar current and direct injury or conduction to the intestine via insulation failure or capacitive coupling.[70] Prevention rests with reusable instrument insulation testing on a regularly scheduled basis. Disposable instruments should never be reused. The uninsulated end of the electrosurgical instrument should be fully visible and in contact with whatever structure is to be cut or coagulated prior to activating current. Unfortunately, due to insulation failure, this does not always prevent electrothermal bowel injury. For this reason bipolar instruments are preferred.

The argon beam coagulator (ABC) is a useful innovation based on gas-mediated electrosurgical dissection, especially in the retroperitoneum.[71] While embolism remains a theoretical risk, the superficial electrical current penetration (0.3–0.9 mm) at lower wattage settings is a predictable and welcome characteristic. In comparison, unipolar cautery is associated with a variable depth of tissue injury, up to 3 mm even with brief exposure. Additionally, the ABC insulation is constructed in such a fashion that capacitive coupling risk is minimized.

Verres needle simple puncture injury to the small intestine, signaled by enteric contents return, is often managed by removing the needle and attempting placement elsewhere. There are no large series to either support or refute this practice, and management rests with the surgeon's experience and specific findings in this situation. Large bowel injury management in a similar fashion has been reported.[72b] This assumes extensive manipulation has not occurred that may have caused a significant laceration.[73] Simple Verres puncture is analogous to the same event occurring at the time of paracentesis with a large-bore needle, which is probably a relatively common occurrence. There is no evidence to support use of prophylactic antibiotics should a simple puncture occur, in the absence of prolonged small-bowel obstruction with feculent bowel contents or extensive injury to the large bowel.

Bowel injuries larger than a Verres needle puncture must be surgically closed. This procedure can be performed via laparoscopy if the surgeon has mastered the necessary skills or via a mini-laparotomy and exteriorization of the injured bowel segment. If an electrosurgical injury appears to be greater than 0.5 cm, it may be prudent to resect the injured area with closure or anastamosis, depending on the size and configuration of the defect. Although it is difficult to gauge the extent of electrosurgical damage, small injuries can be oversewn. If a large enterotomy occurs involving over half of the antimesenteric circumference, or the bowel has been devascularized, a bowel resection is indicated via laparoscopy or laparotomy. Management of all of the above injuries will vary with surgeon's experience, specific findings, and other contributing factors, such as a history of radiation therapy.

A thorough mechanical and antibiotic bowel prep should be considered in any patient scheduled for operative laparoscopy who has had prior abdominal surgery. However, even in cases of minimal but grossly evident fecal intra-operative contamination, colostomy is indicated only if there has been signifi-cant delay in diagnosis, extensive tissue necrosis, gross intraperitoneal infection, or cardiovascular compromise and hypoxemia.[72,74] Copious isotonic peritoneal lavage should be considered when large-bowel injury occurs, and antibiotic therapy initiated with broad-spectrum agents covering mixed GI flora.[75,76]

An often lethal complication is the intraoperatively unrecognized bowel injury. This injury may be due to unappreciated electrosurgical damage or direct operative injury. Forty to 70% of bowel injuries are not recognized during surgery and often become evident only after the patient is discharged.[67b,c] Delay in diagnosis is usually due to a low index of suspicion. These situations are often associated with severe sepsis and death.[67b,c] Thus, initial therapy includes aggressive fluid resuscitation and antibiotic therapy. After effective resuscita-tion, or if the patient fails to rapidly stabilize, exploratory laparotomy with appropriate drainage, repair, and/or diversion should be performed. In a stable patient with a localized process, percutaneous CT-guided drainage is becom-ing the preferred alternative.[77a] This subject is further discussed in Chapter 4. After the inflammation subsides, the patient can be returned to the operating room and definitive surgery performed.

Postoperative ileus is common in women who have undergone either long or extensive operative laparoscopic procedures. It is due to the additive effect of prolonged anesthetic agent exposure, direct bowel manipulation, and possibly chemical peritonitis secondary to carbon dioxide byproducts.[3b,4b] The potential for ileus can be minimized by reducing operative time. However, the physi-ologic events affecting bowel function during laparoscopy are probably more complex than suggested by the above discussion. Animal data indicates that gut inflammatory response, as reflected by blunted serum and gut mucosal IL-6 (interleukin), is minimized by laparoscopy.[67d]

Should the symptoms of ileus fail to abate within 72 hours of bowel rest, a bowel obstruction must be suspected and appropriate radiographic studies per-formed. An extensive discussion regarding the relative merits of plain films versus computerized tomography is presented in Chapter 4.

Urinary Tract Injury

Bladder Injury   A recent literature review reports that injury to the blad-der during gynecologic operative laparoscopy occurs at a rate of 0.02% to 8.3%.[67e] Laparoscopically assisted hysterectomy is associated with the high-est reported rates. Injuries are more common when the bladder is incompletely drained, when the anatomy is distorted due to prior surgery, when inflammatory states or carcinomatosis are present, or when advanced operative procedures are performed. For example, with radical laparoscopic hysterectomy, injury rates approaching 30% have been reported.[77b] Subsequent reports have not substantiated such high rates of injury, reflecting the dynamics of a lengthy learning curve, volume/outcomes relationship, and ever-improving technology in such surgery.[71]

During laparoscopic-assisted vaginal hysterectomy, at the time of vesicouterine reflection development, low posterior bladder-wall injuries can occur. These can be minimized by sharp dissection and attention to detail in dissecting distorted tissue planes that may be the result of prior surgery or inflammatory states.

Risk of Verres needle/trocar injury is reduced by adequate and/or continuous bladder drainage. For longer procedures, a Foley catheter should be introduced and removed at the completion of the procedure. As has been described, appropriate caution and attention to technique must be taken at the time of Verres needle and umbilical sleeve placement. Injury at the time of suprapubic sleeve placement is almost always preventable, since placement can be done under direct visualization.

Fortunately, intraoperatively recognized bladder dome injuries are easily managed. Small defects, especially if extraperitoneal, such as those caused by a Verres needle or 5-mm trocar can be managed solely with 5 to 10 days of bladder drainage. Larger injury repair may be effected laparoscopically, closing the bladder in one or two layers, depending on the extent of injury and the presence or absence of electrosurgical injury.[78] The bladder should be placed at rest and drained completely for approximately 5 days, a point at which 50% of tensile strength has been regained.[79] In patients who have received pelvic radiation, drainage should empirically be continued for a longer period of time. No data exists as to the appropriate length of time for similar healing. However, since the bladder is one of the most rapidly healing tissues in the body, in the absence of such cofactors, prolonged drainage is unwarranted.

Bladder injury unrecognized intraoperatively can cause major postoperative morbidity and usually leads to reoperation.[67f] Approximately half of patients with bladder injuries will not present for many days postoperatively, particularly if an extensive thermal injury was sustained that can cause a delayed rather than immediate cystotomy.[67e] Peritonitis, fevers, ileus, or urine leaking from an incision site may be observed. Intravenous urography and/or cystography will usually confirm an injury and its location. Alternatively, computerized tomography may be employed, as discussed in Chapter 4. Management may be affected by inflammation and scarring, which may mandate repair via laparotomy.

Urachal and Vesicourachal Diverticulum This extremely rare injury is caused by placing a trocar through the diverticular cyst or patent urachus.[80a] The injury can be avoided by recognizing the urachus, assuming it is patent, and angling the suprapubic trocar lateral in such a way as to avoid the structure. Preoperative assessment has been described using ultrasound and contrast studies.[80b] If recognized at the time of surgery, the urachus should be ligated above and below the site of injury. The patient may present postoperatively with urine draining from her umbilical incision. The diagnosis can be confirmed with a cystogram. Treatment may simply entail continuous bladder drainage and confirming closure of the urachus, with repeat cystogram prior to catheter removal.

Ureteral Injuries Although these injuries are rare (less than 0.01–0.2%), there may be a relative increase in occurrence as more complex surgical procedures are performed.[81] The ureter may be injured at the pelvic brim during division of the ovarian vessels; in the broad ligament during lysis of adhesions or ablation of endometriosis/carcinomatosis; or at the level of the uterine artery, as could occur during cardinal ligament division. All of these injuries are preventable by identifying the ureter throughout its retroperitoneal course and dissecting it free from the site of surgery.

Injuries that are intraoperatively identified are associated with the best outcomes. However, these injuries are often recognized postoperatively, at which time the morbidity increases.[82] Ureteral injury should be suspected postoperatively in the presence of fever, leukocytosis, peritonitis, flank pain/tenderness, a urinoma/pelvic mass or hematuria.[77a] Radiographic studies discussed in Chapter 4 should be employed to determine the presence and site of injury. Traditional therapy involves exploratory surgery with primary repair, reimplantation, and interposition techniques. However, selected patients may be successfully managed with ureteroscopy, stent placement, and percutaneous drainage.[83,84] These include patients with minor leaks or partial obstruction due to a kink caused by adjacent absorbable suture placement.

Nerve Injuries

Nerve injuries are extremely rare in gynecologic laparoscopy.[85] Most commonly these are due to stretching or pressure injury (neurapraxia). Rarely, transection of a nerve (neurotmesis) can occur.

Brachial palsy can be due to prolonged steep Trendelenburg position combined with a shoulder brace or hyperabducted arms strapped to an armboard. These injuries can be avoided by placing the arms at the patient's side, avoiding the use of shoulder braces, and ensuring that no undue pressure from equipment occurs. The latter is accomplished with extensive padding and avoiding encroachment on the arm. Physical therapy usually results in good outcomes.

Femoral, sciatic, and peroneal nerve injuries can be due to positioning, hip hyperflexion, and direct pressure. Allen stirrups, which support the knee and foot, in combination with proper positioning limit such injury. If nerve injury is suspected postoperatively due to foot drop or gait disturbance, neurologic evaluation should be sought. Electromyographic and nerve-conduction studies can help isolate the defect. Physical therapy should then be initiated with expected full recovery; however, complete recovery may require several months.

Neurotmesis, or transection of the nerve, is potentially more serious. However, the nerves at risk for this injury are the genitofemoral nerve branches bordering the psoas muscle lateral to the external iliac artery and the obturator nerve that lies deep in the obturator space. Only radical laparoscopic surgery, including pelvic lymph node dissection, exposes these nerves to such injury.

The genitofemoral nerve is composed of several branches, all or some of which may be transected during pelvic lymph node dissection, and are not repaired. Although bothersome, medial thigh dysesthesia may result, but can resolve over time. If the obturator nerve is transected, it should be repaired using microsurgical technique. Despite dual motor innervation, adductor function of the leg may be impaired. With epineurial repair and/or postoperative physiotherapy, recovery is complete in most instances.[85]

Incisional Complications

Wound Infections   Laparoscopy is usually a clean or clean/contaminated operation, depending on the intraperitoneal procedure performed. Therefore, infections are uncommon (0.1–3.0%) (Level I).[35,60,61,86–90] The umbilicus, where the Verres needle and principal sleeve is placed, should be thoroughly cleansed.[60,88] In an effort to minimize the risk of infection, all attempts should be made to maintain aseptic technique. Antibiotics are not used routinely in laparoscopy; they are recommended only for prophylaxis as dictated by open procedure indications as discussed in chapters 9 and 11.

Incision-site infection management includes opening the skin for debridement and administration of appropriate antibiotics in the event of cellulitis. Initial coverage, which should be modified when culture results become available, should include activity against staph species and hemolytic streptococci. Finally, although necrotizing fasciitis is rare after laparoscopy, it may occur and can be difficult to assess due to the small incision size.[59,91] The index of suspicion must remain high in order to initiate timely, aggressive, and effective therapy.

Wound Dehiscence and Incisional Hernias   The incidence of these complications is probably underreported, but is likely between 0.2% and 0.02%.[92,93a] The cause of these wound complications is inadequate closure of a fascial incision. As would be expected, the larger the size of the sleeve used, the more likely that a hernia will occur. The vast majority (86.3%) occur at 10-mm or greater size sleeve sites, and three-quarters of hernias develop at the umbilical site.[93a] Prevention centers on adequate primary closure of the incisional defect. Adequacy of closure is key, since primary fascial closure is completed in 18% to 60% of patients who susequently develop a hernia at 10–12-mm sleeve sites.[92,93a]

Adequate closure can be ensured by placing the sutures under direct laparoscopic visualization at all 10 mm or greater sleeve sites. Also, placing the trocars via a "Z" technique (i.e., offsetting the skin incision and peritoneal entry site) may help reduce the risk of a hernia tract by relying on natural staggered tissue apposition.

In the event of a hernia or wound dehiscence, management should include conventional techniques of surgical evaluation for bowel involvement and hernia repair. Up to 17% of laparoscopic hernias present with evidence of small or large intestine morbidity.[93a]

Postoperative Pain

Although definitive studies have not been performed, the degree of pain that follows a laparoscopic procedure is often not fully appreciated and is multifactorial. Incisional pain may be decreased, but operative site pain will depend on the degree of tissue inflammation, ischemia, and trauma related to the procedure. Also, pain may be due to carbon dioxide mediated peritoneal irritation.[17] For this reason, consideration may be given to small-dose hypobaric lidocaine-fentanyl spinal anesthesia for short duration laparoscopic procedures (Level I).[93b,c] Postural spinal headache may occur, but patient acceptance was shown to be high.

Various series report that 35% to 65% of patients experience shoulder pain.[94a,95] Thorough attempts at deflating the pneumoperitoneum at the procedure conclusion must be undertaken, including valsalva provided by the anesthesiologist, although this does not completely eliminate the problem.[96a] Patients undergoing gasless laparoscopy have similar pain location and duration patterns.[96b] Shoulder tip pain may be reduced by bupivicaine irrigation (10 cc of 0.5% bupivicaine in 500 cc normal saline) to both hemidiaphragms at the end of surgery.[96c–e]

Even though CO_2 is rapidly absorbed, free gas can be demonstrated under the diaphragm for up to 3 days postoperatively, although it is uncommon after 24 hours.[94a–c] A large volume of gas under the diaphragm on an upright chest film more than 24 hours postoperatively should signal the strong possibility of viscus perforation.[94c] Placing a drain into the peritoneal cavity for 6 hours after surgery, especially in a suprahepatic location, may significantly decrease pain severity.[97]

Postoperative analgesic requirements may be reduced but are not eliminated due to the lack of a laparotomy incision. Incisional pain may be reduced if subcutaneous lidocaine or bupivicaine are used at closure.[96d,e] However, conflicting Level-I data exists, supporting preemptive injection as being more effective (Level I).[96f] In general, pain is easier to manage if analgesic therapy is instituted preemptively in the postoperative period. A common regimen may include parenteral nonsteroidal anti-inflammatory drugs, with a narcotic analgesic added as needed.

Postoperative administration of Tramadol (3 mg/kg) was shown in one study to reduce postanesthetic shivering and additional analgesic use, thus reducing postanesthesia recovery time (Level I).[96g] However, administration of narcotics or injectable nonsteroidal agents earlier, at or immediately preceding induction, fails to impact postoperative consumption of analgesics (Level I).[96h,i] A more detailed discussion regarding pain management is offered in Chapter 20.

The patient should be reassured that the pain will subside and that it does not represent an unexpected complication or a failure of the procedure, but rather a physiologic sequela to surgical trauma and pneumoperitoneum.

Postoperative Nausea

Postoperative nausea, dizziness, and emesis is common after laparoscopy, is related to the total amount of CO_2 used, and often prolongs length of stay, thus increasing costs.[34,98a] These effects can persist for 24 hours or more in up to 25% of patients.[98b] Risk factors for nausea and emesis include female gender, anxiety, obesity, history of motion sickness, and performance of the procedure during menses.[99–102] Emesis rates seem to be lowest during the third and fourth weeks of the menstrual cycle.[101]

The emetogenic potential of anesthetic and analgesic agents is variable. Nitrous oxide may also contribute in longer procedures via intestinal dilatation and autonomic effects,[18,334,103,104] but this possibility has not been confirmed by all investigators. Otherwise, the commonly used inhalational agents seem to be equivalent in emetogenic potential.[34]

Epidural anesthesia may be superior to general anesthesia in reducing emesis, but this advantage may be decreased depending on which systemic agents are used.[105] For example, propofol as a systemic agent is associated with very low rates of emesis.[106] In contrast, narcotic analgesics contribute significantly to nausea and emesis.[107]

Several investigators have reported reduction in postoperative nausea and emesis following parenteral ketorolac administered prior to the conclusion of laparoscopy.[108,109] Other intraoperatively administered agents that may prophylactically reduce postoperative nausea by acting centrally are intravenous metoclopramide (0.1–0.2 mg/kg) and IV droperidol (10–20 mcg/kg), and dexamethasone (0.17 mg/kg),[34,110,111a,b] although metaclopramide has higher potential for side effects. Ondansetron, a serotonin antagonist, may be superior to the above agents with minimal side effects (Level I).[112,113a,b] However, this benefit may be marginal with a higher marginal cost and, in the face of evidence that demonstrates that the serotonin metabolite 5-HT3 (5-hydroxy-tryptamine) is not elevated after gynecologic laparoscopy.[113c,d] Finally, transdermal scopolamine applied preoperatively has been reported to be effective.[114] Since the genesis of nausea and emesis is multifactorial, each patient has to be preoperatively evaluated individually and, in some cases, multiple agent regimens should be applied.

LAPAROSCOPIC PROCEDURES DURING PREGNANCY

Surgical procedures performed during pregnancy by any route carry a risk of fetal loss and theoretical first trimester anesthetic exposure-related teratogenesis. Although pelvic and abdominal laparoscopic surgery have become widely accepted in nonpregnant patients, pregnancy has been considered a relative contraindication mostly due to potential for direct trauma, theoretical physiologic concerns, and animal data.

Potential physiologic advantages of an operative laparoscopic approach during pregnancy include decreased postoperative narcotic requirements, diminished postoperative maternal hypoventilation, and more rapid return of bowel function.[115] However, risks include direct trauma from blind trocar and Verres needle introduction, physiologic sequelae due to increased intra-abdominal pressure, and/or direct CO_2 effects.[115–124] The latter two effects may lead to reduced uterine blood flow and/or uterine contractions, which in turn may lead to premature labor and/or fetal acidosis.

Clinically significant reduction in uterine blood as a direct result of pneumoperitoneum is unproven. In an animal model, fetal acidosis, decreased uterine blood flow, and increased intrauterine pressure have been reported during CO_2 pneumoperitoneum. Maternal respiratory alkalosis compensated to a degree and, most importantly, all ewes delivered normal lambs at term gestation.[125,126] Gasless laparoscopy utilizing mechanical methods for abdominal wall elevation has been proposed as an alternative to pneumoperitoneum to eliminate such concerns.[127,128] However, further research into the physiologic effects of laparoscopy during pregnancy is required in order to determine optimal management.

Multiple case reports, small series, and reviews suggest that operative laparoscopy during pregnancy is safe during first, second, and, possibly, third trimesters, depending on the procedure(s) performed.[116,129–139] However, limited clinical data, reports of complications, and animal-model-based physiologic concerns mandate caution until prospective trials prove safety.[126,140]

In the absence of strong Level-I data, the Society of American Gastrointestinal Endoscopic Surgeons (SAGES) offers the following consensus guidelines for operative laparoscopy during pregnancy:[141]

1. When possible, operative intervention should be deferred until the second trimester, when fetal risk is lowest.

2. Since pneumoperitoneum enhances lower extremity venous stasis, already present in the gravid patient, and since pregnancy induces a hypercoagulable state, pneumatic compression devices must be utilized.

3. Fetal and uterine status, as well as maternal end tidal CO_2 and arterial blood gases, should be monitored.

4. The uterus should be protected with a lead shield if intraoperative cholangiography is a possibility. Fluoroscopy should be utilized selectively.

5. Given the enlarged gravid uterus, abdominal access should be attained using an open technique.

6. Dependent positioning should be utilized to shift the uterus off of the inferior vena cava.

7. Pneumoperitoneum pressures should be minimized (to 8–12 mmHg) and not allowed to exceed 15 mmHg.

8. Obstetrical consultation should be obtained preoperatively.

REFERENCES

1. Ott D. Die Direkte Beleuchtung der Bauchhole, der Haranblase, des Dichdarams und des Uterus zu Diagnostichen Zwecken. *Rev Med Tcheque* 1909;2:27–30.

2. Kelling G. Zur Coelioskopie. *Arch Klin Chir* 1923;126:226–229.

3. Jacobaeus HC. Uber die Moglichkeit die Zystoskopie bei Untersuchung seroser Hohlungen anzumenden. *Munch Med Wochenschr* 1911;58:2017–2019.

3b. Holthausen UH, Nagelschmidt M, Troidl H. CO_2 pneumoperitoneum: what we know and what we need to know. *World J Surg* 1999;23:794–800.

3c. Koivusalo AM, Kellokumpu I, Lindgren L. Postoperative drowsiness and emetic sequelae correlate to total amount of carbon dioxide used during laparoscopic cholecystectomy. *Surg Endosc* 1997;11:42–44.

3d. Casati A, Valentini G, Ferrari S, Senatore R, Zangrillo A, Torri G. Cardiorespiratory changes during gynaecological laparoscopy by abdominal wall elevation: comparison with carbon dioxide pneumoperitoneum. *Br J Anaesth* 1997;78:51–54.

3e. Goldberg JM, Maurer WG. A randomized comparison of gasless laparoscopy and CO_2 pneumoperitoneum. *Obstet Gynecol* 1997;90:416–420.

4a. Nunn JF. *Nunn's Applied Respiratory Physiology*. 4th ed. Stoneham, MA: Butterworth, 1993, pp. 219–246.

4b. Taskin O, Buhur A, Birincioglu M, Burak F, Atmaca R, Yilmaz I, Wheeler JM. The effects of duration of CO_2 insufflation and irrigation on peritoneal microcirculation assessed by free radical scavengers and total glutathione levels during operative laparoscopy. *J Am Assoc Gynecol Laparosc* 1998;5:129–133.

4c. Kopernik G, Avinoach E, Grossman Y, Levy R, Yulzari R, Rogachev B, Douvdevani A. The effect of a high partial pressure of carbon dioxide environment on metabolism and immune functions of human peritoneal cells: relevance to carbon dioxide pneumoperitoneum. *Am J Obstet Gynecol* 1998;179:1503–1510.

5. Alexander GD, Brown EM. Physiologic alterations during pelvic laparoscopy. *Am J Obstet Gynecol* 1969;105:1078–1081.

6a. Puri GD, Singh H. Ventilatory effects of laparoscopy under general anesthesia. *Br J Anaesth* 1992;68:211–213.

6b. Ott DE. Carboxyhemoglobinemia due to peritoneal smoke absorption from laser tissue combustion at laparoscopy. *J Clin Laser Med Surg* 1998;16:309–315.

7a. Scott DB, Julian DG. Observations on cardiac arrhythmias during laparascopy. *Br J Med* 1972;1:411–413.

7b. Ware RE, Kinney TR, Casey JR, Pappas TN, Meyers WC. Laparoscopic cholecystectomy in young patients with sickle hemoglobinopathies. *J Pediatr* 1992;120:58–61.

8. Seed TF, Shakespeare TF, Muldoon MJ. Carbon dioxide homeostasis during anaesthesia for laparoscopy. *Anaesthesia* 1970;25:223–231.

9. Wittgen CM, Andrus CH, Fitzgerald SD, Baudendistel LJ, Dahms TE, Kaminski DL. Analysis of the hemodynamic and ventilatory effects of laparoscopic cholecystectomy. *Arch Surg* 1991;126:997–1001.

10. Kalhan SB, Reaney JA, Collins RL. Pneumomediastinum and subcutaneous emphysema during laparoscopy. *Cleveland Clin J Med* 1990;57:639–642.

11. Liu SY, Leighton T, Davis I, et al. Prospective analysis of cardiopulmonary responses to laparoscopic cholecystectomy. *J Laparoendosc Surg* 1991;1:241–244.

12a. McKinstry LJ, Perverseff RA, Yip RW. Arterial and end-tidal carbon dioxide in patients undergoing laparoscopic cholecystectomy. *Anesthesiology* 1992;77(A): 108–112.

12b. Eisehnauer DM, Saunders CJ, Ho HS, Wolfe BM. Hemodynamic effects of argon pneumoperitoneum. *Surg Endosc* 1994;8:315–321.

13a. Mann C, Boccara G, Grevy V, Navarro F, Fabre JM, Colson P. Argon pneumoperitoneum is more dangerous than CO_2 pneumoperitoneum during venous gas embolism. *Anesth Analg* 1997;85(6):1367–1371.

13b. Reichert JA. Argon as distending medium in laparoscopy compared with carbon dioxide and nitrous oxide. *J Am Assoc Gynecol Laparosc* 1996;3:S41.

14. Eger EI, Saidman LJ. Hazards of nitrous oxide anesthesia in bowel obstruction and pneumothorax. *Anesthesiology* 1965;26:61–66.

15a. Taylor E, Feinstein R, White RF, Soper N. Anesthesia for laparoscopic cholecystectomy. Is nitrous oxide contraindicated? *Anesthesiology* 1992;76:541–543.

15b. Neuman GG, Sidebotham G, Negoianu E, Bernstein J, Kopman AF, Hicks RG, West ST, Haring L. Laparoscopy explosion hazards with nitrous oxide. *Anesthesiology* 1993;78:857–859.

16. Sharp JR, Pierson WP, Brady CE. Comparison of CO_2 and N_2O induced discomfort during peritoneoscopy under local anesthesia. *Gastroenterology* 1982;82:453–456.

17. Minoli G, Terruzzi V, Spizzi GC, et al. The influence of carbon dioxide and nitrous oxide on pain during laparoscopy: a double blind, controlled trial. *Gastrointest Endosc* 1982;28:173–175.

18. Lonie DS, Harper NJN. Nitrous oxide anaesthesia and vomiting: the effect of nitrous oxide anaesthesia on the incidence of vomiting following gynaecological laparoscopy. *Anaesthesia* 1986;41:703–708.

19. Versichelen L, Serreyn R, Rolly G, et al. Physiopathologic changes during anesthesia administration during gynecological laparoscopy. *J Reprod Med* 1984;29:697–700.

20. Wilcox S, Vandam LD. Alas, poor Trendelenburg and his position! A critique of its uses and effectiveness. *Anesth Analg* 1988;67:574–577.

21a. Burton A, Steinbrook RA. Precipitous decrease in oxygen saturation during laparoscopic surgery. *Anesth Analg* 1993;76:1177.

21b. Joris J, Kaba A, Lamy M. Postoperative spirometry with laparoscopy for lower abdominal or upper abdominal surgical procedures. *Br J Anaesth* 1997;79:422–426.

22. Motew M, Ivankovich AD, Bieniarz J, et al. Cardiovascular effects and acid base and blood gas changes during laparoscopy. *Am J Obstet Gynecol* 1973;115:1002–1012.

23. Hodgson C, McClelland RMA, Newton JR. Some effects of peritoneal insufflation of carbon dioxide at laparoscopy. *Anaesthesia* 1970;25:382–390.

24. Sibbald WJ, Paterson NAM, Holliday RL, et al. The Trendelenburg position: hemodynamic effects in hypotensive and normotensive patients. *Crit Care Med* 1979;7:218–224.

25. Sing R, O'Hara D, Sawyer MAJ, Parino PL. Trendelenburg position and oxygen transport in hypovolemic adults. *Ann Emerg Med* 1994;23:564–568.

26. Ortega AE, Peters JH, Incarbone R, Estrada L, et al. A randomized prospective comparison of the metabolic and stress hormonal responses of laparoscopic and open cholecystectomy. *J Am Coll Surg* 1996;183:249–256.

27. Aktan A, Buyukgebiz O, Yegen C, Yalin R. How minimally invasive is laparoscopic cholecystectomy? *Surg Laparosc Endosc* 1994;4:18–21.

28. Mealy K, Gallagher H, Barry M, et al. Physiological and metabolic response to open and laparoscopic cholecystectomy. *Br J Surg* 1992;79:1061–1064.

29a. McMahon AJ, O'Dwyer PJ, Cruishank AM, et al. Comparison of metabolic responses to laparoscopic and minilaparotomy cholecystectomy. *Br J Surg* 1993;80:1255–1258.

29b. Kehlet H. Surgical stress response: does endoscopic surgery confer an advantage? *World J Surg* 1999;23:801–807.

29c. Bouvy ND, Marquet RL, Tseng LN, Steyerberg EW, Lamberts SW, Jeekel H, Bonjer HJ. Laparoscopic vs. conventional bowel resection in the rat. Earlier restoration of serum insulin-like growth factor 1 levels. *Surg Endosc* 1998;12:412–415.

29d. Hackam DJ, Rotstein OD. Host response to laparoscopic surgery: mechanisms and clinical correlates. *Can J Surg* 1998;41:103–111.

30. Chiu AW, Chang LS, Birkett DH, Babayan RK. The impact of pneumoperitoneum, pneumoretroperitoneum and gasless laparoscopy on the systemic and renal hemodynamics. *J Am Coll Surg* 1995;181:397–406.

31. Vasilev SA, McGonigle KF. Extraperitoneal laparoscopic paraaortic lymph node dissection. *Gynecol Oncol* 1996;61:315–320.

32. Mansour MA, Stiegmann GV, Yamamoto M, Berguer R. Neuroendocrine stress response after minimally invasive surgery. *Surg Endosc* 1992;6:294–297.

33a. Punnonen R, Viinamaki O. Vasopressin release during laparoscopy: role of increased intra-abdominal pressure. *Lancet* 1982;16:175–176.

33b. Ishizaki Y, Bandai Y, Shimomura K, Abe H, Ohtomo Y, Idezuki Y. Changes in splanchnic blood flow and cardiovascular effects following peritoneal insufflation of carbon dioxide. *Surg Endosc* 1993;7:420–423.

33c. Windberger UB, Auer R, Keplinger F, Langle F, Heinze G, Schindl M, Losert UM. The role of intra-abdominal pressure on splanchnic and pulmonary hemodynamic and metabolic changes during carbon dioxide pneumoperitoneum. *Gastrointest Endosc* 1999;49(Jan):84–91.

33d. Junghans T, Bohm B, Grundel K, Schwenk W, Muller JM. Does pneumoperitoneum with different gases, body positions, and intraperitoneal pressures influence renal and hepatic blood flow? *Surgery* 1997;121:206–211.

34. Watcha MF, White PF. Postoperative nausea and vomiting. *Anesthesiology* 1992;77:162–184.

35a. Hulka JF, Peterson HB, Phillips JM, Surrey MW. American Association of Gynecologic Laproscopists' 1991 membership survey on operative laparoscopy. *J Reprod Med.* 1993;38:569–571.

35b. Hulka JF, Peterson HB, Phillips JM, Surrey MW. American Association of Gynecologic Laproscopists' 1993 membership survey. *J Am Assoc Gynecol Laparosc* 1995;2:133–136.

35c. Jansen FW, Kapiteyn K, Trimbos-Kemper T, Hermans J, Trimbos JB. Complications of laparoscopy: a prospective multicentre observational study. *Br J Obstet Gynaecol* 1997;104:595–600.

35d. Chapron C, Querleu D, Bruhat MA, Madelenat P, Fernandez H, Pierre F, Dubuisson JB. Surgical complications of diagnostic and operative gynaecological laparoscopy: a series of 29,966 cases. *Hum Reprod* 1998;13:867–872.

36. Toub DB, Sedlacek TV, Campion MJ. Acidemia associated with the use of high-flow insufflators during laparoscopy. *Am J Obstet Gynecol* 1994;170:959–960.

37. Ostman PL, Pautle-Fisher FH, Faure EA, et al. Circulatory collapse during laparoscopy. *J Clin Anesthesiol* 1990;2:129–132.

38. Gaff TD, Arbgast NR, Phillips OC, et al. Gas embolism: a comparative study of air and carbon dioxide as embolic agents in the systemic vascular system. *Am J Obstet Gynecol* 1959;78:259–265.

39. Shulman D, Aronson HB. Capnography in the early diagnosis of carbon dioxide embolism. *Can Anaesthesiol Soc J* 1984;31:455–459.

40. Albertine KH. Lung injury and neutrophil density during air embolization in sheep after leukocyte depletion with nitrogen mustard. *Am Rev Respir Dis* 1988;138:1444–1447.

41. Sloan TB, Kimovec MA. Detection of venous air embolism by airway pressure monitoring. *Anesthesiology* 1986;64:645–648.

42. Winter PH, Alvis HJ, Gag M. Hyperbaric treatment of cerebral air embolism during cardiopulmonary bypass. *JAMA* 1971;21(5):1786–1788.

43. Bernard GR, Artigas A, Brigham KL, et al. The American-European Consensus Conference on ARDS: definitions, mechanisms, relevant outcomes and clinical trial coordination. *Am Rev Respir Crit Care Med* 1994;149:818–824.

44. Shah P, Rmakantan R. Pneumoperitoneum and pneumomediastinum: unusual complications of laparoscopy. *J Post Grad Med* 1990;36:31–32.

45. Pascual JB, Baranda MM, Tarrero MT, et al. Subcutaneous emphysema, pseudomediastinum, bilateral pneumothorax and pneumopericardium after laparoscopy. *Endoscopy* 1990;22:59–61.

46. Knos GB, Sung, YF, Toledo A. Pneumopericardium associated with laparoscopy. *J Clin Anesthesiol* 1991;3:56–59.

47. Safran D, Sgambati S, Orlando R III. Laparoscopic surgery in high risk cardiac patients. *Surg Gynecol Obstet* 1993;176:548–554.

48. Harris MNE, Plantevin OM, Crowther A. Cardiac arrhythmias during anaesthesia for laparoscopy. *Br J Anaesthesiol* 1984;56:1213–1216.

49. Myles PS. Bradyarrhythmias and laparoscopy: a prospective study of heart rate changes during laparoscopy. *Aust NZ J Obstet Gynaecol* 1991;31:171–173.

50. Carmichael DE. Laparoscopy-cardiac considerations. *Fertil Steril* 1971;22: 69–70.

51. Doyle DJ, Mark PWS. Laparoscopy and vagal arrest. *Anaesthesia* 1989;44:448.

52. Shifren JL, Adlestein L, Finkler NJ. Asystolic cardiac arrest: a rare complication of laparoscopy. *Obstet Gynecol* 1992;79:840–841.

53. Ganansia MF, Francois TP, Ormezzano X, et al. Atrioventricular Mobitz I block during propofol anesthesia for laparoscopic tubal ligation. *Anesth Analg* 1989;69:524–525.

54. Nord HJ. Complications of laparoscopy. *Endoscopy* 1992;24:693–700.

55. Hulka JF, Socerstrom RM, Corson SL, et al. Complications Committee of the American Association of Gynecologic Laparoscopist: First Annual Report. *J Reprod Med* 1975;10:301–306.

56. Verghese C, Brimacombe JR. Survey of laryngeal mask airway usage in 11,910 patients: safety and efficacy for conventional and nonconventional usage. *Anesth Analg* 1996;82:129–133.

57. Scott DB. Regurgitation during laparoscopy. *Br J Anaesth* 1980;52:559–561.

58a. Moore SS, Green CR, Wang FL. The role of irrigation in the development of hypothermia during laparoscopic surgery. *Am J Obstet Gynecol* 1997;176(3):598–602.

58b. Ott DE, Reich H, Love B, McCorvey R, Toledo A, Liu CY, Syed R, Kumar K. Reduction of laparoscopic induced hypothermia, postoperative pain and recovery room length of stay by preconditioning gas with the Insuflow device: a prospective randomized controlled multi-center trial. *J Soc Laparoendosc Surg* 1998;2:321–329.

59. Deziel DJ, Millikan KW, Economou SG, et al. Complications of laparoscopic cholecystectomy: results of a national survey of 4,292 hospitals and analysis of 77,604 cases. *Am J Surg* 1993;165:9–14.

60. Larson GM, Vitale GC, Casey J, et al. Multipractice analysis of laparoscopic cholecystectomy in 1,983 patients. *Am J Surg* 1992;163:221–226.

61. The Southern Surgeons Club: a prospective analysis of 1518 laparoscopic cholecystectomies. *N Engl J Med* 1991;324:1073–1078.

62. Schwenk W, Bohm B, Junghans T, Hofmann H, Muller JM. Intermittent sequential compression of the lower limbs prevents venous stasis in laparoscopic and conventional colorectal surgery. *Dis Colon Rectum* 1997;40(9):1056–1062.

63a. Pring DW. Inferior epigastric hemorrhage, an avoidable complication of laparoscopic clip sterilization. *Br J Obstet Gynaecol* 1983;90:480–482.

63b. Hulka JF, Levy BS, Parker WH, Phillips JM. Laparoscopic assisted vaginal hysterectomy: American Association of Gynecologic Laparsocopists' 1995 membership survey. *J Am Assoc Gynecol Laparosc* 1997;4:167–171.

64. Gottlieb ME, Chandrasekhar B, Terz JJ, Sherman R. Clinical applications of the extended deep inferior epigastric flap. *Plastic Recon Surg* 1986;78:788–792.

65a. Baadsgaard SE, Bile S, Egeblad K. Major vascular injury during gynecologic laparoscopy. *Acta Obstet Gynecol Scand* 1989;68:283–285.

65b. Saville LE, Woods MS. Laparoscopy and major retroperitoneal vascular injuries (MVRI). *Surg Endosc* 1995;9:1096–1100.

65c. Chapron CM, Pierre F, Lacroix S, Querleu D, Lansac J, Dubuisson JB. Major vascular injuries during gynecologic laparoscopy. *J Am Coll Surg* 1997;185:461–465.

65d. Lam A, Rosen DMB. Laparoscopic bowel and vascular complications: should the Verres needle and cannula be replaced? *J Am Assoc Gynecol Laparosc* 1996;3:S24.

66a. Shackford SR, Sise MJ. Renal and mesenteric vascular trauma. In Bongard FS, Wilson SE, Perry MO (Eds), *Vascular Injuries in Surgical Practice*. Norwalk, CT: Appleton and Lange, 1991, pp. 179–181.

66b. Nassar AH, Htwe T, Hefny, H, Kholeif Y. The abdominal drain: a convenient port for second look laparoscopy. *Surg Endosc* 1996;10:1114–1115.

67a. Alvarez RD. Gastrointestinal complications in gynecologic surgery: a review for the general gynecologist. *Obstet Gynecol* 1988;72:533–540.

67b. Bishoff JT, Allaf ME, Kirkels, W, Moore RG, Kavoussi LR, Schroder F. Laparoscopic bowel injury: incidence and clinical presentation. *J Urol* 1999;161:887–890.

67c. Schrenk P, Woisetschlager R, Rieger R, Wayand W. Mechanism, management, and prevention of laparoscopic bowel injuries. *Gastrointest Endosc* 1996;43:572–574.

67d. Tung PH, Wang Q, Ogle CK, Smith CD. Minimal increase in gut-mucosal interleukin-6 during laparoscopy. *Surg Endosc* 1998;12:409–411.

67e. Ostrzenski A, Ostrzenska KM. Bladder injury during laparoscopic surgery. *Obstet Gynecol Surv* 1998;53:175–180.

67f. Saida MH, Sadler RK, Vancaillie TG, Akbright BD, Farhart SA, White AJ. Diagnosis and management of serious urinary complications after major operative laparoscopy. *Obstet Gynecol* 1996;87:272–276.

68a. Childers JM, Brzechffa PR, Surwit EA. Laparoscopy using the left upper quadrant as the primary trocar site. *Gynecol Oncol* 1993;50:221–225.

68b. Lee PI, Chi YS, Chang YK, Joo KY. Minilaparoscopy to reduce complications from cannula insertion in patients with previous pelvic or abdominal surgery. *J Am Assoc Gynecol Laparosc* 1999;6:91–95.

69. Bruhat MA, Goldchmit R: Minilaparoscopy in gynecology. *Eur J Obstet Gynecol Reprod Biol* 1998;76:207–210.

70. Grosskinsky CM, Ryder RM, Pendergrass HM, Hulka JF. Laparoscopic capacitance: a mystery measured. *Am J Obstet Gynecol* 1993;169:1632–1635.

71. Spirtos NM, Schlaerth JB, Kimball RE, Leiphart VM, Ballon SC. Laparoscopic radical hysterectomy with aortic and pelvic lymphadenectomy. *Am J Obstet Gynecol* 1996;174:1763–1768.

72a. Flint LM, Vitale GC, Richardson JD, Polk H. The injured colon: relationships of management to complications. *Ann Surg* 1981;193:619–623.

72b. Berry MA, Rangraj M. Conservative treatment of recognized laparoscopic colonic injury. *J Soc Laparoendosc Surg* 1998;2:195–196.

73. Birns MT. Inadvertent instrumental perforation of the colon during laparoscopy: nonsurgical repair. *Gastrointest Endosc* 1989;35:54–55.

74. Ridgeway CA, Frame SB, Rice JC, Timberlake GA, McSwain JE Jr, Kerstein MD. Primary repair vs. colostomy for treatment of penetrating colon injuries. *Dis Colon Rectum* 1989;32:1046–1049.

75. Heseltine PNR, Berne TV, Yellin AE. The efficacy of cefoxitin vs. clindamycin/ gentamycin in surgically treated stab wounds of the bowel. *J Trauma* 1986;26:241–244.

76. Rowlands BJ, Ericsson CH, Fischer RP. Penetrating abdominal trauma: the use of operative findings to determine length of antibiotic therapy. *J Trauma* 1987;27:250–255.

77a. Gazelle GS, Mueller PR. Abdominal abscess: imaging and intervention. *Radiol Clin N Am* 1994;32(5):913–932.

77b. Sedlacek TV. Laparoscopic radical hysterectomy: the next evolutionary step in the treatment of invasive cervical cancer. *J Gynecol Tech* 1995;1:223–230.

78. Reich H, McGlynn F. Laparoscopic repair of bladder injury. *Obstet Gynecol* 1990;76:909.

79. Degner DA; Walshaw R. Healing responses of the lower urinary tract. *Veterinary Clin N Am. Small Animal Pract* 1996;26(2):197–206.

80a. McLucas B, March C. Urachal sinus perforation during laparoscopy: a case report. *J Reprod Med* 1990;75:573–574.

80b. Ostrzenski A, Osborne NG, Ostrzenska K, Godette AO. Preoperative contrast ultrasonographic diagnosis of patent urachal sinus. *Int Urogynecol J Pelvic Floor Dysfunct* 1998;9:52–54.

81. Woodland MB. Ureteral injury during laparoscopy-assisted vaginal hysterectomy with the endoscopic linear stapler. *Am J Obstet Gynecol* 1992;167:756–757.

82. Grainger DA, Soderstrom RM, Schiff SF, et al. Ureteral injuries at laparoscopy: insights into diagnosis, management, and prevention. *Obstet Gynecol* 1990;75:839–843.

83. Koonings PP, et al. uerteroscopy: a new asset in the management of postoperative ureterovaginal fistulas. *Obstet Gynecol* 1992;80(3):548–549.

84. Selzman AA, Spirnak JP, Kursh ED. The changing management of ureterovaginal fistulas. *J Urol* 1995;153(3, pt 1):626–628.

85. Vasilev SA. Obturator nerve injury: a review of management options. *Gynecol Oncol* 1994;53:152–155.

86. Atwood SEA, Hill ADK, Murphy PG, et al. A prospective randomized trial of laparoscopic versus open appendectomy. *Surgery* 1992;112:457–501.

87. Peters JH, Gibbons GD, Innes JT, et al. Complications of laparoscopic cholecystectomy. *Surgery* 1991;110:769–778.

88. Pier A, Gotz F, Bacher C, Ibald R. Laparoscopic appendectomy. *World J Surg* 1993;17(1):29–33.

89. Schultz L, Graber J, Pietrafitta J, et al. Laser laparoscopic herniorrhaphy: a clinical trial preliminary results. *J Laparoendosc Surg* 1990;1:41–45.

90. Scott-Conner CEH, Hall TJ, Anglin BL, et al. Laparoscopic appendectomy: initial experience in a teaching program. *Ann Surg* 1992;215:660–668.

91. Sotrel G, Hirsch E, Edelin KC. Necrotizing fasciitis following diagnostic laparoscopy. *Obstet Gynecol* 1983;62S:67S–69S.

92. Kadar N, Reich H, Lui CY, Manko GF, Gimpelson R. Incisional hernias after major laparoscopic gynecologic procedures. *Am J Obstet Gynecol* 1993;168:4193–4195.

93a. Montz FJ, Holschneider CH, Munro MG. Incisional hernia following laparoscopy: a survey of the American Association of Gynecologic Laparoscopists. *Obstet Gynecol* 1994;84(5):881–884.

93b. Vaghadia H, McLeod DH, Mitchell GW, Merrick PM, Chilvers CR. Small dose hypobaric lidocaine-fentanyl spinal anesthesia for short duration outpatient laparoscopy. I. A randomized comparison with conventional dose hyperbaric lidocaine. *Anesth Analg* 1997;84:59–64.

93c. Chilvers CR, Vaghadia H, Mitchell GW, Merrick PM. Small dose hypobaric lidocaine-fentanyl spinal anesthesia for short duration outpatient laparoscopy. II. Optimal fentanyl dose. *Anesthesiol Analg* 1997;84:65–70.

94a. Dobbs FF, Kumar V, Alexander JL, Hull MGR. Pain after laparoscopy related to posture and ring versus clip sterilization. *Br J Obstet Gynaecol* 1987;94:262–266.

94b. Schauer PR, Page CP, Ghiatas AA, Miller JE, Schwesinger WH, Sirinek KR. Incidence and significance of subdiaphragmatic air following laparoscopic cholecystectomy. *Am Surg* 1997;63:132–136.

94c. Toub DB, Zubernis J, Campion MJ, Sedlacek TV. Resolution of free intraperitoneal air after laparoscopy: utility of abdominal radiography in the diagnosis of bowel injury. *J Am Assoc Gynecol Laparosc* 1994;1:S37.

95. Kenefick JP, Leader A, Maltby JR, Taylor PJ. Laparoscopy: blood gas values and minor sequelae associated with three techniques based on isoflurane. *Br J Anaesthesiol* 1987;59:189–194.

96a. Chamberlain G. The recovery of gases insufflated at laparoscopy. *Br J Obstet Gynaecol* 1984;91:367–370.

96b. Guido RS, Brooks K, McKenzie R, Gruss J, Krohn MA. A randomized, prospective comparison of pain after gasless laparoscopy and traditional laparoscopy. *J Am Assoc Gynecol Laparosc* 1998;5:149–153.

96c. Cunniffe MG, McAnena OJ, Dar MA, Clleary J, Flynn N. A prospective randomized trial of intraoperative bupivicaine irrigation for management of shoulder tip pain following laparoscopy. *Am J Surg* 1998;176:258–261.

96d. Zullo F, Pellicano M, Cappiello F, Zupi E, Marconi D, Nappi C. Pain control after microlaparoscopy. *J Am Assoc Gynecol Laparosc* 1998;5:161–163.

96e. Abdolhosseinzadeh M, Asgarieh S, Hajian H. Postoperative pain after lidocaine injection intraperitoneally and subcutaneously for laparoscopic surgery. *J Am Assoc Gynecol Laparosc* 1995;2:S1.

96f. Ke RW, Portera SG, Bagous W, Lincoln SR. A randomized double blinded trial of pre-emptive analgesia in laparoscopy. *Obstet Gynecol* 1998;92:972–975.

96g. De Witte J, Rietman GW, Vandenbroucke G, Deloof T. Postoperative effects of tramadol administered at wound closure. *Eur J Anaesthesiol* 1998;15:190–195.

96h. Windsor A, McDonald P, Mumtaz T, Millar JM. The analgesic efficacy of tenoxicam versus placebo in day case laparoscopy: a randomised parallel double blind trial. *Anaesthesia* 1996;51:1066–1069.

96i. Rasanayagam R, Harrison G. Preoperative oral administration of morphine in day-case gynaecological laparoscopy. *Anaesthesia* 1996;51:1179–1181.

97. Alexander JI, Hull MGR. Abdominal pain after laparoscopy: the value of a gas drain. *Br J Obstet Gynaecol* 1987;94:267–269.

98a. Metter SE, Kitz DS, Young ML, et al. Nausea and vomiting after outpatient laparoscopy: incidence, impact on recovery room stay and cost. *Anesthesiol Analg* 1987;66:S116.

98b. Chung F, Un V, Su J. Postoperative symptoms 24 hours after ambulatory anaesthesia. *Can J Anaesthesiol* 1996;43:1121–1127.

99. Palazzo MGA, Strunin L. Anaesthesia and emesis: etiology. *Can Anaesthesiol Soc J* 1984;31:178–187.

100. Boulton TB, Chir B. Oral chlorpromazine hydrochloride. *Anaesthesia* 1995;10:233–246.

101. Beattie WS, Lindblad T, Buckley DN, Forrest JB. The incidence of postoperative nausea and vomiting in women undergoing laparoscopy is influenced by the day of menstrual cycle. *Can J Anaesthesiol* 1991;38:298–302.

102. Bellville JW. Postanesthetic nausea and vomiting. *Anesthesiology* 1961;22:773–780.

103. Hovorka J, Kortilla K, Erkola O. Nitrous oxide does not increase nausea and vomiting following gynaecological laparoscopy. *Can J Anaesthesiol* 1989;36:145–148.

104. Sengupta P, Plantevin OM. Nitrous oxide and day case laparoscopy: effects on nausea, vomiting, and return to normal activity. *Br J Anaesthesiol* 1988;60:570–573.

105. Bridenbaugh LD. Regional anaesthesia for outpatient surgery—a summary of 12 years experience. *Can Anaesthesiol Soc J* 1983;30:548–552.

106. Gunawardene RD, White DC. Propofol and emesis. *Anaesthesia* 1988;43:65–57.

107. Rising S, Dodgson MS, Steen PA. Isoflurane v fentanyl for outpatient laparoscopy. *Acta Anaesthesiol Scand* 1985;29:251–255.

108. Oh S, Fabrick J, Pagualayan G. Evaluation of toradol for pain control after laparoscopic cholecystectomy. *Anesthesiology* 1992;77:440–443.

109. Calhoun B, Viani B, LaRue D. The effect of ketorolac on patients undergoing laparoscopic cholecystectomy. *Anesthesiology* 1992;77:48–52.

110. Parris WC, Lee EM. Anaesthesia for laparoscopic cholecystectomy. *Anaesthesia* 1991;46:997.

111a. Pandit SK, Kothary SP, Pandit UA, et al. Dose-response study of droperidol and metoclopramide as antiemetics for outpatient anesthesia. *Anesthesiol Analg* 1989;68:798–802.

111b. Rothenberg DM, McCarthy RJ, Peng CC, Normoyle DA. Nausea and vomiting after dexamethasone versus droperidol following outpatient laparoscopy with a propofol based general anesthetic. *Acta Anaesthesiol Scand* 1998;42:637–642.

112. Alon E, Himmelseher S. Ondansetron in the treatment of postoperative vomiting: a randomized double blind comparison with droperidol and metoclopramide. *Anesthesiol Analg* 1992;75:561–565.

113a. Wetchler BV, Sung YF, Duncalf D, Joslyn AF. Ondansetron decreases emetic symptoms following outpatient laparoscopy. *Anesthesiology* 1990;73:A35.

113b. Polati E, Verlato G, Finco G, Mosaner W, Grosso S, Gottin L, Pinaroli AM, Ischia S. Ondasteron versus metaclopramide in the treatment of postoperative nausea and vomiting. *Anesthesiol Analg* 1997;85:395–399.

113c. Borgeat A, Hasler P, Fahti M. Gynecologic laparoscopic surgery is not associated with an increase of serotonin metabolites excretion. *Anesthesiol Analg* 1998;87:1104–1108.

113d. Sniadach MS, Alberts MS. A comparison of the prophylactic antiemetic effect of ondasteron and droperidol on patients undergoing gynecologic laparoscopy. *Anesthesiol Analg* 1997;85:797–800.

114. Baily PL, Streisand JB, Pace NL, et al. Transdermal scopolamine reduces nausea and vomiting after outpatient laparoscopy. *Anesthesiology* 1990;72:977–980.

115. Curet MJ, Allen D, Josloff RK, et al. Laparoscopy in pregnancy. *Arch Surg* 1996;131:546–551.

116. Reedy MB, Galan HL, Richards WE, Preece CK, Wetter PA, Kuehl TJ. Laparoscopy during pregnancy. A survey of laparoendoscopic surgeons. *J Reprod Med* 1997;42:33–38.

117. Arvidsson D, Gerdin E. Laparoscopic cholecystectomy during pregnancy. *Surg Laparosc Endosc* 1991;1:193–194.

118. Pucci RO, Seed RW. Case report of laparoscopic cholecystectomy in the third trimester of pregnancy. *Am J Obstet Gynecol* 1991;165:401–402.

119. Morrell DG, Mullins JR, Harrison PB. Laparoscopic cholecystectomy during pregnancy in symptomatic patients. *Surgery* 1992;112:856–859.

120. Soper NJ, Hunter JG, Petrie RH. Laparoscopic cholecystectomy during pregnancy. *Surg Endosc* 1992;6:115–117.

121. Constantino GN, Vincent GJ, Mukalian CG, et al. Laparoscopic cholecystectomy in pregnancy. *J Laparoendosc Surg* 1994;4:161–164.

122. Posta CG. Laparoscopic surgery in pregnancy: report on two cases. *J Laparoendosc Surg* 1995;4:161–164.

123. Williams JK, Rosemurgy AS, Albrink MH, et al. Laparoscopic cholecystectomy in pregnancy: a case report. *J Reprod Surg* 1995;40:243–244.

124. Martin IG, Dexter SP, McMahon MJ. Laparoscopic cholecystectomy in pregnancy. A safe option during the second trimester. *Surg Endosc* 1996;10:508–510.

125. Curet MJ, Vogt DA, Schob O, Qualls C, Izquierdo LA, Zucker KA. Effects of CO_2 pneumoperitoneum in pregnant ewes. *J Surg Res* 1996;63:339–344.

126. Hunter JG, Swanstrom L, Thornburg K. Carbon dioxide pneumoperitoneum induces fetal acidosis in a pregnant ewe model. *Surg Endosc* 1995;9:272–279.

127. Iafrati MD, Yarnell R, Schwaitzberg SD. Gasless laparoscopic cholecystectomy in pregnancy. *J Laparoendosc Surg* 1995;5:127–130.

128. Akira S, Yamanaka A, Ishihara T, Takeshita T, Araki T. Gasless laparoscopic ovarian cystectomy during pregnancy: comparison with laparotomy. *Am J Obstet Gynecol* 1999;180:554–557.

129. Luxman D, Cohen JR, David MP. Laparoscopic myomectomy in pregnancy. *J Am Assoc Gynecol Laparosc* 1995;2:S28.

130. Dufuor P, Delebecq T, Vinatier D, Haentjens-Verbeke K, Tordjeman N, Prolongeau JF, Monnier JC, Puech F. Appendicitis in pregnancy. Seven case reports. *J Gynecol Obstet Biol Reprod (Paris)* 1996;25:411–415.

131. Barone JE, Bears S, Chen S, Tsai J, Russell JC. Outcome study of cholecystectomy in pregnancy. *Am J Surg* 1999;177:232–236.

132. Geisler JP, Rose SL, Mernitz CS, Warner JL, Hiett AK. Nongynecologic laparoscopy in the second and third trimester pregnancy: obstetric implications. *J Soc Laparoendosc Surg* 1998;2:235–238.

133. Gurbuz AT, Peetz ME. The acute abdomen in the pregnant patient. Is there a role for laparoscopy? *Surg Endosc* 1997;11:98–102.

134. Reedy MB, Kallen B, Kuehl TJ. Laparoscopy during pregnancy: a study of five fetal outcome parameters with use of the Swedish Health Registry. *Am J Obstet Gynecol* 1997;177:673–679.

135. Nezhat FR, Tazuke S, Nezhat CH, Seidman DS, Philips DR, Nezhat CR. Laparoscopy during pregnancy: a literature review. *J Soc Laparoendosc Surg* 1997;1:17–27.

136. Morice P, Louis-Sylvestre C, Chapron C, Dubuisson JB. Laparoscopy for adnexal torsion in pregnant women. *J Reprod Med* 1997;42:435–439.

137. Yuval Y, Soriano D, Goldenberg M, Seidman DS, Oelsner G. Is operative laparoscopy contraindicated in the first trimester of pregnancy? *J Am Assoc Gynecol Laparosc* 1995;2:S61–62.

138. Conron RW Jr, Abbruzzi K, Cochrane SO, Sarno AJ, Cochrane PJ. Laparoscopic procedures in pregnancy. *Am Surg* 1999;65:259–263.

139. Soriano D, Yefet Y, Seidman DS, Goldenberg M, Mashiach S, Oelsner G. Laparoscopy versus laparotomy in the management of adnexal masses during pregnancy. *Fertil Steril* 1999;71:955–960.

140. Amos JD, Schorr SJ, Norman PF, et al. Laparoscopic surgery during pregnancy. *Am J Surg* 1996;171:435–437.

141. Guidelines for laparoscopic surgery during pregnancy. Society of American Gastrointestinal Endoscopic Surgeons. *Surg Endosc* 1998;12:189–190.

PART III

ONCOLOGIC PERIOPERATIVE DECISION MAKING

CHAPTER 13

ENDOMETRIAL AND CERVICAL CARCINOMA

BRADLEY J. MONK, M.D., and ROBERT A. BURGER, M.D.

Hysterectomy is second only to cesarean section as the most frequently performed major operation in the United States. Data from the National Hospital Discharge Survey (NHDS) indicate that approximately 590,000 hysterectomies are performed annually. By the age of 60, over one-third of U.S. women have undergone a hysterectomy. Although hysterectomy rates vary substantially according to geographic area, as well as by patient- and physician-related factors, cervical and corpus cancer remain consistent indications for this procedure (Table 13.1; Level III).[1,2]

Hysterectomies performed for benign indications are associated with much less morbidity and mortality than for indications associated with pregnancy or cancer. For example, the reported mortality rates after hysterectomy increase from 6 to 11 per 10,000 for indications not involving pregnancy or cancer, to 29 to 38 per 10,000 when the indication is associated with pregnancy, and ultimately to 70 to 200 per 10,000 when associated with invasive cancer.[3] Modern surgical management and meticulous perioperative care may limit this morbidity and improve outcome. This chapter summarizes the evidence for modern perioperative evaluation, decision making, and treatment of uterine cervix and corpus cancers.

CURRENT SURGICAL MANAGEMENT OF ENDOMETRIAL CANCER

Endometrial carcinoma is the most common malignancy of the female genital tract in the United States. Annually, approximately 34,900 new cases and 6,000 deaths occur.[4] This is predominantly a disease of affluent, overweight,

Perioperative and Supportive Care in Gynecologic Oncology: Evidence-Based Management,
Edited by Steven A. Vasilev.
ISBN 0-471-24788-X   Copyright © 2000 by Wiley-Liss, Inc.

TABLE 13.1. Indications for Hysterectomy

Indication	Approximate Percent (%)
Uterine leiomyomata	30
Dysfunctional uterine bleeding	20
Endometriosis and adenomyosis	20
Genital prolapse	15
Endometrial hyperplasia	6
CIN, invasive cervical and corpus cancer	6
Other (pain, PID, obstetrical)	3

TABLE 13.2. Conditions Associated with Endometrial Carcinoma

Advanced age (>70 years)
Obesity
Hypertension
Diabetes
Atherosclerotic heart disease

postmenopausal women of low parity, although an increasing proportion of younger patients with endometrial cancer has been reported.[5] The median age at diagnosis is approximately 54 years. Concurrent medical illnesses frequently associated with endometrial malignancies place these patients at significant risk for perioperative morbidity (Table 13.2).

The cornerstone of therapy for endometrial cancer is total abdominal hysterectomy and bilateral salpingo-oophorectomy, with selected pelvic and para-aortic lymph node dissection. This operation should be performed in all cases whenever feasible. In addition, many patients will require some type of adjuvant radiation therapy to help prevent vaginal vault recurrence and/or to sterilize occult disease in the lymph nodes. In contrast to the outcome for patients with cervical cancer, that for patients with cancer of the corpus treated with hysterectomy alone or hysterectomy and radiation is significantly better than for those treated with radiation alone.[5]

CURRENT SURGICAL MANAGEMENT OF CERVICAL CANCER

Although cervical cancer is the third most common gynecologic malignancy in the United States, it is the leading cause of cancer-related death among women worldwide, and according to World Health Organization estimates, more than 400,000 new cases of cervical cancer are diagnosed annually (Level II-1).[6] In the United States, the incidence of cervical carcinoma is substantially higher among minority women and/or those of lower socioeconomic status. Consequently, these individuals have generally not had adequate access to health care and frequently have not been screened for common illness such as diabetes, hypertension, and cardiovascular disease.[7] Therefore, careful attention to nongynecologic symptoms as well as a high index of suspicion of other medical illnesses is critical during the perioperative period when treating patients with cervical cancer. These include diabetes and hypertension, which are common among Hispanic-American and African-American women, respectively. Furthermore, human immunodeficiency virus (HIV) seropositivity has recently been identified as a risk factor of cervical neoplasia, in addition to the more commonly accepted risk factors, such as early age of first intercourse, history of sexual promiscuity, and multigravidity. The median age at diagnosis in the United States is approximately 45 years.

The surgical treatment of invasive cervical cancer can be grouped into four categories based on extent and status of disease (Level II-1).[7,8] First, patients with squamous lesions that are not confluent, invade to ≤3 mm below the basement membrane, and do not exhibit evidence of lymph-vascular space invasion (FIGO [International Federation of Gynecology and Obstetrics] Stage IA1), can be treated with extrafascial hysterectomy alone, with cure rates approaching 100%, since the risk of parametrial and/or lymphatic spread is 1% or less. Disease extent can be accurately assessed only after an excisional procedure has been performed and negative surgical margins obtained. Cold knife cone and large loop excision of the transformation zone (LLETZ) are equally efficacious when the latter is performed by experienced operators who limit thermal artifact and properly orient the specimen, thus simplifying histologic analysis (Level II-1).[8] The decision to perform an extrafascial or radical hysterectomy based on frozen section evaluation of a cone of LLETZ specimens has been associated with inaccuracies when compared to standard histologic review and may lead to inappropriate surgical management (Level II-3).[9–11]

Second, those with more extensive squamous lesions (FIGO Stage IA2), but not more than a FIGO stage IIA, as well as those with FIGO Stage I and IIA adenocarcinomas, are treated with either radical hysterectomy and bilateral pelvic lymphadenectomy, or radiation therapy combining whole-pelvic teletherapy with local brachytherapy. These treatment modalities are recognized as equally efficacious with respect to local control and survival. Surgery is often preferred to radiotherapy in younger women because ovarian function is eliminated and sexual function often is compromised following radiation. In addition, the late complications of radiation are avoided when patients are treated with surgery alone. However, women with early cervical cancer treated with radical surgery may occasionally benefit from a combined approach, including adjuvant radiation, usually with chemotherapy, if surgical margins are compromised or if regional lymphatic spread is present (Level II-3).[7,12]

Compared to less radical therapy, such as extrafascial hysterectomy, patients treated with radical hysterectomy experience increased blood loss and more frequently require transfusions. The estimated average blood loss associated with radical hysterectomy varies with operator experience, patient body habitus and anatomy, as well as lesion size. Averages ranging from 500 to 2,000 ml of blood have been reported, but 800 to 1,200 ml is probably more accurate (Level II-3).[13] In addition, patients undergoing radical hysterectomy are at increased risk of urinary and intestinal tract fistula formation than women treated with extrafascial hysterectomy, although the exact incidence is not known since most cases are not reported. A reasonable noncancer-related fistula rate following radical hysterectomy approximates 1–2% compared to 0.1–0.5% after simple extrafascial hysterectomy. Clearly, the lowest rates of fistula formation occur when injury to the urinary or intestinal tract is immediately detected intraoperatively and properly repaired, since fistulae generally occur only after occult injuries or in patients who have received radiation (Level II-3).[14,15] Probably the most common cause of morbidity following radical hysterectomy is chronic bladder dysfunction, occurring in 30% to 70% of patients.[7] Patients experience a significant reduction in detrusor contractility, and considerable abdominal straining is often required to empty the bladder after radical hysterectomy. In addition, diminished vesical sensation is almost universal.

Third, when primary surgical extirpation is not possible, such as with FIGO Stage IIB to IVA lesions, radiotherapy with chemotherapy becomes the first line of therapy. Commonly, patients receive 4,000 to 6,000 cGy external beam irradiation in 170 to 200 cGy daily fractions followed by two brachytherapy applications, delivering a mean total tumor dose of approximately 8,500 to 9,000 cGy (Level II-2).[16] Cisplatin is used as a radiosensitizer usually at a dose of 40mg/ml intravenously for 6 weekly doses. Theoretically, surgical debulking of grossly involved pelvic or para-aortic nodal metastasis, or extended field radiation treating the para-aortic region when para-aortic disease is documented, combined with standard pelvic irradiation, could improve outcome among patients with metastatic disease (Level II-3).[17]

The fourth category of patients with cervical cancer amenable to surgical therapy includes those with recurrent disease in the central pelvis. These are the only patients with recurrent cervical carcinoma who are potentially curable with surgery. Such patients are offered pelvic exenteration with resection of the bladder, vagina, cervix, uterus, ovaries, fallopian tubes, and rectum, necessitating urinary diversion, as well as fecal diversion and vaginal reconstruction in many cases.[7]

PREOPERATIVE EVALUATION

The goal of the preoperative evaluation is to assess surgical risk and formulate a risk : benefit ratio of surgical management. In addition, careful preoperative assessment of the patient enables preventive measures to be taken that decrease surgical risk and morbidity. Preoperative care begins with a careful history, including the current illness, medical history, surgical history, gynecologic history, family history, social history, and documentation of medications, allergies to medications, and habits. Inherent in this screening evaluation is a complete physical examination and testing to assess organ system function, with particular attention to the cardiovascular, respiratory, renal/urinary, gastrointestinal, immune, and nervous systems. Furthermore, nutritional status is evaluated, as well as risk of infectious, thromboembolic disease, and bleeding complications. Routine preoperative testing is covered in Chapter 8.

Prognostic risk stratification to identify perioperative and long-term cardiac risk in selected patients undergoing gynecologic surgery is part of good clinical practice. Noninvasive cardiac testing may be used selectively in patients undergoing noncardiac surgery to provide useful estimates of short- and long-term risk of cardiac events. Results from noninvasive testing and the magnitude of abnormality should then be used to formulate decisions regarding the need for coronary angiography and subsequent revascularization prior to the planned elective gynecologic operation. Controversy exists regarding the guidelines for ordering noninvasive studies beyond the standard preoperative electrocardiogram (ECG). Exercise variables have been proposed as criteria to screen patients who may benefit from other noninvasive cardiac studies beyond the ECG. Factors associated with significant increased cardiac risk include poor functional capacity and may be an indication for a preoperative exercise ECG. Marked exercise-induced ST segment shift or angina at low workloads, as well as an inability to increase or actually decrease systolic blood pressure with progressive exercise, may be indications for further testing.

Unfortunately, many obese and/or elderly patients are unable to perform an adequate level of exercise to test cardiac reserve, making the exercise ECG uninterpretable. The predictive value for a perioperative event (i.e., death or myocardial infarction) ranges from 5% to 25% for a positive exercise ECG test and 90% to 95% for a negative test. When an exercise ECG is not feasible (approximately 30–50% of patients), pharmacological stress imaging should be used in patients who require further perioperative noninvasive risk stratification. Myocardial perfusion variables predictive of increased cardiac events include severity of the perfusion defect, number of reversible defects, extent of fixed and reversible defects, increased lung uptake of thallium-201, and marked ST segment changes associated with angina during the test. The reported sensitivity and specificity of dobutamine-induced echocardiographic wall motion abnormalities in patients with peripheral vascular disease is similar to myocardial perfusion scintigraphy (Level II-2).[18]

For most gynecologic procedures, a chest radiograph is not routinely recommended unless the patient is over 60 years of age, since the yield in asymptomatic nonsmokers without preexisting pulmonary disease is low and therefore not supported by evidence (Level II-2).[19,20] However, when performing surgery for an invasive gynecologic malignancy, it is important to exclude lung metastasis, although this is also an unusual occurrence and the cost-effectiveness of chest radiographs in asymptomatic women with early gynecologic cancers is not well established (Level II-2).[21] Data on this subject is further reviewed in Chapter 8.

Crossmatching of packed red blood cell units is also not part of the routine evaluation for gynecologic surgery, but due to the potential for vascular injury and rapid blood loss during lymph node dissections and/or radical hysterectomy, preparation for an emergency intraoperative blood transfusion may be considered. Blood ordering practices and perioperative preparation are further addressed in Chapter 8.

Endometrial Cancer

Issues unique to the preoperative evaluation of women with endometrial cancer include the possible role of preoperative radiologic and endoscopic studies to assess the extent of disease. Evidence supporting the routine use of tests that investigate the urologic and intestinal systems, such as intravenous pyelogram (IVP), cystogram, cystoscopy, barium enema (BE), sigmoidoscopy, and colonoscopy, is lacking (21). However, testing for occult fecal blood and a urinalysis are standard tests performed on women over age 50 prior to surgery, although the cost-effectiveness of these tests remains in question (Level II-2).[22–25] Moreover, CT and MRI scanning of the abdomen and pelvis have not been shown to alter treatment strategies among patients with uterine cancer. Preoperative serum CA-125 levels are predictive of extrauterine spread of cancer, but this marker is only prognostic and can be ordered after final histopathologic data are available (among those greater than Stage II) (Level II-3).[26] Perioperative CA-125 levels and other molecular markers, such as HER2/neu, estrogen and progesterone receptor status, P53, and ploidy, are not sufficiently sensitive or specific to alter current surgical or adjuvant therapies.

Endometrial biopsy (EMB) is effective in diagnosing endometrial carcinoma and should be performed in all women with postmenopausal bleeding, asymptomatic postmenopausal women with endometrial cells on Pap smear, women with cells on Pap smear suggestive of adenocarcinoma, and perimenopausal women with intermenstrual bleeding or menorrhagia. EMB and transvaginal ultrasound may also be an important tool in the evaluation of a Pap smear showing atypical glandular cells of undetermined significance or postmenopausal women with pyometria (Level II-3).[27] Classically, a fractional uterine curettage after cervical dilatation (D&C) was the method of choice in diagnosing endometrial cancer. However, since endometrial cancer is now surgically staged, an office EMB is acceptable.[5] The role of hysteroscopy in the diagnosis of endometrial cancer has not been established; furthermore, hysteroscopy may potentially disseminate cancer through fallopian tube transport. Because of this theoretical risk of metastasis, as well as the limited diagnostic value of hysteroscopy, it should only be selectively performed as part of an operative procedure (endometrial ablation or myomectomy) or if an endometrial polyp is strongly suspected and not amenable to D&C alone (Level II-3).[28]

Cervical Cancer

The foundation of the evaluation of an abnormal Pap includes physical examination and colposcopy with directed biposies and endocervical curettage.[7] Therapeutic decisions are then made based on the histologic findings. Cone or LLETZ may be necessary to better define the extent of an occult or minimally invasive cancer as discussed above. Other diagnostic studies have not been proven useful except those judiciously applied in specific cases (i.e., larger or more advanced lesions) to determine hydronephrosis, bladder and rectal involvement, and lymphatic metastasis. By staging convention, all patients with FIGO Stage IB1 or more advanced lesions should at least have a pretreatment intravenous urogram (IVU a.k.a. IVP). Patients with tumors >4 cm (≥FIGO Stage IB2) or individuals with smaller tumors in locations encroaching upon urologic or intestinal structures should be considered for an examination under anesthesia with cystoscopy and proctoscopy.

Barium enema (BE) has little or no role in the routine evaluation of patients with cervical cancer (Level II-2).[29] However, ultrasonography has recently been studied as an alternative to cystoscopy during the evaluation of bladder invasion (Level II-3).[30] Patients not treated surgically who are at significant risk of lymphatic metastasis (i.e., FIGO Stage IB1 or greater) are candidates for radiologic assessment for possible lymphatic metastasis. Ultrasound, CT, magnetic resonance imaging (MRI), and lymphangiography have all been studied as modalities to evaluate for lymphatic spread. Although lymphangiography is not widely available, it appears to be more effective in assessing pelvic and para-aortic nodal status than both MRI and CT scanning. However, CT scanning and MRI, although more costly, are useful in selected patients to assess extent of disease and plan optimal therapy (Level III).[31] The measurement of serum tumor markers in patients with invasive cervical cancer has not been found to be of clear benefit.

INTRAOPERATIVE CONSIDERATIONS

Careful intraoperative management simplifies postoperative care and reduces complications. Prolonged operative time leads to increased operative site infection presumably due to a decrease in tissue perfusion secondary to transient hypothermia (Level II-2).[34] Every effort possible should be made to accomplish a safe and expeditious surgical procedure.

Generally, patients undergoing abdominal hysterectomy (simple or radical) with or without lymph node dissection for cervical or uterine corpus cancer are positioned in the supine position. Alternatively, low lithotomy positioning can be used, but care must be exercised to avoid peroneal nerve injury. This nerve injury occurs commonly after improper patient positioning when the peroneal nerve becomes entrapped between the head of the fibula and the stirrup (Level II-3).[35] Moreover, femoral and/or obturator nerve injuries can be prevented by avoiding hip hyperextension and hip overabduction, respectively (Levels II-3 and III).[36,37]

After positioning, hair at the operative site is removed and the patient is prepped. Clipping of hair is preferred to shaving since shaving predisposes to skin disruption and folliculitis (Level II-2).[38] Iodine preps have traditionally been the standard method of skin preparation, but noniodinated preps, such as those containing cyclochlorhexidene, may be used in iodine-sensitive individuals without an increase in wound complications. Newer iodine-based gel-preps do not require extensive scrubbing like the standard two-step iodine-based preps and have been shown to be effective and time-saving (Levels III and II-1).[39,40] Finally, a transurethral Foley catheter is placed and the patient is draped in a sterile fashion. Adhesive drapes have not been shown to reduce wound complications.[39,40]

Rarely, adequate operative exposure can be obtained through a Pfannenstiel incision. Preferably, a muscle-cutting incision such as a Maylard or Cherney incision or a vertical incision is used for uterine extirpation and lymphadenectomy (Level II-3).[5,7,41] Self-retaining retractors such as the Bookwalter retractor have been shown to reduce the incidence of femoral nerve injury but are costly to purchase.

ROUTINE POSTOPERATIVE ASSESSMENT AND MANAGEMENT

The specific details of postoperative assessment and management depend on the extent and type of operative procedure, the immediate outcome of the procedure, intraoperative complications, and the existence of preoperative comorbidities. The surgeon must also focus on problems unique to the patient's medical condition relative to the radicality of the operation. For example, more frequent assessment of pedal pulses may be necessary after an extensive node dissection in patients with atherosclerosis.

Postoperative Laboratory Tests

Postoperative laboratory evaluation should be tailored to the extent of surgery, specific fluid and electrolyte concerns, and the patient's preoperative condition. With regard to hematologic evaluation, a blood hemoglobin concentration and hematocrit should be obtained within the immediate 24-hour postoperative period for any patient with an estimated intraoperative blood loss greater than 250 cc or an expected postoperative hemoglobin concentration or hematocrit of below 10 g/dl or 30%, respectively. A blood leukocyte count with differential should be obtained and monitored in patients with postoperative fever not responding to conservative management or first-line antibiotic therapy.

Decisions regarding the postoperative evaluation and monitoring of serum chemistries should be made based on the clinical situation. For example, patients undergoing radical hysterectomy, retroperitoneal lymphadenectomy, or exenterative procedures are at risk for electrolyte alterations due to manipulations such as intensive intraoperative fluid resuscitation, surgical muscle injury, nasogastric decompression, and urinary diversion. Therefore, serum electrolytes (sodium, potassium, chloride, bicarbonate) should be assessed within the first 24-hour postoperative period. For patients with ileus or for those maintained without oral intake, electrolytes should be monitored every 48 hours until resolution of ileus or toleration of oral intake. A serum calcium concentration should be obtained on patients transfused with more than 2 units of red blood cells intraoperatively or postoperatively, since ionized calcium is chelated by preservatives in banked blood. Because these patients are at increased risk of ureteral obstruction, a serum creatinine should be obtained on the first postoperative day, since a short-term elevation above baseline may occur with unilateral obstruction. Finally, since diabetes mellitus is common in obese patients with endometrial cancer, such patients should undergo capillary blood glucose monitoring at least four times daily, with insulin therapy instituted to keep blood glucose concentrations below 200 mg/dl, to reduce the risk of postoperative infections, wound complications, fluid imbalance and electrolyte disturbances.

Activity

Venous stasis, atelectasis, and ileus are common morbidities following surgery for cervical and uterine malignancies. Rapid postoperative recovery and the prevention of complications from these conditions rest on early and progressive physical mobilization of the patient. Early ambulation, beginning within the first 24-hour period, is recommended and should be increased daily until discharge. In general, when patients are at bed rest, they should be positioned with the head of the bed elevated to avoid aspiration of secretions and gastric contents, with pneumatic sequential compression stockings in place.

Intake and Output

The frequency of postoperative intake and output monitoring and reporting will depend on the surgery performed and postoperative condition. For a 70 kg adult, the surgeon should be contacted for urine output that falls below 35 cc/hr (0.5 cc/kg/hr). Urine output below this level may be a sign of renal hypoperfusion, which may lead to acute tubular necrosis.

Diet and Nutrition

Most patients undergoing primary operation for endometrial and cervical cancer or even total pelvic exenteration for recurrent disease are nutritionally replete and anabolic at the time of surgery. Therefore, the majority of patients will not require hyperalimentation. Specific indications for hyperalimentation, either by enteral or parenteral route, as well as methods for calculating caloric requirement, are discussed in Chapter 7. In general, oral intake can safely begin on the first postoperative day, once sensorium has normalized, even after retroperitoneal node dissections or anastomoses of the colon and small intestine (Level I).[42] A more conservative approach is recommended for patients who have previously been treated with pelvic and/or abdominal radiotherapy, especially in the presence of an intestinal anastomosis.

Pulmonary Care

Patients undergoing abdominal-pelvic surgery for endometrial and cervical cancer have numerous risk factors for pneumonia. Some of these risk factors include poor respiratory effort due to pain from abdominal incision, anesthesia with endotracheal intubation, decreased clearance of endobronchial secretions, impaired sensorium from analgesics and sedative-hypnotics, obesity, and immobility. In addition to early ambulation, patients should have specific respiratory rehabilitation implemented. Although incentive spirometry has not been found to alter pulmonary volumes and arterial gas values in prospective studies, it has been found to reduce postoperative pulmonary complications such as atelectasis and pneumonia. This protective effect appears to be significant only for moderate and high-risk patients (e.g., those with a history of COPD, reactive airway disease, general anesthesia time greater than 120 minutes; (Level I).[43,44] However, deep breathing alone may be as effective as incentive spirometry in preventing postoperative pulmonary complications among patients at low risk for pulmonary complications, such as those less than 60 years of age with an ASA score equal to 1 (Level I).[44]

Thromboembolic Prophylaxis

Prophylactic measures to reduce the incidence of deep venous thrombosis and pulmonary embolus should be continued through the postoperative period, until the patient is fully ambulatory (Level I).[32,33]

Wound Care

Wound infections are more common in obese patients with a subcutaneous tissue depth ≥3 cm (Level I).[45] Such patients may benefit from a subcutaneous closed drainage system. For example, one prospective, randomized study on 197 obese patients undergoing gynecologic surgery showed that overall wound complication rates decreased from 31% to 20% when drains were placed (Level I).[46] Drains are generally left in place for at least 72 hours until drainage is less than 50 cc in 24 hours.[46]

Some surgeons recommend abdominal binders to improve support of the abdominal wall in obese patients. However, this practice is unstudied and of questionable benefit for pain control or hernia prevention.

On the first postoperative day, dressings should be removed, and if no drainage is present, they may be discontinued. Dressings required for open or draining operative sites should be regularly removed to assess healing and to evaluate the possibility of infection, dehiscence, and seroma formation. Primary closed incisions should be kept clean and dry. Since re-epithelialization occurs within the first 24-hour postoperative period, hygiene can be facilitated by showers or sponge baths beginning on the second postoperative day in order to clear peri-incisional debris, which may contain a high bacterial inoculum. Although exact data are lacking, skin staples/skin sutures are generally removed 3 to 10 days after surgery. Some surgeons prefer delayed staple/skin suture removal (10 to 14 days after surgery) in patients at increased risk of superficial skin separation, such as those who are obese, radiated, malnourished, immuno-suppressed, or diabetic.

Postoperative Bladder Drainage

There are no convincing data to support prolonged bladder drainage following extrafascial hysterectomy as performed for endometrial cancer staging oper-ations. However, prophylactic bladder drainage historically has been recom-mended in women undergoing radical hysterectomy, since bladder denerva-tion and partial devascularization are much more common events, leading to urinary retention, incontinence, ascending urinary tract infection, and vesical fistulae (Level II-3).[47] The incidence and extent of these complications have been thought to correlate directly with patient age, primary tumor size, extent of surgery, and use of adjuvant postoperative radiotherapy, although few stud-ies have been conducted to substantiate these relationships. However, one ret-rospective study of 59 patients following radical hysterectomy suggested that older age and postoperative radiotherapy shorten the interval between surgery and the onset of voiding dysfunction, without an impact on the level of voiding dysfunction (Level II-2).[48]

Bladder drainage has been implemented after radical hysterectomy with the goal of reducing complications such as fistula and those due to neurogenic blad-der. Prolonged indwelling catheterization, either by the transurethral or supra-pubic route, has been a cornerstone of postoperative management after this operation until the acute effects of surgery on voiding function have resolved. However, early postoperative catheter removal, with a strict voiding schedule, and intermittent self-catheterization (ISC) for postvoid residuals (PVR), has also been proposed. Prospective evaluation of this alternative ISC approach has been limited. In one study, compared to 25 historical controls treated with the tra-ditional approach, 8 patients managed with the alternative ISC approach had a lower median indwelling catheter duration (6 days compared to 30 days) with no increase in postoperative complications. This approach appears to be an acceptable alternative to long-term catheterization. There is some evidence that the incidence of lower urinary tract infection can be reduced with suprapubic as opposed to transurethral catheterization (Level II-3).[49] Although intuitive, evidence for prevention of fistulae with prolonged bladder drainage is lacking. Once PVR (approximately <50 ml) and voiding (150–400 ml) volumes are nor-mal, bladder catheterization or drainage is discontinued.

Bladder Rehabilitation

Rehabilitative or "training" techniques have been employed to shorten the dura-tion of urinary retention and reduce the risk of urinary complications. Urody-namic testing has revealed high residual urine volumes and/or stress inconti-nence in the majority of patients following radical hysterectomy who present with voiding dysfunction. In one study of 64 patients receiving early rehabilitative treatment with kinesitherapy and/or pharmacological therapy after bladder catheter removal, functional recovery of the bladder activity was demonstrated in 91% of 50 symptomatic patients (Level II-2).[50] Whether rehabilitative techniques such as kinesitherapy or pharmacologic therapy can be helpful is still unclear, since there are no analytical studies.

DISCHARGE PLANNING

Medication

After extrafascial or radical hysterectomy, as well as other surgical procedures for corpus and cervical cancer, patients are given oral narcotic analgesics (e.g., codeine or oxycodone) with or without acetaminophen once intestinal function returns. Since fluid intake is frequently low and intestinal motility is compromised by narcotic analgesics, oral cathartics such as milk of magnesia may be required to avoid cramping associated with constipation. Hormonal replacement therapy is not contraindicated among cervical cancer patients and is being prospectively evaluated by the Gynecologic Oncology Group in patients after surgery for Stage I and II endometrial cancer. However, retrospective case series have not demonstrated an increased recurrence rate among endometrial cancer patients receiving hormonal replacement when compared to historical controls (Level II-2).[51] Early postoperative hormone replacement may increase the risk of thromboembolic disease, although this controversial area has not been well studied (Level II-2).[52] Thus, many surgeons begin hormonal therapy while the patient is still hospitalized if vasomotor symptoms occur after oophorectomy.

Follow-up

After hysterectomy, patients are generally seen in an outpatient setting 1 to 2 weeks after surgery. Staples are removed if still in place, intestinal function is assessed, signs and symptoms of infection are investigated, and results of surgical and pathologic findings are reviewed. Patients who require wound or drain care (including suprapubic catheters) should be seen weekly until wound or drain care is discontinued. Six weeks after surgery, the vaginal cuff is examined and patients are generally released to return to work unless complications have occurred. Home health consultation is useful when a new permanent central venous catheter, suprapubic catheter, nephrostomy tube, colostomy, or open wound exists.

MANAGEMENT ISSUES UNIQUE TO PELVIC EXENTERATION

Patients with documented centrally recurrent cervical cancer can have long-term survival after an exenterative procedure. Recent reviews indicate that operative mortality is less than 2%, and 5-year cure rates range from 40% to 60% among selected patients (Levels II-3 and III).[53–56] Most gynecologic oncologists would recommend that a pelvic exenteration be performed only when a patient experiences a histologically confirmed recurrence in the central pelvis after radiotherapy for cervical carcinoma. Many of these patients will have also been previously treated with surgery consisting either of a radical hysterectomy or perhaps a surgical staging procedure to assess nodal spread (Level II-3).[57] Patients with long intertreatment intervals and those with smaller central recurrent tumors have a more favorable prognosis than those with a shorter interval following primary radiation, those with persistent disease after radiotherapy, and/or those with large lesions.[53–57] In addition, hydronephrosis and symptoms such as leg or back pain portend an increased risk of cancer outside the surgical field and thus are also poor prognostic factors. Spread to the pelvic side wall and/or multiple lymph node metastasis are generally considered to be contraindications for this radical surgical procedure.

In selected patients with an anterior recurrence, the rectum can be spared by performing an anterior exenteration.[54] Before an exenterative procedure, the patient should undergo an extensive work-up to determine the feasibility of a successful operation. This should include a metastatic survey (CT of the abdomen and pelvis, chest radiograph) and an extensive medical and psychological assessment to ensure the patient's ability to withstand the operative procedure and the prolonged morbidity and body changes that result from this operation. The psychosocial aspects of this subject area are further discussed in Chapter 19.

Randomized studies investigating perioperative techniques to reduce morbidity and mortality after pelvic exenteration have not been performed. Usually, protocols similar to those used for patients undergoing radical hysterectomy are used with careful attention to preoperative testing and bowel preparation, prophylaxis against infection and thromboembolism, as well as intraoperative monitoring. However, because pelvic exenteration is more extensive than radical hysterectomy, and since patients undergoing exenterative surgery have generally previously received pelvic radiation, complication rates are frequently greater than after radical hysterectomy, including ileus, infection, visceral injury, fistula, and hemorrhage requiring tranfusion of blood products.[53–56,58] Preoperative consultation with an enterostomal therapist is helpful for patient education and proper positioning/marking of possible stomas. Also, a majority of patients can undergo immediate reconstruction of the vagina. Multiple flap procedures have been described for this purpose and should be selected carefully depending on the patient's desires and the surgical need to fill the pelvic cavity (Level II-3).[59,60]

RECOGNITION AND MANAGEMENT OF POSTOPERATIVE COMPLICATIONS

Complications such as infection, thromboembolism, and intestinal fistulas are discussed in other sections of this text. However, a few complications unique to the perioperative care of patients with uterine corpus and cervical cancer deserve special consideration.

Ureteral Obstruction

The patient with bilateral ureteral obstruction and uremia secondary to the extension of endometrial or cervical cancer presents a serious dilemma for the clinician. Management should be divided into two subsets of patients: (1) those who have not received prior radiation therapy and (2) those who have recurrent disease after pelvic irradiation. Ureteral obstruction resulting from endometrial cancer differs from obstruction secondary to cervical cancer in that it is more frequently associated with disease outside the pelvis and thus more difficult to cure. In addition, adequate doses of radiation are more difficult to deliver to the corpus than the cervix using standard brachytherapy techniques, thus contributing to the lower rate of pelvic control among endometrial cancer patients following radiation.

The patient with bilateral ureteral obstruction from untreated cancer or from recurrent pelvic disease after surgical therapy should be seriously considered for urinary diversion followed by appropriate radiation therapy. However, since the salvage rate in the latter clinical situation is low, supportive care alone, allowing progressive uremia and demise, must be considered as an alternative to more aggressive therapy in certain cases. If aggressive management is selected, placement of retrograde ureteral stents using cystoscopy should be attempted first. When this is not possible, a percutaneous nephrostomy followed by antegrade stent placement is an alternative (Level II-3).[61–63] A third option is surgical urinary diversion such as a urinary conduit, anastomosing both ureters into an isolated loop of ileum (e.g. Bricker procedure) or creating a continent pouch from a segment of bowel (Level II-3).[64] When necessary, urinary diversion is usually performed before the irradiation is begun, allowing for surgical assessment of disease extent. If extrapelvic disease is discovered at laparotomy, therapy is then altered, since chance of cure is greatly diminished (Level II-3).[65]

The patient with bilateral ureteral obstruction following a full dose of pelvic radiation therapy is a more complicated problem. Fewer than 5% of these patients will have obstruction caused by radiation fibrosis alone, and often this group is difficult to identify (Level II-3).[66] In order to identify patients whose obstruction is a result of recurrent disease, an examination under anesthesia, including cystoscopy and proctoscopy with multiple biopsies, is recommended. When recurrent cancer is absent, simple diversion of the urinary stream can be lifesaving, and therefore all patients must be considerd as possibly belonging to this category until recurrent malignancy is found.

When the presence of recurrent disease has been unequivocally established as the cause of bilateral ureteral obstruction, the decision process becomes difficult and somewhat philosophical. Numerous studies suggest that "useful life" is not achieved by urinary diversion in this subset of patients. Brin et al. (Level II-3)[67] reported on 47 cases (5 with cervical cancer) with ureteral obstruction secondary to advanced pelvic malignancy. The results of this report are discouraging; the average survival time was 5.3 months, with only 50% of the patients alive at 3 months and only 22.7% alive at 6 months. After the diversion, 63.8% of the survival time was spent in the hospital.

Delgato[64] also reported on a group of patients with recurrent pelvic cancer and renal failure who underwent urinary conduit diversion. His results showed no significant increase in survival time. It has been suggested that these patients should never undergo urinary diversion, since a more preferable terminal course (i.e., uremia) is thereby eliminated from the patient's options. Obviously, these decisions should be made in consultation with the family and with the patient if possible. When urinary diversion is performed, an accentuation of the other clinical manifestations of recurrent pelvic cancer (i.e., severe pelvic pain, repeated infections, and hemorrhage) are generally observed, leading to increased suffering. Pain control and progressive cachexia are major management problems. Episodes of massive pelvic hemorrhage are associated with difficult decisions for transfusion. An extension of the inpatient hospital stay is inevitable, and the financial impact on the patient and her family are often considerable.

Urinary Fistula

The bladder is the most common site of urinary tract injury during pelvic surgery and potential complications are almost never life-threatening. When bladder injuries are recognized and immediately repaired, the potential for long-term sequelae is low. In contrast, ureteral injuries, especially if unrecognized, may result in permanent kidney damage or loss. The great majority of ureteral injuries are associated with total abdominal hysterectomies performed for benign indications. However, urologic injuries may also occur when the hysterectomy is performed for a malignant condition. Many ureteral and some bladder injuries are not recognized intraoperatively. Indeed, 70% to 95% of cases go undetected. Thus, the cornerstone to prevention of urinary fistulae is intraoperative recognition and immediate repair.

The exact incidence of accidental urinary tract injury during hysterectomy is difficult to determine because most cases are unreported, but approximates 0.2% to 2.5%. Bladder injuries are approximately five times more common than ureteral injuries. Both ureteral and bladder injuries are also more common when a radical hysterectomy is performed for a carcinoma of the cervix or corpus.

As a general rule, bladder injuries should be repaired when recognized. Late recognition of bladder damage usually is associated with a vesicovaginal fistula that appears 3 to 12 days postoperatively with urine leaking through the vagina. Bladder damage can be avoided during extrafascial or radical hysterectomy by careful incision of the bladder peritoneum, careful separation of the bladder from the uterine cervix and upper vagina, and careful retraction of the bladder during vaginal closure. Risk factors for fistula formation after hysterectomy include prior cesarean section, endometriosis, recent cold knife conization, and previous irradiation therapy. Once a vesicovaginal fistula is suspected, the diagnosis can often be readily made by filling the bladder with a dilute solution of sterile blue fluid (methylene blue in saline) and inspecting the vaginal wall and cuff for leakage. Cystoscopy may also be helpful in determining the site and anatomic location of the fistula. In addition, cystoscopy is important, since foreign material such as sutures in the bladder can be removed during this procedure, perhaps accelerating spontaneous healing.

When a fistula is not immediately obvious, a tampon may be placed in the vagina after methylene blue solution has been instilled into the bladder. After allowing the patient to walk for 10 to 15 minutes, staining of the upper portion of the tampon is highly suggestive of a vesicovaginal fistula. If the tampon is not stained blue but the patient remains wet, a uretero-vaginal fistula is suspected. A uretero-vaginal fistula may also be diagnosed with an intravenous urogram, retrograde pyelography, or IV injection of 5 ml of indigo carmine with observation of blue dye in the vagina.

Previously, many physicians recommended delayed repair of a vesicovaginal fistula for 4 to 6 months after discovery to allow maturation of the fistulous tract. When delayed repair is performed, cure rates have averaged 90%. In addition, delayed surgical closure permits a trial of spontaneous healing with the use of continuous bladder drainage. This has been shown to be successful in approximately 15% to 20% of patients. Spontaneous healing is unlikely except for very small fistulas measuring a few millimeters in diameter. When surgical repair is necessary, repair may be accomplished using either a vaginal or abdominal approach.[68]

Of all injuries to the urinary tract, those involving the ureter are the most difficult to recognize and produce the most serious complications. Untreated ureteral injuries may result in fistula formation or loss of kidney function. The gynecologic surgeon must be vigilant in every operative procedure to identify and locate the ureters, thus taking the necessary steps to avoid iatrogenic ureteral injury. Ureteral injuries generally occur at four locations during gynecologic surgery:

1. At or above the infundibulo-pelvic ligament and near the pelvic brim. This can occur during infundibulo-pelvic ligament ligation or during an aortic lymphadenectomy.

2. Along the lateral pelvic side wall just above the uterosacral ligaments. This site of ureteral injury is most common when a pelvic lymphadenectomy is performed or when the rectovaginal septum is developed during a radical hysterectomy.

3. In the base of the broad ligament where the ureter passes beneath the uterine vessels. This site of ureteral injury is more common when the ureter is dissected out of the cardinal ligament during a radical hysterectomy.

4. As the ureter leaves the cardinal ligament and enters the bladder. This site of injury can occur with both an extrafascial and radical hysterectomy.

Six types of operative ureteral injuries have been described by Thompson:[68] (1) crushing injury from misapplication of surgical clips; (2) ligation with suture; (3) transection (either partial or complete); (4) angulation with secondary, partial, or complete obstruction; (5) ischemia with stripping of the adventitia and depriving a segment of ureter of its blood supply; and (6) resection of a segment of ureter either intentionally in radical surgery for malignancy or unintentionally. Displacement of the ureter by cervical or intraligamentous tumors, inflammatory exudates in the base of the broad ligament, previous pelvic irradiation, endometriosis, postoperative adhesions, and retroperitoneal masses all predispose to ureteral injury.

Ureteral injuries are almost always avoided during extrafascial hysterectomy when dissection is accomplished immediately adjacent to the cervix medial to the ureter. Since a radical hysterectomy requires complete dissection of the terminal ureter, the ureteral blood supply may be compromised, leading to ischemia and necrosis. Thus, a careful retroperitoneal dissection is essential to prevent ureteral injury. As in bladder injuries, intraoperative recognition and immediate repair are critical to fistula prevention. If the ureteral sheath is traumatized during radical hysterectomy, placement of a semipermanent ureteral catheter for 7 to 14 days should be considered while revascularization of the ureter takes place. Perioperative retroperitoneal, closed suction drains should be used liberally when ureteral damage is suspected to prevent urinoma formation, which induces fibrosis.

When the ureter has been partially or completely divided, or is so devitalized by suture or clamping that necrosis is likely to occur, more aggressive management is indicated. The appropriate repair for a severely injured ureter depends on the level of the ureteral injury in the pelvis, the length of the segment traumatized or removed, the mobility of the ureter and bladder, the quality of the pelvic tissues, the condition for which the operation is being performed, and the general condition and anticipated lifetime of the patient. When possible, direct reimplantation of the ureter is often successful using a ureteroneocystostomy. When injury to the pelvic ureter is so extensive that the proximal ureter cannot be brought to the bladder without tension, several techniques are available to reduce the ureteral-vesical gap. These include the Boari bladder flap tube technique and the psoas muscle hitch. If the ureter is transsected above the pelvic brim, the preferred method is either a uretero-ureterostomy or the interposition of an intestinal segment between the injured ureter and the bladder.[68]

When a ureteral injury is not recognized at the time of operation, ureteral damage can be demonstrated by intravenous urogram or retrograde radiographic studies. Once identified, the initial step in management of a ureteral injury is ureteral stent placement. Since retrograde urography allows more accurate delineation of the precise anatomy and can be performed in combination with retrograde ureteral stent placement, this method of diagnosis is preferred to an intravenous study.

If a stent can be successfully placed, the ureter will generally heal spontaneously in the absence of previous radiation. The catheter should be left in place for 14 to 28 days to allow the ureter to heal without stricture formation. After stent removal, a follow-up urogram or ultrasound should be performed at 4- to 6-week intervals to rule out hydronephrosis and stricture. If a ureteral catheter does not pass the obstruction during cystoscopy, ureteroscopy may be considered in an attempt to save an open operative procedure (Level III).[69] Otherwise, either immediate ureteral repair or percutaneous nephrostomy should be performed to preserve remaining renal function. When percutaneous nephrostomy is successful, definite surgery may be deferred for 6 to 12 weeks as many ureteral injuries will resolve with percutaneous nephrostomy alone. Moreover, antegrade ureteral stent placement through the percutaneous nephrostomy may promote spontaneous healing (Level II-3).[70]

Controversy exists as to the management of ureteral obstruction secondary to ureteral ligation discovered in the immediate postoperative period. Early (i.e., 48 to 72 hours after surgery) repair (usually ureteroneocystotomy) is favored by many clinicians, since it may be accomplished before inflammation and scarring occur. Certainly, surgery should be delayed in the patient with significant pelvic infection or in any patient whose medical status is compromised and in whom surgery for ureteral obstruction might pose a significant threat.

Bladder Dysfunction and Urinary Retention

The reported frequency of urinary tract dysfunction following nonradical gynecologic operations is quite variable. Storage function of the lower urinary tract after extrafascial and vaginal hysterectomy, studied by comparing pre- and postoperative urodynamic parameters, is characterized by a significant reduction in maximum cystometric capacity and a decline in bladder compliance. Both findings have been attributed to a decrease in the musculoelastic properties of the detrusor muscle caused by edema and surgical injury. However, neither the decrease in bladder capacity nor the decrease in compliance seem to result in clinical sequelae.

Urodynamic studies of changes in evacuation function following hysterectomy have failed to show any significant changes in detrusor contractility and suggest that lower urinary tract evacuation function remains relatively unaltered by either total abdominal or vaginal hysterectomy. Thus, urinary dysfunction should not be a consequence of an uncomplicated nonradical hysterectomy with or without lymph node sampling when performed for an early invasive cervical cancer or uterine corpus malignancy in women who were previously free of urinary symptoms. Indeed, it has been suggested that urinary tract symptoms after simple hysterectomy should be no more common than after curettage (Level II-1).[71]

The findings observed after radical hysterectomy differ significantly from those observed after extrafascial hysterectomy, apparently because of more extensive nerve injury during radical hysterectomy, which occurs when the cardinal and uterosacral ligaments are divided. Following radical hysterectomy, many women must valsalva to completely empty their bladder due to a significant reduction in detrusor contractility. Severe urinary dysfunction after radical pelvic surgery occurs in as many as 30% to 70% of the patients (Level II-3).[72,73] Following radical hysterectomy, two phases of bladder dysfunction have been described: a hypertonic phase and a hypotonic phase (Level II-3).[74] The first phase occurs immediately postoperatively and is characterized by a high filling pressure and reduced capacity of the bladder. It is generally ascribed to postoperative changes such as edema and hematoma affecting the elastic properties of the bladder, but sympathetic denervation may also be involved. This phase generally resolves spontaneously and is replaced by mild chronic loss of bladder sensation and hypotonicity. In order to limit postoperative urinary dysfunction, some authors recommend modification of the surgical technique of a radical hysterectomy by limiting the dissection to the anterior part of the cardinal ligament, since it is clear that extensive dissection below and lateral to the uterine artery causes bladder denervation. When a severely hypotonic bladder develops, intermittent bladder catheterization may be necessary to empty the bladder completely, avoiding recurrent urinary tract infections.

MANAGEMENT OF COEXISTING PREGNANCY AND CERVICAL CANCER

Carcinoma of the cervix complicates approximately 0.01% of all pregnancies, making it the most common cancer in pregnancy. In deciding on therapy for these malignant neoplasms, the extent of the disease, the patient's attitude toward pregnancy termination, and the gestational age of the fetus, must all be considered. The preponderance of existing evidence suggests that pregnancy does not have a detrimental effect on prognosis from accelerated tumor growth. It was once thought that parturition was associated with the dissemination of viable cells into the lymph-vascular system and increasing the incidence of metastatic spread, but this has not been substantiated by recent studies. In fact, several studies have shown that, stage for stage, the outcome for the pregnant patient with cervical cancer is essentially the same as that for the nonpregnant women (Level II-3).[75,76] However, cesarean delivery may still be preferred to vaginal delivery in patients with large cervical lesions when bleeding and infection from a vaginal delivery might occur.

Vaginal bleeding is the most common symptom seen in carcinoma of the cervix in both the pregnant and the nonpregnant woman. Unfortunately, this symptom usually appears only among those with advanced disease. Since most cervical cancers in pregnancy are early lesions, it is not surprising that Creasman et al. reported that at least 30% of pregnant patients with invasive cervical carcinoma have no symptoms when the diagnosis of cancer is established.[75] When bleeding occurs during pregnancy, this symptom must be investigated and not automatically attributed to the pregnancy. Examination during the first trimester will not lead to miscarriage. Third-trimester bleeding may be adequately assessed in the operating room as a "double setup" procedure if a placenta previa has not been excluded through ultrasonography.

The methods for screening, diagnosis, and treatment of dysplasia and cervical cancer in the pregnant or postpartum woman are the same as in the nonpregnant patient. Frequently, a careful physical examination including visual inspection and cervical biopsy are sufficient to diagnose this malignancy.

The Pap smear is as sensitive and accurate in detecting cervical neoplasia during pregnancy as in the nonpregnant state and should be performed at the first prenatal visit. Half of cervical cancers in asymptomatic pregnant patients will be detected through Pap smear screening.[75] Thus, all Pap smears in pregnancy suggesting a significant abnormality should be investigated with physical examination and colposcopy. If invasion is suspected, a colposcopically directed biopsy should be performed. Cervical biopsies are safe during pregnancy and have not been associated with an increased incidence of pregnancy loss. An endocervical curettage, however, should be avoided. If the cytologic and colposcopic impression suggests only cervical intraepithelial neoplasia (CIN), the pregnancy should be allowed to continue, anticipating a vaginal delivery if indicated. Further evaluation can be postponed until 6 weeks postpartum when the effects of pregnancy on the cervix have resolved.

Occasionally, a Pap smear and/or colposcopic examination will suggest only CIN, but the entire transformation zone will not be visualized. This examination is unsatisfactory and frequently occurs in the first trimester. Repeat colposcopy in the second trimester generally allows eversion of the endocervix, making colposcopy more satisfactory and allowing complete visualization of the transformation zone and cervical lesion. If the cytology shows cancer but the colposcopy does not, repeat Pap smear and colposcopy later in pregnancy (4–6 weeks depending on gestational age) is recommended.

Only lesions suggestive of invasion require biopsy in pregnancy. Similarly, cone biopsy can generally be avoided in pregnancy and should be performed only if invasive disease is suspected or the extent of an early microinvasive lesion requires further evaluation for treatment planning. Cone biopsy is unnecessary if pregnancy termination is not a consideration or if a gross lesion is present. When performed, a "coin" rather than a cone biopsy as described by DiSaia and Creasman, can usually be performed safely without interrupting the pregnancy.[7]

Once the diagnosis of cervical cancer has been established in pregnancy, treatment planning is similar to the nonpregnant patient as already described. However, a delay in treatment may be considered until fetal viability in selected cases. Such a delay, however, may allow cancer progression and worsen prognosis. Interestingly, Sood and colleagues at the University of Iowa reported on 11 patients with early invasive cervical lesions undergoing surgical treatment in the third trimester with a mean planned delay in therapy of 16 weeks. None of these patients with a planned delay in therapy developed recurrent disease and no neonatal morbidity was encountered (Level II-2).[77] Nevertheless, a delay in treatment should be recommended with caution, and criteria for this course of management have not been uniformly established.

Except for increased blood loss, a radical hysterectomy and pelvic lymphadenectomy can be safely performed with the fetus in situ during the first and early second trimester or after cesarean delivery once fetal viability has been established in the late third trimester.[76] Strong consideration of a short delay in therapy should be given if the diagnosis of cancer is made after 24 weeks but before fetal viability and lung maturity (approximately 33 to 36 weeks gestation), in an attempt to avoid neonatal morbidity associated with premature delivery. Using this approach, the maximum delay in treatment would be only 12 weeks (24 to 36 weeks) and would generally be expected to be much shorter.

Radiation therapy is equally efficacious to surgery in treating patients with early-stage cervical cancer in pregnancy and is the treatment of choice in more advanced stages. Before 24 weeks gestation, the pregnancy is disregarded, and the patient is started on whole-pelvic irradiation. If abortion does not occur, excision of the remaining neoplasm by means of a modified radical hysterectomy (Class II) or surgical evacuation of the uterus must follow completion of the external irradiation. Once the uterus is evacuated, radiotherapy can resume. If the uterus has been removed, vaginal vault irradiation may be required to adequately treat the paracolpos. In the event that a hysterectomy has not been performed and the uterus evacuated, standard brachytherapy techniques are applicable to the empty uterus and upper vagina after a 4-week waiting period. If an advanced cancer is detected in the later stages of pregnancy and/or a radical hysterectomy with pelvic lymphadenectomy is not performed at the time of cesarean section, whole-pelvic irradiation may begin immediately after the cesarean incision has healed. Intracavitary irradiation can follow completion of the whole-pelvic irradiation.

Cliby reported four patients with episiotomy site recurrences of squamous cell carcinoma of the cervix at the Mayo Clinic. The cervical cancers were originally diagnosed at delivery or in the immediate postpartum period and had been treated by radical hysterectomy. Episiotomy site recurrences were detected less than 12 weeks after surgery in three patients and at 2 years in one patient. Three patients died of recurrent cancer. One patient was disease-free at 1 year at the time of the report. The authors concluded that vaginal delivery can be associated with this rare but serious complication, and patients who deliver vaginally should be monitored closely for this recurrence (Level II-3).[78]

REFERENCES

1. Lepine LA, Hellis SD, Marchbanks PA, Koonings LM, Morrow B, Kieke BA, Wilcox LS, Hysterectomy surveillance—United States, 1980–1993. *MMWR CDC Surveill Summ* 1997;46:1–15.

2. Steege JF. Indications for hysterectomy: Have they changed? *Clin Obstet Gynecol* 1997;40:878–885.

3. Bachmann GA, Hysterectomy. a critical review. *J Reprod Med* 1990;35:839–862.

4. Parker SL, Tong T, Bolden S, Wingo PA. Cancer statistics, 1997 (published erratum appears in *CA Cancer J Clin* 1997;47(2):68). *CA Cancer J Clin* 1997;47:5–27.

5. DiSaia PJ, Creasman WT. Adenocarcinoma of the uterus. In DiSaia PJ, Creasman WT (Eds), *Clinical Gynecologic Oncology*. St. Louis: Mosby, 1997, pp. 135–167.

6. Kosary CL. FIGO stage, histology, histologic grade, age and race as prognostic factors in determining survival for cancers of the female gynecological system: an analysis of 1973–87 SEER cases of cancers of the endometrium, cervix, ovary, vulva, and vagina. *Semin Surg Oncol* 1994;10:31–46.

7. DiSaia PJ, Creasman WT. Invasive cervical cancer. In DiSaia PJ, Creasman WT (Eds), *Clinical Gynecologic Oncology*, St. Louis: Mosby, 1997.

8. Prendiville W. Large loop excision of the transformation zone. *Clin Obstet Gynecol* 1995;38:622–639.

9. Bennett BB, Stone IK, Anderson CD, Wilkinson EJ. Deep loop excision for pre-hysterectomy endocervical evaluation. *Am J Obstet Gynecol* 1997;176:82–86.

10. Hoffman MS, Collins E, Roberts WS, Fiorica JV, Gunasekaran S, Cavanagh D. Cervical conization with frozen section before planned hysterectomy. *Obstet Gynecol* 1993;82:394–398.

11. Woodford HD, Poston, W, Elkins TE. Reliability of the frozen section in sharp knife cone biopsy of the cervix. *J Reprod Med* 1986;31:951–953.

12. Monk BJ, Cha DS, Walker JL, Burger RA, Ramsinghani NS, Manetta A, DiSaia PJ, Berman ML. Extent of disease as an indication for pelvic radiation following radical hysterectomy and bilateral pelvic lymph node dissection in the treatment of Stage IB and IIA cervical carcinoma (see comments). *Gynecol Oncol* 1994;54:4–9.

13. Monk BJ, Tewari K, Gamboa-Vujicic G, Burger RA, Manetta A, Berman ML. Does perioperative blood transfusion affect survival in patients with cervical cancer treated with radical hysterectomy? *Obstet Gynecol* 1995;85:343–348.

14. Angioli R, Penalver M. Ureteral injury at the time of radical pelvic surgery. *Operative Techniques Gynecol Surg* 1998;3:132–140.

15. Elkins TE. Ureteral injury at the time of abdominal hysterectomy for benign disease. *Operative Techniques Gynecol Surg* 1998;3:108–114.

16. Monk BJ, Tewari K, Burger RA, Johnson MT, Montz FJ, Berman ML. A comparison of intracavitary versus interstitial irradiation in the treatment of cervical cancer. *Gynecol Oncol* 1997;67:241–247.

17. Kim PY, Monk BJ, Chabra S, Burger RA, Vasilev SA, Manetta A, DiSaia PJ, Berman ML. Cervical cancer with paraaortic metastases: significance of residual paraaortic disease after surgical staging. *Gynecol Oncol* 1998;69:243–247.

18. Chaitman BR, Miller DD. Perioperative cardiac evaluation for noncardiac surgery noninvasive cardiac testing. *Prog Cardiovasc Dis* 1998;40:405–418.

19. Ishaq M, Kamal RS, Aqil M. Value of routine pre-operative chest X-ray in patients over the age of 40 years. *JPMA J Pak Med Assoc* 1997;47:279–281.

20. Ritz JP, Germer CT, Buhr HJ. Preoperative routine chest x-ray: expensive and of little value. *Langenbecks Arch Chir Suppl Kongressbd* 1997;114:1051–1053.

21. Lindell LK, Anderson B. Routine pretreatment evaluation of patients with gynecologic cancer. *Obstet Gynecol* 1987;69:242–246.

22. Arant BJ. Screening for urinary abnormalities: worth doing and worth doing well. *Lancet* 1998;351:307–308.

23. Lang CA, Ransohoff DF. What can we conclude from the randomized con-

trolled trials of fecal occult blood test screening? *Eur J Gastroenterol Hepatol* 1998;10:199–204.

24. Simon JB. Fecal occult blood testing: clinical value and limitations. *Gastroenterologist* 1998;6:66–78.

25. Velanovich V. Preoperative laboratory screening based on age, gender, and concomitant medical diseases. *Surgery* 1994;115:56–61.

26. Sood AK, Buller RE, Burger RA, Dawson JD, Sorosky JI, Berman M. Value of preoperative CA-125 level in the management of uterine cancer and prediction of clinical outcome. *Obstet Gynecol* 1997;90:441–447.

27. O'Connell LP, Fries MH, Zeringue E, Brehm W. Triage of abnormal postmenopausal bleeding: a comparison of endometrial biopsy and transvaginal sonohysterography versus fractional curettage with hysteroscopy. *Am J Obstet Gynecol* 1998;178:956–961.

28. Sagawa T, Yamada H, Sakuragi N, Fujimoto S. A comparison between the preoperative and operative findings of peritoneal cytology in patients with endometrial cancer. *Asia Oceania J Obstet Gynaecol* 1994;20:39–47.

29. Russell AH, Shingleton HM, Jones WB, Fremgen A, Winchester DP, Clive R, Chmiel JS. Diagnostic assessments in patients with invasive cancer of the cervix: a national patterns of care study of the American College of Surgeons (see comments). *Gynecol Oncol* 1996;63:159–165.

30. Iwamoto K, Kigawa J, Minagawa Y, Miura H, Terakawa N. Transvaginal ultrasonographic diagnosis of bladder-wall invasion in patients with cervical cancer (see comments). *Obstet Gynecol* 1994;83:217–219.

31. Anonymous National Institutes of Health Consensus Development Conference Statement on Cervical Cancer. April 1–3, 1996. *Gynecol Oncol* 1997;66:351–361.

32. Clarke-Pearson DL, Synan IS, Dodge R, Soper JT, Berchuck A, Coleman RE. A randomized trial of low-dose heparin and intermittent pneumatic calf compression for the prevention of deep venous thrombosis after gynecologic oncology surgery (see comments). *Am J Obstet Gynecol* 1993;168:1146–1153.

33. Fishman A, Altaras M, Klein Z, Aviram R, Beyth Y. Low molecular heparin (Enoxaparin) as an alternative treatment of acute deep venous thrombosis in gynecologic oncology patients. *Eur J Gynaecol Oncol* 1996;17:365–367.

34. Kurz A, Sessler DI, Lenhardt R. Perioperative normothermia to reduce the incidence of surgical-wound infection and shorten hospitalization. Study of Wound Infection and Temperature Group (see comments). *N Engl J Med* 1996;334:1209–1215.

35. Jacobs D, Azagra JS, Delauwer M, Bain H, Vanderheyden JE. Unusual complication after pelvic surgery: unilateral lower limb crush syndrome and bilateral common peroneal nerve paralysis. *Acta Anaesthesiol Belg* 1992;43:139–143.

36. Gombar KK, Gombar S, Singh B, Sangwan SS, Siwach RC. Femoral neuropathy: a complication of the lithotomy position. *Reg Anesth* 1992;17:306–308.

37. Vasilev SA. Obturator nerve injury: a review of management options: *Gynecol Oncol* 1994;53:152–155.

38. Alexander JW, Fischer JE, Boyajian M, Palmquist J, Morris MJ. The influence of hair-removal methods on wound infections. *Arch Surg* 1983;118:347–352.

39. Masterson BJ. Skin preparation. *Clin Obstet Gynecol* 1988;31:736–743.

40. Terry BA. Cost-effective application of the Centers for Disease Control Guideline for Prevention of Surgical Wound Infections. *Am J Infect Control* 1985;13:232–235.

41. Helmkamp BF, Krebs HB, Corbett SL, Trodden RM, Black PW. Radical hysterectomy: current management guidelines. *Am J Obstet Gynecol* 1997;177:372–374.

42. Pearl ML, Valea FA, Fischer M, Mahler L, Chalas E. A randomized controlled trial of early postoperative feeding in gynecologic oncology patients undergoing intra-abdominal surgery. *Obstet Gynecol* 1998;92:94–97.

43. Chumillas S, Ponce JL, Delgado F, Viciano V, Mateu M. Prevention of postoperative pulmonary complications through respiratory rehabilitation: a controlled clinical study. *Arch Phys Med Rehab* 1998;79:5–9.

44. Hall JC, Tarala RA, Tapper J, Hall JL. Prevention of respiratory complications after abdominal surgery: a randomised clinical trial. *Br Med J* 1996;312:148–152.

45. Soper DE, Bump RC, Hurt WG. Wound infection after abdominal hysterectomy: effect of the depth of subcutaneous tissue. *Am J Obstet Gynecol* 1995;173:465–469.

46. Gallup DC, Gallup DG, Nolan TE, Smith RP, Messing MF, Kline KL. Use of a subcutaneous closed drainage system and antibiotics in obese gynecologic patients. *Am J Obstet Gynecol* 1996;175:358–361.

47. Seski JC, Diokno AC. Bladder dysfunction after radical abdominal hysterectomy. *Am J Obstet Gynecol* 1977;128:643–651.

48. Ueda T, Yamauchi T, Kageyama S, Tsuzuki M, Kawakami S, Yonese J, Kawai T. Voiding dysfunction after abdominal radical hysterectomy. Comparison between patients with and without adjuvant irradiation therapy. *Nippon Hinyokika Gakkai Zasshi* 1994;85:1743–1746.

49. Hayasaki M. Studies on the causes and prophylaxis of urinary tract infection following radical hysterectomy for cervical cancer. *Nippon Sanka Fujinka Gakkai Zasshi* 1982;34:2185–2194.

50. Zanolla R, Monzeglio C, Campo B, Ordesi G, Balzarini A, Martino G. Bladder and urethral dysfunction after radical abdominal hysterectomy: rehabilitative treatment. *J Surg Oncol* 1985;28:190–194.

51. Chapman JA, DiSaia PJ, Osann K, Roth PD, Gillotte DL, Berman ML. Estrogen replacement in surgical Stage I and II endometrial cancer survivors. *Am J Obstet Gynecol* 1996;175(5):1195–2000.

52. Whitehead EM, Whitehead MI. The pill, HRT and postoperative thromboembolism: Cause for concern? *Anaesthesia* 1991;46(7):521–522.

53. Barber HR. Pelvic exenteration. *Cancer Invest* 1987;5:331.

54. Hatch KD, et al. Anterior pelvic exenteration. *Gynecol Oncol* 1988;31:205.

55. Jones WB. Surgical approaches for advanced or recurrent cancer of the cervix. *Cancer* 1987;60:2094.

56. Lawhead RA, et al. Pelvic exenteration for recurrent or persistent gynecologic malignancies: a 10-year review of the Memorial Sloan-Kettering Cancer Center experience (1972–1981). *Gynecol Oncol* 1989;33:279.

57. Lagasse LD, et al. Results and complications of operative staging in cervical cancer: experience of the Gynecologic Oncology Group. *Gynecol Oncol* 1980;9:90.

58. Monk BJ, Berman ML, Montz FJ. Adhesions after extensive gynecologic surgery:

clinical significance, etiology, and prevention. *Am J Obstet Gynecol* 1994;170(5, pt 1):1396–1403.

59. Morley GW, Lindenauer SM, Young D. Vaginal reconstruction following pelvic exenteration. *Am J Obstet Gynecol* 1973;116:996.

60. Wheeless CR Jr. Neovagina constructed from an omental J flap and a split thickness skin graft. *Gynecol Oncol* 1989;35:224.

61. Fisher HA, et al. Nonoperative supravesical urinary diversion in obstetrics and gynecology. *Gynecol Oncol* 1982;14:365.

62. Carter J, Ramirez C, Waugh R, et al. Percutaneous urinary diversion in gynecologic oncology. *Gynecol Oncol* 1991;40:248.

63. Coddington CC, Thomas JR, Hoskins WJ. Percutaneous nephrostomy for ureteral obstruction in patients with gynecologic malignancy. *Gynecol Oncol* 1984;18: 339.

64. Delgato G. Urinary conduit diversion in advanced gynecologic malignancies. *Gynecol Oncol* 1978;6:217.

65. Monk BJ, Walker JL, Tewari K, Ramsinghani NS, Nisar Syed AM, DiSaia PJ. Open interstitial brachytherapy for the treatment of local-regional recurrences of uterine corpus and cervix cancer after primary surgery. *Gynecol Oncol* 1994;52(2):222–228.

66. Graham JB, Abab RS. Ureteral obstruction due to radiation. *Am J Obstet Gynecol* 1967;99:409.

67. Brin EN, Schiff M, Weiss RM. Palliative urinary diversion for pelvic malignancy. *J Urol* 1975;113:619.

68. Thompson JD. Operative injuries to the ureter: prevention, recognition, and management. Vesicovaginal fistulas. In Thompson JD, Rock JA (Eds), *Te Linde's Operative Gynecology.* Philadelphia: JB Lippincott, 1992, pp. 749–818.

69. Koonings PP, et al. Ureteroscopy: a new asset in the management of postoperative ureterovaginal fistulas. *Obstet Gynecol* 1992;80(3):548–549.

70. Dowling RA, Corriere JN Jr, Sandler CM. Iatrogenic ureteral injury. *J Urol* 1986;135(5):912–915.

71. Carlson KJ. Outcomes of hysterectomy. *Clin Obstet Gynecol* 1997;40(4):939–946.

72. Sekido N, Kawai K, Akaza H. Lower urinary tract dysfunction as persistent complication of radical hysterectomy. *Int J Urol* 1997;4(3):259–264.

73. Debus-Thiede G, Maassen V, Dimpfl T, Klosterhalfen T, Kindermann G. Late disorders of bladder function after Wertheim operation—an analysis of urodynamic parameters with reference to surgical radicality. *Geburtshilfe und Frauenheilkunde* 1993;53(8):525–531.

74. Iio S, Yoshioka S, Nishio S, Yokoyama M, Iwata H, Takeuchi M. Urodynamic evaluation for bladder dysfunction after radical hysterectomy. *Nippon Hinyokika Gakkai Zasshi. Japan J Urol* 1993;84(3):535–540.

75. Creasman WT, Rutledge FN, Fletcher GH. Carcinoma of the cervix associated with pregnancy. *Obstet Gynecol* 1970;36(4):495–501.

76. Monk BJ, Montz FJ. Invasive cancer complicating intrauterine pregnancy: treatment with radical hysterectomy. *Obstet Gynecol* 1992;80(2):199–203.

77. Sood AK, Sorosky JI, Krogman S, Anderson B, Benda J, Buller RE. Surgical man-

agement of cervical cancer complicating pregnancy: a case-control study (see comments). *Gynecol Oncol* 1996;63(3):294–298.

78. Cliby WA, Dodson MK, Podratz KC. Cervical cancer complicated by pregnancy: episiotomy site recurrences following vaginal delivery. *Obstet Gynecol* 1994;84(2):179–182.

CHAPTER 14

PELVIC MASSES AND OVARIAN CARCINOMA

JOHN B. SCHLAERTH, M.D.

Ovarian cancer is the most significant disease that presents as a pelvic mass, based not only on its frequency in that clinical setting but also on the threat to health and life that it poses. The most important aspect of evaluating a woman with a pelvic mass is the necessity of making decisions without a firm diagnosis, because until a microscopic examination of the tissue from the mass is made, many possibilities exist, including physiologic changes, congenital masses, non-neoplastic lesions, benign and cancerous neoplasms of the ovary, benign and cancerous neoplasms of other pelvic organs, and cancers metastatic to pelvic organs. In this chapter, perioperative decision making regarding the woman with a pelvic mass is viewed from two aspects: where a cancer diagnosis is uncertain and where ovarian cancer is known to be present.

OVARIAN CANCER DIAGNOSIS UNCERTAIN

This clinical grouping is much larger than that in which a certain diagnosis exists and can be further subdivided into patients with pelvic masses at low risk for representing ovarian cancer and patients with pelvic masses at high risk for representing ovarian cancer. There have been several attempts at creating algorithms for managing women with pelvic masses. Most have developed a clinical profile from the history and physical examination, the determination of a serum CA-125 level or other tumor markers, details of an ultrasound examination of the pelvis, and sometimes other factors to triage patients.[1-3] Items in the history that would suggest a noncancerous etiology for a pelvic mass are young age, postmenarchal but premenopausal status, use and length of oral contraceptives in the past, tubal ligation, and parity.

Perioperative and Supportive Care in Gynecologic Oncology: Evidence-Based Management,
Edited by Steven A. Vasilev.
ISBN 0-471-24788-X   Copyright © 2000 by Wiley-Liss, Inc.

On physical examination, small size, mobility, and nonsolid, smooth, uniform character on palpation of the mass generally suggest a benign process. Serum CA-125 levels under 35 U/ml in a premenopausal woman and under 20 U/ml in a postmenopausal woman are reassuring. In young girls and women under age 30, there is risk that an ovarian germ cell cancer may be present. That diagnosis could be anticipated by other tumor markers, namely lactate dehydrogenase, alpha-fetoprotein, and human chorionic gonadotropin.[4] A number of ultrasound characteristics have been shown to indicate high risk for the presence of an ovarian cancer. They include solid areas in the tumor, thickened septa in multilocular cysts, ascites, bilateral ovarian involvement, and large size. Using the color flow Doppler technique, a decreased vascular resistance has been suggested as a high-risk finding for cancer.

Perhaps the best multiple-factor scoring system, summarized in Table 14.1, is that proposed by Jacobs.[1] This Risk of Malignancy Index (RMI) profile integrates the menopausal status, the serum CA-125 level in units per ml, and an ultrasound scoring system. Ultrasound grading assigns 1 point each for (1) multiocular cysts, (2) solid areas, (3) evidence of metastases, (4) ascites, and (5) bilateral lesions. Use of this clinical profile produces a sensitivity of 85% and a specificity of 97% if the RMI is set at 200, and a very high likelihood of representing cancer if the result exceeds 250. The most frequent errors in applying this scoring system occur in young women whose endometriotic pelvic mass or masses produce high levels (potentially over 1,000 U/ml) of CA-125. This would naturally cause the scoring system to reflect a high risk for ovarian cancer, which, in fact, would not be found. The other potential error group is the pre- and postmenopausal women whose ovarian cancers are among the 20% or so that do not produce CA-125.

Ultrasound examinations have provided a new group of female patients for consideration of pelvic mass lesions, and those are newborn girls. Sometimes

TABLE 14.1. Risk of Malignancy Index

RMI = U × M × serum CA-125
U = 0 for ultrasound score of 0, 1 for ultrasound score of 1, 3 for ultrasound score of 2–5
M = 1 if premenopausal, 3 if postmenopausal

RMI Score	Sensitivity (%)	95% CI (%)	Specificity (%)	95% CI	Malignancy Likelihood Ratio Positive	Negative
150	85	71–95	94	87–98	14	16
200	85	71–95	97	91–99	42	15
250	78	62–89	99	95–100	77	22

fetal ultrasound examination detects the presence of a cystic pelvic abdominal mass.[5] Most masses identified antenatally in this manner demonstrate involution over the next month or so following delivery. In premenarcal girls, subclinical cystic masses are identified on occasion by ultrasound done for other reasons. Despite the difficulties in explaining a physiological origin for cystic masses under 8 cm in size, a short period of observation is probably warranted in this group.

During the reproductive years, unilateral cystic masses over 5 cm in size that persist through a menstrual cycle or into the second trimester of pregnancy are unlikely to be physiologic and are best considered for removal.[6] Smaller masses incidentally discovered on ultrasound examinations that persist through 3 or more months may warrant enough clinical suspicion to recommend removal.

Menopausal women with cystic pelvic masses are at significant risk for harboring a benign or malignant ovarian neoplasm. The standard treatment has been to approach such lesions surgically. Recently there has been a growing interest in defining a group of menopausal women whose pelvic masses can be safely observed without surgical intervention. Generally speaking, these women have unilocular pelvic cystic masses less than 5 cm in diameter (although less than 3 cm may represent a safer upper limit) with normal serum CA-125 determinations. There seems to be little risk that such lesions represent or will evolve into ovarian cancers. Similarly, there seems to be little risk if such a mass stays stable over a period of time that increased growth or adnexal accidents such as rupture, hemorrhage, or torsion will occur. Indefinite long-term follow-up with physical examinations ultrasound determinations, and CA-125 determinations is necessary. Although this concept seems to have merit, no one has shown comparative data illustrating whether removal or follow-up is superior.[7]

For patients with a pathologic mass of low malignancy risk, a straightforward elective surgical operation to provide diagnosis and therapy for the mass is indicated. In this group of patients, the very low risk of cancer being present allows for some latitude in surgical planning. An emphasis on minimally invasive surgical maneuvers, including laparoscopically directed surgery, can be employed. Elective decompression of the cystic mass to facilitate removal, preservation of fertility by unilateral oophorectomy, or of ovarian tissue itself by cystectomy are reasonable undertakings in premenopausal women in this setting.[8,9] In postmenopausal women it is still wise to consider a bilateral adnexectomy combined with a hysterectomy as definitive treatment in this low-risk situation. This recommendation has received recent support by an elegant analysis performed by the group at the University of California at San Francisco.[10]

The definition of a pelvic mass at high risk for representing a cancer is arbitrary and debated. The previously cited definition of Jacobs is one attempt to divide high- from low-risk masses. The three important decisions to make in this setting are (1) what further diagnostic work-up should be considered, (2) what intraoperative contingencies need to be planned for, and (3) what preparations for therapy need to be undertaken.[11]

DIAGNOSTIC CONSIDERATIONS

The diagnostic modalities that should have been applied to reach this point are the history and physical examination, a serum CA-125 determination, and an ultrasound examination of the pelvis. In anticipation of major clinical intervention, preoperative testing should be initiated as discussed in Chapters 8 and 9. If the woman is in her childbearing years, pregnancy testing should be undertaken, a recent Pap smear result should be available, and a test for occult blood in the stool should be considered. Aside from testing for occult blood in the stool, further routine evaluation of the intestinal tract in the presence of a high-risk pelvic mass is not justified. However, if significant gastrointestinal symptoms and signs are elicited, they should become a matter of focus and could lead to upper or lower gastrointestinal endoscopy and/or upper gastrointestinal series or barium enema evaluation.[12] Particular clinical scenarios where this could be important would be with a tender, relatively fixed pelvic mass in a woman over the age of 35 where diverticulitis could be a consideration, or the finding of bilateral ovarian masses largely solid in character, which may represent a gastrointestinal (gastric) cancer becoming clinically evident by metastasis to the ovaries (Krukenberg's tumors).

Another clinical question that faces every pelvic surgeon regarding a pelvic mass is whether the mass compromises the lower urinary tract. If the pelvic mass is large, immobile, or there is demonstrated distortion of pelvic organs on examination, then outlining the bladder as it interfaces with the mass and the position and number of ureters in relation to the mass is an important determination. Intravenous urography is a straightforward method of discerning these issues. However, a more elaborate way of defining this mass is with computerized tomography (CT) or magnetic resonance imaging (MRI).[13] Although they are more expensive, they may also provide more information for intraoperative decision making. Particularly important in the setting of the high-risk pelvic mass is the possible demonstration of retroperitoneal lymph node involvement, intraperitoneal metastasis to the omentum, the parietes, the subdiaphragmatic spaces, as well as intrahepatic and intrasplenic lesions.

Preanesthetic tests (a chest X ray and electrocardiogram) as well as provision for blood transfusions are usual hospital requirements prior to major surgery.[14] Assuming a woman is in stable health with adequate cardiopulmonary reserve, following the diagnostic work-up an exploratory laparatomy should be scheduled for the diagnosis and treatment of the pelvic mass. The ideal situation is for the surgery to be undertaken by a team of physicians fully capable of addressing complete removal of the pelvic tumor mass and of addressing the anatomic sites that contain or are at risk for containing metastasis so that a firm diagnostic basis can be provided for further treatment which can then be given in the best situation possible (i.e., little or no residual cancer.)[15–20] Having a surgical team in charge of such patients has ramifications for the diagnostic work-up. This team would make a CT scan relatively superfluous. Except for the rare, deep hepatic parenchymal metastasis, whatever organ involvement or metastatic sites might be detected could be handled by such a surgical team. However, if the surgery must take place without access to a surgical team capable of optimal cytoreduction, information from a CT scan and other extended diagnostic tests could be considered as "screening tests" for possible referral for such surgery. It is important to note, however, that CT is not very good at detecting intra-abdominal metastasis or retroperitoneal lymph node metastasis, especially if they are small in size. As noted, it is uncommon that involvement of solid structures such as the liver or spleen would be encountered in this setting.

PREPARATION FOR SURGERY

Reasonable provisions for this group would include assessing the risk for blood transfusion and anticipating an inpatient hospital stay. A pathologist should be available for specimen examination to include rapid frozen section analysis. A clear plan should be delineated covering the circumstances under which ovarian function or fertility would be terminated, considering age and patient preference. Prophylactic measures should be initiated as discussed in Chapters 9 and 11.

The surgical procedures judged essential to address an ovarian cancer discovered intraoperatively are best defined by the Gynecologic Oncology Group in their surgical procedures manual (Tables 14.2 and 14.3). This manual was developed as a consensus for standardizing research based on intraoperative data regarding ovarian center.

Under certain circumstances, health status will be severely affected by the pelvic mass. The most common direct indicator of a mass markedly affecting health is the presence of clinical ascites. Undertaking surgery in such women can lead to a need for multifocal excavations of large metastatic sites and potential for incomplete removal of metastasis. It is not at all uncommon for such women to reaccumulate ascites rapidly following the surgery. In this setting, oliguria, inconsistent central venous pressures, inconsistent arterial blood pressures, and abdominal distention can cause a confusing clinical picture where heart failure, respiratory failure, internal hemorrhage, and renal failure are not easily sorted out. Preoperative consideration for an intensive care unit with possible central venous or Swan–Ganz catheter monitoring is probably a wise plan for such patients. However, in the only review published addressing this issue specifically, the intraoperative course was more predictive than preoperative condition with respect to extended use of ICU resources beyond 24 hours.[22] Cardiac, pulmonary, renal, or systemic diseases such as diabetes known to be present preoperatively heighten the concern for intra- and postoperative problems. A long anesthetic accompanied by extensive fluid shifts with compromised organ systems can well require extended postoperative endotracheal intubation and respiratory ventilator support.[21,22] Such intervention and risk taking is reasonable in many women with metastatic ovarian cancer because it is

TABLE 14.2. Ovarian Cancer Surgical Staging Procedure

1. The abdominal incision must be adequate to explore the entire abdominal cavity and allow safe cytoreductive surgery. A vertical incision is recommended but not required.
2. The volume of any free peritoneal fluid should be estimated. Free peritoneal fluid is to be aspirated for cytology. If no free peritoneal fluid is present, separate peritoneal washings will be obtained from the pelvis, paracolic gutters, and infradiaphragmatic area. These may be submitted separately or as a single specimen. Patients with Stage III or IV disease do not require cytologic assessment.
3. All peritoneal surfaces including the undersurface of both diaphragms and the serosa and mesentery of the entire gastrointestinal tract will be visualized for evidence of metastatic disease.
4. Careful inspection of the omentum and removal if possible of at least the infracolic omentum will be accomplished. At minimum a biopsy of the omentum is required.
5. If possible, an extrafascial total abdominal hysterectomy and bilateral salpingo-oophorectomy will be performed. If this is not possible, a biopsy of the ovary and sampling of the endometrium must be performed. In selected situations of apparent low-stage disease in a woman desiring reproductive potential, a unilateral salpingo-oophorectomy may be appropriate.
6. If possible, all remaining gross disease within the abdominal cavity is resected.
7. If there is no evidence of disease beyond the ovary or pelvis, the following must be done:
   a. Peritoneal biopsies from
      1. Cul-de-sac
      2. Vesical peritoneum
      3. Right and left pelvic sidewalls
      4. Right and left paracolic gutters
   b. Biopsy and scraping of the right diaphragm
   c. Selective bilateral pelvic and para-aortic node dissection
8. Selective pelvic and para-aortic node dissection must be done in the following situations:
   a. Patients with tumor nodules outside the pelvis that are less than or equal to 2 cm
   b. Patients with Stage IV disease and those with tumor nodules outside the pelvis that are greater than 2 cm do not require node dissection, unless the only nodule greater than 2 cm is a lymph node, in which case it must be biopsied.

Source: Excerpted and modified from the *Gynecologic Oncology Group Surgical Manual.*

widely held that return to health and length of life with subsequent postoperative treatment are directly related to the amount of residual cancer remaining at the end of the surgical operation.

The most common nonvital disability issue that surrounds ovarian cancer surgery is enterostomy or colostomy. Mechanical and antibiotic bowel preparation have allowed for bowel resection and anastomosis to be performed with

TABLE 14.3. Reassessment Laparotomy (Second Look) for Ovarian Cancer

Indications	1. To assess completeness of response to chemotherapy
	2. To resect residual disease
Timing	After therapy, patients exhibiting a complete response or a partial response will undergo a restaging laparotomy.
Incision	The abdominal incision must be adequate to explore the entire abdominal cavity and allow safe cytoreductive surgery. A vertical incision is recommended but not required.
Ascites	If present, ascites must be examined cytologically.
Washings	If ascites is not present, washings must be obtained immediately upon entry into the peitoneal cavity from the pelvis, right and left paracolic gutters, and the subdiaphragmatic space. These may be submitted separately or as a single specimen. Patients who have histologically confirmed persistent disease do not require cytologic assessment.
Exploration	All peritoneal surfaces must be visually examined including direct inspection of the diaphragm. The location and exact size of tumor nodules must be described. Biopsy proof of residual disease is necessary.
	If no tumor is visualized, routine biopsies must be performed from:
	• Right and left pelvic sidewall
	• Cul-de-sac and vesical peritoneum
	• Right and left abdominal gutter peritoneum
	• Undersurface of the right hemidiaphragm (or scraping of the diaphragm may be submitted as an alternative)
	• Residual omentum
	• Adhesive bands, abnormally scarred areas
	• Retroperitoneum: If lymph node dissection was performed at the initial staging procedure and was negative, resampling is not required. If the lymph nodes were positive, or were not done at the time of initial surgery, pelvic and para-aortic node dissection should be performed.
Laparoscopy	Laparoscopic evaluation of the peritoneal cavity is acceptable as a second-look surgery if histologically confirmed persistent disease can be seen and biopsied. If no disease is seen, then exploratory laparotomy is mandatory for purposes of Gynecologic Oncology Group protocol activity.

Source: Excerpted and modified from the *Gynecologic Oncology Group Surgical Manual.*

the high expectation of avoiding enterostomy or colostomy. This practice and the use of gastrointestinal stapling devices have allowed for safe performance of coloproctostomies, which are frequently an issue with large pelvic cancers. In fact, it should be an unusual circumstance in which a permanent intestinal stoma is necessary in the setting of a planned first operation for a metastatic ovarian cancer.

When a woman with a high-risk pelvic mass is medically compromised, a surgical operation of any sort may be too hazardous. Here an extended diagnostic work-up would seem to be indicated because the physician may be forced to act on a presumptive diagnosis, since biopsy information from the tumor mass would require the surgery that is contraindicated. Imaging-guided needle biopsy has been problematic in the evaluation of pelvic masses. Intervening vital structures, masses comprised mostly of cyst fluid, and the risk of intraperitoneal spill of malignant cells are all cited as difficulties, the latter being controversial in terms of clinical implications. In this setting, the choice may be to follow a patient, hoping that her physical situation can be improved so that the surgery could be undertaken in a period of weeks or a few months. This would be most applicable in cases where there is no evidence of metastasis.

In the presence of ascites or metastatic masses, it may be best to proceed with chemotherapy for a presumed ovarian cancer. Recently, interest has developed regarding neoadjuvant chemotherapy, which involves several chemotherapy courses following a surgical operation of modest extent during which the histologic diagnosis of metastatic ovarian cancer has been established. Complete cytoreductive surgery is then performed following response to chemotherapy.[23,24] Whether this approach will prove to be better than the traditional one of a primary definitive surgical attempt followed by chemotherapy is not clear at the present time. There is, however, enough merit from this experience to warrant beginning the chemotherapy in medically compromised patients with presumed metastatic ovarian cancers. Sometimes patients burdened with acute heart failure, the ravages of cerebral vascular accidents, the disabilities of pleural effusions with respiratory compromise, and immobility from ascites may have their general health status improved such that they become, after a short interval of chemotherapy, acceptable surgical candidates. Should that not be the case, for those who respond to the initial courses of chemotherapy, that could continue and represent the sole method of management. As a final point, women who present with a setting likely indicative of ovarian cancer who do not respond to the chemotherapy are unlikely to benefit from any surgical interventions.

OVARIAN CANCER DIAGNOSIS CERTAIN

Following (Initial) Incomplete Surgery

When the primary surgical procedure provides the diagnosis of low malignant potential or invasive carcinoma of the ovary but incomplete staging information, the oncologist must decide whether another surgical operation is warranted to provide necessary information upon which to base further treatment. This situation is especially difficult because there is usually some degree of information available regarding staging. In patients with presumed Stage I neoplasms, information regarding exploration of the abdomen, the status of the omentum, and the clinical status of lymph nodes is usually present to some extent. There are no published or universally agreed upon guidelines regarding which combinations of data suffice in this setting (i.e., exploration, with or without omental biopsy/omentectomy, with or without target biopsies, with or without lymph node removal, with or without peritoneal cytology). Recent reports describe management of such cases with a second laparoscopic staging operation, involving inspection of all accessible peritoneal surfaces, omentectomy, pelvic and para-aortic lymphadenectomies, and peritoneal cytologic washings. This management has the advantage of gathering all of the information in a surgical operation, which is of much less physical impact and total cost than an exploratory laparotomy, and it can probably be applied to most incompletely staged patients.

Some presumably Stage I patients will have enough worrisome factors already known (i.e., the presence of malignant cells in ascitic fluid or high-grade cancers penetrating the tumor capsule) that chemotherapy is warranted.[25] In such patients, a case can be made for deferring the staging surgery until after the completion of chemotherapy, with a reassessment or second-look surgery.

In known metastatic cases, metastatic ovarian cancer is encountered at the initial surgery that was not anticipated. The diagnosis has been established and usually some therapeutic intervention has taken place. Often an adnexectomy or hysterectomy/adnexectomy, or even surgical correction of a bowel obstruction with or without an intestinal stoma, has been performed. In many cases, the intraperitoneal metastases are left largely unaddressed.

To the extent that the initial surgery was minor in scope (e.g., mini-laparotomy or laparoscopy), recovery is prompt and uncomplicated, and a major cytoreduction seems possible, it is best to proceed in a medically fit patient, with a definitive surgery prior to chemotherapy. If the initial surgery is followed by slow recovery, complications, or the identification of unresectable metastases, delaying the cytoreductive surgery and beginning chemotherapy seems prudent. This clinical setting is another scenario for neoadjuvant chemotherapy consideration.[23,24]

During Postoperative Chemotherapy

Up to 20% of patients with metastases will exhibit progression of their disease during chemotherapy. Surgical intervention in an attempt to salvage the situation risks significant morbidity. There is little evidence that survival can be affected in this group by further surgery.[26]

Following Postoperative Chemotherapy

Patients whose measureable disease has remained stable at the conclusion of primary chemotherapy should also be considered refractory to such chemotherapy, although the clinical situation may have less immediate peril. Since these patients represent a minority of the refractory patient population, little is known regarding the impact of surgical intervention. Relatively healthy individuals, who have a few large isolated metastases noted on imaging studies or examination, may represent an exception. Surgical intervention may be considered if these are judged amenable to complete resection.

Persistence of disease following postoperative chemotherapy can represent either a partial response or stable disease at the end of planned chemotherapy. In the absence of clinically measurable disease, persistence can also be inferred by a serum CA-125 level that has failed to normalize during treatment.[27] In these situations, a second-look laparotomy for diagnostic purposes is superfluous. Resistance to first-line chemotherapeutic agents is clear and elective cytoreductive surgery is futile, with the possible exception of isolated disease resection as already noted. This group of patients is most similar to those with refractory disease, although the threat to health and life is less immediate. Elective therapeutic interventions should generally be medical, not surgical. This area requires further study and will likely evolve as a result of development of more effective primary and secondary salvage chemotherapy regimens.

Persistence can also be determined by finding residual cancer at the time of second-look laparotomy. Of all the postchemotherapy scenarios, this is the one where an aggressive surgical approach can best be justified, because at the time of discovery a significant proportion of the surgical risks have already been taken. Also, the disease burden for cytoreduction is usually modest, in that it is subclinical. This usually means a partial response has been achieved and salvage therapy can be applied in an optimal residual disease setting.

Whether the knowledge gained regarding disease status and/or the tumor removal at second look laparotomy translates to a survival advantage is debated. Retrospective analyses have spoken strongly both for[28] and against[29] an advantage, but are severely limited in drawing meaningful conclusions due to study design. Other prospective studies including randomized trials have failed to show an advantage,[30–32] but are also burdened by problems with study design and questionable chemotherapeutic choices for both initial and salvage regimens. Thus, the bulk of available data rests with conflicting Level II and minimal Level I evidence.

There seems to be general agreement that (1) some positive second-look patients will experience prolonged (i.e., greater than 5 years) survival, and (2) large-volume disease at second look is an ominous finding. What is not clear is the relative impacts of therapies at and subsequent to the second look and what subgroups of patients and tumor types stand to benefit most from the second look.[33]

Many patients with metastatic ovarian carcinoma will complete first-line chemotherapy and present no evidence of their cancer (i.e., physical examination is normal, serum tumor markers have normalized, and imaging studies reveal no abnormalities). Performing a laparatomy on patients with previously documented metastatic disease but with a normal physical examination and serum CA-125 will demonstrate persisting cancer in approximately 50% (Table 14.2).[34,35]

Barter's collective review suggests CTs add little precision to decision making because of a false negative rate of 28% and a false positive rate of 6%.[34]

There is little evidence that MRI or sonography are superior to CT imaging for evaluation of persistence.[36] The role of spiral CT scanning is yet to be investigated.

Newer approaches employing radioisotope labeled monoclonal antibodies such as indium labeled TAG-72 may offer promise for the future. But current experience suggests the sensitivity of this method to be about 60%, not equal to the sensitivity of second-look laparatomy.[37] Currently, this modality seems most useful where there is already strong evidence that occult cancer is present.

Thus, it seems that second-look laparotomy at this point offers the best information regarding disease status. Two groups of patients are derived from this endeavor: those with no evidence of disease and those with persistent cancer. In the group of women with no evidence of persisting disease (approximately 50%), approaches such as no further therapy, consolidation therapy by continuing the same chemotherapy, or consolidation therapy by changing treatment have been tried. Interest in continuing treatment in some form is supported by long-term follow-up of patients with negative second-look, which suggests recurrences rates may eventually approach 50%.[38,39] It is important to note also that in this group where at least 50% will experience extended disease-free survival, serious postoperative complications are uncommon. Surgical mortality is estimated to be 0.1%.[40] Significant morbidities include ileus and infections, each occurring with an incidence as high as 15%.[41]

Second-look laparoscopy has been suggested as a means to reduce morbidity and total costs, with no loss in reliability as opposed to laparotomy.[42] There is no long-term information on the outcome of negative second-look laparoscopy. There have also been concerns voiced concerning possible increased morbidity from laparoscopy because of extensive adhesions, which limit exposure and conceal visceral injury.[43,44] In the other 50% of women who harbor persistent disease, management decisions can be made on a sound basis and without delay. There is also the opportunity for secondary cytoreduction during reassessment surgery as mentioned previously.[45]

Women being followed after chemotherapy may have a sequence of follow-up tumor markers, may have internal scans, and will have interval physical examinations, all of which can elicit findings suggestive of recurrence. Patients with evidence of asymptomatic recurrence of ovarian cancer should be considered for surgical intervention. This becomes more of a consideration if the appearance of the putative recurrence is late (i.e., longer than 6 months from chemotherapy), if it is unifocal or is confined to a region, and if there are no significant adverse sequelae from the initial surgery and chemotherapy. The same principles for cytoreductive surgery apply in this setting as they would in the initial surgical setting for properly selected patients. The goals may include increased disease-free interval and quality-adjusted life-year (QALY) gain after completion of therapeutic intervention.

Most symptomatic recurrences of ovarian cancer are related to obstruction of the intestinal tract. Exploratory laparotomy will usually be performed in the hope that a decisive surgical maneuver can be done to overcome the obstruction, either by bypass, resection and anastomosis, or creation of an intestinal stoma.[45] This situation occurs often enough that it is worthwhile to consider, as long as the limitations of such an approach are clearly understood. The likelihood of creating multiple enterotomies during dissection, of not relieving the obstruction, of creating a stoma with a significantly shortened intestinal tract, or of settling for placement of a gastrostomy or jejunostomy tube for dainage only is very high. Worst of all, coalescent metastases affecting most or all of the intestinal tract are often encountered such that the result may be damaged bowel segments and an unrelieved obstruction. These are all sobering realities to such surgery. Marginal analysis (i.e., high morbidity and cost for one additional unit of benefit) of this situation suggests that few patients will benefit overall. Therefore, highly individualized patient selection that may result in an acceptable outcome must be addressed. It is critical to appreciate that these decisions are made in the face of no real alternative other than terminal care. Medical management of bowel obstruction in this setting, with or without chemotherapy and intravenous hyperalimentation, is even less effective.[46]

Randomized controlled trials are lacking in areas related to primary, much less secondary, cytoreductive surgery and the associated scenarios already described. However, given the spectrum of clinical management problems, it is unlikely that all questions will be answered at Level I certainty. Thus, patient management should be based on individual assessment of risk and cost to benefit, with an emphasis on clinical trial participation.

REFERENCES

1. Jacobs I, Oram D, Fairbanks J, Turner J, Frost C, Grudzinskas JG. A risk of malignancy index incorporating CA-125, ultrasound, and menopausal status for the accurate preoperative diagnosis of ovarian cancer. *Br J Obstet Gynecaeol* 1990;97:922–929.

2. Lerner JP, Timor-Tritsch IE, Federman A, Kitao MA. Transvaginal ultrasonographic characterization of ovarian masses with an improved weighted scoring system. *Am J Obstet Gynecol* 1994;170:81–85.

3. Finkler NJ, Benacerraf B, Lavin PT, Wojciechowski C, Knapp RC. Comparison of serum CA-125 clinical impression and ultrasound in the preoperative evaluation of ovarian masses. *Obstet Gynecol* 1988;72:659–671.

4. Schwartz PE. The role of tumor markers in the preoperative diagnosis of ovarian cysts. *Clin Obstet Gynecol* 1993;36(2):384–394.

5. Miller DM, Blake JM, Stringer DA, Hara H, Babiak C. Prepubertal ovarian cyst formation: five years experience. *Obstet Gynecol* 1993;81:434–438.

6. NIH Consensus Conference. Ovarian cancer screening treatment and follow-up. *JAMA* 1995;276:491–498.

7. Goldstein SR. Conservative management of small postmenopausal cystic masses. *Clin Obstet Gynecol* 1993;36:395–401.

8. Hasson HM. Laparoscopic management of ovarian cysts. *J Reprod Med* 1990;35:863–867.

9. Granberg S. Relationship of macroscopic appearance to the histologic diagnosis of ovarian tumors. *Clin Obstet Gynecol* 36(2):363—374.

10. Grover CM, Kupperman M, Kahn JG, Washington AE. Concurrent hysterectomy at bilateral salpingo-oophorectomy: benefits, risks, and costs. *Obstet Gynecol* 1996;88:907–913.

11. Society of Gynecologic Oncologists Clinical Practice Guidelines. *Oncology* 1998;12(1):129–133.

12. Saltzman AK, Carter JR, Fowler NM, Carlson JW, Hartenback EM, Julian SE, Carson LT, Twiggs LB. The utility of preoperative screening colonoscopy in gynecologic oncology. *Gynecol Oncol* 1995;56:181–186.

13. Buist MR, Golding RP, Burger CW, Vermorken JB, Kenemaus P, Schutler MJ, Baak JPA, Heitbrink MA, Falke THM. Comparative evaluation of diagnostic methods in ovarian carcinoma with emphasis on CT and MRI. *Gynecol Oncol* 1994;52:191–198.

14. Brooks S. Preoperative evaluation of patients with suspected ovarian cancer. *Gynecol Oncol* 1994;55:580–590.

15. Nguyen HN, Averette HE, Hoskins W, Penalver M, Sevin B, Steren A. National Survey of Ovarian Carcinoma. Part V. The impact of physicians' specialty on patients' survival. *Cancer* 1993;72(12):3663-3670.

16. Eisenkop SM, Spirtos NM, Montag TW, Nalick RH, Wang HJ. The impact of subspecialty training on the management of advanced ovarian cancer. *Gynecol Oncol* 1992;47:203–209.

17. Liu PC, Benjamin I, Morgan MA, King SA, Mikuta JJ, Rubin SC. Effect of surgical debulking on survival in Stage IV ovarian cancer. *Gynecol Oncol* 1997;64:4–8.

18. Le T, Krepart GV, Lotocki RJ, Heywood MS. Does debulking surgery improve survival in biologically aggressive ovarian carcinoma. *Gynecol Oncol* 1997;67:208–214.

19. Munkarah AR, Hallum AV, Morris M, Burke TW, Levenback C, Atkinson EN, Wharton JF, Gershenson DM. Prognostic significance of residual disease in patients with stage IV epithelial ovarian cancer. *Gynecol Oncol* 1997;64:13–17.

20. Curtin JP, Malik R, Venkatraman E, Barakat RR, Hoskins WJ. Stage IV ovarian cancer: impact of surgical debulking. *Gynecol Oncol* 1997;64:9–12.

21. Van Le L, Fakhry S, Walton LA, Moore DH, Fowler WC, Rutledge R. Use of APACHE II scoring system to determine mortality of gynecologic oncologic patients in the intensive care unit. *Oncol Gynecol* 1995;85:53–59.

22. Amir M, Shabot M, Karlan BY. Surgical intensive care unit care after ovarian cancer surgery: an analysis of indications. *Am J Obstet Gynecol* 1997;176:1389–1393.

23. Shapiro F, Schneider J, Markman M, Reichman BS, Venkatraman G, Barakat R, Al Madrones L, Spriggs D. High intensity intravenous cyclophosphamide and cisplatin, interim surgical debulking and intraperitoneal cisplatin in advanced ovarian carcinoma: a pilot trial with ten year followup. *Gynecol Oncol* 1997;67:39–45.

24. Vanderburg Mel, VanLent M, Buyse M, Kobiersk A, Colombo N, Favalli G, LaCave AJ, Nardi M, Renard J, Pecorelli S. The effect of debulking surgery after induction chemotherapy on the prognosis in advanced epethelial ovarian cancer. *N Eng J Med* 1995;10:629–634.

25. Schilder RJ, Boente MP, Corn BW, Lanciano RM, Young RC, Ozols RF. The management of early ovarian cancer. *Oncology* 1995;9:171–182.

26. Morris M, Gershenson DM, Wharton JT. Secondary cytoreductive surgery in epithelial ovarian cancer: nonresponders to first line therapy. *Gynecol Oncol* 1989;33:1–5.

27. Markman M. CA-125: an evolving role in the management of ovarian cancer. Editorial. *J Clin Oncol* 1996;14:1411–1412.

28. Friedman RL, Eisenkop SM, Wang HJ. Second look laparotomy for ovarian cancer provides reliable prognostic information and improves survival. *Gynecol Oncol* 1997;67:88–94.

29. Chambers SK, Chambers KTR, Koboris EL, et al. Evaluation of the role of second look surgery in ovarian cancer. *Obstet Gynecol* 1988;71(3):404–408.

30. Leusley D, Lawton F, Blackledge G, et al. Failure of secondlook laparotomy to influence survival in epithelial ovarian cancer. *Lancet* 1988;2:599–602.

31. Rajji KS, McKinna JA, Becker GH et al. Second look operations in the planned management of advanced ovarian carcinoma. *Am J Obstet Gynecol* 1982;144:650–654.

32. Fiorentino MV, Nicoletta MO, Tumolo S, et al. Uselessness of surgical second look in epithelial ovarian cancer: a randomized study. *Proc ASCO* 1994;13:259.

33. Bookman MA, Ozols RF. Factoring outcomes in ovarian cancer. *J Clin Oncol* 1996;14:325–327.

34. Barter JF, Barnes WA. Second look laparotomy. In Rubin SC, Sutton GP (Eds), *Ovarian Cancer.* New York: McGraw-Hill, 1993, pp. 269–300.

35. Rubin SC. Second look laparotomy. In Markman M, Hodkins WJ (Eds), *Cancer of the Ovary.* New York: Raven Press, 1993, pp. 179–186.

36. Copeland LJ, Vaccarello L, Lewandowski GS. Second look laparotomy in epithelial ovarian cancer. *Obstet Gynecol Clin N Am* 1994;21(1):155–166.

37. Surwit EA, Childers JM, Krag DN, et al. Clinical assessment of immunoscintigraphy in ovarian cancer. *Gynecol Oncol* 1993;48:285–292.

38. Copeland LJ, Gershenson DJ. Ovarian cancer recurrences in patients with no macroscopic tumor at second look laparotomy. *Obstet Gynecol* 1986;68:873–877.

39. Rubin SC, Hogkins WN, Saigo PE, et al. Prognostic factors for recurrence following negative second look laparotomy in ovarian cancer patients treated with platinum-based chemotherapy. *Gynecol Oncol* 1991;42:137–141.

40. Barter F, Barnes WA. Second look laparotomy. In Rubin SC, Sutton GP (Eds), *Ovarian Cancer.* New York: McGraw-Hill, 1993, pp. 269–300.

41. Gallup DG, Talledo OE, Dudzinski MR, et al. Another look at the second assessment procedure for ovarian epithelial carcinoma. *Am J Obstet Gynecol* 1987;157:590–594.

42. Childers JM, Laug J, Surwit EA, Hatch KD. Laparoscopic surgical staging of ovarian cancer. *Gynecol Oncol* 1995;59:23–33.

43. Friedman RI, Eisenkop SM, Wang HJ. Second look laparotomy for ovarian cancer provides reliable prognostic inforamtion and improves survival. *Gynecol Oncol* 1997;67:88–94.

44. Rome R, Fortune DW, Aust NZ. The role of second look laparotomy in the management of patients with ovarian carcinoma. *J Obstet Gynecol* 1988;28:318–322.

45. Rubin SE, Lewis JJ. Second look surgery in ovarian carcinoma. *Crit Rev Oncol Hematol* 1988;8:75–91.

46. Abu-Rustum NR, Barakat RR, Venkatraman E, Spriggs D. Chemotherapy and total parenteral nutrition for advanced ovarian cancer with bowel obstruction. *Gynecol Oncol* 1997;64:493–495.

CHAPTER 15

MOLAR GESTATION

STEVEN A. VASILEV, M.D., M.B.A., and C. PAUL MORROW, M.D.

Mortality and severe complications due to molar pregnancy are rare in the United States today, largely because of early recognition and timely treatment.[1] Moreover, this early recognition and improved postevacuation follow-up has resulted in earlier diagnosis of the malignant sequelae of molar gestation, choriocarcinoma, and invasive mole.

This chapter addresses molar gestation–related perioperative problems and their evidence-based management. With few exceptions, the conditions discussed arise in patients with complete rather than partial molar gestation. Often, coexisting problems arise and may be due to multiple etiologies. For example, cardiorespiratory insufficiency has been blamed on trophoblastic embolization, cardiogenic and noncardiogenic pulmonary edema, thyrotoxicosis, and iatrogenic fluid overload.[2] Hematologic, endocrinologic, neurologic, and infectious complications occur in up to 70% of patients.[3] Central to all these problems is the presence and relative volume of molar tissue in utero. The goal is early diagnosis and expeditious evacuation of the molar gestation, along with supportive and preventive measures. Guidelines for evacuation are summarized in Table 15.1.

TROPHOBLASTIC EMBOLIZATION AND CARDIORESPIRATORY INSUFFICIENCY

Sudden hypoxemia or tachypnea with associated tachycardia occurs in 2% to 11% of molar gestations. This incidence increases to 27% in patients who present with a molar pregnancy exceeding 16 weeks gestation.[2,4–6] Although this condition most often spontaneously resolves, maternal deaths have been reported.[2] Most often, the acute cardiorespiratory insufficiency is clinically as-

Perioperative and Supportive Care in Gynecologic Oncology: Evidence-Based Management,
Edited by Steven A. Vasilev.
ISBN 0-471-24788-X   Copyright © 2000 by Wiley-Liss, Inc.

TABLE 15.1. Management Guidelines for Molar Pregnancy Evacuation

Therapeutic Goals

1. Complete and expeditious uterine evacuation.
2. Prevent volume overload and cardiorespiratory compromise.
3. Avoid or be prepared to treat massive hemorrhage.
4. Recognize and provide supportive care for pregnancy-induced hypertension and hyperthyroidism.

Evidence-Based Management Guidelines

1. Establish *IV access* (16–18 gauge angiocath) running isotonic crystalloid (Level II-2).
2. *Laboratory:* CBC, quantitative beta-HCG routine (Level I); coagulation screen (fibrinogen, PT, PTT, platelet count, Fibrin Split Products) in high-risk patients (Level II-2).
3. *Blood bank:* 2 units of PRBC type and cross or type and screen for greater than or less than 14–16-week gestation, respectively (also depending on pre-evacuation blood indices) (Level II-2).
4. Correct severe preevacuation anemia, avoiding hypervolemia.
5. *Chest X ray* if greater than 14–16 weeks uterus (Level II-1).
6. *Pulse oximetry,* arterial blood gas if severe anemia or hypotension (Level II-1).
7. *Central-line cordis* if uterus is greater than 14–16 weeks gestation for rapid fluid infusion capability; pulmonary artery catheter if high risk/clinically unstable (Level II-2).
8. *MgSO4* if superimposed PIH (Level I).
9. *Beta blockade* for evidence of thyroid storm (Level I).
10. Carefully use *suction/curettage*, without preevacuation uterine sounding, followed by large-curette, sharp, gentle curettage (Level II-1).
11. Begin *oxytocin* infusion at curettage and continue for 24 hours or until vaginal bleeding subsides (methergine if no contraindication as alternative) (Level III).
12. Match intake and output, discounting sanguinous molar tissue.
13. Laparotomy tray in the OR.
14. *Hysterectomy* if competed childbearing (Level II-2).
15. If clinical *hyperthyroidism* suspected, treat with beta blockade and iodides as indicated and evacuate (Level II-3).
16. Observe carefully for evidence of respiratory distress.

cribed to trophoblastic embolization. While the etiology is more likely multifactorial, there are many reports of presumed or documented pulmonary trophoblastic deportation. Some result in cardiac failure and death.[7–12] However, the occurrence of clinical embolism, well documented or not, approximates only 3%.[7–12] Thus, it is doubtful that this is the main cause of cardiorespiratory insufficiency in these patients.

According to data from autopsy and central catheterization series, the magnitude of trophoblastic deportation varies markedly. The term *embolism* should be reserved for clinically significant deportation.[7–14] Trophoblastic embolization appears to occur most often in patients with a large-for-dates uterus, particularly if the uterine size exceeds 16 to 20 weeks.[2,3]

Trophoblastic deportation has been associated temporally with uterine manipulation.[11] However, because all methods of evacuation increase uterine activity, this factor is not highly controllable. Suction dilatation and curettage, which increases uterine activity indirectly, has become a standard for molar evacuation (Level II-1).[15] Most molar pregnancies can be safely evacuated by suction curettage.[16,17] However, if a fetus and mole gestation are slated for termination, a dilatation and evacuation (D&E) may be required as a supplement under some circumstances. Although D&E is widely considered to be statistically the safest method of termination for a fetus greater than 16 weeks gestation, there is no evidence that directly supports this approach in the case of combined fetus-mole pregnancies.[18] A recommendation to perform a D&E in this situation is purely by extrapolation, and several caveats are in order. First of all, the safety of this approach depends on the orientation of the molar pregnancy in utero and the degree of fetal gestational development. Pre- and intraoperative ultrasonography may be instrumental in preventing or decreasing complications. Second, if the fetus is trisomic, its growth is usually quite retarded such that suction evacuation is adequate. Third, the evacuation of a large fetus-mole gestation is often incited or accompanied by pregnancy-induced hypertension (PIH) and its comorbidities and sequelae. In the presence of such a clinical presentation, hysterotomy may be advised as an alternative.

Oxytocin or prostaglandin induction as the primary evacuation method is far less desirable because of a potential for increased deportation and sudden uncontrolled hemorrhage.[3] Furthermore, tissue is often retained so that curettage is still required in addition to the induced evacuation. However, the perioperative addition of oxytocin at the initiation of suction curettage may cause contraction of the myometrium around venous sinusoids as the uterus is emptied. This may decrease the degree of deportation[3,10] and decrease blood loss.

Hysterectomy, usually with the molar pregnancy in situ, may be considered in patients without significant medical complications from the molar gestation who are hemodynamically stable and who do not desire further fertility (Level II-2).[19] This approach reduces the risk of malignant sequelae from 20% to approximately 3.5%.[19–22] Whether trophoblastic embolization risk is decreased remains controversial.

Invasive monitoring data in patients undergoing molar evacuation refute trophoblastic embolization as a common cause of acute cardiorespiratory insufficiency. When embolization occurs, symptoms are likely dose related as opposed to being anaphylactoid in nature.[13,14] Despite the findings of transient cardiorespiratory dysfunction and pulmonary edema, several small series failed to identify unequivocally the presence of circulating trophoblastic cells in patients with pulmonary complications.[13,14] Therefore, pulmonary insufficiency associated with hydatidiform mole is more likely due to factors other than trophoblastic deportation as discussed below (Level II-3).

PULMONARY EDEMA

Etiologic factors contributing to pulmonary edema may include (1) cardiac depression by anesthetic agents, (2) preexisting dilutional anemia, (3) iatrogenic fluid overload, (4) thyrotoxicosis, (5) PIH, and (6) heart failure due to either trophoblastic embolization or preexisting cardiopulmonary disease.

General anesthesia with nitrous oxide, fentanyl, or other narcotics can transiently depress ventricular performance.[23] Limited data in patients with molar gestations greater than 16-week size, monitored perioperatively with pulmonary artery catheters, confirm this effect.[13,14] A low colloid osmotic pressure (COP) to pulmonary capillary wedge pressure (PCWP) gradient combined with aggressive volume resuscitation, in the presence of depressed myocardial function, may exacerbate the development of pulmonary edema.[24]

Relative or dilutional anemia due to plasma volume expansion may exist in molar gestation, just as in normal pregnancy, becoming more pronounced in the second trimester (Level II-1).[25-27] This is a physiologic response that acts to provide a reserve for hemorrhage, among other protective effects.[28] Due to the hypervolemia, a large patient can lose up to 2 L of blood at delivery without serious sequelae.[29] One notable exception is seen in patients with coexisting PIH in which a hypovolemic state may be present (Level II-1).[30,31] This may be reflected by hemoconcentration and a falsely "normal" hematocrit determination.

Estimated "blood loss" at evacuation of a molar pregnancy includes sanguinous molar tissue, which should not be included in the estimate of circulating blood volume loss. While preexisting severe anemia may be corrected with packed red blood cells (PRBC), any attempt to replace potentially overestimated losses with whole blood or other large-volume infusion in an already hypervolemic state will increase the likelihood of developing pulmonary edema. Patients with PIH or hypertension, in whom there may be an increase in systemic vascular resistance (SVR) and a contracted blood volume, tolerate acute volume loads even less well.[13]

An inverse relationship between the intrinsic work capability of the left heart, measured by left ventricular stroke work index (LVSWI) and SVR, has been documented in eclamptic patients.[32] Therefore, if uncertainty exists as to volume status, especially in those already symptomatic or with coexisting severe PIH, use of a pulmonary artery catheter should be considered (Level II-2).[33]

Thyrotoxicosis can contribute to pulmonary edema as a known cause of high-output cardiac failure.[34] The adverse effect of thyrotoxicosis would be especially important in patients with already limited cardiac reserve from the aforementioned factors. Reported cases in which cardiac failure or acute dyspnea complicated hyperthyroidism have resolved spontaneously after evacuation. Several of these patients were being treated medically for hyperthyroidism for a prolonged time period with a known molar gestation in situ. Their adverse outcome emphasizes the need to evacuate a molar gestation as soon as possible rather than to attempt protracted medical treatment.

Several small series have reported molar pregnancy complicated by acute respiratory distress syndrome (ARDS). ARDS may coexist with or be complicated by sepsis, disseminated intravascular coagulation (DIC), PIH, and pneumothorax.[4,6]

Risk factors for the development of pulmonary edema in molar pregnancy have been summarized by Morrow.[5] These include advancing patient age, advanced molar gestation, theca-lutein cysts, large uterine size, hypertension, extensive uterine hemorrhage, and anemia. Evaluation of pulmonary edema in these patients should begin with the recognition of risk factors and the maintenance of a high index of suspicion. Conversely, a high index of suspicion for molar gestation should be maintained when a woman of childbearing age presents with pulmonary edema. In one case report, a patient with infiltrates due to pulmonary edema was mistakenly treated for presumed pneumonia for a week prior to the discovery of a molar gestation.[2]

In light of the above factors and syndromes, laboratory determinations and preoperative preparation should be expeditious. The evaluation should include a complete blood count (CBC), serum electrolytes, and a urinalysis, including a test for protein as part of screening for PIH. Thyroid function tests may be sent, but evacuation should not be delayed pending results. A chest X ray should be obtained for all patients. Findings may include pulmonary infiltrates or effusions with variable appearance (Level II-1).[6] Those in the high-risk group for pulmonary complications or with symptoms of respiratory insufficiency should have pulse oximetry measurements taken. In a hemodynamically unstable patient with poor peripheral perfusion, arterial blood gas measurements may be indicated if the Hb is <3 g/dl or hypotension exists at <30 mmHg (Level II-1).[35,36] Finally, a central venous pressure (CVP) or pulmonary artery catheter should be considered in especially high-risk or symptomatic patients. Central venous pressure monitoring may be sufficient in some patients. However, the extensive added information made possible by flow-directed catheters far outweighs the slight additional risk from placement, making its use preferable in most high-risk or unstable instances (Level II-2).[37,38]

ANEMIA

The consequences of dilutional or relative anemia have already been discussed. Its development is due to an increase in plasma volume out of proportion to red blood cell production, resulting in a hypervolemic state.[25,26] Increasing levels of circulating beta human chorionic gonadotropin (beta-HCG) do not suppress bone marrow production of red cells as initially suspected.[26] In most patients, a bone marrow evaluation reveals normoblastic cells.[26] However, dietary deficiencies in iron or folate may result in mixed anemia indices. Development of morning sickness or hyperemesis gravidarum may further affect adequate nutrition. Acute and chronic blood loss can also contribute or may be a major factor if excessive. Except in rare instances of DIC, hemolysis is not a significant factor.[26]

If correction of severe anemia is required, replacement should generally be with packed red cells slowly infused, to avoid fluid overload. The decision to transfuse should be based on symptoms and findings and not on any absolute hemoglobin or hematocrit values, which may be misleading in view of pregnancy-related dilutional anemia. Furthermore, hemoglobin/hematocrit values provide no information regarding tissue oxygenation or oxygen-carrying capacity. Thus, several physiologic tissue oxygenation indicators proposed as transfusion triggers for normovolemic anemia are an oxygen extraction ratio (O_2ER) > 50% and blood lactate > 4 mmol/L.[39] In hypovolemic anemia, volume resuscitation is indicated, but transfusion to a normotensive endpoint may actually promote continued blood loss.[40] The key is early and adequate resuscitation with appropriate volume in order to stave off persistent microvascular hypoperfusion as manifested by the no-reflow phenomenon.[41]

COAGULOPATHY

Deaths have been reported due to DIC complicating molar pregnancy.[42] Although not yet isolated, factors released by hydatidiform moles are known to have thromboplastic and fibrinolytic activity.[43] In vitro studies have shown procoagulant activity in molar vesicle fluid at the level of factor X.[44] This activity is similar to that described for amniotic fluid. Spillage of these factors into uterine maternal blood spaces may account for focal necrosis and uterine bleeding.[44,45]

Prostanoids produced by various tumors may cause platelet aggregation and activation of coagulation cascades.[46] However, even though vesicular fluid contains thromboxane and prostacyclin in high concentrations, plasma levels of these substances remain low.[46] Therefore, a systemic effect is unlikely. The coexistence of ARDS and DIC has been documented, and deposition of platelets on damaged pulmonary epithelium has been reported, but a cause-and-effect relationship has not been established.[47]

The evaluation of high-risk molar gestation patients should include a coagulation screen (Level II-3). Results may include a decreased platelet count, prolonged clotting time, prolonged partial thromboplastin time (PTT), or prolonged prothrombin time (PT). Confirmatory studies with fibrin degradation products and fibrin split products should not delay evacuation, which remains the cornerstone of therapy. Sepsis as an etiology for DIC should also be considered, appropriate cultures taken, and antibiotics started as indicated. Finally, use of oxytocin immediately before suction evacuation may decrease the release of thromboplastins and reduce the risk of coagulopathy (Level II-3).[10]

PREGNANCY-INDUCED HYPERTENSION/ECLAMPSIA

PIH occurs in 12% to 50% of molar pregnancies. However, only 57 cases of eclampsia have been reported, with 7 fatalities. In a review of these cases,

Newman[48] noted that completeness of records and diagnostic accuracy was variable. Several salient features can be gleaned from these reports, which emphasize the need for early evacuation. In most cases, multiple seizures were noted, 70% of which occurred before evacuation. Prolonged delay in evacuation of the molar gestation was common. All three components of the classic PIH triad (elevated blood pressure, proteinuria, and edema) were present in most patients. These patients usually met "severe PIH" criteria by blood pressure or proteinuria, although decreased platelets were documented in only one patient.

There are also many reports that detail atypical presentation, with hypertension as the only finding. Acosta-Sison and colleagues[49] noted that 100% of the hypertensive patients in their series had an enlarged uterus, at or above the umbilicus. They emphasized the importance of tumor volume and uterine size rather than weeks of amenorrhea as a risk factor. Paradoxically, PIH incidence in patients with molar pregnancy is higher in multiparous women.

Any pregnant patient presenting in the second trimester with evidence of PIH should be promptly evaluated with ultrasound for the presence of a molar gestation.[20] If PIH is diagnosed, appropriate prophylactic measures with magnesium sulfate should be initiated. Any delay in evacuation will contribute to increased morbidity and mortality.

HYPERTHYROIDISM

Since first noted by Tisne in 1955, there have been numerous reports of hyperthyroidism in patients with molar gestation.[50–56] Chemically, hyperthyroidism is evidenced by an elevated free thyroxine index (FTI) and an increased plasma free T_4 level. Clinical evidence may include agitation and sinus tachycardia or atrial fibrillation, which may progress to thyroid crisis evidenced by fever, severe agitation, and high-output heart failure. Left untreated, this condition can in turn progress to coma and fatal hypotension.

Fortunately, clinical hyperthyroidism is rare in molar pregnancy, and the etiology of thyroid hyperfunction remains unclear. The level of thyroid-stimulating hormone (TSH) is low or normal in these patients, and a secondary thyroid-stimulating factor has not been isolated. Initially beta-HCG was reported as being the causative factor,[51] but this has not been substantiated in larger clinical studies.[52] Some in vitro evidence supports the fact that beta-HCG binds to TSH receptors in the human thyroid gland.[53,54] However, the methodology has been questioned, and others have reported contraindicating data.[55] Because the thyroid-stimulating activity of beta-HCG has been estimated at 1/4,000 that of TSH, it may have an effect in very high concentration. Higher beta-HCG levels, seen with large molar gestations, are more often associated with pronounced hyperthyroidism. Upon evacuation, clinical and laboratory evidence of hyperthyroidism quickly resolves.

If clinically suspected, evacuation should not be delayed in awaiting confirmatory thyroid function tests or in an attempt to medically control thyroid hyperfunction. Beta blockade with intravenous propranolol, initially 1 mg every 5 minutes until tachyarrhythmia is controlled, can be adjusted to 20–120 mg four times/day. Additionally, sodium or potassium iodide may be administered intravenously (500–1,000 mg every 12 hours) to block release of thyroxine and thus reduce the circulating levels of triodothyronine. In the event of iodine allergy, lithium (300 mg PO every 8 hours) may be used as a substitute. Prior to evacuation, administration of propylthiouracil (PTU) and awaiting its effects on thyroid hormone synthesis is unwarranted (Level II-3).

HYPEREMESIS GRAVIDARUM

The presence of hyperemesis in the pregnant patient after the first trimester should arouse suspicion for the presence of hydatidiform mole. This late occurrence of severe nausea and emesis may be related to elevated beta-HCG levels and hyperthyroidism, although the relationship has not been completely elucidated.[56–58] Excessive emesis and poor dietary intake secondary to nausea lead to electrolyte imbalance and dehydration, which should be treated as indicated.

ENDOMYOMETRITIS

Infection of molar tissue and endomyometritis complicate up to 20% of molar gestations evacuated electively and up to 56% of those requiring suction evacuation.[3] The mechanism is probably an ascending bacterial invasion through an open cervical os in the presence of chronic bleeding. Instrumentation for evacuation increases the risk. Extrapolation from elective and spontaneous abortion data suggests that broad-spectrum antibiotics sufficient to cover both gram-negative and anaerobic bacteria should be administered if infection is suspected.[59] Based on similar elective abortion data, prophylactic intravenous antibiotics should be administered in high-risk cases and could be considered for all cases (Level I).[60] Evacuation should be performed as soon as therapeutic levels of antibiotics are established.

POSTEVACUATION DELAYED BLEEDING

Follow-up after evacuation of a molar gestation includes beta-HCG titers and routine examinations as discussed elsewhere (Level I).[20,21] During such follow-up, recurrence of vaginal bleeding more often represents development of malignant sequelae rather than retained molar trophoblastic tissue. This is usually reflected by an abnormal HCG regression curve. Of course, if the bleeding occurs soon after the initial evacuation, incomplete suction curettage could be suspected and recurettage may be indicated. This scenario can often be avoided by a very minimal and careful sharp curettage with a large curette following the initial suction evacuation.

When delayed bleeding occurs, a pelvic ultrasound may be misleading in creating the impression of a uterus full of molar contents. Recurettage in this situation is usually ill advised, as the risks of perforation outweigh the minimal potential benefits (Level II-2).[61,62] Such patients require evaluation for chemotherapy initiation.

Finally, as the beta-HCG level normalizes, delayed bleeding may simply represent resurgence of normal menses. Thus, in the face of a normal regression curve with delayed bleeding, an extensive work-up leading to possible recurettage is unwarranted (Level I).[20,21,62]

REFERENCES

1. Soto-Wright V, Bernstein M, Goldstein DP, Berkowitz RS. The changing clinical presentation of complete molar pregnancy. *Obstet Gynecol* 1995;86(5):775.

2. Twiggs LB, Morrow CP, Schlaerth JB. Acute pulmonary complications of molar pregnancy. *Am J Obstet Gynecol* 1979;135:189.

3. Schlaerth JB, Morrow CP, Montz FJ, dAblaing G. Initial management of hydatidiform mole. *Am J Obstet Gynecol* 1988;158(6):1299.

4. Orr JW, Austin JM, Hatch KD, et al. Acute pulmonary edema associated with molar pregnancies: a high risk factor for development of persistent trophoblastic disease. *Am J Obstet Gynecol* 1980;136:412.

5. Morrow CP, Kletzky DA, DiSaia JJ, et al. Clinical and laboratory correlates of molar pregnancy and trophoblastic disease. *Am J Obstet Gynecol* 1977;128:424.

6. Huberman RP, Fon GT, Bein ME. Benign molar pregnancies: pulmonary complications. *Am J. Radiol* 1982;138:71.

7. Trotter RF, Tieche HL. Maternal death due to pulmonary embolism of trophoblastic cells. *Am J Obstet Gynecol* 1956;71:1114.

8. Lipp RG, Kindschi JD, Schmitz R. Death from pulmonary embolism associated with hydatidiform mole. *Am J Obstet Gynecol* 1962;83:1644.

9. Kohorn EI, McGinn RC, Gee BL, et al. Pulmonary embolization of trophoblastic tissue in molar pregnancy. *Obstet Gynecol* 1978;51(suppl):165.

10. Kohorn EI, Richard CM, Bernard LG, et al. Pulmonary embolisation of trophoblastic tissue in molar pregnancy. *Scand J Clin Lab Invest* 1978;23:191.

11. Wagner D. Trophoblastic cells in the blood stream with normal and abnormal pregnancy. *Acta Cytol* 1968;12:137.

12. Kohorn EI. Clinical management and the neoplastic sequelae of trophoblastic embolization associated with hydatidiform mole. *Obstet Gynecol Surv* 1987;42:484.

13. Hankins GD, Wendell GD, Snyder RR, et al. Trophoblastic embolization during molar evacuation: central hemodynamic observations. *Obstet Gynecol* 1987;69:368.

14. Cotton DB, Bernstein SG, Read JA, et al. Hemodynamic observations in evacuation of molar pregnancy. *Am J Obstet Gynecol* 1980;138:6.

15. Brandes JM, Grunstein S, Peretz A. Suction evacuation of the uterine cavity in hydatidiform mole. *Obstet Gynecol* 1966;28:689.

16. Goldstein DP, Berkowitz RS. Current management of complete and partial molar pregnancy. *J Reprod Med* 1994;39:139–143.

17. Berkowitz RS, Goldstein DP, DuBeshter B, et al. Management of complete molar pregnancy. *J Reprod Med* 1987;32:634–638.

18. Grimes DA, Cates W Jr. The composite efficacy and safety of intraamniotic prostaglandin F2a and hypertonic saline for second trimester abortion. *J Reprod Med* 1979;22:248–252.

19. Bahar AM, el-Ashnei MS, Senthilsel van A. Hydatidiform mole in the elderly: hysterectomy or evacuation. *Int J Obstet Gynecol* 1989;23:233–237.

20. Morrow CP, Curtain JP, Townsend DE (Eds). *Synopsis of Gynecologic Oncology*, 4th ed. New York: Churchill Livingstone Inc., 1993, p. 317.

21. Soper JT, Lewis JL, Hammond CB. *Gestational Trophoblastic Disease in Principles and Practice of Gynecologic Oncology*, Hoskins WJ, Perez CA, Young RC (eds). Philadelphia: Lippincott-Raven Publishers, 1997, p. 1050.

22. Curry SL, Hanmard CB, Tyrey L, et al. Hydatidiform mole. Diagnosis, management, and long term follow up of 347 patients. *Obstet Gynecol* 1975;45:1.

23. Stoelting RK, Gibbs PS, Creasser CW, et al. Hemodynamic and ventilatory responses to fentanyl, fentanyl-droperidol, and nitrous oxide in patients with acquired valvular disease. *Anesthesiology* 1975;42:319.

24. Rackow EC, Fein IA, Leppo J. Colloid somotic pressure as a prognostic indicator of pulmonary edema and mortality in the critically ill. *Chest* 1977;72:709.

25. Chesley LC. Plasma and red cell volumes during pregnancy. *Am J Obstet Gynecol* 1972;112:440.

26. Pritchard JW. Blood volume changes in pregnancy and puerperium IV. Anemia associated with hydatidiform mole. *Am J Obstet Gynecol* 1965;91:621.

27. Liley AW. Clinical and laboratory evidence of variations in maternal plasma volume in pregnancy. *Int J Gynaecol Obstet* 1970;8:358.

28. Goodlin RC. Why treat "physiologic" anemia of pregnancy? *J Reprod Med* 1982;27:639.

29. Pritchard JA. Changes in the blood volume during pregnancy and delivery. *Anesthesiology* 1965;26:393.

30. Benedetti TJ, Twiggs LB, Morrow CP. Pre- and postevacuation metabolic studies of hydatidiform mole and severe pregnancy induced hypertension. *J Reprod Med* 1980;25:133.

31. Soffronoff EC, Kaufmann BM, Connaughton JF. Intravascular volume determinations of pregnancy. *Am J Obstet Gynecol* 1977;127:4.

32. Hankin GDV, Wendel GD Jr, Cunningham FG, et al. Longitudinal evaluation of hemodynamic changes in eclampsia. *Am J Obstet Gynecol* 1984;150:506.

33. Cotton DB, Gonik B, Dorman K, et al. Cardiovascular alterations in severe pregnancy induced hypertension: relationship of central venous pressure to pulmonary capillary wedge pressure. *Am J Obstet Gynecol* 1985;151:762.

34. Higgins HP, Herschmann JM, Kenimer JG, et al. The thyrotoxicosis of hydatidiform mole. *Ann Intern Med* 1975;83:307.

35. Severinghaus JW, Spellman MJ. Pulse oximeter failure thresholds in hypotension and vasoconstriction. *Anesthesiology* 1990;73:532.

36. Jay GD, Hughes L, Renzi FP. Pulse oximetry is accurate in acute anemia from hemorrhage. *Ann Emerg Med* 1994;24:32.

37. Scott WL. Complications associated with central venous catheters. *Chest* 1988;91:1221.

38. Patel C, Labby V, Venus B, et al. Acute complications of pulmonary artery catheter insertion in critically ill patients. *Crit Care Med* 1986;14:195.

39. Levy P, Chavez RP, Crystal GJ, et al. Oxygen extraction ratio: a valid indicator of transfusion need in limited coronary vascular reserve? *J Trauma* 1992;32:769–774.

40. American College of Physicians. Practice strategies for elective red blood cell transfusions. *Ann Int Med* 1992;116:403–406.

41. Consensus Conference. Perioperative red blood cell transfusion. *JAMA* 1988;260:2700–2703.

42. Tsakok FHM, Koh S, Ilancheran A, et al. Maternal death associated with hydatidiform molar pregnancy. *Int J Gynaecol Obstet* 1983;21:485.

43. Tsakok FHM, Ratnam SS, Chew SC, et al. Thromboplastic and fibrinolytic activity of hydatidiform molar tissue and vesicular fluid. *J Obstet Gynecol* 1977;86:233.

44. Kaplan SS, Szulman AE, Surti U. Effect of hydatidiform molar vesicular fluid on blood coagulation. *Am J Obstet Gynecol* 1985;153:703.

45. Roy AC, Karim MM, Kottegoda SR, et al. Thromboxane A_2 and prostacylin levels in molar pregnancy. *Br J Obstet Gynaecol* 1984;91:908.

46. Honn KV, Bockman RS, Marnett LJ. Prostaglandins and cancer: a review of tumor initiation through tumor metastasis. *Prostaglandins* 1981;21:833.

47. Bone RC, Francis PB, Pierce AK. Intravascular coagulation associated with adult respiratory distress syndrome. *Am J Med* 1976;61:585.

48. Newman RB, Eddy GL. Association of eclampsia and hydatidiform mole: case report and review of the literature. *Obstet Gynecol Surv* 1988;43:185.

49. Acosta-Sison H. The relationship of hydatidiform mole to pre-eclampsia and eclampsia. A study of 85 cases. *Am J Obstet Gynecol* 1956;71:1279.

50. Tisne L, Barzalotto J, Steverson C. Estudio de funcion tirodea durante el estado gravido-puerperal con el yodo radioactive. *Bolietin de la Sociedad Chilena de Obstetricia y Ginecologia* 1955;20:246.

51. Kenimer JG, Hershman JM, Higgins HP. The thyrotropin in hydatidiform moles is human chorionic gonadotropin. *J Clin Endocrin Metab* 1975;40:480–489.

52. Amir SM, Osathanonah R, Berkowitz RS, et al. Human chorionic gonadotropin and thyroid function in patients with hydatidiform mole. *Am J Obstet Gynecol* 1984;150:723.

53. Silverberg J, O'Donnell J, Sugeronya A, et al. Effect of human thyroid tissue in vitro. *J Clin Endocrinol Metab* 1978;46:420.

54. Carayon P, Lefort G, Nisula B. Interaction of human chorionic gonadotropin and human luteinizing hormone with human thyroid membranes. *Endocrinology* 1980;106:1907.

55. Amir SM, Kane P, Osathanodh R. Divergent responses by human and mouse thyroid

to human chorionic gonadotropin in vitro. *Program of the 64th Annual Meeting of the Endocrine Society*, 1982, Abstract 1222.

56. Ngowngarmratana S, Sunthornthepvarakul T, Kanchanawat N. Thyroid function and human chorionic gonadotropin in patients with hydatidiform mole. *J Med Assoc Thailand* 1997;80(11):693–697.

57. Soules MR, Hughes CL Jr, Garcia JA, et al. Nausea vomiting of pregnancy: role of human chorionic gonadotropin and 17-hydroxyprogesterone. *Obstet Gynecol* 1980;55:696.

58. Tareen AK, Baseer A, Jaffry HF, Shafiq M. Thyroid hormone in hyperemesis gravidarum. *J Obstet Gynaecol* 1995;21(5):497–501.

59. Burkman RT, Atienza MF, King TM. Culture and treatment in endometritis following elective abortion. *Am J Obstet Gynecol* 1977;128:556.

60. Henriques CU, Wilken-Jensen C, Thorsen P, Moller BR. A randomised controlled trial of prophylaxis of post-abortal infection: ceftriaxone versus placebo. *Br J Obstet Gynaecol* 1994;101(7):610.

61. Schlaerth JB, Morrow CP, Rodriguez M. Diagnostic and therapeutic curettage in gestational trophoblastic disease. *Am J Obstet Gynecol* 1990;162:1465.

62. Lao TTH, Lee FHC, Yeung SSL. Repeat curettage after evacuation of a hydatidiform mole. *Acta Obstet Gynecol Scand* 1987;66:306.

CHAPTER 16

PERIOPERATIVE ISSUES IN THE MANAGEMENT OF VULVAR CANCER

KATHRYN F. McGONIGLE, M.D. and LEO D. LAGASSE, M.D.

Perioperative issues surrounding the care of patients with vulvar malignancy have evolved rapidly over the last few decades. Improvements in surgical technique, less radical surgery, improved perioperative management, and better antibiotic therapies have dramatically decreased complications associated with the treatment of vulvar cancer. These changes have been associated with a reduction of both immediate and delayed morbidity, shorter hospital stay and recovery time, and less interference with body image and sexual function.

Treatment of vulvar cancer depends on the stage at presentation, histologic type, size of lesion, location of the primary lesion on the vulva relative to the midline and relative to anatomic structures including the urethra, bladder, anus, and rectum. In addition, treatment is influenced by the status of regional lymph nodes. The focus of this chapter is not on specific management of patients based on these factors but on perioperative issues in patients with vulvar cancer. Surgery is the primary treatment for vulvar cancer, particularly early-stage disease. Radiation therapy and/or chemotherapy are sometimes used prior to or after surgical treatment, depending on the extent of disease, and may be pivotal in optimizing chance for cure. However, their use is commonly associated with an increased risk of perioperative complications.

LESS RADICAL SURGERY

Over the last several decades numerous modifications in surgical technique have been incorporated into the management of vulvar cancer. The classic approach to vulvar cancer, regardless of size or location of the primary lesion, was radical

Perioperative and Supportive Care in Gynecologic Oncology: Evidence-Based Management,
Edited by Steven A. Vasilev.
ISBN 0-471-24788-X   Copyright © 2000 by Wiley-Liss, Inc.

vulvectomy with bilateral inguinal-femoral lymphadenectomy using an en bloc technique. This approach for the treatment of vulvar cancer and its regional lymphatics was initially proposed by Basset in 1912 and successfully implemented by Taussig and Way several decades later.[1,2] Subsequently, the modified Basset procedure (butterfly incision) was introduced. This incision involved the removal of 2–3 cm of skin over the groin from the anterior-superior iliac spine to the pubic tubercle and crossing anteriorly and inferiorly to the inguinal ligament incorporating the underlying lymphatic tissue along with the radical vulvectomy specimen.

These extensive en bloc procedures were associated with appreciable morbidity and prolonged hospitalizations with wound complication rates that approached 60%.[3] In one series, the modified Basset procedure was associated with impairment of primary wound healing in 85%, varying degrees of lymphedema in 69%, and thrombophlebitis in 9% of patients.[4] Operative mortality was also high, in the range of 2.6% to 5.7%.[5,6] Because of the substantial morbidity and prolonged hospitalization associated with the en bloc procedures, gynecologic cancer surgeons have been inspired to examine modifications to this classic surgical approach to vulvar cancer. The acceptance of these modifications and incorporation into the care of vulvar cancer patients has been based on multiple observational and nonrandomized studies demonstrating a reduction in morbidity without demonstrating a reduction in patient cure.

As early as 1940, Taussig suggested that radical vulvectomy and inguinal lymphadenectomy be performed through three separate incisions.[1] This technique was not accepted into the general management of vulvar cancer until many decades later when gynecologic cancer surgeons described performing a three-incision technique. Compared with the en bloc incision in historical controls, a significant reduction in morbidity was observed.[7–9] In one series, there was a reduction in groin breakdown from 70% using the en bloc technique to 20% using the three-incision technique.[10] In another study, wound breakdown decreased from 64% to 38%, wound infection decreased from 21% to 14%, and lymphocyst formation decreased from 28% to 14%.[11] The reduction in perioperative morbidity was not associated with an obvious increase in skin bridge or local recurrences.[9,11] Numerous studies suggest that more conservative surgery has been associated with a marked reduction in hospital stay, blood loss, operating time, blood transfusion, and other perioperative morbidity.[4,10–12] Modifications of surgery for vulvar cancer were initially performed in a very select group of patients with early vulvar cancer, but over time these techniques have been more widely applied to patients with larger and more extensive and invasive primary vulvar cancers. These observations have been made based on Level III evidence.

As the surgical management of vulvar cancer evolved, further modifications were introduced. A prospective nonrandomized, noncontrolled Gynecology Oncology Group (GOG) study treated Stage I vulvar cancer patients with modified radical hemivulvectomy and ipsilateral superficial inguinal lymphadenectomy.[13] Compared with historical controls, the authors noted an increased failure in the vulva, but 8 of 10 patients were salvaged by a second operation. They also noted recurrences in both the contralateral groin and ipsilateral groin among 9 of 121 patients. Acute and long-term complications were lower than historical controls. Wound separation, hematoma, or infection occurred in 28.9% of 121 patients and only 19% developed lymphedema, the majority of cases being mild. Compared with historical controls, there was a significantly increased risk of recurrence, but not death. The authors suggested this modified surgical approach is an appropriate alternative to the traditional radical operation for selective vulvar cancer patients.[13] More recently, further modifications have occurred, including radical local excision of the primary vulvar lesion with a 1–2 cm margin and unilateral inguinal-femoral lymphadenectomy for the more invasive lateralized lesion.[14] Since there are no randomized prospective studies, it is possible that the more conservative approach is associated with a slightly higher risk of local recurrence. These observations have been made based on Level III evidence.

Way's classic technique of inguinal-femoral lymphadenectomy included removal of superficial groin nodes with sartorius muscle fascia, cribiform fascia over the femoral vessels, adductor longus fascia, and pectineus muscle fascia. Over the last several decades, investigators have found that preservation of the fascia lata is a satisfactory method for groin lymphadenectomy, without obvious evidence of compromising the patient's survival. Another proposed modification of the groin dissection is omission of the deep femoral node dissection in the absence of groin metastases in superficial inguinal nodes. Some have suggested that the risk of lymphedema and infection may be reduced with this approach, but this is unproven.[15] The safety of this modification has been seriously questioned. In a prospective noncontrolled GOG study, 4 women among 121 vulvar cancer patients died after recurrence in the groin subjected to superficial lymphadenectomy with negative superficial nodes. These and similar reported cases suggest possible involvement of femoral nodes in the absence of superficial groin involvement.[13] Patients with groin recurrences have a dismal prognosis, with greater than 80% mortality. Because of this and the absence of compelling evidence that eliminating the deep groin dissection results in a decrease in morbidity, this approach has not gained widespread approval.[16,17] These observations are made based on Level III evidence.

A further surgical modification is the elimination of pelvic lymphadenectomy in the majority of patients with vulvar cancer. Because pelvic node involvement is exceedingly rare in the absence of positive groin nodes, it has been suggested that pelvic lymphadenectomy be reserved for patients with involvement of groin nodes only.[4,18] Subsequently, data from a randomized prospective GOG study suggested there may be little to no role of pelvic lymphadenectomy in vulvar cancer patients. In this study, patients undergoing groin and pelvic lymphadenectomy fared worse that those treated with radiation therapy. As a result, the authors suggested that even in the setting of involved groin nodes, pelvic lymphadenectomy should not be performed, but rather the patient should be treated with postoperative pelvic and groin irradiation.[5]

Although some have reported no increased morbidity from the addition of pelvic lymphadenectomy to radical vulvectomy and bilateral groin dissection, others have not verified this possibility.[6,19–21] One study suggested that operative mortality could be reduced by 2% if pelvic lymphadenectomy were omitted and another study found that major complications were twice as common in patients undergoing pelvic lymphadenectomy.[6,20,21] There is a growing body of evidence suggesting that involvement of the pelvic lymph nodes is associated with a dismal chance of survival not improved by pelvic lymphadenectomy. The role of pelvic lymphadenectomy in the management of vulvar cancer appears to be limited. Indications may include patients with prior radiation therapy to the pelvis or other contraindications to pelvic radiation therapy. These observations have been made based on Level I[5] and II evidence.

For patients with advanced or recurrent vulvar cancer, the ultraradical surgical approach (exenterative surgery) to the treatment of advanced vulvar cancer has historically been associated with a 7% postoperative mortality in combined series. Furthermore, the loss of organ function and impairment of sexual function is significant.[10] Based on favorable results in uncontrolled series and in other solid tumors (head and neck cancer and anal carcinoma), the GOG has studied the use of chemotherapy in conjunction with radiation therapy to reduce the radicality of surgery required for patients with advanced (T3 and T4) vulvar cancers.[22] In many cases, organ preservation has been possible when treatment otherwise would have necessitated pelvic exenteration. The use of radiation therapy in the management of advanced vulvar cancer is further discussed at the end of this chapter.

SENTINEL LYMPH NODE BIOPSY

A further modification of surgery being examined for vulvar cancer patients is the use of intraoperative lymphatic mapping techniques to identify the first draining lymph node (the sentinel node) in the regional lymphatic basin. Numerous published studies of patients with solid malignancies support the efficacy of these techniques in identifying the sentinel node and its potential to better select a group of patients that may benefit from formal nodal dissection.[23–26]

The most common techniques involve the use of isosulfan blue dye or [99m]technicium-labeled sulfur colloid (lymphoscintigraphy). Using isosulfan blue dye, 2–4 ml of 2.5% dye is injected into the tissue around the perimeter of the primary vulvar cancer. After a short period of time (5–10 min), the ipsilateral groin is explored. Blue-stained lymphatics are identified and dissected to the sentinel node, which is then removed. Using lymphoscintigraphy, [99m]technicium-labeled sulfur colloid is similarly injected around the perimeter of the tumor. Following injection (approximately 30 min), imaging of the injection site and draining node basin is performed. With this technique, a "hot node" is identified as one with increased focal radiotracer uptake using a hand-held gamma probe.

Most reported experience with sentinel lymph node biopsy is in patients with breast cancer and malignant melanoma. Overall, studies suggest tht the sentinel lymph node is successfully identified in 68% to 98% of cases using the isosulfan blue dye technique.[25,27] Using a combination of isosulfan dye and [99m]technicium-labeled sulfur colloid, the success of sentinel lymph node identification may be improved, with identification in 98% of cases.[26,28–30] The false negative rate (defined as a negative sentinel lymph node while a higher node is positive) has been reported to be between 0% and 5% in most series of breast cancer patients.[25,27,31]

Although experience with lymphatic mapping in vulvar cancer is somewhat limited compared with other solid tumors, there are some data. In an uncontrolled series, the use of intraoperative lymphatic mapping was examined in 21 patients with vulvar cancer using isosulfan blue dye. The sentinel lymph node was identified in 86% of patients and 66% of groins (8 of 11 had bilateral groin dissections). After removal of the sentinel node, formal groin dissection was performed. In no cases was a nonsentinel node positive if the sentinel node was negative. There were no complications related to the injection of dye.[32]

In another study, intraoperative lymphoscintigraphy was used in 10 patients with vulvar cancer who underwent inguinal-femoral lymphadenectomy. Three patients were found to have groin node metastases and in no case was a non-sentinel node positive when the sentinel node was negative. In a third study the combined use of lymphatic mapping with isosulfan blue dye and lymphoscintigraphy was examined in 6 patients with vulvar cancer.[34] Sentinel nodes were identified in all 6 patients, but in 1 of 7 groins the sentinel node was not blue but "hot." There was minimal morbidity associated with sentinel lymphadenectomy. No patient developed numbness or edema and one patient developed a small groin seroma that resolved. These preliminary data suggest that lymphatic mapping may have similar efficacy in vulvar cancer patients as in other solid malignancies. However, because of limited Level III data in vulvar cancer, lymphatic mapping techniques should not be routinely used, except in the setting of a research study.

COMPLICATIONS OF THERAPY

Early Complications

Wound Breakdown or Cellulitis   By far the most common and serious complications associated with the surgical treatment of vulvar cancer, particularly with the en bloc classical surgical procedures, have been infectious. The large size of the wounds, reduction in residual vascular supply, and the shearing forces during flexion and extension of the lower extremities compromise wound healing and result in suboptimal adherence of tissue to the underlying structures. The result is accumulation of lymphatic fluid, skin and soft tissue infection, and possible necrosis of the compromised cutaneous flaps.[4] Efforts to reduce complications have primarily focused on less radical surgery. Other perioperative treatment modalities, including the use of groin suction catheters for evacuation of subcutaneous fluid and debris, selective use of sartorius muscle flaps, and improved antibiotics, have led to a decrease in infectious complications.

Perioperative morbidity from wound breakdown may be significant, and in rare cases, death may occur as a result of sepsis.[22] The risk of wound breakdown after surgery for vulvar cancer is directly related to the extent of the surgery and underlying disease processes that may impair wound healing. With the classic en bloc radical vulvectomy and bilateral inguinal-femoral lymphadenectomy, wound breakdown was as high as 60% to 70%.[35] With the three-incision technique of radical vulvectomy and groin dissection, the risk of wound breakdown was reduced to approximately 20%.[10] The risk has been even further reduced with more conservative surgical modifications limiting the amount of resection, such as radical hemivulvectomy or radical local excision. The risk of breakdown is also related to surgical technique and is clearly increased with tension on the wound. Factors that may impair wound healing and increase infectious complications include diabetes mellitus, peripheral vascular disease, history of parenteral drug use, chronic malnutrition, steroid use, or alcoholism. Optimizing glucose control in the diabetic patient is important to minimize risk of infectious complications. Prior radiation therapy to the groins and/or vulva also significantly increases risk for wound breakdown. These issues are further discussed in the section on "Wound Healing."

Some researchers have suggested using hyperbaric oxygen therapy following radical vulvectomy to improve wound healing.[36] In a nonrandomized prospective study, the authors noted a reduction in wound breakdown for patients undergoing radical vulvectomy with lymph node dissection and hyperbaric oxygen therapy compared with historical controls. There are no randomized prospective data on the use of hyperbaric oxygen in this setting. Because of limited Level III research, its use to reduce wound complications in vulvar cancer patients should be considered experimental.

In one large retrospective series, the risk of complications in the groin did not correlate with the extent of the vulvar surgery and similarly the addition of groin lymphadenectomy did not increase the risk of vulvar complications.[37] Sparing of the saphenous vein did not appear to affect postoperative groin wound breakdown or cellulitis occurring in 24% of patients in whom the vessel was sacrificed compared with 18% whose vein was spared.[38] Sartorius muscle transposition may decrease the risk of groin wound complications in vulvar cancer patients. A retrospective analysis of the effect of sartorius transposition on wound morbidity following inguinal-femoral lymphadenectomy through separate incisions suggested there may be some benefit on risk of wound infection. In this study, the incidence of groin cellulitis or wound breakdown was less in patients undergoing sartorius transposition than those who did not have the procedure performed, 41% vs. 66%, respectively ($p = 0.33$).[38] Also reported is anecdotal success using the sartorius transposition in the treatment of infected groin wounds with vascular grafts after reconstructive vascular surgery.[39–41] However, its use in vulvar cancer patients after groin wound infection has not been described. Selective use of sartorius muscle transposition after groin dissection may be appropriate based on limited Level III data.

For the vulvar wound, drains are not routinely used and perioperative care consists of keeping the wound clean and dry. Cleansing with warm saline or water should be started approximately 24 hours postoperatively. After cleaning the wound, excess moisture is removed with a towel. Since the vulva tends to be a very moist area, moisture is minimized by use of a heating lamp or blow dryer. Drying should be performed two to three times daily and after bowel movements, depending on the size and location of the wound. The groins are routinely drained and the drains are not removed until there is less than 30–40 cc/day of drainage. Particularly in the immediate postoperative period, it is essential that the groin flaps remain adherent to the underlying tissues. This is accomplished using compression dressing and drains and may prevent a fluid collection that could lead to an abscess or lymphocyst formation, or increase the risk of flap necrosis. Either wall suction or bulb suction is appropriate, but if bulb suction is used, vigilance to maintain continued suction is essential. Some have suggested that wall suction might be preferable, particularly in the first 2 to 3 postoperative days. When evidence of either groin or vulvar infection occurs, such as drainage, induration, or erythema, the wound must be inspected to exclude an abscess collection and broad-spectrum antibiotics should be instituted. If an abscess is present, it should be drained and the wound opened.

Wound Healing   In general, wound healing mechanisms may be divided into four phases: early, intermediate, later, and a final phase. The early phase includes changes occurring over the initial 3 days after a surgical incision. The change in the tensional or compressional state of the tissue is immediately communicated to local connective tissue cells. There are also mechanisms of hemostasis including vasoconstriction and retraction mediated through the sympathetic nervous system and possibly prostaglandins. In addition, immediately following the production of a wound, the coagulation cascade is initiated and clot formation occurs. In addition to its role in the clotting cascade, fibrin serves as a lattice to facilitate adhesion, migration, and phagocytic processes of leukocytes during inflammation. It also provides a scaffold for subsequent angiogenesis. Platelet aggregation is initiated primarily by exposure of subendothelial collagen. Finally, inflammation occurs during the early phase of wound healing and is the key modulator of the healing process. Inflammation is associated with initial vasoconstriction, followed by a more prolonged vasodilation of postcapillary venules. During this phase, there is a cellular response with an inflammatory cell influx of neutrophils, monocytes, macrophages, and lymphocytes for scavenging the wound. Mediators of inflammation are also released from the plasma and tissues, including kinins, complements, histamine, serotonin, prostaglandins, fibronectin, lysosomal proteases, and lymphokines.[41–43]

During the intermediate phase of wound healing, fibroblast migration and proliferation occur. In addition, angiogenesis is stimulated by the release of growth factors, low oxygen tension, high lactate, and a low pH. Epithelialization occurs by mobilization, migration, mitosis, and differentiation. Epithelial cells immediately adjacent to the wound mobilize. Cellular migration is visible at 24 hours following injury. During cellular migration, fixed basal cells adjacent to the wound begin mitosis, resulting in resurfacing of the wound. As the new epithelial layer becomes complete and begins to thicken, normal cellular differentiation from basal to surface layers resumes. The stratification of epithelial layers occurs within 48 to 72 hours.[41–43]

During the later phase of wound healing, collagen synthesis occurs. This process does not begin for 3 to 5 days after the surgical incision. Collagen is a fibrous protein and is the major component of scar tissue. The formation of glycosaminoglycan occurs and functions to act as a "glue" to the subepithelial tissues. Wound contraction as part of the later phase of healing plays a minimal role in the healing of a surgically created linear incision.[41–43]

During the final phase of wound healing, scar remodeling occurs. Collagen synthesis and collagen degradation are in a finely controlled state of equilibrium during normal tissue repair. The tensile strength of a wound can be correlated with collagen synthesis only up to 45 days after injury. Despite no increase in net collagen synthesis, cutaneous scars continue to increase in breaking and tensile strength for months. Tensile strength results from collagen cross-linking. Even in optimal circumstances, wound strength never reaches that of normal skin.[41–43]

There are numerous factors that may adversely affect wound healing. In vulvar cancer patients, bacterial infection is the most common and is defined as the presence of greater than 10^5 organisms per gram of tissue in a wound where clinical signs of infection are present. At this level, wound healing may be inhibited or complicated because of competition for nutrition or destruction of cells by bacterial toxins, increased collagen lysis, decreased tissue oxygen tension, and a continued presence of an inflammatory reaction.[44] Other factors in patients with vulvar cancer that may impair wound healing include alcoholism, diabetes, glucocorticoids, hematoma formation, severe malnutrition, older age, prior radiation therapy, cigarette smoking, and suboptimal surgical technique.

Chronic alcohol use is associated with slower wound healing and slower collagen accumulation. The use of glucocorticoids is associated with a decrease in the inflammatory response, less collagen formation, and delay in angiogenesis. These effects are seen whether steroids are used topically or given systemically and are markedly potentiated by even mild malnutrition.[45] Although there have been no carefully controlled human trials that clearly demonstrate the deleterious effect of therapeutic steroid doses on wound healing, retrospective data suggest that many episodes of nonhealing have been associated with steroid use. Based on Level III data, we recommend that steroid administration be limited to those clinical situations in which it is absolutely necessary.

The diabetic has many problems that predispose to wound healing complications, including neuropathy (more mechanical trauma), microangiopathy, and an increased risk of infection.[46–48] One factor implicated in poor wound healing is the impaired circulation secondary to large- and small-vessel occlusive disease. Diabetics have been found to have five times the risk of infection in clean incisions than nondiabetics. Well-controlled diabetics are more resistant to wound infection than poorly controlled diabetics. In the poorly controlled diabetic, a major component of this phenomenon is the impaired inflammatory response caused by hyperglycemia. In addition, all aspects of leukocyte function are impaired, especially phagocytosis.[47] Hyperglycemia is also associated with a general suppression of both humoral and cellular immunity. In animal models, these immunologic defects can largely be reversed by good control of blood glucose, but relevant human data are not available.[47] In addition, collagen accumulates at a slower rate and breaking strength is diminished. Insulin may improve the decrease in collagen synthesis.[48]

Massive loss of body weight and malnutrition impairs wound healing. Protein depletion and vitamin deficiencies may impair collagen synthesis.[49,50] Malnutrition has long been implicated in poor wound healing. In animal models, loss of 15% to 20% of lean body mass can result in a decrease in wound breaking strength and colonic bursting pressure. A prospective randomized trial of preoperative total parenteral nutrition in patients with gastrointestinal malignancies reported a significant reduction in postoperative morbidity and mortality.[49] Another study that evaluated the pooled results of prospective randomized trials of perioperative total parenteral nutrition in cancer patients concluded that its use can reduce the incidence of major surgical morbidity and mortality, at the expense of an increased risk of infection.[50] At present it is generally agreed that nutritional support may have a beneficial effect on wound healing in nutritionally depleted patients, but has no such effect in well-nourished patients and may even increase risk of complications. Parenteral nutrition should be used selectively in patients with documented malnutrition. This recommendation is based on Level I through Level III evidence.

Older age is associated with slower wound healing than in younger patients.[51] Cigarette smoking impairs wound healing, probably by several mechanisms. Smoking is associated with decreased tissue oxygenation due to elevated carboxyhemoglobin levels. Endothelial changes and increased platelet adhesiveness occur and can lead to additional limitation of local blood flow. It is not entirely clear how nicotine impairs wound healing.[52]

The effect of prior radiation therapy in the wound healing process can be seen in all aspects of the repair process. The problems with wound healing and ulceration after radiation have been historically related to relative ischemia of the irradiated tissue due to an obliterative endarteritis of the microvasculature with resulting reduction in blood supply.[53] More recent experiments suggest that the change is due to a diminished transcutaneous oxygen pressure, although this is controversial.[54] Radiation also affects cells of the hematopoietic system, which might account for the delayed inflammatory process. It also affects cells that participate in wound remodeling and repair. Radiation has a direct effect on structural collagen with a marked reduction in tensile strength. As a result, radiated wounds have a higher risk of wound dehiscence, wound infection, and overall delay in wound healing.[55,56] Data from animal studies suggest that many of the adverse effects of radiation on wound healing may be reversed by the administration of high doses of vitamin A. However, only anecdotal evidence is available in humans.[57]

Finally, meticulous surgical technique is required to minimize the risk of wound complications. Delicate tissue handling, particularly the delicate skin flaps in the groin dissection, is essential. Meticulous hemostasis, asepsis, minimizing the amount of foreign bodies (sutures), and avoiding dead space are also important. Hematoma increases the likelihood of bacterial infection, since neutrophils do not migrate effectively into an avascular hematoma and a small inoculum of bacteria in a hematoma could multiply without limitation by host defense mechanisms. These clinical observations on wound healing have been made based on Level III evidence.

Necrotizing Soft Tissue Infections and Necrotizing Fascitis Necrotizing soft tissue infections may occur in the vulva or groin after surgical treatment of vulvar cancer or in a patient who has not recently had surgery. Management is similar regardless of events preceding the patient's presentation. Necrotizing soft tissue infections after radical vulvar surgery may present initially with only localized mimimal pain and a deceptively benign appearance, but usually an infectious process is obvious in the wound.[58–61] Local signs of infection such as edema, erythema, crepitis, or bullae may or may not be present. Signs of deep tissue infection may be evident such as cyanosis or bronzing of the skin. Induration is common and crepitance may be present with a gas-producing organism. As the inflammatory process progresses, thrombosis of the perforating vessels to the skin may occur, resulting in breakdown of the overlying skin and sometimes associated paresthesias. The fascia and muscle may become involved. Systemic manifestations of sepsis may develop concurrently, but bacteremia is rarely identified. Wound culture usualy reveals a polymicrobial infection, particularly in infections occurring postoperatively. Organisms that are commonly isolated include *Bacteroides*; coliforms; *Klebsiella*; *Proteus*; Group A β-hemolytic *Streptococcus*, *Staphylococcus*, and *Peptostreptococcus*; and *Clostridia*.[62,63]

Because the patient may present either with an obvious vulvar wound infection or with minimal cutaneous manifestations or a necrotizing soft tissue infection, a high index of suspicion is needed in order to make an early diagnosis. Certainly, if the patient with an apparent cellulitis fails to respond to standard therapy with appropriate antibiotics and wound care, a suspicion of a more extensive infection should be considered. Radiologic studies are seldom helpful in making the diagnosis of a necrotizing soft tissue infection.[64]

Whenever the diagnosis is considered, management initially consists of aggressive resuscitative measures and broad-spectrum antibiotic therapy, prior to proceeding to the operating room for surgical exploration. Some have suggested the use of frozen tissue sections to help make the diagnosis.[65] Surgical exploration and debridement should not be delayed, even if the patient remains in septic shock, since the sepis will not resolve until excision of the infected tissue is performed.[64]

Surgical exploration of the vulvar wound should be thorough and include direct visual examination of the underlying muscle and fascia. The presence and extent of undermining and a manifestation of subcutaneous and fascial necrosis should be assessed. All necrotic tissue, including muscle or fascia, is excised until healthy viable tissue is seen.[66] The wound is packed open and kept moist with saline and is reexplored in the operating room daily until progression of necrosis has ceased. Depending on the primary focus and extent of the necrotizing infection, there may be involvement of the anal sphincter and/or urethra, but if possible these are preserved. Patients with disruption of the anal sphincter or colonic perforation require diversion of stool.[64]

Untreated necrotizing soft tissue infections will progress to extensive tissue necrosis, florid sepsis and death. The overall mortality rate for patients with all types of necrotizing soft tissue infections is approximately 38%.[58] In general, the literature supports the association of factors that contribute to death, including diabetes mellitus, increased age, delay in diagnosis, and failure to control infection at first operation (i.e., inadequate debridement). Delay of surgical intervention is consistently a factor associated with increased mortality.[64] One study of 33 male and female patients with necrotizing fasciitis found that the time from diagnosis of an infectious process to operative intervention was higher for those who died, 11.7 days, compared with 6.0 days for those who survived.[67] Similarly, McHenry et al. found that in 65 patients with necrotizing soft tissue infections, the average time from admission to operation was 90 hours in nonsurvivors and 25 hours in survivors ($p = 0.0002$).[68]

Observational clinical and animal studies have suggested that hyperbaric oxygen therapy may be beneficial in the treatment of necrotizing soft tissue infections.[69–71] Several mechanisms are postulated by which hyperbaric oxygen may improve wound healing and a detailed discussion of these is beyond the scope of this chapter.[62,72–74]

Animal models of necrotizing soft tissue infection using intramuscular injection of *Clostridia* have shown an advantage of hyperbaric oxygen when used early after inoculation, with less tissue loss and decreased mortality rates.[75,76] Limited data on the use of hyperbaric oxygen in humans with recrotizing soft tissue infections are available, and there has never been a controlled, randomized prospective study in humans. Riseman et al. examined the use of hyperbaric oxygen therapy for necrotizing fasciitis in a retrospective fashion in 29 patients treated either with or without hyperbaric oxygen. The first group of patients received surgical therapy and antibiotics and the second group also received hyperbaric oxygen therapy. Patients treated with hyperbaric oxygen were more seriously ill but had a significantly lower mortality, 23%, compared with 66% in the group not receiving hyperbaric oxygen therapy.[70] Preservation of tissue may be a significant benefit of hyperbaric oxygen therapy in the treatment of necrotizing fasciitis. Riseman et al. found that in addition to a reduction in mortality, the addition of hyperbaric oxygen significantly reduced the number of debridements required to achieve wound control.[70] Others have demonstrated a reduction in amputation rate from 75% to 20% among patients with necrotizing soft tissue infections of the extremity.[77]

There are serious potential complications of hyperbaric oxygen therapy and its administration is complex. Baratrauma may aggravate sinusitis and cause tympanic membrane rupture, pneumothorax, or air embolism. Oxygen may be toxic to the lungs or central nervous system and reversible visual changes may occur. In the hemodynamicaly unstable patient, the hyperbaric oxygen chamber makes resuscitation difficult. Patient claustrophobia may limit its practical use.[64] Patients with diabetes require particularly close monitoring with hyperbaric oxygen since dextrose metabolism is enhanced. As a result, patients may be more susceptible to hypoglycemic seizures.[78] These observations on the use of hyperbaric oxygen in patients with necrotizing soft tissue infections are based on Level III evidence, and its use in clinical practice should be considered experimental.

Osteomyelitis Pubis   After surgery for vulvar cancer, partial necrosis or osteomyelitis of the pubic bone is a rare but serious infection that usually results from a contiguous focus of infection weeks or months after a surgical procedure. Associated morbidity is significant and rarely may lead to fulminant sepsis and death.[37] In one large series of patients undergoing radical vulvectomy, the rate of osteomyelitis was 2%.[12] In a series of four patients who developed osteomyelitis of the pubic bone after radical vulvectomy, the mean hospital stay was increased by 5.6 weeks.[79] The patients presented 2 to 4 months after surgery with pain and tenderness over the pubic symphysis, difficulty ambulating, and evidence of infection in the pubic or vulvar area. Plain X-ray films showed abnormalities of the pubic bone in all cases. In a review of the literature, the infecting organism was *Staphylococcus aureus* in 60% of cases, and in the other 40%, gram-negative organisms were etiologic.[79] Management includes wound and bone cultures, drainage and debridement, and intravenous antibiotics. The more serious cases involving bone necrosis require surgical resection of the necrotic bone.

Femoral Vessel Rupture or Hemorrhage   Femoral vessel rupture with hemorrhage is a rare but serious complication of groin dissection. Groin wound breakdown is more common in patients undergoing more radical surgery, and when the groin breaks down, femoral vessels may be exposed, increasing the risk of vessel rupture, a potentially catastrophic event.[80] Rarely, femoral vessel rupture may result in perioperative death in patients with vulvar cancer.[22] One retrospective study suggested that sartorius muscle transposition may be associated with a decreased risk of this occurrence.[35] In patients with groin wound breakdown, rupture of a femoral vessel occurred on 4 occasions among 50 patients (9%) who did not have sartorius muscle transposition after inguinal-femoral lymphadenectomy. In 3 cases, there was rupture of the artery, and in

1 case, rupture of the vein. No femoral vessel rupture occurred in over 200 patients who underwent sartorius muscle transposition.[35] Some of the disadvantages of sartorius muscle transposition include an increase in operative time, risk of femoral nerve injury, and lower-extremity pain with associated limitation of mobility.

In an effort to evaluate the effectiveness of alternative surgical techniques to protect the femoral vessels after inguinal-femoral lymphadenectomy, authors have examined the use of dura mater grafts and artificial dura film to cover the femoral vessels.[81,82] The use of dura mater to cover the femoral vessels was examined in 20 patients who underwent inguinal-femoral lymphadenectomy. Among 38 groins, the 3 groin wounds that broke down healed satisfactorily without exposing the femoral vessels. The authors suggest that coverage of the femoral vessels with dura mater is a safe and effective alternative to sartorius muscle transposition.[81] In contrast, the use of artificial dura film to cover femoral vessels in 11 patients was associated with an inacceptable complication rate, with 9 of 11 patients experiencing infectious complications. In the 3 patients who suffered groin breakdown, removal of the dura film was necessary.[82] Sartorius muscle transposition or placement of dura mater to cover the femoral vessels may decrease the risk of femoral vessel rupture, but data are very limited and only Level III evidence is available. We recommend the use of sartorius muscle transposition in selective cases in patients at high risk for infectious morbidity after inguinal-femoral lymphadenectomy.

Thromboembolic/Arterial Occlusion Deep venous thrombosis and pulmonary embolism are major complications following gynecologic cancer surgery. Using ^{125}I fibrinogen leg counting to detect deep vein thrombi, studies have shown that 17% to 45% of patients develop thrombosis after surgery for gynecologic cancer.[83,84] In a retrospective review of 281 patients with early uterine or cervical cancer, Clarke-Pearson et al. found that clinically significant thromboemboli were encountered in 7.8% of patients postoperatively.[85] Approximately 1% to 2.5% of patients with a gynecologic malignancy will die from a postoperative pulmonary embolism.[85,86] Radical surgery for vulvar cancer appears to be a significant risk factor for the development of postoperative venous thrombosis. In a prospective analysis, authors examined variables associated with postoperative deep venous thrombosis in 411 patients undergoing gynecologic surgery using ^{125}I fibrinogen leg counting.[83] Seventy-two (17.5%) of the 411 patients developed ^{125}I fibrinogen evidence of postoperative deep venous thrombosis. Frequency of deep venous thrombosis was highest in patients undergoing radical vulvectomy with inguinal lymphadenectomy and pelvic exenteration, occurring in 32% and 88% of patients, respectively. Patients undergoing radiation therapy prior to surgery also appear to be at an increased risk of postoperative thromboembolic disease.[85]

Risk of postoperative thrombosis in gynecologic oncology patients is reduced by the use of intermittent pneumatic calf compression devices instituted in the operating room and continued for the first 5 postoperative days.[87] Low-dose perioperative heparin has also been shown to reduce the risk of thrombosis, but its use may increase the risk of bleeding and lymphocyst formation.[88,89] The patient must be followed closely for evidence of venous thrombosis throughout the postoperative recovery period. The routine use of intermittent pneumatic compression devices in patients undergoing surgery for vulvar cancer is recommended based on Level I evidence. The use of prophylactic heparin therapy should be considered on a case-by-case, acknowledging there may be some increased risk of perioperative complications.

Lower-extremity arterial occlusion after radical vulvar surgery is a rare but serious event.[90] Predisposing factors may be a prior history of thromboembolic disease and groin infection after surgery. Limited Level III evidence supports these observations. Following inguinal-femoral lymphadenectomy for vulvar cancer, the patient should be examined for presence of pulses or signs of arterial ischemia that may represent femoral artery thrombosis, particularly in the first 24 hours postoperatively.[91] Treatment consists of anticoagulation and sometimes vascular thrombectomy.

Lymphocyst   Formation of a lymphocyst in the groin is a potential complication of inguinal-femoral lymphadenectomy. A lymphocyst is a lymph-filled space without a distinct epithelial lining. Lymphocysts occur after inguinal-femoral lymphadenectomy in 2% to 28% of cases.[11,12,15,20,92] Piver et al. suggested that prophylactic mini-dose heparin may be associated with an increase in occurrence of inguinal lymphocysts after radical vulvectomy and inguinal lymphadenectomy, occurring in 43% of those receiving heparin versus 0% of those not receiving heparin.[89] Other factors that have been found to be associated with the development of pelvic lymphocysts, but whose association with inguinal lymphocysts has not been examined, include previous radiation therapy, lymph node metastases, and pregnancy.[93–97] The risk of lymphocyst formation does not appear to be related to the extent of the vulvar surgery.[37] Furthermore, sparing of the saphenous vein did not appear to affect the occurrence of lymphocyst formation.[38]

The formation of lymphocysts cannot always be avoided, even with meticulous surgical technique and optimal perioperative care. Modification of groin dissection with a three-incision technique compared with an en bloc procedure was not found to reduce this complication.[98] Inguinal drains placed at the time of surgery and compression dressings in the first 24 hours after surgery are thought to decrease the risk of lymphocyst formation. It has been suggested that added protection against lymphocyst formation is given by leaving the drain in place after discontinuing the suction, allowing it to be advanced slowly over several days.[91]

Inguinal lymphocysts can cause a significant amount of discomfort. The median time for their development has been reported to be 7.5 days after lymphadenectomy.[89] Although small lymphocysts usually resolve spontaneously, persistent large lymphocysts may contribute to thigh and leg edema, are prone to become infected, or cause necrosis of the overlying skin.[91] Thus, large and/or symptomatic lymphocysts should be treated. Information about the management of inguinal lymphocysts is scant compared with pelvic lymphocysts. The management of pelvic lymphocysts has involved percutaneous drainage, sclerotherapy, and if unsuccessful, laparotomy and marsupialization.[99–102] Most inguinal lymphocysts should be managed, at least initially, by drainage.[103] In most cases, daily aspiration of lymphocyst fluid may result in resolution, but there is a significant risk of infection. Anecdotal experience with insertion of a rubber drain for approximately 7 days and use of antibiotic therapy has successfully resulted in resolution of inguinal lymphocysts. If these methods are ineffective, sclerotherapy should be considered. Bleomycin sclerotherapy has been used to successfully manage inguinal lymphocysts.[104] The sclerosing action of antibiotics is thought to be secondary to induction of an inflammatory reaction. Although not reported for inguinal lymphocysts, Gilliland and colleagues have successfully used 10% povidone-iodine solution for sclerosis of pelvic lymphocysts.[105] It has also been suggested that absolute ethanol may be used as a sclerosing solution. Rarely, open drainage is necessary and will result in slow healing of groin lymphocysts.[91] The muscle paddle of a myocutaneous flap may be used to fill dead space after open drainage of a lymphocyst and will readily accept a skin graft.[106] These observations and recommendations are based on Level III evidence.

Delayed Complications

Lymphedema   Lymphedema is a common and particularly problematic long-term complication of groin dissection. Its frequency after inguinal-femoral lymphadenectomy generally varies from 7% to 19%.[10–13,15] Lymphedema occurs to some degree in almost every patient, commonly temporarily. Patients receiving radiation therapy to the groin in addition to surgical dissection are at an increased risk of lymphedema. In addition, concurrent pelvic node dissection, obesity, postoperative deep venous thrombosis, and varicosities increase the risk of lymphedema after groin dissection.[91] Some have suggested fitting the patient for knee-length antiedema stockings either before surgery or in the early postoperative period to decrease the occurrence of lymphedema, but there are no studies to document the efficacy of this practice.[91]

It has been suggested that preservation of the long saphenous vein decreases the risk of postoperative lymphedema, but there are no data to support the efficacy of this therapy. In a retrospective study of wound morbidity after inguinal-femoral lymphadenectomy through separate incisions, lymphedema occurred in 36% of patients who had preservation of the saphenous vein compared with 21% in whom the vessel was sacrificed.[38] Similarly, Lin et al., in a retrospective study of patients undergoing groin dissection, found that lymphedema occurred in 17% of patients who had preservation of the long saphenous vein versus 13% in whom the vein was sacrificed.[98] In the same study, the authors noted that omission of the deep femoral node dissection was not of significant benefit in reducing lower-extremity edema. Furthermore, they found that performance of an en bloc or three-incision technique did not affect the occurrence of lymphedema in patients undergoing groin dissection, occurring in 13% and 15% respectively.[98] The extent of vulvar surgery was not found to influence the risk of lymphedema,[37] and the incidence of lymphedema was not greater in patients developing groin necrosis, lymphocysts, or vulvar complications compared with those without complications.[37]

Available medical and surgical treatment of lymphedema is unsatisfactory. Management consists of elevation of legs, the use of thigh-high stockings, and in more severe cases, the use of mechanical stockings to compress the edema out of the lower extremities. The patient should be instructed to avoid standing still for any period of time and to avoid exposure to hot weather.[91] Prompt antibiotic treatment of cellulitis is important. Within approximately 2 years, collateral lymphatic pathways usually become established and there may be an improvement of lymphedema. Formation of these pathways may take a significantly longer period of time in radiated tissues. Surgical intervention may be necessary for complications of severe chronic lymphedema. These observations and recommendations are based on Level III evidence.

Hernia and Prolapse Hernia formation after radical vulvar surgery with inguinal-femoral lymphadenectomy may occur, which is usually perineal, vaginal, inguinal, or femoral. After completion of the inguinal node dissection, the external inguinal ring and the femoral canal should be examined for evidence of looseness and presence of a hernia sac. If the inguinal ring is not snug, it is tightened with permanent sutures, or for the femoral canal, sutures are placed between the inguinal ligament and the lacunar ligament to tighten the femoral canal. Care must be taken to avoid compromising the diameter of the femoral vein.[91] A rare but serious complication of a strangulated femoral hernia has been reported in a patient undergoing laparoscopic pelvic lymphadenectomy after groin node dissection.[80] It is possible that the increased abdominal pressure associated with insufflation of gas into the peritoneal cavity was a predisposing factor in this case.

Rectocele, cystocele, and uterine prolapse have been reported to complicate vulvectomy in 5% to 25% of patients.[107–109] Calame et al. found that 17% of 58 patients undergoing surgery for vulvar cancer developed some form of pelvic floor defect, with surgical repair required in most.[109] Magrina et al. examined complications in 225 patients with vulvar cancer undergoing radical versus modified radical surgery.[37] Cystocele and rectocele formation occurred in 16% and 12% of patients undergoing radical vulvar surgery compared with 2% and 1% of patients in the modified surgical group. Stress urinary incontinence occurred in 16% of patients in the radical surgery group compared with 8% of patients undergoing modified radical vulvar surgery. The authors suggest that radical extirpation of the labia and perineum, the advancement of the vaginal walls to effect closure, and the resulting tension of the vulvar wound may contribute to these occurrences.[37] These complications are typically late, but can appear within a few weeks of surgery or even in the immediate postoperative period. It has been suggested that they occur predominantly in patients with pre-existing pelvic floor defects and may be aggravated by tension on the vagina from the operative closure. One expert recommended that a perinorrhaphy be routinely performed after radical vulvectomy to reduce the risk of this occurrence, but the efficacy of this approach is unproven.[91] These observations are based on Level III evidence.

Urinary or Stool Incontinence   Excision of the distal portion of the urethra as part of radical excision of a vulvar cancer may result in stress or total incontinence.[107] As a general rule, up to 2 cm of the distal urethra can be resected without producing incontinence, and anecdotal experience suggests that more of the posterior wall of the urethra can be removed than the anterior wall. When the functional length of the urethra is inadequate or marginal, incontinence may be avoided by combining the meatal resection with plication of the urethra and bladder neck or by performing a retropubic bladder neck suspension.[91] Care must be taken with closure of skin surrounding the urethra, since the position of the urethra and urinary stream may be distorted. Leaving a small area of open tissue anterior to the urethra may minimize this occurrence.[91] When distortion of the urinary stream occurs, the patient may respond to urethral dilation postoperatively or surgical correction may be necessary. These observations are based on Level III evidence.

After partial or total excision of the anal sphincter, stool incontinence may occur and diverting colostomy may be necessary. For posterior vulvar lesions, in order to get a minimum 1 cm margin, shaving off the anterior portion of the anal sphincter may be required. This can usually be performed without producing anal incontinence. However, about 10% of women have a very thin perineal body, severely limiting the depth of resection that can be performed without damaging the integrity of the sphincter.[91] When necessary, the entire anterior quadrant of the external and sphincter and perineal body can be removed as a wedge without necessarily producing fecal incontinence, particularly when there is good levator tone. In such cases, the patient should be instructed to institute constipating measures postoperatively. Plication of the levator muscles may improve continence of stool, but incontinence of flatus will almost invariably occur. In some cases, surgical repair of the external sphincter can be performed with some symptomatic relief.[91] These observations are based on Level III evidence.

Radiation Necrosis and Fistula   Radionecrosis of the vulva is an uncommon event in the modern management of vulvar cancer because the disease is primarily treated surgically and because of improved radiation techniques. The vulvar skin is, however, notoriously less tolerant of radiation therapy than skin covering other areas of the body, and as a result, it is subject to an increase in complications. Reasons may include moisture, friction, nonflat surface, and a larger proportion of end arteries than in other areas of skin. Patients exposed to low-energy radiation therapy, an older technique that delivered most of the energy to the skin or slightly below the skin, were found to have a significant increased risk of radiation skin complications. In contrast, modern megavoltage radiotherapy is less commonly associated with radionecrosis of skin and the injury tends to be much deeper than that seen with low-energy radiation therapy. These are further discussed in the "Radiation Therapy" section.

Minor chronic radiation-induced injury to the skin is manifested by hyperpigmentation, dryness, telangiectasias, induration, decreased resilience, thinning of epidermis, and loss of normal adnexal structures.[110–112] The most serious chronic effects on skin and soft tissues are related to slowly progressive fibrosis and an obliterative vasculitis.[113] As a result, subcutaneous tissues become progressively ischemic and viability of overlying epithelium cannot be maintained.[110] Bacterial overgrowth in ischemic soft tissues may result in frank tissue necrosis.[110] The result is a radionecrotic wound and usually presents 6 to 18 months after completion of radiation, although a latent period of up to 20 years may occur.[113,114] Radionecrotic wounds demonstrate little ability to contract or epithelialize and may slowly increase in size as ischemia progresses and bacterial contamination continues.[114]

When radionecrosis involves the lower genital tract, the patient is commonly in severe pain and suffers from a foul discharge. Traditional initial conservative therapy consists of narcotic analgesics, antibiotics, load debridement, and intensive local care.[115] However, conservative therapy rarely leads to resolution of the radionecrosis. Such treatment was not associated with even partial healing in any of 12 patients with vaginal or vulvar radionecrosis.[116] Systemic antibiotics may be of limited value in the initial treatment of radionecrotic wounds because of poor tissue perfusion, but may be of greater value during definitive wound closure.

Treatment of chronic radionecrotic wounds begin with control of pain and correction of underlying systemic factors that may be contributing to poor wound healing, such as poor nutrition, diabetes, and smoking. Radical surgical excision of the radionecrotic wound is usually necessary. When surgical debridement is undertaken, all necrotic tissue should be removed down to a bleeding base.[110,111] If bone is infected and exposed within the wound, removal of either the outer cortex or entire bone may be necessary.[106,117] In the chronic wound that is poorly drained, grossly infected, or very large, staged surgical excision may be necessary.[118] In such cases, superficial debridement of necrotic material to promote wound drainage should be performed initially. Recurrent cancer should be excluded by performing biopsies of nonnecrotic tissue at the edge of the ulcer. Depending on the site of the radionecrotic lesion, urinary or fecal diversion may be required. In some cases, necrosis may progress to form a fistula.

Definitive closure of the radionecrotic wound should usually be performed immediately after excision. Delaying closure until there is adequate growth of granulation tissue over the wound base usually fails, since capillary or fibroblastic proliferation does not normally occur in the radiation-damaged tissue. The result is continued ischemia and bacterial regrowth, which leads to further wound breakdown.[110] Radiated tissues are not pliable and will not tolerate even very minimal tension on the wound or disruption will occur.[114] In rare cases, primary closure may be appropriate, but usually well-vascularized tissue must be used and brought in to close the ischemic defects.[119] Simple skin grafting is commonly inadequate for coverage of the wound, since soft tissues may have a poor blood supply. Split-thickness skin grafting for radiation ulcer treatment had a 100% complication rate in nine cases, defined as the need for further surgery. The complication rate for local full-thickness flaps was similarly very high.[119] As a result, myocutaneous flaps are usually necessary.

Techniques of wound coverage of the vulva are similar to those discussed in the section on "Vulvar Reconstruction." In general, they include random-pattern skin flaps, myocutaneous flaps, or free flaps. Complete excision of radiation-damaged tissue so that a myocutaneous flap can be sewn into normal tissue both on the underside and at the periphery must be emphasized.[119] Complications of healing, even with a myocutaneous flap, may occur, because after excision of the ulcer the radiated bed may accept the myocutaneous flap poorly. These observations and recommendations concerning the radionecrotic wound are based on Level III evidence.

Pentoxifylline is a drug that has been used anecdotally to improve healing of radionecrotic wounds. Pentoxifylline is a methylxanthine derivative that produces dose-related hemorrheologic effects, lowers blood viscosity, improves erythrocyte flexibility, and increases tissue oxygenation. Twenty-six patients with late radiation complications of the head and neck were treated with oral pentoxifylline. Nine of 12 patients with soft tissue necrosis completely healed. Five patients with mucosal pain had resolution of their symptoms. Radiation fibrosis improved in 67% of patients.[120] In another series, 12 patients with 15 sites of late-radiation necrosis of soft tissues were treated with pentoxifylline. Thirteen of 15 (87%) of the necroses had healed completely, and 1 was partially healed. Furthermore, the time course of healing was significantly less than the duration of nonhealing prior to pentoxifylline: 9 weeks versus 30 weeks on average.[121] These anecdotal data suggest that pentoxifylline may accelerate healing of radiation-associated soft tissue necrosis and reverse some late radiation injuries. Since the risks associated with administration of the drug are minimal, its use in patients with radionecrotic wounds should be considered despite the lack of randomized prospective evidence supporting its efficacy.

The use of hyperbaric oxygen has been studied with some anecdotal success in treatment of radionecrosis of some head and neck radionecrotic wounds.[122,123] The experience of using hyperbaric oxygen for radionecrotic wounds at other locations has been more limited.[116,124] As a result, its use in radionecrotic wounds of the vulva cannot be recommended outside of a research study.

VULVAR RECONSTRUCTION

Despite the more conservative surgical approach to vulvar cancer that is common practice today, there are still cases where primary closure of the skin may not be possible. This is more commonly problematic with a large lesion or one in an unfavorable location for closure. In some cases, although closure may be technically feasible, risk of breakdown may be unacceptably high because of tension on the suture line, or scarring and disfigurement of the vulva may be excessive. In such cases, reconstruction of the vulva should be performed using local tissues such as skin flaps, or myocutaneous flaps, usually at the time of the original surgery.

The random-pattern skin flap is relatively simple and useful for closure of a wound that is not too large. These flaps are at risk for ischemia, since they lack an anatomically identifiable vascular pedicle and rely on a dermal-subdermal vascular plexus between skin and fascia. Their marginal vascular supply requires that these flaps be short, with a maximum length-to-width ratio of 2 : 1, or flap necrosis will occur.[106,118] In addition, they should be avoided in the irradiated patient, since the proximity of the flap donor site to the wound makes radiation damage likely within the flap itself.[106,114]

Local advancement flaps such as the rhomboid flap may be used to cover a vulvar wound that otherwise would be closed under significant tension. The flap derives its blood supply from the underlying subcutaneous vascular network. The flap must maintain a 1.0–1.5 cm layer of attached subcutaneous tissue. Unilateral or bilateral flaps may be used. Burke et al. described the use of rhomboid flaps in 13 patients who underwent extensive vulvar resections.[125] Two of 13 had minor wound disruptions and there were no other early or delayed complications. With this technique, approximately 15% to 20% of patients may have minor separation of wounds, with rare cases of major wound disruption (<5%).[126,127] Others have used the Z-plasty full-thickness pedicle flap for similar indications. Close attention to the design of the flap is necessary, since the base of the flap should be twice as long as the length of the flap to ensure adequate blood supply to the distal flap.[91]

The axial-pattern skin flap is formed by a longitudinally oriented vascular pedicle traveling superficially to the deep fascia.[106,128] Adding a random flap to the end of an axial flap results in an improved blood supply that allows for a significant increase in the length : width ratio of the flap of up to 4 : 1.[118] One example of an axial flap is the groin flap, based on the superficial circumflex iliac artery.[128] Unfortunately, its vascular pedicle is frequently ligated during the course of genitourinary surgery, limiting its usefulness in vulvar reconstruction.[106]

Mayer et al. described the use of bilateral axial pedicle skin flaps based on the superficial external pudendal artery to successfully close a vulvar defect.[129] Skin-fascial flaps such as the gluteal thigh flap provide another option for wound coverage and are formed by large paddles of skin and deep fascia supplied by vascular pedicles that branch from major extremity or truncal vessels.[106,130] This flap is useful for closure of perineal and sacral defects.

Myocutaneous flaps are based on the vascular pedicle of a major muscle that is elevated and transposed together with its overlying skin paddle to an adjacent site.[131–135] Depending on the size of the defect, its location, and prior radiation history, this may be the technique of choice to close vulvar or groin wounds. Because of its excellent blood supply from an anatomically distinct vascular pedicle, this type of flap tends to be more resistant to infection and quite durable. Myocutaneous flaps may be either transposition flaps or free flaps. Muscle-perforating vessels allow survival of the skin that is transferred with the muscle.[136] Variations of the myocutaneous flap include creation of a muscle flap by deletion of the skin island.

Selection of the myocutaneous flap is based on its reliability, location to the defect, potential disability from donor muscle loss, and other anatomic factors.[136] The gracilis muscle flap is commonly used for repair of wounds of the perineum and groin.[137] It is supplied by the medial circumflex branch of the profunda femoris artery, and the flap may be rotated medially and superiorly. The skin island is raised from the proximal or middle thigh. Since the adductor longus and magnus muscles remain intact, there is no functional impairment in the leg.[106] The rectus abdominus muscle is a very versatile flap with a dual blood supply from both the superior and inferior epigastric arteries, and as a result, it may be transposed in either direction. Its skin island may be harvested in a transverse or longitudinal orientation, and when used to cover vulvar or groin defects, it is based on the deep inferior epigastric artery.[91,135,138–141] Many surgeons' experience with the rectus abdominus flap has been more favorable than with the gracilis myocutaneous flap. The flap is more reliable and provides quality surface restoration and revascularization of the wound.

The rectus femoris muscle, supplied primarily by the descending branch of the lateral circumflex femoral artery, can be used for groin wounds with little or no loss of function in the ipsilateral leg.[106] Other myocutaneous flaps include the gluteus maximus flap, best suited for covering defects in the posterior vulva and perineum, and the tensor fascia lata muscle flap, used primarily for covering a predominantly anterior defect.[91] A free pedicle flap allows for closure of a wound distant from the flap donor site through microvascular reanastomosis of its vascular pedicle to vessels in proximity to the recipient wound.[142] This is rarely performed for closure of vulvar wounds, since local myocutaneous flaps tend to be readily available.

RADIATION THERAPY

Traditionally, radiation therapy has been considered to have a limited role in the primary management of vulvar cancer. Radiation techniques used in the past were associated with poor survival and severe acute skin reactions were common. Vulva and perineal tissues were thought to be intolerant of radiation therapy. With the introduction of megavoltage external-beam equipment, and the judicious use of electrons or interstitial brachytherapy, there has been an overall improvement in vulvar tissue tolerance to radiation therapy. As a result, radiation therapy is used more commonly to treat vulvar cancer.[143–145]

Even with modern radiation techniques, interruption of radiation therapy to the vulva is often necessary in the third or fourth week to relieve symptoms of severe moist desquamation of the perineal region. In addition, delay of therapy is common due to symptoms of cystitis or proctitis.[146] Overall, radiation therapy should be used selectively for vulvar cancer because of complications of radiation fibrosis, lymphedema, skin ulceration, and other severe morbidity.

Radiation therapy plays a role in treatment of patients with vulvar cancer in a variety of ways: (1) to decrease locoregional failures after surgery in patients undergoing radical local excision and bilateral inguinal-femoral lymphadenectomy with close surgical margins or involved inguinal lymph nodes: (2) to serve as an alternative to inguinal or pelvic lymph node dissection in patients with clinically negative nodes; (3) to reduce the extent of surgery required in patients with Stage III and IV disease (e.g., a lesion that extends to vital structures such as the anus, rectum, proximal urethra, or bladder; (4) to treat patients before surgery for locally extensive tumors that may be considered inoperable initially (e.g., fixed groin nodes); and (5) to treat recurrent disease.[146,147] In patients receiving preoperative radiation therapy, less radical surgery may be performed to resect the disease or unresectable nodes may be rendered resectable. In patients with recurrent vulvar cancer, radiation therapy has been used with limited success.[148-150] Treatment-related morbidity may be significant, including rectovaginal fistula; proctitis; rectal stricture; bone, vaginal, or skin necroses; and groin abscess.[146]

The use of chemotherapy synchronous with radiation therapy to treat locally advanced vulvar cancer has stemmed from its success in patients with locally advanced anal and head and neck cancers. Concurrent radiation therapy and chemotherapy for carcinoma of the anus yields an 80% complete response rate and 75% cure rate for lesions less than 8 cm in diameter, results similar to those obtained with surgery, but with preservation of a functional anus.[151] These excellent preliminary results have led investigators to utilize this technique for locally advanced vulvar cancer to improve treatment outcome and reduce need for ultraradical surgery.[152-154]

Leiserowitz et al. studied the use of chemoradiation therapy in 23 patients with locally advanced squamous cell carcinoma of the vulva with clinically uninvolved groin nodes. Subsequent groin surgery was not performed. No patient failed in the groin and there were no cases of lymphedema, vascular insufficiency or neurological injury, or aseptic necrosis of the femur.[155] Moore et al. reported preliminary results of a Phase II prospective GOG study of preoperative chemoradiation for advanced vulvar cancer.[22] Seventy-three patients with T3 or T4 primary tumors were treated with concurrent cisplatin/5-fluorouracil and radiation therapy followed by surgical excision of the residual primary tumor plus inguinal-femoral lymph node dissection. At the time of surgery, 33 of 71 (46.5%) patients had no visible vulvar cancer. For patients with residual cancer, complete resection was almost always possible, except in 2.8% of patients. Toxicity was acceptable.[22] This and other studies suggest that preoperative chemoradiotherapy in advanced squamous cell carcinoma of the vulva is feasible and may reduce the need for more radical surgery, including pelvic exenteration. The use of this technique is recommended based on Level II and III evidence.

REFERENCES

1. Taussig FJ. Cancer of the vulva: an analysis of 155 cases (1911–1940). *Am J Obstet Gynecol* 1940;40:764.

2. Way S. The anatomy of the lymphatic drainage of the vulva and its influence on the radical operation for carcinoma. *Ann R Coll Surg. Engl* 1948;3:187.

3. Morley GW. Infiltrative carcinoma of the vulva: results of surgical treatment. *Am J Obstet Gynecol* 1976;124:874.

4. Podratz KC, Symmonds RE, Taylor WF, Williams TJ. Carcinoma of the vulva: analysis of treatment and survival. *Obstet Gynecol* 1983;61:63–74.

5. Homesley HD, Bundy BN, Sedlis A, et al. Assessment of current International Federation of Gynecology and Obstetrics staging of vulvar carcinoma relative to prognostic factors for survival (a Gynecologic Oncology Group study). *Am J Obstet Gynecol* 1991;164:998–1004.

6. Aalders JG, Christensen H, Kolstad P. Squamous cell carcinoma of the vulva: a review of 424 patients, 1956–1974. *Gynecol Oncol* 1980;9:271–279.

7. Ballon SC, Lamb EJ. Separate incisions in the treatment of carcinoma of the vulva. *Surg Gynecol Obstet* 1975;140:81–84.

8. Flannelly GM, Foley ME, Lenehan PM, Kelehan P, Murphy JF, Stronge J. En bloc radical vulvectomy and lymphadenectomy with modifications of separate groin incisions. *Obstet Gynecol* 1992;79:307–309.

9. Hacker NF, Leuchter RS, Berek JS, Castaldo TW, Lagasse LD. Radical vulvectomy and bilateral inguinal lymphadenectomy through separate groin incisions. *Obstet Gynecol* 1981;58:574–579.

10. Cavanagh D, Fiorica JV, Hoffman MS, Roberts WS, Bryson SCP, LaPolla JP, Barton DPJ. Invasive carcinoma of the vulva. Changing trends in surgical management. *Am J Obstet Gynecol* 1990;163:1007–1015.

11. Hopkins MP, Reid GC, Morley GW. Radical vulvectomy—the decision for the incision. *Cancer* 1993;72:799–803.

12. Sutton GP, Miser MR, Stehman FB, Look KY, Ehrlich CE. Trends in the operative management of invasive squamous carcinoma of the vulva at Indiana University, 1974–1988. *Am J Obstet Gynecol* 1991;164:1472–1481.

13. Stehman FB, Bundy BN, Dvoretsky PM, Creasman WT. Early Stage I carcinoma of the vulva treated with ipsilateral inguinal lymphadenectomy and modified radical hemivulvectomy: a prospective study of the Gynecology Oncology Group. *Obstet Gynecol* 1992;79:490–497.

14. Heaps JM, Fu YS, Montz FJ, Hacker NF, Berek JS. Surgical-pathologic variables predictive of local recurrence in squamous cell carcinoma of the vulva. *Gynecol Oncol* 1990;38:309–314.

15. Burke TW, Stringer CA, Gershenson DM, Edwards CL, Morris M, Wharton JT. Radical wide excision and selective inguinal node dissection for squamous cell carcinoma of the vulva. *Gynecol Oncol* 1990;38:328–332.

16. Hacker NF, Nieberg RK, Berek JS, et al. Superficially invasive vulvar cancer with nodal metastases. *Gynecol Oncol* 1983;15:65–77.

17. Hacker NF, Berek JS, Lagasse LD, Nieberg RK, Leuchter RS. Individualization of treatment for stage I squamous cell vulvar carcinoma. *Obstet Gynecol* 1984;63:155–162.

18. Hacker NF, Berek JS, Lagasse LD, Leuchter RS, Moore JG. Management of regional lymph nodes and their prognostic influence in vulvar cancer. *Obstet Gynecol* 1983;61:408–412.

19. Krupp PJ, Bohm JW. Lymph gland metastases in invasive squamous cell cancer of the vulva. *Am J Obstet Gynecol* 1978;130:943.

20. Figge DC, Gaudenz R. Invasive carcinoma of the vulva. *Am J Obstet Gynecol* 1974;119:382.

21. Morris JM. A formula for selective lymphadenectomy. *Obstet Gynecol* 1977;50:152.

22. Moore DH, Thomas GM, Montana GS, Saxer A, Gallup DG, Olt G. Preoperative chemoradiation for advanced vulvar cancer: a phase II study of the Gynecologic Oncology Group. *Int J Rad Oncol Biol Phys* 1988;42:79–85.

23. Kelemen PR, VanHerle AJ, Giuliano AE. Sentinel lymphadenectomy in thyroid malignant neoplasms. *Arch Surg* 1998;133:288–292.

24. Stadelmann WK, Javaheri S, Cruse CW, Reintgen DS. The use of selective lymphadenectomy in squamous cell carcinoma of the wrist: a case report. *J Hand Surg* 1997;22:726–731.

25. Cox CE, Haddad F, Bass S, Cox JM, Ku NN, Berman C, Shons AR, Yeatman T, Pendas S, Reintgen DS. Lymphatic mapping in the treatment of breast cancer. *Oncology* 1998;12:1283–1298.

26. Leong SP, Steinmetz I, Habib FA, McMillan A, Gans JZ, Allen RE, Moritz ET, el-Kadi M, Epstein HD, Kashani-Sabet M, Sagebiel RW. Optimal selection sentinel lymph node dissection in primary malignant melanoma. *Arch Surg* 1997;132:666–672.

27. Flett MM, Going JJ, Stanton PD, Cooke TG. Sentinel node localization in patients with breast cancer. *Brit J Surg* 1998;85:991–993.

28. O'Hea BJ, Hill AD, El-Shirbiny AM, Yeh SD, Rosen PP, Coit DG, Borgen PI, Cody HS. Sentinel lymph node biopsy in breast cancer: initial experience at Memorial Sloan-Kettering Cancer Center. *J Am Coll Surg* 1998;186:423–427.

29. Gershenwald JE, Tseng C-H, Thompson W, Mansfield PF, Lee JE, Bouvet M, Lee JJ, Ross MI. Improved sentinel lymph node localization in patients with primray melanoma with the use of radiolabeled colloid. *Surgery* 1998;124:203–210.

30. Cox CE, Pendas S, Cox JM, Joseph E, Shons AR, Yeatman T, Ku NN, Lyman GH, Berman C, Haddad F, Reintgen DS. Guidelines for sentinel node biopsy and lymphatic mapping of patients with breast cancer. *Ann Surg* 1998;227:645–651.

31. Giuliano AE, Jones RC, Brennan M, Statman R. Sentinel lymphadenectomy in breast cancer. *J Clin Oncol* 1997;15:2345–2350.

32. Levenback C, Burke TW, Morris M, Malpica A, Lucas KR, Gershenson DM. Potential applications of intraoperative lymphatic mapping in vulvar cancer. *Gynecol Oncol* 1995;59:216–220.

33. DeCesare SL, Fiorica JV, Roberts WS, Reintgen D, Arango H, Hoffman MS,

Puleo C, Cavanagh D. A pilot study utilizing intraoperative lymphscintigraphy for identification of the sentinel lymph nodes in vulvar cancer. *Gynecol Oncol* 1997;66:425–428.

34. Terada KY, Coel MN, Ko P, Wong JH. Combined use of intraoperative lymphatic mapping and lymphscintigraphy in the management of squamous cell cancer of the vulva. *Gynecol Oncol* 1998;70:65–69.

35. Cavanagh D, Roberts WS, Bryson SCP, Marsden DE, Ingram JM, Anderson WR. Changing trends in the surgical treatment of invasive carcinoma of the vulva. *Surg Gynecol Obstet* 1986;162:164–168.

36. Reedy MB, Capen CV, Baker DP, Petersen WG, Kuehl TJ. Hyperbaric oxygen therapy following radical vulvectomy: an adjunctive therapy to improve wound healing. *Gynecol Oncol* 1994;53:13–16.

37. Magrina JF, Gonzalez-Bosquet J, Weaver AL, Gaffey TA, Webb MJ, Podratz KC, Cornella JL. Primary squamous cell cancer of the vulva: radical versus modified radical vulvar surgery. *Gynecol Oncol* 1998;71:116–121.

38. Paley PJ, Johnson PR, Adcock LL, Cosin JA, Chem MD, Fowler JM, Twiggs LB, Carson LF. The effect of sartorius transposition on wound morbidity following inguinal-femoral lymphadenectomy. *Gynecol Oncol* 1997;64;237–141.

39. Gomes MN, Spear SL. Pedicled muscle flaps in the management of infected aortofemoral grafts. *Cardiovasc Surg* 1994;2:70–77.

40. Perez-Burkhardt JL, Gonzalez-Fajardo JA, Carpintero LA, Mateo AM. Sartorius myoplasty for the treatment of infected groins with vascular grafts. *J Cardiovasc Surg* 1995;36:581–585.

41. Cohen IK, Diegelman RF, Lindblad WJ. *Wound Healing–Biochemical and Clinical Aspects.* Philadelphia: WB Saunders, 1992.

42. Forrest L. Current concepts in soft tissue connective tissue wound healing. *Br J Surg* 1983;70:133–140.

43. Nemeth AJ. *Wound Healing. Dematologic Clinics.* Philadelphia: WB Saunders, 1993.

44. Thomson PD, Smith DJ. What is infection? *Am J Surg* 1994;167:7S–11S.

45. Peacock EE. *Wound Repair*, 3rd ed. Philadelphia: WB Saunders, 1984, p. 128.

46. Duncan HJ, Faris IB. Skin vascular resistance and skin perfusion pressure as predictors of healing of ischemic lesions of the lower limb: influences of diabetes mellitus, hypertension, and age. *Surgery* 1986;99:432.

47. Robertson HD, Polk HC. The mechanism of infection in patients with diabetes mellitus: a review of leukocyte malfunction. *Surgery* 1974;75:123.

48. Yue DK, McLennan S, Marsh M, et al. Effects of experimental diabetes, uremia, and malnutrition on wound healing. *Diabetes* 1987;36:295.

49. Müller JM, Brenner U, Dienst C, et al. Preoperative parenteral feeding in patients with gastrointestinal carcinoma. *Lancet* 1982;1:68.

50. Klein S, Simes J, Blackburn GL. Total parenteral nutrition and cancer clinical trails. *Cancer* 1986;58:1378.

51. Eaglstein WH. Wound healing and aging. *Clin Geriatr Med* 1989;5:183.

52. Sherwin MA, Gastwirth CM. Detrimental effects of cigarette smoking on lower extremity wound healing. *J Foot Surg* 1990;29:84–87.

53. Wolbach SB. Summary of the effects of repeated roentgen ray exposure upon human skin, antecendent to the formation of carcinoma. *Am J Roentgenol* 1925;13:139–143.

54. Mustoe TA, Porras-Reyes BH. Modulation of wound healing response in chronic irradiated tissues. *Clin Plast Surg* 1993;20:466–472.

55. Bailey AJ, Tromans WJ. Effects of ionizing radiation on the ultrastructure of collagen fibrils. *Radiat Res* 1964;23:145.

56. Grant RA, Cox RW, Kent CM. The effects of gamma radiation on the structure of native and cross-linked collagen fibers. *J Anat* 1973;115:29.

57. Levenson SM, Gruber CA, Returra G, et al. Supplemental vitamin A prevents the acute radiation-induced defect in wound healing. *Ann Surg* 1984;200:494.

58. Ahrenholz DH. Surgical spectrum. Clinical skin and soft tissue infection. *Physicians World Communications [Monograph]*, West Point, PA: Merke Sharpe, and Dohme, 1988, pp. 16–24.

59. Baxter CR. Surgical management of soft tissue infections. *Surg Clin N Am* 1972;52:1483.

60. Dellinger EP. Severe necrotizing soft-tissue infections. *JAMA* 1981;246:15–17.

61. Kaiser RE, Cerra FB. Progressive necrotizing surgical infections—a unified approach. *J Trauma* 1981;21:349.

62. Bakker DJ. Clostridial myonecrosis. In Davis JC, Hunt TK (Eds), *Problem Wounds. The Role of Oxygen.* New York: Elsevier, 1988, p. 153.

63. Baskin LS, Carroll PR, Cottolica EV, et al. Necrotizing soft tissue infections of the perineum and genitalia: bacteriology, treatment, and risk assessment. *Br J Urol* 1990;65:524.

64. Sutherland ME, Meyer AA. Necrotizing soft-tissue infections. *Surg Clin N Am* 1994;74:591–606.

65. Stamenkovic I, Lew PD. Early recognition of potentially fatal necrotizing fasciitis. The use of frozen-section biopsy. *New Engl J Med* 1984;310:1689–1693.

66. Wilson B. Necrotizing fasciitis. *Am Surg* 1970;172:957.

67. Pessa ME, Howard RJ. Necrotizing fasciitis. *Surg Gynecol Obstet* 1985;161:357–361.

68. McHenry CR, Piotrowski JJ, Petrinic D, Malangoni MA. Determinants of mortality of necrotizing soft-tissue infections. *Ann Surg* 1995;221:558–563.

69. Grim PS, Gottlieb LJ, Boddie A, et al. Hyberbaric oxygen therapy. *JAMA* 1990;263:2216.

70. Riseman JA, Zamboni WA, Curtis A, Graham DR, Konrad HR, Ross DS. Hyperbaric oxygen therapy for necrotizing fasciitis reduces mortality and the need for debridements. *Surgery* 1990;108:847–850.

71. Rudge FW. The role of hyperbaric oxygenation in the treatment of clostridial myonecrosis. *Military Med* 1993;158:80–83.

72. Forman HJ, Thomas MJ. Oxidant production and bactericidal activity of phagocytes. *Annu Rev Physiol* 1986;48:669.

73. Nylander G, Lewis D, Nordstrom H, et al. Reduction of postischemic edema with hyperbaric oxygen. *Plast Reconstr Surg* 1985;76:596.

74. Knighton DR, Silver JA, Hunt TK. Regulation of wound healing angiogen-

esis; effect of oxygen gradients and improved oxygen concentration. *Surgery* 1981;89:262.

75. Hill GB, Osterhout S. Experimental effects of hyperbaric oxygen on selected clostridial species: II: In vivo studies in mice. *J Infect Dis* 1972;125:26.

76. Holland JA, Hill GB, Wolfe WG, et al. Experimental and clinical experience with hyperbaric oxygen in the treatment of clostridial myonecrosis. *Surgery* 1975;77:75.

77. Jackson RW, Waddell JP. Hyperbaric oxygen in the management of clostridial myonecrosis (gas gangrene). *Clin Orthop* 1973;96:271–276.

78. Love TL, Schnure JJ, Lankin EC, Lipman RL, Lecocq FR. Glucose intolerance in man during prolonged exposure to a hyperbaric-hyperoxic environment. *Diabetes* 1975;20:282–285.

79. Hoyme UB, Tamimi HK, Eschenbach DA, Ramsey PG, Figge DC. Osteomyelitis pubis after radical gynecologic operations. *Obstet Gynecol* 1984;63:47S–51S.

80. Magrina JF, Tahery MM, Heppell J, Cornella JL. Femoral hernia: a complication of laparoscopic pelvic lymphadenectomy after groin node dissection. *J Laparoendosc Adv Surg Tech* 1997;7:191–193.

81. Fiorica JV, Roberts WS, LaPolla JP, Hoffman MS, Barton DPJ, Cavanagh D. Femoral vessel coverage with dura mater after inguino femoral lymphadenectomy. *Gynecol Oncol* 1991;42:217–221.

82. Finan MA, Fiorica JV, Roberts WS, Hoffman MS, Gleeson N, Barton DPJ, Cavanagh D. Artificial dura film for femoral vessel coverage after inguinal femoral lymphadenectomy. *Gynecol Oncol* 1994;55:333–335.

83. Clarke-Pearson DL, DeLong ER, Synan IS, Coleman RE, Creasman WT. Variables associated with postoperative deep venous thrombosis: a prospective study of 411 gynecology patients and creation of a prognostic model. *Obstet Gynecol* 1987;69:146–150.

84. Crandon AJ, Koutts J. Incidence of postoperative deep vein thrombosis in gynecologic oncology. *Aust NZ J Obstet Gynecol* 1983;23:216–219.

85. Clarke-Pearson DL, Jelovsek FR, Creasman WT. Thromboembolism complicating surgery for cervical and uterine malignancy: incidence, risk factors, and prophylaxis. *Obstet Gynecol* 1983;61:87–94.

86. Jones HW III. Treatment of adenocarcinoma of the endometrium. *Obstet Gynecol Surv* 1975;30:147–169.

87. Clarke-Pearson DL, Synan IS, Hinshaw WM, Coleman RE, Creasman WT. Prevention of postoperative venous thromboembolism by external pneumatic calf compression in patients with gynecologic malignancy. *Obstet Gynecol* 1984;63:92–98.

88. Clarke-Pearson DL, Synan IS, Dodge R, Soper JT, Berchuck A, Coleman RE. A randomized trial of low-dose heparin and intermittent pneumatic calf compression for the prevention of deep venous thrombosis after gynecologic oncology surgery. *Am J Obstet Gynecol* 1993;168:1146–1154.

89. Piver MS, Malfetano JH, Lele SB, Moore RH. Prophylactic anticoagulation as a possible cause of inguinal lymphocyst after radical vulvectomy and inguinal lymphadenectomy. *Obstet Gynecol* 1983;62:17–21.

90. Levenback C, Burke TW, Rubin SC, Curtin JP, Wharton JT. Arterial occlu-

sion complicating treatment of gynecologic cancer: a case series. *Gynecol Oncol* 1996;63:40–46.

91. Morrow CP, Curtin JP (Eds). *Gynecologic Cancer Surgery.* New York: Churchill Livingstone, 1996, pp. 329–377, 381–450.

92. Rutledge F, Smith JP, Franklin EW. Carcinoma of the vulva. *Am J Obstet Gynecol* 1973;106:1117–1130.

93. Dodd GD, Rutledge F, Wallace S. Postoperative pelvic lymphocyst. *Am J Roentgenol* 1970;108:312–323.

94. Mori N. Clinical and experimental studies on so-called lymphocyst which develops after radical hysterectomy in cancer of uterine cervix. *J Jpn Obstet Gynecol Soc* 1955;2:178–182.

95. Gray MJ, Plentl AA, Taylor HC. The lymphocyst: a complication of pelvic lymph node dissection. *Am J Obstet Gynecol* 1958;75:1059–1062.

96. Rutledge F, Dodd GD, Kasilag FB. Lymphocyst, a complication of radical pelvic surgery. *Am J Obstet Gynecol* 1959;77:1165–1175.

97. Ferguson JH, Maclure JG. Lymphocele following lymphadenectomy. *Am J Obstet Gynecol* 1961;82:783–791.

98. Lin JY, DuBeshter B, Angel C, Dvoretsky PM. Morbidity and recurrence with modifications of radical vulvectomy and groin dissection. *Gynecol Oncol* 1992;47:80–86.

99. Mann W, Vogel F, Patsuer B, Chalas E. Management of lymphocysts after radical gynecologic surgery. *Gynecol Oncol* 1987;33:248–250.

100. Choo YC, Wong LC, Wong KP, Ma HK. The management of intractable lymphocyst following radical hysterectomy. *Gynecol Oncol* 1986;24:309–317.

101. Conte M, Panic PB, Guariglia L, Scambia G, Greggi S, Mancuso S. Pelvic lymphocele following radical paraaortic and pelvic lymphadenectomy for cervical carcinoma: incidence, rate and percutaneous management. *Obstet Gynecol* 1990;76:268–271.

102. Ostrowski MJ. Intracavitary therapy with bleomycin for the treatment of malignant pleural effusion. *J Surg Oncol Suppl* 1989;1:7–13.

103. Daly JW, Pomerance AJ. Groin dissection with prevention of tissue loss and postoperative infection. *Obstet Gynecol* 1979;53:395–398.

104. Khorran O, Stern JL. Bleomycin sclerotherapy of an intractable inguinal lymphocyst. *Gynecol Oncol* 1993;50:244–246.

105. Gilliland JD, Spies JB, Brown SB, et al. Lymphoceles: percutaneous treatment with povidone-iodine sclerosis. *Radiology* 1989;171:227.

106. Mathes SJ, Hurwitz DJ. Repair of chronic radiation wounds of the pelvis. *World J Surg* 1986;10:269–280.

107. Reid GC, DeLancey JO, Hopkins MP, Roberts JA, Morley GW. Urinary incontinence following radical vulvectomy. *Obstet Gynecol* 1990;75:852–858.

108. Ansink AC, vanTinteren M, Artsen EJ, Heinz AP. Outcome, complications and follow-up in surgically treated squamous cell carcinoma of the vulva 1956–1982. *Eur J Obstet Gynecol Reprod Biol* 1991;42:137.

109. Calame RJ. Pelvic relaxation as a complication of the radical vulvectomy. *Obstet Gynecol* 1980;55:716.

110. Luce EA. The irradiated wound. *Surg Clin N Am* 1984;64:821–829.

111. Robinson DW. Surgical problems in the excision and repair of radiated tissue. *Plast Reconstr Surg* 1975;55:41–49.

112. Cox JD, Byhardt RW, Wilson JF, et al. Complications of radiation therapy and factors in their prevention. *World J Surg* 1986;10:171–188.

113. Kinsella TJ, Bloomer WD. New therapeutic strategies in radiation therapy. *JAMA* 1981;245:1669–1674.

114. Reinish JF, Pucket CL. Management of radiation wounds. *Surg Clin N Am* 1984;64:795–802.

115. Williams JA Jr, Clarke D, Dennis WA, Dennis EJ, Smith ST. The treatment of pelvic soft tissue radiation necrosis with hyperbaric oxygen. *Am J Obstet Gynecol* 1992;167:412–416.

116. Roberts WS, Hoffman MS, LaPolla JP, Ruas E, Fiorica JV, Cavanagh D. Management of radionecrosis of the vulva and distal vagina. *Am J Obstet Gynecol* 1991;164:1235–1238.

117. Arnold PG, Pairolero PC. Surgical management of the radiated chest wall. *Plast Reconstr Surg* 1986;77:605–612.

118. Lynch DJ, Whitte RR IV. Management of the chronic radiation wound. *Surg Clin N Am* 1982;62:309–319.

119. Rudolph R. Complications of surgery for radiotherapy skin damage. *Plast Reconstr Surg* 1982;70:179–183.

120. Futran ND, Trotti A, Gwede C. Pentoxifylline in the treatment of radiation-related soft tissue injury: preliminary observations. *Laryngoscope* 1997;107:391–395.

121. Dion MW, Hussey DH, Doornbos JF, Vigliotti AP, Wen BC, Anderson B. Preliminary results of a pilot study of pentoxifylline in the treatment of late radiation soft tissue necrosis. *Int J Radiat Oncol Biol Phys* 1990;19:401–407.

122. Mainous EG, Hart GB. Osteoradionecrosis of the mandible: treatment with hyperbaric oxygen. *Arch Otolaryngol* 1975;101:173–177.

123. Farmer JC, Shelton DL, Angelillo, et al. Treatment of radiation-induced tissue injury by hyperbaric oxygen. *Ann Otol Rhinol Laryngol* 1978;87:707–715.

124. Shupak A, Shoshani O, Goldenberg I, Barzilai A, Moskuna R, Bursztein S. Necrotizing fasciitis: An indication for hyperbaric oxygenation therapy? *Surgery* 1995;118:873–878.

125. Burke TW, Morris M, Levenback C, Gershenson DM, Wharton JT. Closure of complex vulvar defects using local rhomboid flaps. *Obstet Gynecol* 1994;84:1043–1047.

126. Barnhill DR, Hoskins WJ, Metz P. Use of the rhomboid flap after partial vulvectomy. *Obstet Gynecol* 1983;62:444–447.

127. Helm CW, Hatch KD, Partridge EE, Shingleton HM. The rhomboid flap for repair of the perineal defect after radical vulvar surgery. *Gynecol Oncol* 1993;50:164–167.

128. McGregor IA, Jackson IT. The groin flap. *Br J Plast Surg* 1972;25:3–16.

129. Mayer AR, Rodriguez RL. Vulvar reconstruction using a pedicle flap based on the superficial external pudendal artery. *Obstet Gynecol* 1991;78:964–968.

130. Ponten B. The fasciocutaneous flap: its use in soft tissue defects of the lower leg. *Br J Plast Surg* 1981;34:215–220.

131. Brown RG, Jurkiewicz MJ. Reconstructive surgery in the cancer patient. *Curr Probl Cancer* 1977;2:3–73.

132. McCraw JB, Dibbell DG, Carraway JH. Clinical definition of independent myocutaneous territories. *Plast Reconstr Surg* 1977;60:341–352.

133. Vasconez LO, McCraw JB (Eds). Myocutaneous flaps. *Clin Plast Surg* 1980;7:1–134.

134. Mathes SJ, Nahai F. *Clinical Applications for Muscle and Myocutaneous Flaps.* St. Louis: CV Mosby, 1982.

135. Tobin GR, Day TG. Vaginal and pelvic reconstruction with distally based rectus abdominis myocutaneous flaps. *Vaginal Pelvic Reconstr* 1988;81:62–70.

136. Tobin GR. Myocutaneous and muscle flap reconstruction of problem wounds. *Surg Clin N Am* 1984;64:667–681.

137. Ballon SC, Donaldson RC, Roberts JA, Lagasse LD. Reconstruction of the vulva using a myocutaneous graft. *Gynecol Oncol* 1979;7:123–127.

138. Pursell SH, Day TG, Tobin GR. Distally based rectus abdominis flap for reconstruction in radical gynecologic procedures. *Gynecol Oncol* 1990;37:234–238.

139. deHaas WG, Miller MJ, Temple WJ, Kroll SS, Schusterman MA, Reece GP, Skibber JM. Perineal wound closure with the rectus abdominis musculocutaneous flap after tumor ablation. *Ann Surg Oncol* 1995;2:400–406.

140. McAllister E, Wells K, Chaet M, Norman J, Cruse, W. Perineal reconstruction after surgical extirpation of pelvic malignancies using the transpelvic transverse rectus abdominal myocutaneous flap. *Ann Surg Oncol* 1994;1:164–168.

141. Bare RL, Assimos DG, McCullough DL, Smith DP, DeFranzo AJ, Marks MW. Inguinal lymphadenectomy and primary groin reconstruction using rectus abdominus muscle flaps in patients with penile cancer. *Urology* 1994;44:557–561.

142. Daniel RK, Taylor GI. Distant transfer of an island flap by microvascular anastomoses: a clinical technique. *Plast Reconstr Surg* 1973;52:111–117.

143. Backstrom A, Edsmyr F, Wicklund H. Radiotherapy of carcinoma of vulva. *Acta Obstet Gynecol Scan* 1972;51:109–115.

144. Daly JW, Million RR. Radical vulvectomy combined with elective node irradiation for TXN0 squamous carcinoma of the vulva. *Cancer* 1974;34:161–165.

145. Frankendal B, Larsson LG, Westling P. Carcinoma of the vulva. *Acta Radiol (Stock h)* 1973;12:165–174.

146. Perez CA, Grisby PW, Galakatos A, Swanson R, Camel HM, Kao M-S, Lockett MA. Radiation therapy in management of carcinoma of the vulva with emphasis on conservation therapy. *Cancer* 1993;71:3707–3716.

147. Boronow RC, Hickman BT, Reagan MT, Smith A, Steadham RE. Combined therapy as an alternative to exenteration for locally advanced vulvovaginal cancer. II. Results, complications and dosimetric and surgical considerations. *Am J Clin Oncol* 1987;10:171–181.

148. Tilmans AS, Sutton GP, Look KY, Stehman FB, Erlich CE, Hornback NB. Recurrent squamous carcinoma of the vulva. *Am J Obstet Gynecol* 1992;167:1383–1389.

149. Piura B, Masotina A, Murdoch J, Lopes A, Morgan P, Monaghan J. Recurrent squamous cell carcinoma of the vulva: a study of 73 cases. *Gynecol Oncol* 1993;48:189–195.

150. Hopkins MP, Reid GC, Morley GW. The surgical management of recurrent squamous cell carcinoma of the vulva. *Obstet Gynecol* 1990;75:1001–1005.

151. Hussain M, Al-Sarraf M. Anal carcinomas: new combined modality treatment approaches. *Oncology* 1988;2:42.

152. Koh W-J, Wallace HJ, Greer BE, et al. Combined radiotherapy and chemotherapy in the management of local-regionally advanced vulvar cancer. *Int J Radiat Oncol Biol Phys* 1993;26:809.

153. Russel AH, Mesic JB, Scudder SA, et al. Synchronous radiation and cytotoxic chemotherapy for locally advanced or recurrent squamous cancer of the vulvar. *Gynecol Oncol* 1992;47:14–20.

154. Thomas G, Dembo A, DePetrillo A, et al. Concurrent radiation and chemotherapy in vulvar carcinoma. *Gynecol Oncol* 1989;34:263.

155. Leiserowitz GS, Russell AH, Kinney WK, Smith LH, Taylor MH, Scudder SA. Prophylactic chemoradiation of inguinofemoral lymph nodes in patients with locally extensive vulvar cancer. *Gynecol Oncol* 1997;66:509–514.

PART IV

ONCOLOGIC THERAPY COMPLICATIONS MANAGEMENT

CHAPTER 17

BOWEL COMPLICATIONS MANAGEMENT AND RADIATION ENTERITIS

KATHRYN F. McGONIGLE, M.D.

CLINICAL OVERVIEW

Complications of radiotherapy for gynecologic malignancies most commonly concern the gastrointestinal tract.[1] The risk of developing acute or chronic gastrointestinal complications is dependent on both patient and treatment factors. Patient factors that increase risk include adhesions from prior abdominal surgery or infection, poor nutritional state, asthenic habitus, advanced disease status, and anemia. Associated medical problems such as diabetes, hypertension, or rheumatologic diseases also increase the risk of complications.[2–10] Treatment-associated factors that influence radiation complications for an organ relate to the radiation therapy technique, total dose, and proportion of organ irradiated.[11–13] Synchronous chemotherapy, while enhancing therapeutic effect, also increases risk.

Because of differing treatment volumes and dose rates, complications from external beam radiation differ from those occurring after intracavitary or interstitial therapy.[2,8,14] Acute small-bowel enteritis is more common with external beam radiation therapy. Risk of long-term complications is higher with an increase in total dose, higher dose per fraction, and larger portal size (e.g., whole-abdomen vs. whole-pelvic radiation therapy). The use of lateral ports (in addition to anteroposterior ports), which spare the rectum and bladder, and careful use of techniques for blocking vital organs may decrease complications. High-beam energies from linear accelerators commonly used in the United States today are better tolerated than lower-energy radiation because of a better depth-dose distribution.[2]

Perioperative and Supportive Care in Gynecologic Oncology: Evidence-Based Management,
Edited by Steven A. Vasilev.
ISBN 0-471-24788-X   Copyright © 2000 by Wiley-Liss, Inc.

In contrast to external beam radiation, brachytherapy methods are more likely to produce an inhomogeneous dose distribution, potentially delivering a high dose to a small area. Thus, intracavitary radiation more commonly may result in localized injury (e.g., portion of rectosigmoid colon, bladder, or small bowel). Consequently, the risk of complications depends more on "hot spots" than total dose. Parameters influencing the dose distribution include type of applicator used, geometry of application, and arrangement of radioactive sources.[2,3] Optimizing dosimetry can be complex, particularly in cases of unfavorable patient and tumor anatomy. Careful planning utilizing modern radiation oncology techniques may decrease the risk of damage to normal surrounding organs.[2-3]

MECHANISM AND ETIOLOGY OF RADIATION GASTROINTESTINAL INJURY

Acute Radiation Enteritis

Acute radiation enteritis generally corresponds to bowel symptoms occurring within 2 weeks of commencing radiation therapy and persisting for 1 month or less after therapy is completed. Acutely, radiation therapy has its greatest effect on cells with a rapid turnover. Thus, radiation damage to the rapidly dividing bowel mucosal cells accounts for the majority of symptoms occurring in patients with acute radiation enteritis.[15,16] Normally, the cells in the crypts of the bowel divide and provide a continuous supply of cells that move up the villi, differentiate, and become functioning cells. The cells at the top of the folds of the villi are slowly but continuously sloughed off and replaced.

Shortly after radiation therapy is started, crypt degeneration appears. Later, the tips of the villi are sloughed away by normal processes but fail to be replaced because no cells are available from the depopulated crypts. The result of this early toxicity on the gastrointestinal tract is the syndrome of acute radiation enteritis, with the most common symptom being diarrhea. The diarrhea results from malabsorption of bile acids, increased fecal fat excretion, and more rapid small-intestinal and whole-gut transit.[17] In more severe cases, vomiting, anorexia, weight loss, abdominal pain, and bleeding may occur. In most cases, acute radiation enteritis is a self-limiting disorder because the great capacity of the surviving stem cells to regenerate allows significant recovery of the bowel mucosa after completion of radiation.[15,16,18]

Chronic Radiation Enteritis

Chronic complications of radiotherapy occur in 3% to 12% of patients treated for gynecologic malignancies and are generally severe in less than one-half of these.[1,4,11,19-21] The late changes of radiation therapy in the gastrointestinal tract are generally seen in tissues where cellular turnover is slow, such as connective tissues and their supportive elements (e.g., blood vessels, nerves) in the intestines. Radiation causes a progressive cell depletion, obliterative vasculitis of small vessels in the bowel wall, with diffuse collagen deposition, atrophy, and fibrosis of the intestines. Eventually, ischemia, mucosal ulceration, infarction, and necrosis of the bowel wall may occur.[15,16,22,23]

In a prospective longitudinal study, the effect of radiation on gastrointestinal function was examined. At 1 to 2 years after completion of irradiation, there was an increase in the frequency of bowel actions, less bile acid absorption, and more rapid small-intestinal transit compared with that of baseline studies and normal subjects.[17] The degenerative process may be accelerated by superimposed infection. The most common chronic symptom resulting from the atrophic, ulcerated bowel mucosa is diarrhea, which may result in malabsorption syndromes. Because of the types of radiation ports used for gynecologic malignancies, the ileum is generally more severely affected than the jejunum. The terminal ileum is responsible for absorption of bile salts and vitamin B_{12}. The result is inadequate micelle formation and decreased fat absorption, as well as a lack of absorption of vitamin B_{12}, possibly leading to anemia.[24] In addition to a malabsorption syndrome, gastrointestinal bleeding, obstruction, stricture formation, fistula, or perforation may occur.

The symptoms of chronic radiation enteritis require a significant degree of cell depletion, and the changes often occur slowly. As a result, chronic radiation enteritis is an insidious, progressive disease often with a long latent period.[25] The clinical manifestations of chronic radiation enteritis usually occur 6 to 24 months after completion of radiation therapy, but may develop as late as 31 years after therapy.[20,22] The syndrome may be temporary, lasting from months to years, or may remain permanently. Thus, the diagnosis is often difficult and careful work-up is necessary to differentiate it from recurrent or other disease processes. Results of physical examination, laboratory and radiologic studies are frequently nonspecific. Often, a definite diagnosis is not made until the time of surgical exploration.[25] Any patient with even mild symptoms of chronic radiation enteritis is at risk of developing a serious complication.[20,25] The occurrence of significant acute radiation enteritis has been correlated with a nearly threefold increase in risk for subsequent chronic sequelae.[19,23] However, the absence of a severe acute syndrome in up to 75% of patients who develop chronic radiation enteritis suggests there may be independent but overlapping mechanisms.[19]

The total dose of pelvic radiation is the most important factor in the occurrence of severe, chronic radiation-related complications. In one study, complications occurred in 3% of women after 4,000 cGy and 10% after 5,000 cGy whole-pelvic radiation.[26] Radiation tolerance is defined as the amount of radiation that a particular organ can receive without developing a serious complication and varies from organ to organ and from tissue to tissue. Relative to other organs, the bowel has an intermediate level of radiation tolerance. In most patients, between 4,000 and 5,000 cGy can be tolerated by the small bowel and a slightly higher dose by the large bowel. For small bowel, the TD_5 (radiation dose in cGy at which approximately 5% of all patients will develop a significant complication in that organ by 5 years) is 4,250 cGy and the TD_{50} (same value for a 50% complication rate) is 6,250 cGy.[27]

Although the small bowel is less tolerant of radiation than the large bowel, the effect of the administered radiation dose is decreased by its mobility within the peritoneal cavity. Bowel immobilized by adhesions or scarring from previous surgery, pelvic infection, or tumor is at higher risk of injury. This risk is probably related to the actual presence of adhesions, as well as the decreased mobility of small bowel involved in adhesions, resulting in the bowel being relatively fixed and receiving a higher proportion of the administered dose during radiation. The ileum, relatively fixed near the pelvic brim because of its short mesenteric attachment to the cecum, is the most common site of small-bowel radiation injury.[28] These observations are supported by Level III evidence.

Radiation therapy for gynecologic malignancies predominantly affects the small bowel and rectum, although any portion of the bowel in the radiation field may be damaged. Involvement of multiple levels of the gastrointestinal tract is common.[20] In one study, the approximate proportion of bowel injuries for small bowel, rectum, colon, and combination large and small bowel were 40%, 30%, 15%, and 15%, respectively.[29] The morbidity and mortality of chronic radiation enteritis is related to the location of injury, with small-bowel injuries associated with a four times greater mortality compared with colorectal injuries.[29,30] Not uncommonly, nonintestinal organs are also involved (e.g., a complex fistula involving the small bowel, bladder, and vagina).[31]

RADIATION ENTERITIS TREATMENT

Acute Radiation Enteritis

Symptoms of acute radiation enteritis may be severe, depending on how much bowel is affected and the degree of tissue damage. Initial treatment of diarrhea from acute radiation enteritis is aimed at symptomatic relief with diet modification and increasing fluid intake. In general, diets should be low residue, free of gluten, protein, and lactose. Antiemetics provide symptomatic relief of nausea and vomiting. Diarrhea unresponsive to dietary measures usually responds to opiate-like drugs or other antidiarrheal medications. Sulfasalazine has been used anecdotally to treat diarrhea during pelvic radiation therapy that does not respond to standard methods. The therapeutic action is probably related to prostaglandin synthesis inhibition.[32]

In approximately 10% to 20% of patients receiving external pelvic radiation, symptoms of acute radiation enteritis may be severe enough to require a rest period from radiation and/or alteration in the radiation treatment plan.[33] Patients who sustain more than 10% loss of body weight should be treated with intravenous hydration and possibly parenteral nutrition.[34,35] In most cases, symptoms improve with supportive care and a short rest period from radiation therapy, usually 1 week or less. If a patient has symptoms that fail to respond to conservative therapy or to resolve within 2 weeks after completion of radiation therapy, work-up for other etiologies of diarrhea should be considered. Patients rarely require surgery for acute radiation–related bowel injury.[36] The interventions discussed are supported at Level III evidence.[33–36]

Although unusual in patients treated with whole-pelvic radiation alone, in those receiving concurrent chemotherapy, neutropenia, thrombocytopenia, or anemia may occur. The combination sometimes results in sepsis. Bloody diarrhea or frank gastrointestinal bleeding may occur. Initial management consists of supportive care with fluid resuscitation and possibly antibiotics, blood or platelet transfusion. In these cases, discontinuing chemotherapy and a rest period from radiation may be required.

Chronic Radiation Enteritis

Patients with chronic complications of radiation therapy require careful medical evaluation, treatment, and sometimes surgical therapy. Because the pathophysiology of chronic radiation enteritis is poorly understood, the medical management is somewhat empiric and success with most treatments has been anecdotal. A significant proportion of symptoms due to chronic radiation enteritis will resolve spontaneously or improve with time. One group found that 55% of cases of severe chronic radiation proctitis resolved with conservative management within 2 years, either because the condition remitted (33%) or the patient died of disseminated malignant disease (22%).[37] The natural history is similar for other types of chronic radiation enteritis, suggesting that conservative management should be employed for up to 2 years, and abandoned in those cases when severity of symptoms dictates the need for more immediate surgical therapy.

Others have suggested using a methylxanthine derivative, pentoxifylline, in patients with radiation injuries. It is a hemorrheologic agent that improves blood flow through narrowed microvasculature. It is used clinically to treat a variety of vasculo-occlusive disorders by increasing red blood cell deformability in small capillaries and stimulating prostacyclin release. Dion et al. described the use of pentoxifylline in the treatment of late radiation soft tissue necrosis.[38] Although the series was uncontrolled, 87% of patients had complete healing in 9 weeks while receiving pentoxifylline compared with 30 weeks of nonhealing prior to its use. The administration of this drug to reverse the effects of radiation enteritis or to decrease the occurrence of serious complications has not been described. Because one of the prevailing injuries of radiation tissue damage is vascular injury, a drug that increases blood flow in small vessels may be useful in alleviating symptoms of radiation injury and deserves further investigation.

Chronic Radiation Diarrhea   Patients with radiation enteritis have both an overall decreased amount of functional bowel and a reduction of functional mucosa in specific areas of bowel, resulting in malabsorption. Conservative modalities for treatment of chronic radiation enteritis are similar to those discussed for the acute syndrome. Depending on the severity and characteristics of the symptoms, medical treatment varies from pharmacological manipulation to diet alteration, or possibly total parenteral nutrition. Drugs to decrease bowel hypermotility, such as antispasmodics and anticholinergics, have been used, as well as broad-spectrum antibiotics to treat overgrowth of infectious organisms. In select cases, administration of specialized low-fat, low-residue, gluten or lactose-free diets have also been helpful.[39] Bile acid malabsorption in the ileum results in unabsorbed bile acids in the colon. Secretion of salt and water occurs, resulting in diarrhea.[40] Bile sequestering agents have been utilized with some success by reducing the amount of bile acids in the colon. Elemental diets or total parenteral nutrition have also been used either on a chronic basis or as an adjunct to a surgical procedure.[39]

Recently, authors have studied the effects of loperamide-N-oxide, a peripheral opiate agonist precursor, given in a double-blinded randomized order in patients with diarrhea caused by chronic radiation enteritis. Compared with placebo, treatment with loperamide-N-oxide was associated with a reduced frequency of bowel actions, slower small intestinal and total gut transit, and improved absorption of bile acids.[41] Others have used octreotide with anecdotal success to manage chronic radiation enteritis.[42] The multiple types of medical interventions for chronic radiation diarrhea are supported by Levels I[41] and III evidence.[39,42]

Gastrointestinal Bleeding Chronic gastrointestinal bleeding after radiation therapy for gynecologic malignancies generally occurs as a result of damage to the bowel mucosa, resulting in atrophic friable tissue that bleeds easily with minimal trauma. Severity of bleeding may range from guaiac-positive stools to massive hemorrhage. In some cases, focal injury may be the etiology for the bleeding, but usually diffuse injury to the bowel is causal. The lower gastrointestinal tract is the most common source of the bleeding, so part of the initial work-up should include a sigmoidoscopy. Sigmoidoscopy commonly reveals multiple telangiectasia, which may be actively bleeding.[43] If radiation changes are not consistent with the patient's symptoms, a full gastrointestinal evaluation is necessary to evaluate for other causal factors. Endoscopic examination should be performed with care because the radiated colon is quite rigid and easily perforated. In general, biopsy should be avoided, since even a seemingly superficial biopsy can result in perforation or fistula because of the radiated bowel's marginal vascular supply.[44] This management is supported by Level III evidence.

In most cases, bleeding resolves spontaneously, without surgical therapy. Patients should be instructed to avoid constipation because large, firm stools may irritate the fragile, radiated bowel mucosa, causing further bleeding. Mild stool softeners may be necessary on a chronic basis. Because recurrence of symptoms is common, patients should be monitored closely for many years. For isolated damage to the rectum or rectosigmoid colon, management with a low-residue diet and steroid suppositories has met with limited success.[20,45]

Kochhar et al. performed a prospective, randomized, double-blind controlled trial of oral sulfasalazine plus rectal steroids versus rectal sucralfate in patients with radiation-induced proctosigmoiditis.[46] Patients had symptoms of rectal bleeding, tenesmus, and diarrhea. At 4 weeks, both groups showed significant clinical improvement and endoscopic healing. However, the patients treated with sucralfate enemas showed a significantly better response as assessed clinically, but not endoscopically. Another study evaluated the efficacy of enemas of 5-aminosalicylic acid, the active component in sulfasalazine, to improve chronic radiation proctitis. No clinical or endoscopic improvement was noted after 2 to 6 months of treatment in four patients.[47] The use of pharmaceuticals as medical management for gastrointestinal bleeding from chronic radiation enteritis is supported by Levels I[46] and III evidence.[20,45,47]

If bleeding persists or is massive, localization with technetium sulfur colloid scintigraphy or ^{99m}Tc-labeled red blood cells should be considered.[48] Technetium sulfur colloid scintigraphy requires that bleeding be very rapid at examination while the ^{99m}Tc-labeled red blood cell scan permits identification of as little as 500 cc in 24 hours. These studies are more sensitive than angiography in identifying colonic bleeding because selective angiography requires bleeding to be at the rate of at least 0.5–1.0 ml/min at the time of the examination.[49] If a bleeding site is identified, the use of an intra-arterial vasoconstrictor may arrest bleeding.[50] Alternatively, embolization with Gelfoam particles or autologous clotted blood can be performed.[51] These procedures have limited usefulness in the radiated patient because bleeding is rarely localized and active bleeding is necessary at the time of examination.

Endoscopic Nd:YAG laser therapy to the bleeding area of rectosigmoid mucosa has been used anecdotally in radiated patients and is reasonable to consider prior to surgical intervention.[52] Electrocoagulation of radiated bowel mucosa in general should be performed with care because of the risk of perforation or fistula. Jensen et al. described the successful use of a heater probe or bipolar electrocoagulation, using low settings. Multiple treatments may be required, but significant palliation of symptoms may result.[43] These managements are supported by Level III evidence.[43,49–52]

In cases where bleeding from radiation injury is severe or recurrent, surgical therapy may be necessary. Rarely, a localized area of bowel may be involved, and in such cases, resection with reanastomosis may be appropriate. Bleeding is usually from the hemorrhagic mucosa of the rectosigmoid colon, and the passage of stool commonly irritates the radiated bowel, causing bleeding. Consequently, formation of a colostomy by diverting stool away from the damaged segment will often result in a significant improvement or resolution of symptoms. In a series of 18 patients with severe protosigmoiditis, 16 had diverting colostomies and the bleeding was controlled in 14 of the 16 patients.[31] The colostomy is usually considered permanent because it does not prevent progression of damage in the defunctionalized bowel and reanastomosis of the bowel is generally associated with recurrence of symptoms. If symptoms persist after colostomy formation, resection of the involved bowel is usually necessary, but has a higher surgical morbidity than colostomy alone. Surgical interventions are supported by Level III evidence.[31]

Stricture Formation and Obstruction   Stricture formation or obstruction can occur in either the large or small bowel. Obstruction of the small intestine as a result of radiation therapy is the most frequent form of chronic obstructive radiation enteritis and may occur as a result of adhesions of devascularized bowel or from stricture formation. Colonic stricture usually occurs in the rectosigmoid colon, approximately 8 to 10 cm from the anal verge, and often is a result of a "hot spot" during intracavitary or interstitial radiation therapy.[20] As in the small bowel, stricture formation may lead to obstructive symptoms. Even in the absence of frank total obstruction, significant morbidity including tenesmus and obstipation may ensue.

Small-bowel obstruction in the irradiated patient is more likely to result in serious complications, such as strangulation and perforation, than in the nonirradiated patient. These changes may occur more rapidly in the radiated patient whose bowel is marginally vascularized with chronic ulceration and mucosal damage. The degree of radiation bowel injury is commonly greater than what is expected based on the patient's clinical picture. In general, there are fewer ill effects in patients with colonic obstruction than in those with obstruction of the small bowel. This is because obstruction of the radiated colon does not usually result in strangulation. In addition, fluid and electrolyte loss progresses more slowly in colonic obstruction because the large intestine is principally a storage organ, whereas the small bowel has an important absorptive and secretory function.[53]

Often, the degree of distension of the small intestine in colonic obstruction depends on the competency of the ileocecal valve. In patients with a competent valve, there may be little or no small-bowel distension. Rarely, colonic obstruction in these patients behaves as a closed-loop obstruction.[54] The cecum is the most common site of perforation because of its spherical shape and thin wall.[44,55] If the cecum is distended to 9–11 cm, perforation is imminent and an emergency decompressing colostomy is necessary.[56] The ileocecal valve is believed to be competent in 40% to 60% of nonradiated patients; however, radiation therapy may increase the valve's competence. These observations are supported by Level III evidence.

Symptoms of small- or large-bowel obstruction in the radiated patient can be slowly progressive or develop acutely. Partial obstructive symptoms may be insidious, with limited nausea, with or without vomiting, and only slightly crampy pain and modest distension and postprandial bloating. The patient may have repeated episodes of exacerbations and remissions of obstruction or may present acutely with a high-grade obstruction. The radiated patient may be less likely to present with classic signs of peritonitis, and in such cases, a high index of suspicion is required to minimize morbidity.[57] These clinical observations in the irradiated patient are supported by Level III evidence.

Radiologic evaluation is essential in the diagnosis of the irradiated patient with a bowel obstruction and may demonstrate which areas of bowel are most severely affected and whether the obstruction involves multiple areas of bowel. Such studies are often useful to help make the decision about whether to proceed with surgery or attempt medical therapy. Patients with perforation, high-grade obstruction, or multiple recurrent obstructions should undergo surgical therapy.[58] This recommendation is supported by Level III evidence. If possible, a mechanical and antibiotic bowel prep should be performed to decrease the risk of complications of bowel anastomosis or resection. Rarely, limited adhesiolysis will relieve an obstruction in this group of patients. For the remaining patients, resection or bypass is indicated. An alternative to surgical bypass is isolation of the damaged bowel by division proximally and distally and formation of a mucous fistula.[58] The pros and cons of bypass versus resection are discussed later in this chapter.

The patient with rectal stenosis or stricture from chronic radiation injury can rarely be treated with gentle dilation.[20] In more severe cases causing obstruction, surgical therapy is necessary. If the area of obstruction is isolated, resection with reanastomosis may be appropriate. In contrast, if the strictured area is long or radiation damage is diffuse throughout a significant length of colon, the patient is best treated with a colostomy alone, without resection.

Short-Bowel Syndrome Resection or bypass of large portions of irradiated small bowel may result in a short-bowel syndrome. In some cases, because of severe radiation injury, such as distal bowel obstruction, fistula, or in order to protect a more distal anastomosis, a small-bowel ostomy is necessary on a temporary or permanent basis. Most absorption takes place in the duodenum and the first 90 cm of jejunum. With less than 90 to 120 cm of bowel remaining for absorption, maintenance of a positive nitrogen balance and normal carbohydrate absorption is difficult.[59]

The type of malabsorption syndrome depends on the level of small-bowel ostomy or type and amount of bowel resected, jejunum versus ileum. Secretions from proximal jejunal ostomies are very liquid, high in bicarbonate, and can cause metabolic acidosis. Fluid and electrolyte loss can be massive. Resection of a large length of jejunum will seriously impair absorption of fat, calcium, and folic acid. In contrast, if a large length of ileum has been removed or bypassed, vitamin B_{12} and bile salt absorption will be impaired. In the radiated patient, damage to ileum is much more likely than jejunal injury, and as a result, the need for ileal resection or bypass is more common. Overall, the short-bowel syndrome presents a special management problem.[59]

Adaptation in the short-bowel syndrome can be divided into three phases.[60] Functional adaptation results in a compensatory hypertrophy of the intestinal mucosa. Therefore, complete adaptation may take a long period of time. In phase I of adaptation, there is massive diarrhea from failure of water and bile salt absorption, and rapid transit time. Furthermore, the resection of a massive amount of small bowel frequently results in gastric hypersecretion of both fluid and hydrochloric acid. One complication is peptic ulceration with hemorrhage.

Thus, all patients who have had large amounts of bowel resected should be maintained on histamine H_2 blockers permanently. After massive bowel resection, the patient will normally need to be maintained on parenteral nutrition and fluid replacement administered parenterally for a minimum of 2 to 4 months. Oral feeding should be minimized because it tends to seriously aggravate the diarrhea; however, there is evidence that small amounts of oral intake are beneficial in accelerating adapatation of the bowel. Adaptation requires that food be in contact with the bowel mucosa. Exposure of the bowel to glutamine, bile salts, and pancreatic enzymes is important in adaptation.

Phase 2 usually occurs after 2 to 4 months and is recognized by a reduction of diarrhea to approximately 2 liters daily or less. This period usually extends for 9 months to a year. Parenteral nutrition will likely continue to be necessary, but oral feeding should slowly be initiated and caloric intake increased.[61] As oral intake increases, diarrhea will necessarily worsen.

Oral feedings should preferably be initiated with substances that require minimal hydrolysis and are easily absorbed. Such refined preparations as Vivonex® have been useful, because they contain simple sugars and amino acids.[62] However, because these solutions are hypertonic, diarrhea may actually be aggravated. The amount of fat absorbed is proportional to the amount presented to the absorptive surface. Therefore, the maximal intake of fat that does not cause symptoms is desirable. Regardless of which segment of small bowel was removed, the diet should be high in protein. Frequent feedings (six or more times daily), are usually recommended. Oral amino acids, vitamins A, D, K, and B-complex, as well as calcium, iron, and magnesium, may usually be given orally.

Supplementation of the diet by medium-chain triglycerides has been beneficial to patients in reducing diarrhea (steatorrhea) and helping to stabilize weight by improving fat absorption. Because weight gain may be slight and diarrhea may be a problem despite diet manipulation, drugs to decrease intestinal motility are sometimes useful. These include diphenoxylate hydrochloride (5.0 mg two or three times daily), anticholinergics (propantheline, 15–30 mg two or three times daily), and/or tincture of opium (10 drops two or three times daily).[60] Treatment with cholestyramine, a bile salt–binding resin, may ameliorate the diarrhea caused by the effect of unabsorbed bile acids upon the colon.[63] Only about one-third of nonradiated patients with short-bowel syndrome will eventually be able to discontinue parenteral support. This proportion is even lower in irradiated patients. The clinical observations of short-bowel syndrome are supported by Level III evidence.

For periods of up to 12 months postoperatively, the remaining segment of intestine will show progressive improvement in absorptive capacity, associated with elongation and dilatation of the mucosal villi. In phase 3 the patient is stable and has controllable diarrhea on a low-fat diet. Supplemental vitamins and parenteral B_{12} injections are necessary. The patient is also subject to a high frequency of oxalate nephrolithiasis.[60] These observations and recommendations are supported by Level III evidence.

Perforation Spontaneous perforation, a rare complication of pelvic radiation therapy, may occur in a segment of bowel devascularized from radiation-associated vasculitis.[64] More commonly, distal obstruction predisposes the more proximal, dilated bowel to strangulate and perforate. Acute perforation of the small or large intestine regardless of etiology requires prompt surgical therapy. Prior to proceeding with surgery, the patient should be stabilized medically. With undue delay, septic shock may develop and is associated with a very high mortality.[53]

In general, for either a small- or large-bowel perforation of radiated bowel, surgical therapy should be conservative and resection with primary anastomosis avoided.[36] For the patient with a large-bowel perforation, exteriorization of the involved segment of bowel with or without surgical resection is the optimal procedure. For the patient with a small-bowel perforation, exterioration and isolation of the involved segment should usually be performed as well as bypass of the proximal small bowel to a more distal segment of bowel (distal small bowel or colon).

The bowel distal to the anastomosis should be closely examined because perforation or anastomotic breakdown is commonly associated with distal obstruction. In most circumstances, areas of obstruction should be left as a defunctionalized loop. If the defunctionalized segment is too long, resection may be indicated to reduce morbidity resulting from a closed-loop obstruction or a severe overgrowth syndrome from minimal transit in the long segment. Expert surgical clinical judgment is necessary to minimize morbidity in such a case. In general, the perforated segment should be resected as part of another surgical procedure or left as a mucous fistula. These recommendations and observations are made based on Level III evidence.

Fistula Fistula formation as a result of radiation therapy may occur in either the large or small bowel and may concurrently involve almost any organ, including the skin, vagina, perineum, bladder, or colon.[20,65,66] Similar to perforation, bowel fistulas may occur as a result of bowel obstruction distal to the fistula site or because of devascularized bowel from radiation injury.[65] The reported incidence of rectal fistula following radiation therapy ranges from 1.4% to 5.2%.[67] Enterovaginal fistulas are more commonly associated with radiation injury than enterocutaneous fistulas. Piver and Lele reported on 43 patients with gynecologic cancer who presented with a small-bowel fistula.[65] The major cause of the fistulas was cancer in 20 patients and radiation injury in 12 patients. Enterovaginal fistulas were almost always caused by radiation, whereas entercutaneous fistulas resulted from radiation injury in only 1 patient. Therefore, it is important to exclude recurrent cancer in radiated patients developing a fistula outside of the postoperative period, especially in cases of enterocutaneous fistula.

In most circumstances, radiologic characterization of the fistulous tract should be performed using a water-soluble agent.[65] This recommendation is made based on Level III evidence. In some cases, the fistulous tract may be safely evaluated using barium and may result in a more informative radiologic study. Thorough radiologic evaluation of the upper and lower gastrointestinal tracts avoids the problem of unsuspected distal colonic obstruction or simultaneous enteric and colonic fistulas, not uncommon in the radiated patient. It may also disclose an unsuspected abscess cavity and give an indication of the amount of functional intestine.

Management of radiated fistulas is particularly difficult, due to local vascular impairment and poor ability of tissue repair. For the small-bowel fistula, although fistula output may decrease during bowel rest and hyperalimentation, radiation-induced fistulas occurring outside the operative period almost never heal by this approach.[68,69] Surgical therapy should be performed if the patient is medically fit. In contrast, the small-bowel fistula developing postoperatively in a radiated patient may warrant conservative medical management because a small portion will close. Appropriate patient selection for this management depends on the amount of the fistula output, location of the fistula in the bowel, and its characteristics in radiologic studies.

High-output fistulas are variably defined in the literature as daily output greater than 100 cc to greater than 1,000 cc. In general, high-output fistulas tend to be more proximal in the bowel, more commonly require surgical therapy, and have a higher associated morbidity and mortality. The primary management of the patient with a small-bowel fistula is to control fistula output. This is done initially by eliminating oral intake and proximal decompression. Nasogastric suctioning is used in all patients with high-output and proximal fistulas, but is usually not necessary for more distal fistulas.

Continued fistula losses need to be carefully measured and replaced. If the fistula has a high output, is in communication with a large abscess cavity, or has a very short fistulous tract, it is unlikely to close spontaneously. Furthermore, if a distal obstruction is demonstrated, the small-bowel fistula will not close, even with prolonged use of parenteral nutrition, and surgical release of the distal obstruction is necessary.[65,70–73] This statement is made based on observations from multiple studies and Level III evidence.

In patients with a proximal small-bowel fistula where conservative management is deemed appropriate, the patient should ingest only small amounts orally and be treated with prolonged (2–4 weeks) parenteral nutrition therapy. In general, restriction of oral intake is not beneficial in the patient with a large-bowel or distal low-output small-bowel fistula. These recommendations are made based on Level III evidence.

In cases of small-bowel fistula, administration of somatostatin, a naturally occurring amino acid peptide that exhibits strong inhibitory effects on gastrointestinal, pancreatic, and biliary secretion, should be considered. These effects result in decreased fistula output, and several studies suggest it may be useful for both high- and low-output fistulas, and may facilitate the closure of enterocutaneous fistulas when used in conjunction with parenteral nutrition and prolonged bowel rest.[74–79] In a randomized study of 40 patients, Torres et al. reported that intravenous somatostatin (250 U/hr) in nonirradiated bowel produces a higher rate of fistula closure (58% vs. 81%), a more rapid fistula closure (13.9 days vs. 20.4 days), and a reduction in morbidity (35% vs. 69%).[79] It is not known whether these results can be extrapolated to the irradiated patient. Based on this and other studies, it appears that somatostatin may accelerate the rate of fistula closure, but does not increase the success rate of closure. The recommendation to use somatostatin in selected cases of small-bowel enterocutaneous fistulas is based on Levels I[79] and III evidence.[74–78]

With successful conservative management, fistula closure usually occurs between 11 and 33 days of treatment in nonirradiated patients, but may take longer in radiated bowel. If the fistula has not healed in approximately 4 to 6 weeks or significant fistula output (over 200 cc daily) persists, medical therapy has failed. When medical therapy fails or is not appropriate, surgical therapy should be undertaken cautiously. In the patient unable to undergo surgery with a high-output fistula, prolonged administration of parenteral nutrition may be necessary. Low-output fistulas can be managed by maintaining drainage of the fistulous tract and prescription of a low-residue diet. In the case of enterocutaneous fistulas, small-bowel contents rapidly digest the skin because of high levels of pancreatic enzymes. Protection of the skin is essential and is usually best obtained by application of an ileostomy or colostomy appliance around the cutaneous opening.[71] In cases where it is not possible to arrange an appliance over a fistula, such as with an enterovaginal fistula, a suction catheter may be used to minimize skin irritation. These recommendations are based on Level III evidence.

The patient with a large-bowel fistula rarely presents with significant medical disorders and dehydration because of the more solid nature of large-bowel contents. In most cases, the rectum has fistulized to the vagina, and constant leakage of stool on the vulva is irritating and can result in excoriation of the skin. Protective ointment should be applied to the vulvar skin and the patient prescribed a clear liquid diet prior to proceeding with surgical diversion. After radiologic studies to confirm the absence of a concurrent small-bowel fistula, diverting colostomy should be performed. This gives immediate palliation and also is the best permanent solution for many patients. In addition, it allows time for radiation effects to subside so that careful evaluation for disease recurrence can be made. If the fistula tract is small, it may close spontaneously after the fecal stream is diverted, but the problem usually recurs if intestinal continuity is restored.[20] Permanent colostomy is necessary unless surgical repair of the fistula is performed.

Techniques for repair of radiation-induced rectovaginal fistula have involved interposing well-vascularized tissue such as omentum, gracilis muscle, or a turned-down loop of proximal sigmoid colon to plug the ischemic defect in the anterior rectal wall.[20,81] Resection with restoration of continuity by the colo-endoanal anastomosis or abdominal-anal pull-through has also been performed, but experience is limited.[82–86] For the low rectovaginal fistula, the bulbocavernosus muscle has been used successfully.[87] Patients may require repeated operative procedures to achieve fistula closure.

Depending on the site of the colonic fistula, there may be an advantage to complete excision and replacement with well-vascularized nonirradiated colon.

Complete healing of the fistula repair should be confirmed radiologically prior to colostomy take-down, usually many months after the initial surgery. In some cases, the severity of radiation damage does not allow restoration of bowel continuity. Recommendations for management of the large bowel fistula are based on Level III evidence.

General Surgical Principles in the Radiated Intestine

Disabling symptoms may necessitate surgery in 10% to 20% of patients with chronic radiation enteritis.[88] Surgical intervention is indicated in patients with high-grade or persistent bowel obstruction, perforation, fistula, or abscess not drainable percutaneously, and in some cases with severe or chronic gastrointestinal bleeding due to radiation enteritis. Surgical intervention for radiation bowel injury carries a significant risk of postoperative morbidity and a 20% to 50% risk of mortality has been reported in the older literature.[89] Although modern surgical and critical care management has decreased this risk, morbidity remains high. Furthermore, results of surgical therapy are less likely to result in resolution of symptoms compared with the nonirradiated patient. In a study of patients who underwent surgery for bowel obstruction from chronic radiation enteritis, nearly 50% of patients had persistent severe symptoms, most of which were related to prior radiation treatment.[90] Studies have found that up to 50% of patients with radiation enteritis requiring surgery will need to undergo additional surgery to correct the radiation damage or because of complications from the initial operative procedure.[20,44]

The radiated bowel is much less forgiving than the nonirradiated bowel to surgical manipulation.[91,92] Close attention to basic surgical principles is even more essential to avoid complications. Prior to surgery, the patient's radiation history should be carefully reviewed. Patients who require emergency surgery should be treated preoperatively by controlling sepsis, correcting metabolic abnormalities and acid-base imbalances, assuring adequate fluid status, and by supporting them with hyperalimentation, as indicated.

During surgery, extensive adhesiolysis should be avoided. Lysis of adhesions in irradiated intestine may result in serosal denudation with focal devascularization of marginally vascularized intestine or inadvertent minute openings into the intestine. Areas of devascularized intestine may not be readily apparent visually. As a result, postoperative perforations or fistula formation may occur in the absence of surgical enterotomy.[93,94]

Bowel segments with obstruction, associated perforation, fistula, or abscess formation require either resection or bypass. In general, the surgeon should preserve as much bowel as can safely be done and avoid extensive resections and multiple anastomoses. Because of an obliterative vasculitis of small vessels, associated edema, and inflammation in the bowel wall, the radiated bowel does not heal as well as normal bowel. The risk of an anastomotic leak in radiated bowel is substantially higher than that in nonirradiated bowel, and mortality rates approach 50% when this occurs.[25]

Anastomoses should be tension-free and performed in bowel that has the least evidence of radiation damage. Signs of significant radiation injury include a pale gray-white, smooth surface, thickened edematous bowel wall, strictures, and mesenteric shortening. It is sometimes difficult macroscopically to determine which area of bowel is free of radiation damage, and gut that appears grossly normal may ultimately be noted to be damaged when examined microscopically. The use of flouroscein or frozen section have not been reliable in this setting.[93,95]

The ascending, transverse, and descending colon are usually free of radiation-induced lesions, depending on the type of port employed for radiation.[64] If possible, one of these segments of large bowel should be employed in the anastomosis. The use of the transverse colon for anastomosis also has theoretical advantages because of the rich blood supply from the middle colic artery. Formation of an anastomosis in at least one segment of nonirradiated bowel significantly decreases risk of anastomotic failure by improving blood supply to the anastomosis.

Avoidance of anastomoses in watershed vascular areas of the bowel may be important in the radiated patient. Sudeck's point refers to the reduction of splanchnic blood supply of the sigmoid colon between the last sigmoid artery and the superior mesenteric artery.[96] Although the importance of the watershed area of Sudeck's is controversial in nonradiated patients, it may be more important in patients whose bowel has been radiated. These observations and recommendations are made based on Level III evidence.

A tension-free anastomosis is extremely critical in radiated bowel, and even seemingly minimal tension may lead to anastomotic breakdown. Because radiation enteritis is a diffuse process commonly involving multiple portions of bowel, it is not uncommon for a more distal segment of bowel to also be obstructed. This could result in an anastomotic breakdown postoperatively.[65] Therefore, prior to performing the anastomosis, the presence of a distal obstruction should be excluded. This recommendation is based on Level III evidence.

The radiated bowel has a marginal blood supply, and the use of a metal stapling device is recommended if technically possible. This device has the theoretical advantage of minimizing the interruption of blood flow at the bowel edges that might occur with a hand-sewn anastomosis, because staples are more evenly placed. In contrast, some argue that stapling instruments should be avoided in radiated bowel that is edematous and thickened. Overall, there is no evidence that an anastomosis using a stapling device in radiated bowel is at higher risk of anastomotic leakage than a hand-sewn anastomosis. In a prospective randomized study of 132 patients undergoing colorectal anastomoses in nonirradiated colon, manually constructed and stapled anastomoses were found to have no difference in clinical anastomotic leak rates, morbidity, or postoperative mortality.[97]

There has long been a debate over the most appropriate surgical management of the obstructed segment of radiated small bowel, and an extensive discussion of the pros and cons is beyond the scope of this chapter. The debate concerns whether resection and primary anastomosis is associated with less morbidity than a bypass of the involved segment.[44,66,68,89,98–101] Because most radiated patients have generalized bowel damage, many argue that bypass is more appropriate.

There are two main drawbacks to bypassing the diseased segment of bowel. First, progression of damage in the bypassed segment may occur, resulting in necrosis, perforation, and fistulization months or years after the bypass procedure.[84,89,99] Second, bacterial overgrowth in the defunctionalized loop can occur in about half of cases, with bacterial concentrations up to 10^{11}/cc.[99] This overgrowth results in bile acid deconjugation, impaired micelle formation, and fat malabsorption, contributing to diarrhea.[101–103] Other bacterially mediated disturbances of fat, protein, carbohydrate absorption and metabolism likely occur because rarely does bile acid deconjugation alone explain the severe malabsorption observed.[104,105] Although short-term treatment with a broad-spectrum antibiotic is often successful, occasionally the patient requires long-term treatment. Emergence of drug-resistant organisms is not uncommon, so rotation of antibiotics is necessary. In addition, deficiencies of vitamin B_{12} caused by bacterial competition for dietary vitamin B_{12} may occur, preventing its absorption by intestinal cells and leading to pernicious anemia.[106]

The drawbacks to resection and primary anastomosis are that it usually requires a much more extensive surgical procedure, longer surgical time with more extensive dissection of adhesions, and an increased risk of anastomotic breakdown or fistula formation. Furthermore, shortening of the intestine may occur, potentially increasing the radiation-induced ischemia by division of mesenteric blood vessels, or possibly leading to development of a short gut syndrome.[92,107] In rare cases, usually after whole-abdominal or extended-field radiation therapy, the entire small bowel is encased in a fibrous cocoon, and dissection and relief of obstruction are impossible. The only therapy for such patients is lifelong parenteral nutrition.[58]

Analysis of data in the literature regarding optimal surgical treatment for radiated patients with a small-bowel obstruction is difficult, because for most series the resection and bypass groups are not comparable. In general, treatment should be individualized: Certain patients are best treated with resection and primary anastomosis, while others should undergo bypass. Short, isolated segments of intestine that cause obstruction are best resected. In cases where bowel is obviously nonviable, resection is mandatory. Long segments of strictured small intestine, particularly those involved in dense interloop and pelvic adhesions, are probably best treated by bypass. When there is concern about the anastomosis or gross stool contamination, proximal diversion should be performed. These recommendations are based on Level III evidence.

In the nonirradiated patient with a bowel obstruction, the indications for resection versus bypass may differ. In the patient with incurable cancer and carcinomatosis, bypass or small-bowel ostomy may be indicated to minimize surgical morbidity. In general, such patients are unlikely to live long enough to experience symptoms related to overgrowth syndrome resulting from intestinal bypass. In general, cases where the patient's life expectancy is long (greater than a few years) and the patient is physically able to undergo the surgical procedure, resection should be performed rather than bypass. These recommendations are based on Level III evidence.

Laboratory evidence suggests that perioperative administration of vitamin A facilitates the healing of both small- and large-bowel anastomoses after radiation therapy.[108] Although the effectiveness of this treatment in humans is unknown, some have suggested using it in high-risk patients because of the low risk of side effects. A postoperative intravenous dose of 50,000 IU/day for 5 days, reduced to 20,000 IU/day thereafter has been recommended.[58]

A common indication for the diverting colostomy in the irradiated patient is protection of a more distal anastomosis in irradiated bowel. The decision to perform a diverting colostomy should be individualized. It may be prudent to perform with a low rectal anastomosis (<7 cm), particularly in those patients previously exposed to very high doses of radiation. The diverting colostomy is also used to divert the fecal stream proximal to a fistula or distal bowel severely affected by radiation protosigmoiditis. Patients with gastrointestinal hemorrhage from severe radiation protosigmoiditis may have improvement of symptoms by diverting bowel contents away from the friable bowel mucosa. A diverting colostomy is also indicated in cases of gross contamination, sepsis, or perforation or to emergently decompress the distended obstructed colon.

Restoration of bowel continuity is appropriate in selected cases. When used to protect a more distal anastomosis, colostomy closure should be performed not sooner than 6 or longer than 12 weeks. Prolonged delay of colostomy closure may be associated with an increased risk of stricture in the anastomosis.[58] Because a proximal colostomy does not prevent progression of radiation changes in the defunctionalized bowel, closure may result in recurrence of symptoms in the distal bowel.[29] These recommendations are based on Level III evidence.

Sloughing of stomata, retraction, and ulceration are common in irradiated exteriorized intestine. If possible, stoma formation should be performed in bowel and skin free of radiation damage. Ample intestine should be exteriorized and careful attention to the blood supply of the exteriorized bowel is essential. This decreases the risk of stenosis and skin reaction, and improves healing.[92,109] These recommendations are based on Level III evidence.

Postoperatively, adequate nutritional support should be provided. Most patients requiring surgical therapy for radiation enteritis have had chronic symptoms and as a result are malnourished prior to surgery. Furthermore, the radiated bowel is often fibrotic, thickened, and has decreased functional peristalsis relative to normal bowel. Mucosal damage from radiation results in impaired absorption. These factors, in conjunction with slow anastomotic healing, often result in significant delays in oral feeding after surgery. Thus, parenteral nutrition is generally required to provide nutritional support in the postoperative period.

The classic teaching has been that early feeding could result in significant morbidity, worsening ileus, and should be avoided.[110] Recently, data on the gut's immunologic and hormonal activities have led to a questioning of this teaching. Although instituting full alimentation in the immediate postoperative period may be detrimental, small amounts may actually be trophic to the gut. The intestinal tract atrophies without use, in stress states, and during parenteral feeding.[111] Enteral feeding can maintain mucosal integrity and restore villus height.

Glutamine is a primary fuel used by the intestinal tract and is absent from currently available amino acid solutions and many enteral diets. The small intestine is the principal organ of glutamine consumption, extracting approximately 20% to 30% of circulating glutamine in the postabsorptive state. Gut glutamine requirements are increased during critical illness, and studies suggest that glutamine may be essential for the maintenance of gut metabolism, structure, and function.[112] Glutamine, when administered in parenteral formulae, reverses atrophy and increases gut immune function.[113] Enteral glutamine may also provide similar beneficial effects.[114] These observations and recommendations are based on Level III evidence.

PREVENTIVE METHODS TO DECREASE RISK OF ACUTE AND CHRONIC GASTROINTESTINAL COMPLICATIONS

The therapeutic ratio for radiation treatment of malignancies can be determined by examining dose-response curves for tumor and for normal tissues (Fig. 17.1).[115] The farther apart the two curves are, the higher is the therapeutic index. For radiation treatment of most malignant gynecologic diseases, the therapeutic index is quite narrow. As a result, the occurrence of radiation enteritis is common and a certain amount of toxicity to normal tissues must be accepted in order to obtain tumor control. Most authorities agree that an acceptable rate of serious complications is approximately 5%. Risk is most acceptable in patients with advanced malignancies where there is no alternative therapy and inadequate radiation would not control the tumor volume. In contrast, for patients with less advanced disease or when surgical therapy is an alternative to treatment, morbidity from radiation therapy is less acceptable.

If there are no alternatives to radiation therapy, methods of radiation administration that may decrease the risk of intestinal injury include decreasing total dose, decreasing the dose per fraction, using lateral fields in addition to anteroposterior fields, and properly using blocks as well as individualizing dosimetry.[116,117] Other methods that have been used to decrease intestinal injury include minimizing the amount of bowel within the radiation field, altering diet, and administering protective pharmacologic agents. These observations and recommendations are based on Level III evidence.

Because of the narrow therapeutic index, reduction of total dose is usually not feasible because it would result in an unacceptably high rate of persistent dis-

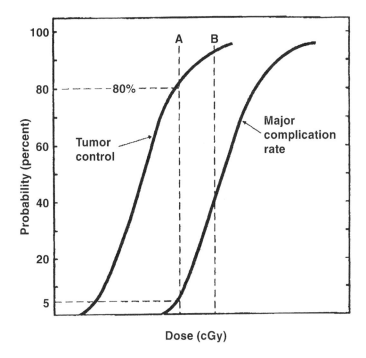

FIGURE 17.1. Theoretical sigmoid dose-response curves for tumor control and major complication rate. The farther apart the two curves, the higher the therapeutic ratio.

ease or recurrence. In most institutions, the dose per fraction of external-beam radiation is limited to 180–200 cGy. Higher doses result in an unacceptably high rate of late complications.[3]

There have been significant changes in radiation therapy equipment and modalities since the early 1970s, which allow more individualization of therapy. External-beam radiation treatment has been made more precise using computer-assisted planning and multiple cross-firing radiation areas from a linear accelerator. During intracavitary radiotherapy, dose and volume of radiated intestine can be minimized with computerized calculations of dosages. In addition, afterloading systems allow more accurate placement of the radiation source.[2] In patients requiring surgery for staging or treatment planning, complications may be significantly reduced if the retroperitoneal approach is used rather than the transperitoneal approach.[118] These observations and recommendations are based on Level III evidence.

Both surgical and radiation techniques have been developed to minimize the amount of bowel in the radiation field. Radiation methods include positioning during treatment to shift the bowel out of the pelvis using Trendelenburg and/or prone positioning, as well as using bladder distension.[119,120] The success of treatment positioning is restricted to position-tolerant patients with mobile small bowel. In one prospective study, pretreatment contrast studies of the small bowel were performed in 140 patients to identify those at high risk for small-bowel injury while undergoing radiation therapy for gynecologic cancers. Radiation dosimetry, patient positioning, and bladder distension were modified. No instances of significant small-bowel injury occurred in the 37 high-risk patients after a median follow-up of 3 years.[121] These observations and recommendations are made based on Levels II-3[121] and III evidence.[119,120]

Surgical methods have also been developed to reduce the risk of small-bowel radiation injury. The use of the omentum to exclude the small bowel from the pelvis out of the radiation field has been described.[122,123] The omentum is pulled over the small intestine anteriorly and secured to the retroperitoneum, the ascending and descending colons, and the pelvic peritoneum, respectively. However, this technique is not possible in certain cases where the omentum is surgically absent, anatomically too small to encompass the viscera, or involved in adhesions and unable to be mobilized as an intact structure. Furthermore, because the omentum is not a fixed structure, the intestines may settle into the pelvis with time. In some cases, the omental sling fails to retain all the loops of the small bowel, and some fall into the pelvis.

The use of anterior parietal peritoneal flaps to reduce radiation injury has been described by Vasilev et al. in six patients who underwent radical hysterectomy and pelvic lymphadenectomy for cervical cancer.[124] Flaps were sewn to the posterior parietal peritoneum at the pelvic brim or higher and functioned as bowel slings. Small-bowel loops were effectively excluded from the pelvic area as documented by radiologic studies. No complications occurred in these patients, with a median follow-up period of 16 months. Devereux et al. described a technique in rats using a polyglycolic acid mesh sling.[125] Small bowel was noted to be successfully excluded from the pelvis when mesh absorption was complete (in all rats after 60 days). No complications of infection or bowel obstruction occurred. The same investigators reported the use of a polyglycolic acid mesh in seven patients with pelvic malignancies requiring bowel resection and postoperative radiation therapy. After a minimum follow-up of 4 months, no patient suffered from acute radiation enteritis and there was no evidence of infection or obstruction.[121]

Sugarbaker described the use of a silicone rubber breast implant to fill the pelvic cavity.[126] A sheet of plastic mesh was sutured to the brim of the pelvis to ensure that the pelvic inlet remained closed. Because the silicone rubber is of water density, its absorption of radiation is similar to that of tissue and no unusual adjustments of radiation dosimetry are required. This procedure may result in a slight reduction of bladder capacity. In addition, the risk of infectious complications or rupture is unknown. In view of the ban in silicone breast implants, it is unlikely that this method will be clinically used in the future. Others have recommended suture of the posterior wall of a distended urinary bladder to the anterior, lateral, and posterior peritoneum or rectosigmoid colon.[127] During radiation, the bladder is acutely distended, elevating the bowel out of the radiation field. These techniques require major surgery for implementation and some require another surgery for removal. These observations and recommendations are based on Level III evidence.

The administration of elemental diets during radiation therapy has been studied to evaluate their ability to provide readily available nutrients and selectively inhibit gastric and pancreatic secretions, possibly resulting in a reduction of ischemic injury. The use of these specialized diets has generally been unsuccessful in decreasing the risk of acute or chronic radiation enteritis.[35,128] Some have advocated using parenteral hyperalimentation without oral supplements during abdominal-pelvic irradiation, allowing the irradiated bowel to be kept at rest, free of intestinal irritation.[35] This may theoretically diminish the injurious effect of radiation in the small intestine by the diversion of pancreatic secretions and bile.[129,130]

Kinsella et al. prospectively examined the use of nutritional support during pelvic irradiation for primary pelvic malignancies in 17 of 32 patients with a prior history of weight loss.[34] Study patients received intravenous hyperalimentation and controls were maintained on their regular diets. Study patients tolerated therapy well by functional and nutritional measurements without a treatment break. Others have demonstrated the use of parenteral nutrition to be associated with fewer side effects compared with those receiving a normal diet.[131,132] In general, studies of nutritional support during radiation therapy have demonstrated no reduction in radiation complications. These observations are based on Level III evidence.

Although a great deal of work has been done with chemical and pharmacologic radioprotective agents, no drugs are in common use today and none have been approved for clinical use.[92] In some patients refractory to these treatments, a bile salt–sequestrating agent may be helpful, although most reports are anecdotal.[133,134] Because of reports suggesting the usefulness of sulfasalazine to treat diarrhea occurring acutely during pelvic radiotherapy, its active moiety, 5-aminosalicylic acid (5-ASA), has been studied for the prevention of acute radiation enteritis. Unfortunately, double-blinded placebo-controlled European trials have failed to demonstrate any improvement in diarrhea in patients receiving 5-ASA prophylactically while undergoing radiation therapy.[135,136] These observations are based on Levels I[135,136] and III evidence.[92,133,134]

REFERENCES

1. Montana GS, Fowler WC. Carcinoma of the cervix: analysis of bladder and rectal radiation dose and complications. *Int J Radiat Oncol Biol Phys* 1989;16:95–100.

2. Choi K, Aziz H, Rotman M. Complications in the radiotherapeutic management of gynecological cancers. In: Nori D, Hilans BS, eds. *Radiation therapy of gynecologic cancer.* New York: Alan R. Liss, Inc., 1987:239–249.

3. Fletcher GH. *Textbook of radiotherapy.* Philadelphia: Lea and Febiger, 1980:144–146, 720–773.

4. Kottmeier HL, Gray MJ. Rectal and bladder injuries in relation to radiation dosage in carcinoma of the cervix. *Am J Obstet Gynecol* 1961;82:74–82.

5. LoIudice T, Baxter DO, Balint J. Effects of abdominal surgery on the development of radiation enteropathy. *Gastroenterology* 1977;73:1093–1097.

6. Potish RA. Importance of predisposing factors in the development of enteric damage. *Am J Clin Oncol* 1982;5:189–194.

7. Shibata HR, Freeman CR, Roman TN. Gastrointestinal complications after radiotherapy for carcinoma of the uterine cervix. *Can J Surg* 1982;25:64–66.

8. Unal A, Hamberger AD, Seski JC, Fletcher GH. An analysis of the severe complications of irradiation of carcinoma of the uterine cervix: treatment with intracavitary radium and parametrial irradiation. *Int J Radiat Oncol Biol Phys* 1981;7:999–1004.

9. VanNagell JR, Maruyama Y, Parker JC, Dalton WL. Small bowel injury following radiation therapy for cervical cancer. *Am J Obstet Gynecol* 1974;118:163–167.

10. VanNagell JR, Parker JC, Jr., Maruyama Y, Utley J, Luckett P. Bladder or rectal injury following radiation therapy for cervical cancer. *Am J Obstet Gynecol* 1974;119:727–732.

11. Montana GS, Fowler WC, Varia MA, Walton LA, Mack Y, Shemanski L. Carcinoma of the cervix, stage III. Results of radiation therapy. *Cancer* 1986;57:148–154.

12. Montana GS, Fowler WC, Varia MA, Walton LA, Mack Y. Analysis of results of radiation therapy for Stage II carcinoma of the cervix. *Cancer* 1985;55:956–962.

13. Lanciano RM, Martz K, Montana GS, Hanks GE. Influence of age, prior abdominal surgery, fraction size, and dose on complications after radiation therapy for squamous cell cancer of the uterine cervix. A patterns of care study. *Cancer* 1992;69:2124–2130.

14. Esche BA, Crook MJ, Horiot JC. Dosimetric methods in the optimization of radiotherapy for carcinoma of the uterine cervix. *Int J Radiat Oncol Biol Phys* 1987;13:1183–1192.

15. Quastler H. The nature of intestinal radiation death. *Rad Res* 1956;4:303–320.

16. Tarpila S. Morphological and functional response of human small intestine to ionizing irradiation. *Scand J Gastroenterol Suppl* 1971;6(suppl 12):9–52.

17. Yeoh E, Horowitz M, Russo A, Muecke T, Robb T, Maddox A et al. Effect of pelvic irradiation on gastrointestinal function: a prospective longitudinal study. *Am J Med* 1993;95:397–406.

18. Jervis HR, Donati RM, Stromberg LR, Sprinz H. Histochemical investigation of the mucosa of the exteriorized small intestine of the rat exposed to x-radiation. *Strahlentherapie* 1969;137:326–343.

19. Bourne RG, Kearsley JH, Grove WD, Roberts SJ. The relationship between early and late gastrointestinal complications of radiation therapy for carcinoma of the cervix. *Int J Radiat Oncol Biol Phys* 1983;9:1445–1450.

20. DeCosse JJ, Rhodes RS, Wentz WB, Reagan JW, Dworken HJ, Holden WD. The natural history and management of radiation induced injury of the gastrointestinal tract. *Ann Surg* 1969;170:369–384.

21. Deitel M, Vasic V. Major intestinal complications of radiotherapy. *Am J Gastro-enterol* 1979;72:65–70.

22. Baker DG, Krochak RJ. The response of the microvascular system to radiation: a review. *Cancer Invest* 1989;7:287–294.

23. Buchler DA, Kline JC, Peckham BM, Boone ML, Carr WF. Radiation reactions in cervical cancer therapy. *Am J Obstet Gynecol* 1971;111:745–750.

24. Reeves RJ, Cavanaugh PJ, Sharpe KW, Thorne WA, Winkler C, Sanders AP. Fat absorption studies and small bowel x-ray studies in patients undergoing Co^{60} teletherapy and/or radium application. *Am J Roentgenol* 1965;94:848–851.

25. Deitel M, To TB. Major intestinal complications of radiotherapy. Management and nutrition. *Arch Surg* 1987;122:1421–1424.

26. Hamberger AD, Unal A, Gershenson DM, Fletcher GH. Analysis of the severe complications of irradiation of carcinoma of the cervix: whole pelvis irradiation and intracavitary radium. *Int J Radiat Oncol Biol Phys* 1983;9:367–371.

27. Fajardo L. *Pathology of radiation injury.* New York: Masson, 1982.

28. Smith DH, DeCosse JJ. Radiation damage to the small intestine. *World J Surg* 1986;10:189–194.

29. Russell JC, Welch JP. Operative management of radiation injuries of the intestinal tract. *Am J Surg* 1979;137:433–442.

30. Covens A, Thomas G, DePetrillo A, Jamieson C, Myhr T. The prognostic importance of site and type of radiation-induced bowel injury in patients requiring surgical management. *Gynecol Oncol* 1991;43:270–274.

31. Smith JP, Golden PE, Rutledge FN. The surgical management of intestinal injuries following irradiation for carcinoma of the cervix. In: *Cancer of the uterus and ovary.* University of Texas M.D. Anderson Hospital and Tumor Institute at Houston: Year Book Medical Publishers Inc., 1969:241.

32. Mennie AT, Dalley V. Aspirin in radiation-induced diarrhea. *Lancet* 1973;1:1131.

33. Yeoh EK, Horowitz M. Radiation enteritis. *Surg Gynecol Obstet* 1987;165:373–379.

34. Kinsella TJ, Bloomer WD. Tolerance of the intestine to radiation therapy. *Surg Gynecol Obstet* 1980;151:273–284.

35. Donaldson SS. Nutritional support as an adjunct to radiation therapy. *J Parenter Enteral Nutr* 1984;8:302–310.

36. Schofield PF, Holden D, Carr ND. Bowel disease after radiotherapy. *J R Soc Med* 1983;76:463–466.

37. Allen-Mersh TG, Wilson EJ, Hope-Stone HF, Mann CV. The management of late radiation-induced rectal injury after treatment of carcinoma of the uterus. *Surg Gynecol Obstet* 1987;164:521–524.

38. Dion MW, Hussey DH, Doornbos JF, Vigliotti AP, Wen BC, Anderson B. Preliminary results of a pilot study of pentoxifylline in the treatment of late radiation soft tissue necrosis. *Int J Radiat Oncol Biol Phys* 1990;19:401–407.

39. Deitel M, Syed AK. Elemental diets in management of clinical nutritional problems. *Mod Med Can* 1974;29:471.

40. Donaldson RM, Corrigan H, Natsios G. Malabsorption of Co^{60} labeled

cyanocobalamin in rats with intestinal diverticula. II: Studies on contents of the diverticula. *Gastroenterology* 1962;43:282–290.

41. Yeoh EK, Horowitz M, Russo A, Muecke T, Robb T, Chatterton BE. Gastrointestinal function in chronic radiation enteritis-effects of loperamide-N-oxide. *Gut* 1993;34:476–482.

42. Baillie-Johnson HR. Octreotide in the management of treatment-related diarrhoea. *Anti-Cancer Drugs* 1996;Suppl 1:11–15.

43. Jensen DM, Jutabha R, Machicado GA, Cheng S, CURE Hemostasis Group. Prospective study of patients with severe rectal bleeding from radiation telangiectasia. *Gastrointestinal Endoscopy* 1994;40:abst #320.

44. Hatcher PA, Thomson HJ, Ludgate SN, Small WP, Smith AN. Surgical aspects of intestinal injury due to pelvic radiotherapy. *Ann Surg* 1985;201:470–475.

45. Kochhar R, Mehta SK, Aggarwal R, Dhar A, Patel F. Sucralfate enema in ulcerative rectosigmoid lesions. *Dis Colon Rectum* 1990;3:49–51.

46. Kochhar R, Patel F, Dhar A, et al. Radiation-induced proctosigmoiditis. Prospective, randomized, double-blind controlled trial of oral sulfasalazine plus rectal steroids versus rectal sucralfate. *Dig Dis Sci* 1991;36:103–107.

47. Baum CA, Biddle WL, Miner PB, Jr. Failure of 5-aminosalicylic acid enemas to improve chronic radiation proctitis. *Dig Dis Sci* 1989;34:758–760.

48. Orecchia PM, Hensley EK, McDonald PT, Lull RJ. Localization of lower gastrointestinal hemorrhage. Experience with red blood cells labeled in vitro with technetium 99m Tc. *Arch Surg* 1985;120:621–624.

49. Baum S. Angiography and the gastrointestinal bleeder. *Radiology* 1982;143:569–572.

50. Baum S, Rösch J, Dotter CT, Ring EJ, Athanasoulis C, Waltman AC, Courey WR. Selective mesenteric arterial infusions in the management of massive diverticular hemorrhage. *N Engl J Med* 1973;288:1269–1272.

51. Matolo NM, Link DP. Selective embolization for control of gastrointestinal hemorrhage. *Am J Surg* 1979;138:840–844.

52. Viggiano TR, Zighelboim J, Ahlquist DA, Gostout CJ, Wang KK, Larson MV. Endoscopic Nd : YAG laser coagulation of bleeding from radiation proctopathy. *Gastrointest Endosc* 1993;39:513–517.

53. Hardy JD ed. *Hardy's textbook of surgery.* Philadelphia: J.B. Lippincott Company, 1988:477.

54. Ulin AW, Grotzinger PJ, Shoemaker WC. Experimental closed loop obstruction of the entire colon. *AMA Arch Surg* 1955;71:775–779.

55. Gatch WD, Trusler HM, Lyons RE. Effects of gaseous distention of obstructive bowel: incarceration of the intestine by gas traps. *AMA Arch Surg* 1927;14:1215–1219.

56. Lowmen RM, Davis L. An evaluation of cecal size in impending perforation of the cecum. *Surg Gynecol Obstet* 1956;103:711–718.

57. Cross MJ. Frazer RC: Surgical treatment of radiation enteritis. *Ann Surg* 1992;58:132.

58. Morrow CP, Curtin JP, eds. *Gynecologic Cancer Surgery.* New York: Churchill Livingston, 1996:252–265.

59. Tilson MD. Pathophysiology and treatment of short bowel syndrome. *Surg Clin North Am* 1980;60:1273–1284.

60. McQuarrie DG. Bowel obstruction following abdominal operations. In: McQuarrie DG, Humphrey EW, eds. *Reoperative General Surgery.* St. Louis: Mosby Year Book, 1992:292–326.

61. Sheldon GF. Role of parenteral nutrition in patients with short bowel syndrome. *Am J Med* 1979;67:1021–1029.

62. Bury KD, Stephens RV, Randall HT. Use of a chemically defined, liquid, elemental diet for nutritional management of fistulas of the alimentary tract. *Am J Surg* 1971;121:174–183.

63. Hofmann AF, Poley JR. Role of bile acid malabsorption in pathogenesis of diarrhea and steatorrhea in patients with ileal resection. I. Response to cholestyramine or replacement of dietary long chain triglyceride by medium chain triglyceride. *Gastroenterology* 1972;62:918–934.

64. Galland RB, Spencer J. Spontaneous postoperative perforation of previously asymptomatic irradiated bowel. *Br J Surg* 1985;72:285.

65. Piver MS, Lele S. Enterovaginal and enterocutaneous fistulae in women with gynecologic malignancies. *Obstet Gynecol* 1976;48:560–563.

66. Schmitt EH, Symmonds RE. Surgical treatment of radiation induced injuries of the intestine. *Surg Gynecol Obstet* 1981;153:896–900.

67. Brintnall ES. Surgical treatment of post-irradiation rectal stricture and rectovaginal fistula. *AMA Arch Surg* 1953;67:346–352.

68. Smith DH, Pierce VK, Lewis JL, Jr. Enteric fistulas encountered on a gynecologic oncology service from 1969 through 1980. *Surg Gynecol Obstet* 1984;158:71–75.

69. Reber HA, Roberts C, Way LW, Dunphy JE. Management of external gastrointestinal fistulas. *Ann Surg* 1978;188:460–467.

70. Aguirre A, Fischer JE, Welch CE. The role of surgery and hyperalimentation in therapy of gastrointestinal-cutaneous fistulae. *Ann Surg* 1974;180:393–401.

71. Rose D, Yarborough MF, Canizaro PC, Lowry SF. One hundred and fourteen fistulas of the gastrointestinal tract treated with total parenteral nutrition. *Surg Gynecol Obstet* 1986;163:345–350.

72. Allardyce DB. Management of small bowel fistulas. *Am J Surg* 1983;145:593–595.

73. Halasz NA. Changing patterns in the management of small bowel fistulas. *Am J Surg* 1978;136:61–65.

74. Borison DI, Bloom AD, Pritchard TJ. Treatment of enterocutaneous and colocutaneous fistulas with early surgery or somatostatin analog. *Dis Colon Rectum* 1992;35:635–639.

75. Geerdsen JP, Pedersen VM, Kjaergård HK. Small bowel fistulas treated with somatostatin: preliminary results. *Surgery* 1986;100:811–814.

76. Nubiola P, Badia JM, Martinez-Rodenas F, Gil MJ, Segura M, Sancho J et al. Treatment of 27 postoperative enterocutaneous fistulas with the long half-life somatostatin analogue SMS 201-995 [published erratum appears in Ann Surg 1990 Feb;211(2):246]. *Ann Surg* 1989;210:56–58.

77. Scott NA, Finnegan S, Irving MH. Octreotide and gastrointestinal fistulae. *Digestion* 1990;45(Suppl 1):66–71.

78. Spiliotis J, Briand D, Gouttebel MC, Astre C, Louer B, Saint-Aubert B et al. Treatment of fistulas of the gastrointestinal tract with total parenteral nutrition and octreotide in patients with carcinoma. *Surg Gynecol Obstet* 1993;176:575–580.

79. Torres AJ, Landa JI, Moreno-Azcoita M, Arguello JM, Silecchia G, Castro J et al. Somatostatin in the management of gastrointestinal fistulas. A multicenter trial. *Arch Surg* 1992;127:97–100.

80. Pricolo VE, Shellito PC. Surgery for radiation injury to the large intestine. *Dis Colon Rectum* 1994;37:675–684.

81. Graham JB. Vaginal fistulas following radiotherapy. *Surg Gynecol Obstet* 1965;120:1019–1030.

82. Bricker EM, Johnston WD, Patwardhan RV. Repair of postirradiation damage to colorectum: a progress report. *Ann Surg* 1981;193:555–564.

83. Bricker EM, Kraybill WG, Lopez MJ. Functional results after postirradiation rectal reconstruction. *World J Surg* 1986;10:249–258.

84. Cuthbertson AM. Resection and pull-through for rectovaginal fistula. *World J Surg* 1986;10:228–236.

85. Gazet JC. Parks' coloanal pull-through anastomosis for severe, complicated radiation proctitis. *Dis Colon Rectum* 1985;28:110–114.

86. Parks AG, Allen CLO, Frank JD, McPartlin JF. A method of treating post-irradiation rectovaginal fistulas. *Br J Surg* 1978;65:417–421.

87. White AJ, Buchsbaum HJ, Blythe JG, Lifshitz S. Use of the bulbocavernosus muscle (Martius procedure) for repair of radiation-induced rectovaginal fistulas. *Obstet Gynecol* 1982;60:114–118.

88. Haddad GK, Grodsinsky C, Allen H. The spectrum of radiation enteritis. Surgical considerations. *Dis Colon Rectum* 1983;26:590–594.

89. Galland RB, Spencer J. Surgical aspects of radiation injury to the intestine. *Br J Surg* 1979;66:135–138.

90. Galland RB, Spencer J. The natural history of clinically established radiation enteritis. *Lancet* 1985;1:1257–1258.

91. Berman ML, Lagasse LD, Watring WG, Moore JG, Smith ML. Enteroperineal fistulae following pelvic exenteration: a 10-point program of management. *Gynecol Oncol* 1976;4:368–374.

92. Morgenstern L, Thompson R, Friedman NB. The modern enigma of radiation enteropathy: sequelae and solutions. *Am J Surg* 1977;134:166–172.

93. Galland RB, Spencer J. Surgical management of radiation enteritis. *Surgery* 1986;99:133–139.

94. Cram AE, Pearlman NW, Jochimsen PR. Surgical management of complications of radiation-injured gut. *Am J Surg* 1977;133:551–553.

95. Caraveo J, Trowbridge, AA, White RR. Gangrene of the bowel. *Surg Clin North Am* 1979;59:869.

96. Corman ML, ed. *Colon and rectal surgery.* Philadelphia: Lippincott Company, 1989:717.

97. Docherty JG, McGregor JR, Akyol AM, Murray GD, Galloway DJ. Comparison of manually constructed and stapled anastomoses in colorectal surgery. *Ann Surg* 1995;221:176–184.

98. Anseline PF, Lavery IC, Fazio VW, Jagelman DG, Weakley FL. Radiation injury of the rectum: evaluation of surgical treatment. *Ann Surg* 1981;194:716–724.

99. Smith ST, Seski JC, Copeland LJ, Gershenson DM, Edwards CL, Herson J. Surgical management of irradiation-induced small bowel damage. *Obstet Gynecol* 1985;65:563–567.

100. Swan RW, Fowler WC, Jr., Boronow RC. Surgical management of radiation injury to the small intestine. *Surg Gynecol Obstet* 1976;142:325–327.

101. Donaldson RM. Studies on the pathogenesis of steatorrhea in the blind-loop syndrome. *J Clin Invest* 1965;44:1815–1825.

102. Kim YS, Spritz N, Blum M, Terz J, Sherlock P. The role of altered bile acid metabolism in the steatorrhea of experimental blind loop. *J Clin Invest* 1966;45:956–962.

103. Tabaqchali S. The pathophysiological role of small intestinal bacterial flora. *Scand J Gastroenterol* 1970;(Suppl 6):139–163.

104. Goldstein F. Mechanisms of malabsorption and malnutrition in the blind loop syndrome. *Gastroenterology* 1971;61:780–784.

105. Tabaqchali S, Booth CC. Jejunal bacteriology and bile-salt metabolism in patients with intestinal malabsorption. *Lancet* 1966;2:12–15.

106. Toskes PP, Deren JJ. Vitamin B_{12} absorption and malabsorption. *Gastroenterology* 1973;65:662–683.

107. Dencker H, Holmdahl KH, Lunderquist A, Olivecrona H, Tylen U. Mesenteric angiography in patients with radiation injury of the bowel after pelvis irradiation. *Am J Roentgenol Radium Ther Nucl Med* 1972;114:476–481.

108. Chapman R, Foran R, Dunphy JE. Management of intestinal fistulas. *Am J Surg* 1964;108:157–164.

109. Palmer JA, Bush RS. Radiation injuries to the bowel associated with the treatment of carcinoma of the cervix. *Surgery* 1976;80:458–464.

110. Ballon SC. Effective early postoperative nutrition by defined formula diet via needle-catheter jejunostomy. *Gynecol Oncol* 1982;14:23–32.

111. Johnson LR, Copeland EM, Dudrick SJ, Lichtenberger LM, Castro GA. Structural and hormonal alterations in the gastrointestinal tract of parenterally fed rats. *Gastroenterology* 1975;68:1177–1183.

112. Klimberg VS, Salloum RM, Kasper M, Plumley DA, Dolson DJ, Hautamaki D et al. Oral glutamine accelerates healing of the small intestine and improves outcome after whole abdominal radiation. *Arch Surg* 1990;125:1040–1045.

113. Hwang TL, O'Dwyer ST, Smith RJ et al. Preservation of small bowel mucosa using glutamine enriched parenteral nutrition. *Surg Forum* 1987;38:56.

114. Alverdy JC. Effects of glutamine-supplemented diets on immunology of the gut. *J Parenter Enteral Nutr* 1990;14:109S–113S.

115. Fletcher GH. Clinical dose-response curves of human malignant epithelial tumours. *Br J Radiol* 1973;46:1–12.

116. Pourquier H, Dubois JB, Delard R. Cancer of the uterine cervix: dosimetric guidelines for prevention of late rectal and rectosigmoid complications as a result of radiotherapeutic treatment. *Int J Radiat Oncol Biol Phys* 1982;8:1887–1895.

117. Ellis F, Sorensen A, Lescrenier C. Radiation therapy schedules for opposing parallel fields and their biological effects. *Radiology* 1974;111:701–707.

118. Berman ML, Lagasse LD, Watring WG, Ballon SC, Schlesinger RE, Moore JG et al. The operative evaluation of patients with cervical carcinoma by an extraperitoneal approach. *Obstet Gynecol* 1977;50:658–664.

119. Green N, Iba G, Smith WR. Measures to minimize small intestine injury in the irradiated pelvis. *Cancer* 1975;35:1633–1640.

120. Caspers RJL, Hop WC. Irradiation of true pelvis for bladder and prostatic carcinoma in supine, prone or Trendelenburg position. *Int J Radiat Oncol Biol Phys* 1983;9:589–593.

121. Kavanah MT, Feldman MI, Devereux DF, Kondi ES. New surgical approach to minimize radiation-associated small bowel injury in patients with pelvic malignancies requiring surgery and high-dose irradiation. A preliminary report. *Cancer* 1985;56:1300–1304.

122. DeLuca FR, Ragins H. Construction of an omental envelope as a method of excluding the small intestine from the field of postoperative irradiation to the pelvis. *Surg Gynecol Obstet* 1985;160:365–366.

123. Logmans A, vanLent M, vanGelt AN, Olofsen-VanAcht M, Koper PC, Wiggers T et al. The pedicled omentoplasty, a simple and effective surgical technique to acquire a safe pelvic radiation field; theoretical and practical aspects. *Radiother Oncolol* 1994;33:269–271.

124. Vasilev SA, McGonigle KF, Spencer-Smith EL. Intestinal peritoneal sling as an adjunct to radical pelvic operation and pelvic irradiation. *J Am Coll Surg* 1995;180:568–572.

125. Devereux DF, Kavanah MT, Feldman MI, Kondi E, Hull D, O'Brien M et al. Small bowel exclusion from the pelvis by a polyglycolic acid mesh sling. *J Surg Oncol* 1984;26:107–112.

126. Sugarbaker PH. Intrapelvic prosthesis to prevent injury of the small intestine with high dosage pelvic irradiation. *Surg Gynecol Obstet* 1983;157:269–271.

127. Freund H, Gunderson L, Krause R, Fischer JE. Prevention of radiation enteritis after abdominoperineal resection and radiotherapy. *Surg Gynecol Obstet* 1979;149:206–208.

128. Bounous G. Protection of the gastrointestinal mucosa by elemental diets. *Clin Invest Med* 1980;3:237–244.

129. Copeland EM, Daly JM, Dudrick SJ. Intravenous hyperalimentation, bowel rest, and cancer. *Crit Care Med* 1980;8:21–28.

130. Morgenstern L, Hiatt N. Injurious effect of pancreatic secretions on postradiation enteropathy. *Gastroenterology* 1967;53:923–929.

131. Kinsella TJ, Malcolm AW, Bothe A, Jr., Valerio D, Blackburn GL. Prospective study of nutritional support during pelvic irradiation. *Int J Radiat Oncol Biol Phys* 1981;7:543–548.

132. Solassol C, Joyeux H, Dubois JB. Total parenteral nutrition (TPN) with complete nutritive mixtures: an artificial gut in cancer patients. *Nutr Cancer* 1980;1:13–18.

133. Heusinkveld RS, Manning MR, Aristizabal SA. Control of radiation-induced diarrhea with cholestyramine. *Int J Radiat Oncol Biol Phys* 1978;4:687–690.

134. Niaz SK, Sandrasegaran K, Renny FH, Jones BJ. Postinfective diarrhoea and bile acid malabsorption. *J Royal Col Phys London* 1997;31:53–56.

135. Baughan CA, Canney PA, Buchanan RB, Pickering RM. A randomized trial to assess the efficacy of 5-aminosalicylic acid for the prevention of radiation enteritis. *Clin Oncol (Royal College of Radiologists)* 1993;5:19–24.

136. Resbeut M, Marteau P, Cowen D, Richaud P, Bourdin S, Dubois JB et al. A randomized double blind placebo controlled multicenter study of mesalazine for the prevention of acute radiation enteritis. *Radiother Oncol* 1997;44:59–63.

CHAPTER 18

CHEMOTHERAPY COMPLICATIONS

LEE S. ROSEN, M.D., and GARY J. SCHILLER, M.D., F.A.C.P.

Many advances in the chemotherapy of solid malignancies have occurred since the first drugs were developed during and shortly after the Second World War. In addition to the development of new agents, research seeks new uses and combinations of existing drugs. Diseases uniformly fatal in 1980 are now often curable. Techniques of dose escalation followed by autologous peripheral stem cell or bone marrow transplantation are also promising. There remains a great deal of room for improvement in the treatment of several malignancies. However, knowledge of the potential side effects of the various agents allows for their safe administration.

Cancer chemotherapy has a role in a variety of situations (Level I and Level II evidence). Perhaps a fundamental distinction should be made between treatment given with the intent to cure and the intent to palliate. If the goal of treatment is to cure, every effort must be made to deliver drugs in their appropriate dose and on an appropriate schedule. Patients and their physicians are often willing to tolerate more side effects in such situations. However, if the goal is palliation, other issues can take precedence. For example, toxicities that can interfere with quality of life (severe nausea and vomiting or repeated inpatient hospital stays) may not be acceptable. Doses are often reduced or delayed because of side effects. As always, careful discussion of options with the patient defines the treatment plan. Goals of therapy can change back and forth through the course of the illness.

This chapter presents the more common side effects of cancer chemotherapy. It is organized by system, rather than by drug, to aid the clinician in the diagnosis and treatment of the major toxicities. There is also discussion of the use of chemotherapy during pregnancy, and in the patient with malignant pleural and peritoneal effusions.

Perioperative and Supportive Care in Gynecologic Oncology: Evidence-Based Management,
Edited by Steven A. Vasilev.
ISBN 0-471-24788-X   Copyright © 2000 by Wiley-Liss, Inc.

ALLERGY AND HYPERSENSITIVITY REACTIONS

Hypersensitivity reactions have been seen with nearly every antineoplastic drug, largely reported in case report format as Level III evidence. However, a few drugs warrant special mention either because reactions are common or because these reactions are a major form of treatment-related toxicity. In general, the management of allergies is the same for chemotherapy as with any other drug. Patients who experience mild cutaneous reactions can be treated topically with corticosteroid creams, or if systemic, with antihistamines or antipyretics. Usually, the drug can be used again if absolutely necessary in the treatment plan. Anaphylactic reactions are treated aggressively with antihistamines, corticosteroids, epinephrine, and oxygen. In these cases, the drug should not be used again.

Taxol

In initial therapeutic trials, many patients suffered severe life-threatening hypersensitivity reactions to this drug.[1] The drug vehicle, Cremophor EL, is thought to be the cause.[2] Prophylactic administration of antihistamines (e.g., diphenhydramine 50 mg), H2-antagonists (e.g., ranitidine 150 mg or cimetidine 600 mg), and corticosteroids (e.g., dexamethasone 20 mg) immediately prior to each treatment is now routine (Level III evidence). Three-hour infusions of the drug are now safe, but patients must be observed carefully for signs of allergic reaction. Ten percent of patients still react in some way to the administration of this drug.[3]

L-Asparaginase

Most allergic reactions to this drug are also type I hypersensitivity phenomena. Ten percent to 20% of patients receiving L-asparaginase as part of combination chemotherapy experience symptoms ranging from a rash to anaphylaxis. Test doses and intradermal skin tests, though commonly employed, are not effective, owing to high rates of false positives and false negatives.[4] Supportive medications should always be available during use of this drug.

Anthracyclines

A "flare reaction" is seen with intravenous infusions of these agents.[5] It consists of erythema, pruritus, and urticaria at the local infusion site. This is thought to be a type I hypersensitivity reaction even though it may mimic extravasation injury. Patients can be treated with local measures and the drug can be continued.

Bleomycin

A rare reaction, consisting of high fevers (> 40°C), is not thought to be dose-related. The syndrome is thought to be related to release of endogenous pyrogens and can progress to hypotension and death.[6] Patients with non-Hodgkin's lymphoma are thought to be more susceptible.[7]

Other Agents

Cisplatin and carboplatin cause hypersensitivity reactions in up to 5% of treated patients.[8] Symptoms include anxiety, pruritus, cough, dyspnea, angioedema, rashes, and hypotension, but deaths have never been reported. VM-26 or teniposide also has a 5% to 15% incidence of type I hypersensitivity reactions, which are worse with rapid intravenous infusion of the drug.

CARDIOVASCULAR TOXICITY

Chemotherapy can affect the heart in a number of ways. Reactions can be acute or chronic, mild or deadly. Fortunately, tests exist to monitor patients and prevent some of the more long-term reactions. This section discusses a number of clinical conditions: acute myocarditis/pericarditis, chronic cardiomyopathy, arrhythmias, ischemic heart disease, and a radiation recall myocarditis.

Acute Myocarditis/Pericarditis

Anthracyclines, particularly daunorubicin, can cause a subacute myocarditis/ pericarditis syndrome (there is Level II evidence for this). Cardiotoxicity begins within days or weeks of infusions, is not dose-related, and the incidence is quite rare.[9] Patients may experience sharp chest pains and signs of congestive heart failure. Because of its narrower therapeutic index in terms of myelosuppression and lack of superior efficacy compared to other anthracyclines, daunorubicin is rarely used to treat solid tumors.

Chronic Cardiomyopathy

Cardiomyopathy is by far the most common manifestation of chemotherapy's cardiotoxicities. The anthracycline antibiotics (doxorubicin or adriamycin, daunorubicin, mitoxantrone, and to a lesser extent, idarubicin) account for most cases, but other drugs such as high-dose cyclophosphamide and mitomycin C can damage the heart as well (Level II).[10,11] Mitomycin C, dacarbazine (DTIC), cyclophosphamide, etoposide, vincristine, and bleomycin all can enhance doxorubicin-induced cardiomyopathy.[12,13]

Doxorubicin-induced cardiomyopathy has been well studied. The incidence is quite low (0.1–1.2%) until cumulative doses of 450 mg/m^2 are achieved.[14]

Above 550 mg/m^2 the risk is 10% to 50%. Modifying these risks are other factors such as drug scheduling to allow lower peak plasma levels, and more frequent lower doses or continuous infusions.[15] A prior history of mediastinal radiation, older age or childhood, and malnutrition are all adverse risk factors. Preexisting heart disease or hypertension are thought to be risk factors as well, but this has not been well documented. Clinical trials using doxorubicin usually preclude patients with preexisting heart failure. It seems logical that patients with known ischemic or other types of heart disease should avoid anthracyclines if possible, and if not, they at least should be monitored quite closely.[16]

Most patients beginning a course of anthracycline antibiotics should have a baseline cardiac evaluation (Level III evidence, at best). Both multiple-gated acquisition (MUGA) scans and echocardiograms are helpful in assessing ejection fraction. Once cumulative doses of 450 mg/m^2 of doxorubicin or 160 mg/m^2 of mitoxantrone are reached, ejection fraction should probably be assessed prior to each dose. In the more critically ill patient, such evaluation regardless of cumulative dose would seem appropriate. Endomyocardial biopsy is the gold standard for measuring early cardiotoxicity and could be considered if circumstances merit a pathologic diagnosis. Although some physicians reserve assessment for patients with symptoms, we recommend assessment of left ventricular ejection fraction prior to initiating therapy with an anthracycline and at 300 mg/m^2. Cardio-protectant drugs such as dexrazoxane may be indicated at cumulative doxorubicin doses above 300 mg/m^2 (Level II).

Chemotherapy-induced cardiomyopathy is usually a subacute or chronic process. Patients routinely present with signs of congestive heart failure such as dyspnea, orthopnea, cough, tachycardia, wheezing, volume overload, increased jugular venous pressure, bipedal edema, hepatomegaly, or cardiomegaly. Symptoms can be exacerbated by volume overload, infection, or anemia. The diagnosis is confirmed by assessment of ejection fraction or invasive hemodynamic monitoring. Conventional treatment of congestive heart failure, consisting of afterload reduction with ACE-inhibitors, diuretics, and digitalis, works in this setting too. However, these patients have a lower threshold for developing digitalis toxicity.[17] Dexrazoxane, an EDTA-analog that chelates a generated hydrogen peroxide–iron complex, may help reduce the incidence of cardiomyopathy. Heart muscle lacks the catalase enzyme to detoxify the free radicals generated by anthracyclines.[18] Liposomal doxorubicin delivery is being investigated to reduce cardiotoxicity as well.[19] In any case, in the event of cardiac insufficiency, the inciting agent should be withheld. Development of doxorubicin-induced cardiomyopathy has a 27% to 60% mortality rate.[20]

Cyclophosphamide cardiomyopathy has a similar clinical picture. It appears to be more common in doses typically used in bone marrow or stem cell transplant protocols and is not cumulative. Here, the onset can be more acute and whatever recovery is seen within the first few weeks is often maintained. Treatment is still the treatment of congestive heart failure. Pathologically, this drug causes cardiac necrosis, which of course can be life-threatening.[21] The syndrome is exacerbated by concurrent radiation, and the use of anthracyclines or carmustine (BCNU).

Arrhythmia

Several drugs can cause cardiac rhythm disturbances, most of which do not require stopping the medication (Level III). Cisplatin has been associated with transient electrocardiogram (EKG) changes, such as atrial fibrillation, supraventricular tachycardias, and bundle branch blocks.[22] Taxol can also produce dysrhythmias during infusions. These do not necessarily recur on repeated infusions and cardiac monitoring is not routinely used.[23] Biologic therapies (alpha-interferon and interleukin-2) can lead to rhythm changes mostly by altering intravascular fluid balance.[24]

Most rhythm disturbances associated with chemotherapeutic agents go unnoticed. Patients who become symptomatic can be evaluated by EKG monitoring and treated supportively. Severe episodes, though quite rare, should lead to discontinuing the chemotherapeutic drug.

Ischemic Heart Disease

A few drugs have been associated with a Prinzmetal's type angina, which rarely can lead to myocardial infarction. 5-FU (1.6% incidence, 12.5% mortality), vincristine (3 reported cases), and etoposide (1 reported case) can cause chest pain, and EKG changes associated with ischemia and myocardial infarction.[25,26] Treatment is supportive care and withdrawal of the drug. The incidence of these effects is increased in patients with preexisting coronary artery disease, but because events are so rare, no special precautions are taken prior to initiation of drug therapy.

Radiation Recall

Prior or concurrent use of radiation exacerbates anthracycline cardiotoxicity (Level II). One study demonstrated a 1.6 higher risk if more than 600 rads were previously delivered to the cardiac apex.[27] Mitoxantrone and Actinomycin D can also produce a radiation recall phenomenon.[28,29]

Extravasation Injuries

Certain drugs, if extravasated, are extremely toxic to surrounding soft tissues. Central venous catheters can reduce the incidence of such reactions but do not eliminate it entirely. If extravasation is suspected, the drug should be stopped immediately and the site evaluated carefully. The drugs listed below require special attention. Prompt evaluation and perhaps surgical excision are required.

Anthracyclines

The incidence of extravasations of these drugs is reported to be from 0.5% to 6%, regardless of the type of catheter used.[30] The "flare reaction," a type of hypersensitivity, is often confused for extravasation but need not be managed similarly. Patients in whom the drug leaks into the soft tissues will almost immediately develop pain and swelling at the site. There is usually no blood return at the site, and if not attended to promptly, the site will ulcerate. The physician should try to aspirate as much drug as possible through the suspected line. Prompt surgical excision is often needed, for once ulcerated, the area needing excision can be much larger. Many studies have suggested antidotes to these extravasations, but most have shown no significant improvements. Corticosteroids injected locally may have some effect. Cold packs and the topical application of dimethyl sulfoxide (DMSO; 50% solution, 1.5 cc) every 6 hours for 14 days can reduce the chance of extensive tissue necrosis.[31]

Mechlorethamine

Extravasations of this drug should also be promptly evaluated for surgical excision. Sodium thiosulfate can be used as an antidote. The physician can dilute 4 cc of 10% sodium thiosulfate with 6 cc of sterile water and inject 2 cc into the site for each mg of drug extravasated.[32]

Vinca Alkaloids

Both vincristine and vinblastine can cause severe extravasation injuries. Hyaluronidase, 150 units diluted in 1–3 cc of normal saline, can be injected locally to minimize tissue damage. Warm packs are then applied without pressure.[33]

Gastrointestinal Toxicity

Nearly all agents will cause some gastrointestinal complaints in nearly all patients. Fortunately, several medications exist to ameliorate these problems. This section discusses nausea and vomiting, mucositis, diarrhea and constipation, bleeding, radiation enhancement, and nutritional concerns.

Nausea and Vomiting This side effect is almost universal and many patients are keenly aware of this potential to be uncomfortable. Vomiting is mediated by a center in the lateral reticular formation of the medulla close to the chemoreceptor trigger zone in the area postrema of the fourth ventricle.[34] Chemotherapy drugs, radiation, uremia, and increased intracranial pressure can all lead to vomiting. Chronic vomiting itself can cause dehydration, weakness, malnutrition, electrolyte imbalances, esophageal tears, or wound dehiscences.

Many antiemetic agents are available, with newer ones in clinical trials

(Levels II and III evidence). Most seek to alter neurotransmitters near the chemoreceptor trigger zone in the brain. Available drugs include phenothiazines (e.g., haloperidol, prochlorperazine), substituted benzamides (e.g., metoclopramide), cannabinoids (e.g., ∂-9-THC or Marinol), benzodiazepines (e.g., lorazepam), serotonin receptor antagonists (e.g., ondansetron, granisetron), and corticosteroids.[35] Most chemotherapy-associated nausea can be prevented with proper premedication and judicious use of treatment following chemotherapy administration. Each patient's regimen should be individualized based on her own pattern of symptoms. Side effects of antiemetics, such as dystonic reactions and sedation, can be treated appropriately. Concomitant use of the antihistamine diphenhydramine with high doses of metoclopramide can prevent many dystonic reactions. With severe nausea and vomiting, physicians should rule out other causes besides chemotherapy side effects, such as intracranial tumors or gastrointestinal obstruction. We recommend the prophylactic use of granisetron or ondansetron for highly emetogenic chemotherapy such as cisplatin, carmustine, Decarbazine, or an anthracycline. Drugs with less emetogenic potential such as the antimetabolites may be given with prophylactic metoclopramide or prochlorperazine.

Mucositis   By affecting the most rapidly dividing cells in the body, chemotherapy is toxic to tumors and the lining of the gastrointestinal tract. Patients frequently develop mucositis that can occur anywhere from the mouth to the anus. Conditions include stomatitis, cheilosis, glossitis, esophagitis, gastritis, and colitis. The mouth sores in particular can be debilitating, leading to malnutrition and cachexia. Drugs particularly toxic to the oral mucosa include methotrexate, the antitumor antibiotics (anthracyclines, Actinomycin D, mitoxantrone, mitomycin C), 5-fluorouracil, and the Vinca alkaloids (Level II and III).[36] All drug-induced mucositis is exacerbated by concurrent radiotherapy. There can even be a radiation recall phenomenon in pretreated patients. Concurrent administration of leucovorin ("rescue") alleviates some of methotrexate's effects. Inappropriate dosing in patients with renal or hepatic dysfunction or in patients with potential drug reservoirs, such as pleural effusions or ascites, exacerbates the mucositis. Treatment ranges from local supportive measures to high narcotic doses. Topical anesthetics (e.g., viscous lidocaine) and warm saline rinses are helpful. Physicians should monitor carefully for malnutrition, considering parenteral feeding if prolonged mucositis is expected. Superinfection with *Candida* is also quite common and can be treated with an antifungal agent (e.g., nystatin or fluconazole).

Diarrhea/Constipation   Disorders of gastrointestinal motility are seen with chemotherapy treatment. Patients can develop diarrhea (even bloody) from drug-induced mucositis. Resulting dehydration or malabsorption often requires intravenous hydration or feeding. Treatment ranges from mild over-the-counter medications to prescription-strength diphenoxylate atropine or tincture of opium. Octreotide has been studied in severe chemotherapy-induced diarrhea;

50–100 mcg subcutaneously twice daily often eliminated the need for hospitalization or intravenous rehydration (Level II).[37]

Autonomic dysfunction can lead to constipation or ileus. Vincristine commonly causes decreased bowel motility and some patients are hospitalized for obstructions. These reactions are rarely fatal.[38] Patients being treated with this drug could be placed on stool softeners prophylactically.

Gastrointestinal Bleeding/Perforation   Tumors themselves can lead to gastrointestinal bleeding. Chemotherapy-induced severe thrombocytopenia will rarely cause hemorrhage. Lymphoma patients with small-bowel disease have a higher risk of perforation in areas responding to treatment.[39]

Radiation Recall   As with other organ systems, certain drugs can elicit radiation recall. Treatment with anthracyclines or Actinomycin D enhances toxicity from prior radiation.[40] Concurrent treatment enhances toxicity as well. Oral cavity radiation produces mucositis and a sicca-like syndrome while abdominal radiation can lead to severe diarrhea, gastrointestinal bleeding, and fistula formation.[41]

Nutrition   Both chemotherapy agents and tumors themselves can lead to malnutrition and cachexia. Attention to nutritional status is essential while treating the cancer patient. Mucositis, nausea, vomiting, and diarrhea can enhance weight loss. Loss of the sense of taste from many drugs is common as well. Calorie supplementation with rich foods or commercial products is a first step. Appetite stimulants such as megestrol acetate (Megace, available in elixir format) or ∂-9-THC (Marinol) have been shown to increase weight (Level I).[42a,42b] Finally, tube enteral feeding and hyperalimentation are available methods for the extremely malnourished patient. Marinol should be used, however, with some care, especially if lorazepam or other benodiazepines are given.

HEPATOTOXICITY

Many patients undergo chemotherapy treatment with some degree of hepatic dysfunction. Drugs that are metabolized by the liver must be dosed appropriately. Other drugs actually cause hepatotoxicity. Issues discussed in this section include liver function test abnormalities, cirrhosis, dosing in patients with liver disease, and hepatic veno-occlusive disease.

Liver Function Test Abnormalities

Cancer patients have many reasons to have liver function test abnormalities. These include drug and toxin effects, metastases, preexisting liver disease, infections, and other comorbid conditions. Baseline screening is essential. The spectrum of clinical manifestations ranges from silent laboratory abnormalities to hepatic necrosis and cirrhosis. Drug effects should be diagnoses of exclusion.

The nitrosourea agents commonly alter liver function tests (incidence of 26%).[43] Ara-C is also a frequent cause of transient and asymptomatic changes.[44] In neither case should the drug be stopped for mild changes. In one study of gestational trophoblastic disease patients, methotrexate had a 14% incidence of transaminase elevation and increased lactic dehydrogenase (LDH).[45] This effect is reversible; however, with chronic therapy (e.g., rheumatologic diseases), the drug can cause fibrosis or cirrhosis.[46] Etoposide, alpha-interferon, actinomycin D and vincristine (the latter two especially with concurrent hepatic radiotherapy) are also associated with transient and reversible changes in liver function tests.[47–49]

Only a few drugs can cause symptomatic hepatotoxicity. Platinum in standard doses is associated with steatosis and cholestasis.[50] Rare patients treated with DTIC can have a syndrome of acute hepatic failure leading to circulatory shock and death.[51]

Dosing in Patients with Hepatic Dysfunction

An understanding of which drugs are metabolized by the liver is helpful in making dosing decisions. The anthracyclines (e.g., doxorubicin, daunorubicin, mitoxantrone) and the vinca alkaloids are mainly cleared in the hepatic circulation. In patients with bilirubin levels greater than 1.5, doses of these drugs should be reduced at least 50%. Cyclophosphamide, methotrexate, and 5-fluorouracil should be dose-reduced in patients with bilirubin levels greater than 3.0. Hepatotoxic drugs should be avoided where possible, with attention paid to non–chemotherapy drugs given to patients. If such drugs must be used, they should be dosed appropriately and the patients followed expectantly. If hepatic metastases are the cause of the dysfunction, chemotherapy can actually improve liver function.

Veno-Occlusive Disease of the Liver

This syndrome is a nonthrombotic obliteration of small intrahepatic veins by reticulin and collagen thickening.[52] Patients present with right upper quadrant pain, ascites or unexplained weight gain, jaundice, and hepatomegaly. Radionuclide scanning or computerized tomography (CT) is helpful in diagnosis, and liver biopsy can be confirmatory. Many agents can cause this syndrome—conventional doses of carboplatin, DTIC, actinomycin D, and ara-C and high doses of busulfan, cyclophosphamide, BCNU, and mitomycin C. Various drug combinations, particularly those used to condition for bone marrow transplantation, have also been implicated.[53] The offending agents should be stopped immediately and patients supported. The mortality rate of patients with veno-occlusive disease of the liver ranges from 10% to 50%.[54]

HEMATOLOGIC TOXICITY

Both chemotherapy drugs and underlying malignancies can affect the hematopoietic system and clotting mechanisms, making it difficult to assess the relative contribution of treatment to hematologic problems. Some reactions are typical to chemotherapy and are discussed in this section, along with a general discussion of the management of marrow toxicity and bleeding.

Bone Marrow Suppression

Nearly all chemotherapy drugs suppress the bone marrow. Tumor involvement of the marrow itself can produce a similar picture that could paradoxically improve with treatment. Myelosuppression due to chemotherapy is often a dose-limiting side effect and plays a significant role is determining drug combinations, drug scheduling, and dosing. Only a few drugs such as alkylating agents and nitrosoureas affect all cell lines simultaneously. The drugs, in a predictable fashion, produce myelosuppression, allowing for repeated dosing on schedule.[55] Host factors can influence the severity of myelosuppression as well. Hepatic or renal dysfunction, the presence of effusions or ascites, and bioavailability may produce prolonged exposure to high levels of the drug. Genetic enzyme systems affecting drug metabolism, changes in serum albumin, or concomitant medication can also change toxicity profiles.[56]

Anemia is usually a late side effect of chemotherapy drugs, owing to the relatively long red cell life span of 120 days. In the short term, this is effectively managed with red cell transfusions. If chronic anemia becomes a problem during or after repeated courses of chemotherapy, erythropoietin can be used (Level I). Doses of 5,000–10,000 units subcutaneously three to five times weekly are helpful, but it takes 1 to 2 weeks before the drug begins to work. Routine use of this agent is quite costly, requires concurrent iron and folate therapy, and may not work in patients with high levels of the circulating endogenous hormone.[57] As with other conditions, other causes of anemia must be ruled out before ascribing it to chemotherapy toxicity. We recommend checking an erythropoietin level in cancer patients with anemia (Hgb $\leq$ 9.0 gb/L). If the level is below 100 and other causes of anemia have been excluded, the patient may benefit from a 2- to 4-week trial of erythropoietin.

Thrombocytopenia occurs with most drugs, but may be delayed and protracted following treatment with nitrosourea and busulfan.[58] Low platelets may produce mild petechiae or life-threatening parenchymal hemorrhages. Transfusion guidelines for thrombocytopenia in a nonbleeding patient are quite controversial. Most now agree that the risk of severe bleeding increases below a platelet count of 10,000 mm^{-3}.[59] Patients become allosensitized to repeated transfusions and may require HLA-matched platelets. The use of the staph A immunoabsorption column has been tried for alloimmunized platelet transfusion-refractory patients.[60] Surgery should be avoided in patients with platelet counts less than 50,000 mm^{-3}.[61] Future research into platelet growth such as thrombopoietin may be promising. A new drug, interleukin-11, has been licensed for chemotherapy-induced thrombocytopenia.

Neutropenia is almost universal with cytotoxic chemotherapeutic agents. Drug doses often need to be modified or scheduling delayed in response to neutropenia, particularly in heavily treated patients. The advent of recombinant neutrophil growth factors such as G-CSF and GM-CSF has revolutionized chemotherapy administration (Level I). These agents, administered subcutaneously on a daily basis, shorten the duration and often the severity of neutropenia in most patients.[62] Their use is warranted in heavily pretreated patients or in patients who have had previous complications attributable to neutropenia (fevers, etc.). Routine use is not cost-effective.[63] Use in the febrile neutropenic patient has not been firmly established. However, in critically ill neutropenic patients, use of growth factors can be considered. In experimental models, the use of growth factors has been shown to improve healing and hasten recovery.[64] No randomized trial has been done to date documenting the effectiveness of routine use in the infected patient. Side effects include fever, bone pain, exacerbation of inflammatory conditions, and a capillary leak syndrome caused by neutrophil pooling in the pulmonary vasculature.[65] We recommend the use of either G-CSF or GM-CSF for patients whose neutrophil count predictably falls below $500–1,000 \text{ mm}^{-3}$ and who have had an episode of febrile neutropenia during a previous cycle of chemotherapy.

Hemolytic Uremic Syndrome

Mitomycin C can cause a syndrome of microangiopathic hemolytic anemia, thrombocytopenia, and renal dysfunction. In 4% to 15% of patients, cumulative doses greater than 60 mg of the drug may produce mortality in as many as 50% of patients.[66] Conventional management involves supportive measures, plasmapheresis, and the use of a Staphylococcus protein A immunoabsorption column.[67]

Coagulopathy

Few drugs actually produce symptomatic coagulopathy, but bleeding problems may develop as a result of underlying malignancy, sepsis, or drug-induced thrombocytopenia. L-asparaginase, used for acute lymphocytic leukemia, is associated with an increased risk of thromboses despite a paradoxical hypofibrinogenemia.[68,69]

INFECTIOUS DISEASE COMPLICATIONS OF CHEMOTHERAPY

Nearly all chemotherapy drugs are myelosuppressive. White blood counts will drop and cause immune suppression. In addition, many drugs can interfere with proper leukocyte functioning.[70] The prevention of potentially fatal outcomes due to infection involves patient education, search for offending organisms, observation for secondary infection, and broad empiric coverage. The major issues in this arena are discussed in this section along with a brief mention of line infections and the use of hematopoietic growth factors.

Neutropenia is the single most important risk factor for infection.[71] Though risk is greatest when patients have less than 100 neutrophils per cubic millimeter, it is still quite high with levels less than 500 neutrophils per cubic millimeter. Other risk factors include the duration of neutropenia, phagocyte dysfunction (worse with certain malignancies and with chemotherapy administration), altering natural defense barriers (breaks in the skin or mucous membranes), and the status of the patient's immune system.[72] Toxicity profiles of most drugs are known, so approximate risks and timing of neutropenia can be predicted. Patients who are heavily pretreated with cytotoxic agents will become neutropenic faster and remain so longer. Inappropriate dosing in patients with renal or hepatic dysfunction will exacerbate hematologic toxicity as well.

Treating any patient with cytotoxic or immunosuppressive agents requires careful education about infectious disease prevention. All patients should be instructed to avoid contact with others who may have infections. Those coming into contact with the patient or who may prepare their food should observe careful hand-washing techniques. This is true in both the inpatient and the outpatient setting. Patients should seek prompt medical attention whenever they have a single fever of $38.5°C$ or greater or three measurements of $38°C$ or greater in a 24-hour period. Proper cultures should be taken and intravenous antibiotics to cover a broad range of infections should begin immediately (see below).

Predominant infections in neutropenic patients during the 1960s and 1970s were gram-negative aerobic organisms (especially *Pseudomonas aeruginosa*, *Escherichia coli*, and *Klebsiella pneumoniae*) and gram-positive organisms (e.g., streptococcus and *Staphylococcus aureus*).[73] In the more recent past, incidence of *Pseudomonas* infection has decreased and infection with coagulase-negative staphylococcus, alpha-hemolytic streptococcus, and *Enterobacter* has increased.[74] Efforts to reduce incidence of infection with protected environments in hospitals, such as laminar flow rooms, have been largely abandoned owing to their expense and relative lack of efficacy.[75] Gut decontamination with antibiotic prophylaxis is also controversial, with most reserving its use for the dose intensification or bone marrow transplant setting.[76]

The work-up of the febrile neutropenic patient requires careful history and physical examinations daily. As one infection clears, another can develop, requiring the modification of the treatment plan. Multiple cultures of appropriate sites, including peripheral blood, urine, sputum, and stool, are taken where appropriate. Neutropenic patients will not have a peripheral blood leukocytosis or pyuria in most cases. Radiographic examinations are directed to suspected sites of infection. Ultrasound or CT examination of the abdomen can be helpful in looking for potential abscess sites and lumbar puncture, or CT/MRI of the brain demonstrates infection there. Patients should be promptly hospitalized for the initiation of broad-spectrum antibiotics. Ideally, antibiotics are begun as soon as the patient arrives at the hospital or clinic rather than waiting for lengthy evaluation or test results.

Initial choice of antibiotics should be suitable for expected infections. This depends greatly on community organisms and sensitivities. Most agree that an extended-spectrum penicillin and third-generation cephalosporin or aminoglycoside are the best choices.[77] Adding vancomycin empirically offers no survival advantage unless there is a high prevalence of methicillin-resistant *Staphylococcus aureus* (MRSA) in the community.[78] Antibiotics should continue until the patient defervesces and has evidence of a rising neutrophil count. Those in whom a source of infection is identified should probably be treated longer. Even when a culture becomes positive, the physician should hesitate to narrow antibiotic coverage. Patients who remain neutropenic are susceptible to secondary infections, which can be fatal if coverage is too narrow.[79]

The cause of fever is not identified in 60% to 70% of cases.[80] In those whose fever persists on broad-spectrum antibiotics, coverage should be broadened. Vancomycin is helpful in those with indwelling catheters. Antifungal therapy is started after 5 to 7 days of prolonged fever. Despite its toxicity, amphotericin B remains the best choice, though studies are being done to evaluate liposomal delivery of the drug or use of fluconazole.[81,82] Antiviral therapy is helpful in those with culture-positive or suspected herpes virus or cytomegalovirus infection.

Line Infections

Indwelling catheters are frequently used in patients undergoing chemotherapy. Their use allows for easier drug administration, laboratory testing, and the minimization of extravasation injury. However, lines destroy the natural skin barrier against infection. Both neutropenic and nonneutropenic patients are at increased risk of infection. The most common organisms are those of normal skin flora—coagulase-negative staphylococcus, *Staphylococcus aureus*, corynebacteria, and gram-negative organisms.[83] *Candida* is a potential problem as well. Cultures from the line as well as the peripheral blood are taken if infection is suspected. Most line infections are safely treated with antibiotics given through the line. In multilumen catheters, the antibiotic should be rotated among the different ports in case only one is infected proximally.[84]

At times, line infections cannot be eradicated. If this is the case, the catheter should be promptly removed. *Candida* infections carry a high risk of dissemination and catheters should be removed.[85] Tunnel infections require catheter removal regardless of the offending organism[86] The type of catheter does not affect the infection rate, so choice depends on purpose of use or patient preference.[87]

Use of Growth Factors

The development of hematopoietic growth factors has helped to decrease the number of patients hospitalized for neutropenic fevers. Cumulative dose and on-time scheduling are improved as well. Agents such as granulocyte colony-stimulating factor (G-CSF) and granulocyte-macrophage colony-stimulating factor (GM-CSF) decrease the incidence of neutropenia and shorten its duration (Level I).[88] One of these agents should be given with subsequent cycles when a patient has had a neutropenic fever or when drug scheduling has to be altered because of severe myelosuppression. It has not been shown to be cost-effective to administer growth factors routinely in all patients getting chemotherapy. Any patient who has been heavily pretreated with cytotoxic agents or who requires prompt treatment and is already leukopenic is a candidate for growth factor use. Neither GCSF nor GM-CSF has beneficial effects on red blood cell or platelet counts.

Neurotoxicity

Several chemotherapy drugs can cause neurologic problems. Their spectrum is quite broad, ranging from transient, mild reactions to severe disabilities. One of the biggest problems in this arena is determining the origin of neurologic conditions in the cancer patient. Complications of cancers themselves affect the central nervous system (CNS). Primary CNS tumors, metastases from other sites, infections caused by immunosuppression, and paraneoplastic syndromes all affect this system. Vascular disease, coagulopathy, and thrombocytopenia-induced hemorrhage all occur. Interactions between various drugs, chemotherapeutic and others, and comorbid conditions can combine to affect the CNS as well.

With newer treatment modalities, newer neurologic sequelae are occurring.[89] Multiagent chemotherapy and multimodality therapy can lead to synergistic effects on the CNS. High-dose therapies, bypassing some of their systemic toxicities with the use of growth factors, bring out previously unseen neurologic damage. Chemotherapy agents directed toward the CNS (intracarotid, intrathecal, or direct intracranial delivery methods) have different toxicity profiles, too.

This section deals with some of the more common effects on the central nervous system. Peripheral neuropathy, encephalopathy, cerebellar toxicity, ototoxicity, and psychiatric effects are discussed. The potential complications of intrathecal therapy are detailed as well.

Peripheral Neuropathy

Peripheral neuropathies occur commonly with chemotherapy use. Three often-used drugs, vincristine, cisplatin, and taxol, cause some form of damage in most patients. Unless disabling, the development of symptoms is not a cause for stopping the drug. Neurotoxicity is dose related and eventually the treatment plan will need to be modified. Vincristine, a plant-derived Vinca alkaloid, causes an almost universal peripheral neuropathy. Patients complain of numbness or tingling in the extremities. Physical exam first reveals loss of the ankle deep tendon reflex, which progresses to complete areflexia, distal symmetric sensory loss, motor weakness, and muscle atrophy. Up to 30% of patients will also have some form of autonomic neuropathy manifested with ileus, urinary retention, impotence, or postural hypotension.[90] Neurotoxicity is reversible, though recovery can take a long time. Steroids and the coadministration of oral glutamic acid have been used to treat the symptoms in a number of patients with only limited success.[91]

Cisplatin is associated with a similar distal symmetric polyneuropathy, though its incidence is more rare.[92] It is dose related and cumulative. Concurrent administration of vincristine and etoposide can exacerbate the nervous system effects.[93] Cisplatin is not used in dose intensification protocols because of this neurotoxicity. Carboplatin causes less damage to the CNS. Taxol is another agent that produces a dose-limited peripheral polyneuropathy. It often requires change in the treatment plan for an affected patient. 5-Fluorouracil and hexamethylmelamine are more rarely associated with these side effects.

Encephalopathy

Altered mental status is a vague symptom. Infections, metabolic disturbances, tumors, and drugs all can cause a panencephalopathy. Other causes must be ruled out before ascribing symptoms to drug effects. Nevertheless, many chemotherapy agents produce diffuse neurologic signs. High-dose methotrexate (doses greater than 1 g/m^2) can produce an acute stroke-like syndrome. Patients can have confusion, seizures, or hemiparesis and in 15% of cases they become comatose.[94] These doses are used in some sarcoma therapy protocols. Inappropriate dosing in the patient with renal failure can lead to the same constellation of symptoms, owing to inadequate drug excretion. With prolonged used of even lower doses, patients can have permanent personality changes or dementia due to leukoencephalopathy. High doses of 5-fluorouracil and BCNU produce rare cases of encephalopathy.[95,96]

Ifosfamide also causes a dose- and schedule-related encephalopathy. Patients can become disoriented and somnolent in response to high doses of the drug, continuous infusions, or inappropriate dosing with renal insufficiency.[97] Five percent of patients who receive continuous infusions of the drug can become comatose and develop seizures, cerebellar abnormalities, or cranial neuropathies.[98] Treatment of all these reactions is stopping the drug and supportive care.

Other drugs associated with encephalopathic reactions are the biologic therapies, interferon and interleukin-2, and hexamethylmelamine.[99,100] The use of cisplatin in a patient with CNS disease requires special mention as well. Fluid shifts from excess hydration, diuretic use, and metabolic disturbances can cause encephalopathy, leading to herniation and death.

Cerebellar Toxicity

High-dose ara-C (particularly greater than 18 $g/m^2/cycle$) is frequently associated with cerebellar toxicity. Onset of symptoms can occur immediately after drug infusion or several days later.[101] Patients develop nystagmus, ataxia, dysarthrias, and rarely can have seizures or become comatose. Symptoms usually spontaneously improve within 1 week and resolve 1 or 2 weeks after that. Treatment consists of stopping the drug and supportive care. 5-Fluorouracil also can produce a rapid-onset ataxia, nystagmus, dysarthria, and diplopia. This condition is dose related, rare, and reversible.[102]

Ototoxicity

Cisplatin, and to a lesser extent, carboplatin, cause irreversible ototoxicity.[103] A sensorineural hearing loss due to loss of cochlear hair cells is common, dose related, and cumulative (Level II). Children and patients receiving concurrent cranial radiation appear to be at greater risk. Patients with a baseline hearing loss or those receiving extended courses of the drug should be monitored often with audiograms. If hearing loss develops, the drug should be stopped. The concurrent use of other ototoxic medications should be avoided.

Psychiatric Effects

As with encephalopathy, psychiatric disturbances are common in cancer patients undergoing chemotherapy. The diseases themselves, intracranial tumors or infections, and other medications can produce mind-altering effects. Prolonged hospitalization, particularly in the elderly, quite often produces a delirium.

Steroids are used as cytotoxic agents, antiemetic prophylaxis, or therapy for a chemotherapy side effect. As in any population, steroids can cause mood elevation or depression, insomnia, and resting tremors. Increasing or decreasing the steroid dose can exacerbate the mood swings as well.

Antiemetic therapy, particularly the phenothiazines (haloperidol or Compazine) and the substituted benzamide metoclopramide, has a high dose-related incidence of dystonic reactions. Concurrent or therapeutic use of antihistamines usually eliminates the problem. Delirium is treated with sedatives or phenothiazines.

Side Effects of Intrathecal Therapy

Three drugs, methotrexate, ara-C, and to a lesser extent, thiotepa, are the most commonly used intrathecal agents. They are generally well tolerated. Methotrexate can cause an acute chemical meningitis.[104] Patients develop fever, headache, and nuchal rigidity, and a cerebrospinal fluid leukocytosis is also detected. Treatment is conservative once infection has been eliminated as the cause. A delayed or progressive leukoencephalopathy is seen.[105] Ara-C and thiotepa similarly cause an acute chemical meningitis, with a similar constellation of symptoms.[106,107] Both drugs cause reactions less commonly than with methotrexate. Rarely, all three drugs cause a myelopathy with intrathecal administration.[108,109]

PULMONARY TOXICITY

Several drugs can affect the lungs. These reactions can be mild or life-threatening and can occur immediately after drug delivery or several years later. This section discusses four quite common reactions: interstitial pneumonitis/pulmonary fibrosis, noncardiogenic pulmonary edema, hypersensitivity pneumonitis, and a radiation recall phenomenon.

Interstitial Pneumonitis/Pulmonary Fibrosis

Chemotherapy-induced pneumonitis can be acute or occur months to years after treatment (Level II). Typically, patients will present with dyspnea on exertion, a nonproductive cough, and perhaps a fever. Further evaluation usually reveals an interstitial infiltrate on chest X ray, although alveolar airspace disease can occur. Abnormal pulmonary function tests consist of decreased vital capacity, decreased lung volumes, and a decreased diffusing capacity of carbon monoxide (DLCO).[110] When a patient presents with these symptoms and signs, it is often difficult to differentiate between drug-induced or radiation-induced pneumonitis, infection, pulmonary hemorrhage from drug-induced thrombocytopenia, and progressive or metastatic disease. The work-up, which can lead to open lung biopsy, depends on the severity and timing of symptoms and the goals of therapy.

Bleomycin is associated with a subacute or chronic pneumonitis that can progress to fatal pulmonary fibrosis. It can be idiosyncratic or dose dependent, with incidence markedly increasing above lifetime doses greater than 450 units.[111] Approximately 10% of patients treated with this drug develop pulmonary sequelae (range 0–50%) and mortality is thought to be 1% to 2%.[112] Other risk factors include age greater than 70, prior chest radiation, concurrent use of high oxygen concentrations, renal dysfunction, and bolus intravenous infusional use. Patients with lymphoma, for unknown reasons, appear to be more susceptible.[113]

The nitrosoureas, particularly BCNU, can cause dose-related pneumonitis as well. There is a 30% to 50% incidence at doses greater than 1,500 mg/m^2 (usually reserved for dose-intensification programs) and 20% incidence at lower doses.[114] Concurrent use of high-dose cyclophosphamide may potentiate pulmonary complications at lower doses as well.[115] Other alkylating agents such as chlorambucil (14 reported cases) and busulfan (incidence) can cause pneumonitis.[116,117] Busulfan is often used in conditioning regimens for autologous and allogeneic bone marrow and peripheral stem cell transplantation. Since pulmonary symptoms may occur long after the initial drug exposure (6 weeks to 3 years on average), clinicians need to follow patients expectantly. Mitomycin C can produce a non-dose-related pneumonitis (incidence 3–36%) that may occur after the first dose or up to 1 year afterward.[118] There appears to be an interaction with cyclophosphamide, radiation, and high concentrations of oxygen. Because of the high risk of pulmonary toxicity with specific agents, researchers have tried to develop early detection programs. For bleomycin, screening of pulmonary function tests has not proven useful.[119] Periodic DLCO (diffusion capacity of carbon monoxide) testing has been helpful in some settings, though not sensitive in most.[120,121] After giving these drugs, patients could be placed on an exercise program (however limited) and instructed to report immediately any change in exercise tolerance. The physician should be cautious with any surgical procedure in a patient who has received a pulmonary-toxic drug. To the extent feasible, high concentrations of oxygen should be avoided as they can exacerbate an undiagnosed pneumonitis.

Clinically, most types of chemotherapy-induced pneumonitis look similar and diagnosis and treatment are the same. In an immediate drug reaction, the drug should be stopped and steroids given. However, most cases of pneumonitis will mimic sepsis or disease progression. Infection should be ruled out rapidly, with appropriate cultures or serologies. Bronchoalveolar lavage (BAL) with biopsy can be helpful. In the immunocompromised patient, infection with rarer organisms such as cytomegalovirus, *Pneumocystis carinii*, *Legionella*, and fungi should be considered. If patients worsen on broad-spectrum antibiotics and BAL is nondiagnostic, an open-lung biopsy can be considered. Chemotherapy-induced pneumonitis is a diagnosis of exclusion and many tests are done to ensure a patient is not infected. The eventual treatment, once a diagnosis is suspected or confirmed, is corticosteroids. Doses range from 1 mg/kg of prednisone as an outpatient to high intravenous doses in the rapidly failing inpatient. Steroids are to be continued for at least a few months, with slow tapering. The pneumonitis can progress to fibrosis and permanent damage (if not death) if diagnosis is delayed or even despite aggressive treatment. Lung transplantation has even been employed successfully in one case.[122]

Noncardiogenic Pulmonary Edema

With all the intravenous hydration that chemotherapy patients often receive, this diagnosis is difficult to make, but a few drugs actually do produce non-cardiogenic pulmonary edema, presumably via a capillary leak phenomenon. Ara-C, used mainly in the treatment of hematologic malignancies, can produce pulmonary edema as well as pleural, pericardial, and peritoneal effusions.[123] Occurring 2 to 21 days after treatment, symptoms include cough, dyspnea, or even respiratory failure. The overall incidence ranges from 5% to 30% and is dose-related. Adult respiratory distress syndrome (ARDS) develops in 16% of cases, and mortality is 10%.[124] High doses of solumedrol may improve the condition, but oftentimes supportive care alone is all that works.[125] Cyclophosphamide and methotrexate have rarely been associated with a capillary leak syndrome.[126,127]

GM-CSF, a neutrophil growth factor often used with chemotherapy, can produce pulmonary edema, pleural and pericardial effusions. Symptoms can begin 2 to 6 hours after the first dose and are caused by a pooling of neutrophils in the pulmonary vasculature.[128]

Biologic therapy with interleukin-2 quite commonly causes a life-threatening syndrome of respiratory failure, hypotension, pulmonary and peripheral edema (Level II).[129] Careful attention to fluid status and strict hemodynamic monitoring can help prevent the need for mechanical ventilation. If respiratory failure supervenes, patients must be supported until the drug wears off.

Hypersensitivity Pneumonitis

Methotrexate, used for many tumors including sarcomas and gestational trophoblastic disease, is also used for rheumatologic conditions. In less than 1% (range 1–8%) of treated patients, a hypersensitivity pneumonitis develops.[130] Patients develop cough, dyspnea, and pleuritic chest pain of rapid or gradual onset. Chest X ray reveals peripheral pulmonary consolidation, hilar or paratracheal adenopathy (mimicking sarcoidosis), and infrequent diffuse nodular-interstitial pneumonitis (20% of cases).[131] Open-lung biopsy reveals eosinophilic infiltrates. Steroids can be helpful in the treatment; however, this does not imply that the pneumonitis is allergic as patients can be safely rechallenged with the drug.[132] If another treatment can be used, the methotrexate should be discontinued. Rarely, bleomycin and procarbazine can cause the same clinical picture.[133,134]

Radiation Recall

Anthracyclines (particularly doxorubicin [Adriamycin] and daunorubicin) and actinomycin D (used often for gestational trophoblastic disease) can produce lung toxicity with prior or concurrent radiation.[135] The symptoms can range from mild cough and dyspnea to ARDS and can extend beyond the radiation field. Treatment is mainly supportive, but steroids may also be useful.

RENAL TOXICITY

Chemotherapy can affect the kidneys in several ways. In addition, patients may have some kidney damage before even starting treatment. Careful baseline monitoring and precautions taken along the way can mitigate many potential problems. This section discusses acute renal failure, electrolyte abnormalities, uric acid nephropathy and tumor lysis syndrome, hemorrhagic cystitis, and the syndrome of inappropriate antidiuretic hormone (SIADH).

Acute Renal Failure

Many drugs are nephrotoxic. Others, excreted through the kidneys, will remain active longer in the circulation and produce enhanced systemic toxicity if patients have underlying renal dysfunction. Transient rises in serum creatinine commonly occur and chronic renal failure may result. Baseline assessment of renal function is required prior to initiating a chemotherapy regimen. Glomerular filtration rate (GFR), though often estimated with a serum creatinine level, is best assessed by a 24-hour urine collection for creatinine clearance. Serum creatinine levels are often inaccurate in the elderly and the malnourished.[136] Proximal tubular function can be assessed via the urinalysis dipstick measurements of pH, glucose, and protein. Distal tubular function and renal tubular acidoses are assessed via total urine volume.[137]

Cisplatin is a frequently used nephrotoxic drug that can produce acute and chronic renal failure, proximal and distal tubular defects (Levels II and III). Without adequate pretreatment hydration, patients can develop an acute and usually reversible oliguria, azotemia, and increase in serum creatinine. The more chronic and potentially irreversible complication, a decrease in glomerular filtration rate (GFR), can be initially undetectable.[138] Various methods have been tried to prevent the nephrotoxicity of cisplatin; none are uniformly successful. Amifostene and thiol compounds, such as sodium thiosulfate, can be given concurrently with high intra-arterial or intraperitoneal platinum doses to protect the kidneys. Sodium thiosulfate cannot be used with routine intravenous platinum as it inactivates the drug.[139,140] Avoiding use of other nephrotoxic medications where possible, such as aminoglycoside antibiotics and nonsteroidal anti-inflammatory drugs, is critical. Carboplatin a related agent with similar antitumor profile is much less nephrotoxic but more myelosuppressive.[141]

Adequate hydration should precede any administration of cisplatin. Depending on the given dose, 1–2 L of normal saline followed by mannitol or Lasix should suffice. The drug itself is usually diluted in large amounts of fluid and 1–2 L of normal saline is supplemented with potassium, and magnesium is given afterward. Patients should be encouraged to drink adequate fluids, which should be no problem with proper antiemetic use. In patients with existing renal failure, cisplatin should be avoided. If carboplatin or other agents are not useful, cisplatin can be used in reduced doses. Fifty-percent dosing is recommended for patients with creatinine clearances of 30–60 ml/min.[142] Patients with single kidneys are not at increased risk for developing nephrotoxicity.[143] In those with renal failure caused by an obstructing mass, treatment can actually improve renal function. Should renal failure develop as a result of cisplatin, the drug should be stopped and the patient supported. Dialysis may be necessary but often will not reverse the renal dysfunction.

Other drugs that are potentially nephrotoxic are high doses of nitrosourea (BCNU/CCNU). They may produce renal failure months to years after treatment.[144] Interleukin-2, presumably via an induced prerenal azotemia, can cause acute and chronic renal failure.[145] Mitomycin C, particularly in cumulative doses greater than 60 mg/m^2, can lead to acute renal failure via a drug-induced vasculitis. This hemolytic uremic syndrome is treated with plasma exchange and supportive care. Mild proximal tubular defects can be seen with ifosfamide and do warrant stopping the drug.[146] Methotrexate is not directly nephrotoxic but is excreted by the kidney.[147] The drug may precipitate in an acidic environment, producing tubular obstruction. In patients with decreased renal function, methotrexate's effects are potentiated. Dialysis is useful to support patients but will not eliminate the drug.

Electrolyte Abnormalities

Again, cisplatin is the most common offender. Hypomagnesemia, apparently caused by a proximal tubular defect, can be symptomatic in up to 10% of patients.[148] Severe hypomagnesemia can lead to hypocalcemia or hypokalemia as well. Careful monitoring of electrolytes around infusion days usually eliminates serious problems.

Uric Acid Nephropathy/Tumor Lysis Syndrome

Certain rapidly growing tumors and tumors exquisitely sensitive to chemotherapy lead to excess uric acid production. The uric acid can precipitate in the distal tubules, particularly with acidified urine. The ensuing nephropathy presents clinically as uremia and sometimes acute renal failure. A large tumor mass or large cell burden of a highly proliferative non-Hodgkin's lymphoma or acute leukemia can be associated with spontaneous uric acid nephropathy. Treatment can cause a tumor lysis syndrome with the first cycle of chemotherapy.[149] Solid tumors rarely can cause a tumor lysis syndrome as well.[150]

The best treatment for tumor lysis is prevention by vigorous hydration and alkalization of the urine. Allopurinol is used prior to therapy initiation to inhibit uric acid synthesis. Once tumor lysis occurs, signs of nephropathy such as hyperkalemia, hyperphosphatemia, hyperuricemia, and hypocalcemia may require dialysis to support patients through the acute episode.

Hemorrhagic Cystitis

Ifosfamide and cyclophosphamide are associated with hemorrhagic cystitis. The mechanism is thought to be a toxic effect on the bladder by one of the drug's metabolites, acrolein.[151] Symptoms include pain, dysuria, hesitancy, and urgency. Patients can have gross or microscopic hematuria, leading to significant blood loss. Again, prevention is the best treatment. Either continuous bladder irrigation for up to 24 hours after the completion of the drug with a triple-lumen Foley catheter or the systemic use of Mesna (sodium 2-mercaptoethane sulfonate) is effective (Level I). In a study comparing the two means of protection, no significant difference was seen in the frequency or severity of cases of hemorrhagic cystitis.[152] Mesna is obviously more practical and can be given intravenously or orally in doses equal to the chemotherapy drug dose. Patients should be encouraged to increase fluid intake around times of drug administration. Urinalyses can be checked to monitor for microscopic hematuria. The drug should be stopped in patients who develop symptoms and bladder fulguration is available for uncontrolled bleeding or clots.

Syndrome of Inappropriate Antidiuretic Hormone (SIADH)

Both cyclophosphamide and vincristine rarely cause SIADH manifested by hyponatremia and decreased urine output.[153,154] Serum and urine osmolarity will be out of balance. Stopping the drug usually eases the problem. For vincristine, fluid restriction is also helpful. However, fluid restriction for a patient receiving cyclophosphamide can lead to hemorrhagic cystitis. If hyponatremia due to excess SIADH persists, a work-up for otherwise occult hypothyroidism and hypoadrenal cortisolism is in order.

CHEMOTHERAPY USE DURING PREGNANCY

Fortunately, malignancies occur only rarely during pregnancy. The most common tumors are those that can occur in young women—lymphoma, leukemia, melanoma, and carcinomas of the cervix, breast, ovary, thyroid, and colon.[155] Decisions to treat malignancies involve ethical considerations and careful attention to the curability of the tumor. This section discusses generally the effects of chemotherapy on both the mother and the fetus rather than treatment recommendations for particular tumors (generally Level III evidence).

Doll et al. has examined extensively the incidence of chemotherapy effects during pregnancy.[156] Single-agent regimes cause severe congenital malformations in 17% of first-trimester-treated patients. This figure jumps to 25% for combination regimens. When folate antagonists (e.g., methotrexate) were excluded, only 6% of fetuses were affected by single agents. In the second and third trimester, only 3 of 110 pregnancies studied had congenital abnormalities. But during these periods, growth retardation and impaired physical and mental development are more common. Toxicities of the individual drugs, myelosuppression, and secondary alopecia can be transmitted across the placenta. Chemotherapy and radiation can cause primary premature ovarian failure, leading to future sterility as well.

When cure is a reasonable goal, treatment must be initiated as soon as possible. Delays could lead to maternal death, as in acute leukemias, or to disease spread, which could reduce chances for cure. If the mother's ethical system allows, abortion should be considered if chemotherapy is needed during the first trimester. If not, antimetabolites (e.g., Ara-C, 5-fluorouracil, and hydroxyurea) and folate antagonists (e.g. methotrexate) are to be avoided. Doxorubicin and the Vinca alkaloids are perhaps less teratogenic. Used later in the pregnancy, single-agent chemotherapy is safer than combination treatment.[157,158]

Intraperitoneal and oral chemotherapy agents should be avoided during pregnancy, owing to erratic absorption. Drugs that can accumulate in extracellular spaces (e.g., methotrexate) should not be used either. At least 3 to 4 weeks should be allowed between the last treatment and delivery to ensure sufficient red blood cell and platelet recovery.[158]

Breast-feeding should be discouraged in mothers receiving chemotherapy. Drugs are identified in the breast milk and therefore can transmit their toxicities.[159]

CHEMOTHERAPY FOR PLEURAL EFFUSIONS

Pleural effusions can be the first manifestation of malignancy or the first sign of a recurrence. When diagnosed, 75% of patients with pleural effusions will have respiratory symptoms.[160] Initial management is a diagnostic thoracocentesis. Symptomatic patients will require drainage of the effusion either via large-volume thoracocentesis or chest tube placement. Chemical pleurodesis can be helpful with recurrent symptomatic effusions, though often fluid will reaccumulate anyway. At times, chemotherapy or radiotherapy directed at the underlying malignancy can be helpful as well. This section reviews the use of chemical pleurodesis in treating malignant pleural effusion. Further technical considerations are covered in Chapter 3.

Tetracycline/Doxycycline

These antibiotics are commonly used as sclerosing agents. Tetracycline, in doses of 500 mg-1 g diluted in 30–50 cc of normal saline has a 45% complete response rate.[161] Adverse side effects are pain on injection through the chest tube and fever. However, the agent is no longer available in many centers, owing to halted drug production. Doxycycline, a related agent, is administered in doses of 500 mg diluted in 30–50 cc of normal saline. Prophylactic lidocaine injected through the chest tube can prevent associated pain. Indwelling time is 2–6 hours with the patient lying flat. Complete response rates of 50–72% have been reported, but patients may require up to four separate doses.[162]

Bleomycin

This antitumor agent has been used effectively for chemical pleurodesis in doses of 1 mg/kg. Indwelling time is similarly 2–6 hours with patients lying flat. Side effects include pain, fever, and nausea. As there is up to a 45% absorption into the circulation, patients who have been pretreated with bleomycin or who have underlying pulmonary disease should be watched carefully.[163] Elderly patients should receive no more than 40 mg at a time. Complete response rates of 548 have been reported with this agent. In the only study randomizing patients with pleural effusions to receive either tetracycline or bleomycin, the latter agent was significantly better. Recurrence rates at 30 days were 67% with tetracycline and 36% for bleomycin ($p = 0.023$), and at 90 days, 53% and 30%, respectively ($p = 0.047$).[164] Bleomycin is significantly more expensive, however (average wholesale price $1,104 vs. $86–$403 for doxycycline).[165]

Talc

Administration of talc via thoracoscopy or a "talc slurry" via the chest tube is also effective chemical pleurodesis. A total of 2.5–10 g of talc in 250 cc of normal saline was administered to 165 patients, with a 93% complete response rate. Side effects were pain, fever, and 3 reports of an acute respiratory distress–like syndrome.[166]

Prophylactic local anesthesia is required. However, talc costs approximately $12 per administration. Given similar efficacy and significant cost advantage, it may represent the agent of choice.[167]

Other Chemotherapeutic Agents

Many other drugs have been used for chemical pleurodesis with varying degrees of success. Cisplatin, 100 mg/m^2, given along with adequate intravenous hydration and sodium thiosulfate, showed only a 16% complete response rate. Side effects were severe, including nausea and vomiting, myelosuppression, and local pain.[168] 5-Fluorouracil, 2–3 g, was used in 35 patients. There was a 66% chance of improvement, with few, if any, side effects.[169] Mitoxantrone, 25–30 mg intrapleurally, was associated with a 50% to 75% response rate, with a 37% recurrence rate within 3 months.[170]

INTRAPERITONEAL CHEMOTHERAPY

Peritoneal effusions occur with many malignancies, particularly with cancers of the ovary and gastrointestinal tract and with peritoneal mesotheliomas. Control of ascites is usually with medical management—diet control, diuretics, and abdominal paracenteses. Occasionally, the use of intraperitoneal chemotherapy can be helpful as well. This section discusses briefly the rationale behind this type of chemotherapy use.

Intraperitoneal administration of chemotherapy seeks to deliver higher concentrations of drug without major systemic side effects. The delivered drug should also exert its antitumor effects for a longer period of time than if the drug were given intravenously. The choice of drug depends on several principles outlined by Markman.[171] Each drug should demonstrate sensitivity against a tumor and a dose-response relationship. The pharmacokinetics of the drug should allow it to remain within the peritoneum without significant systemic absorption. Local side effects should be minimal and the patient should have no mechanical barriers to peritoneal administration of the drug. Those with multiple adhesions or prior abdominal surgeries are often not candidates for intraperitoneal drug use. Thus, CT or nuclear medicine scans are often helpful in defining anatomy.

It appears that the best candidates for intraperitoneal drug use are those with responsive but minimally residual disease. Extensive tumor bulk does not respond as well. Patients with high-grade ovarian cancers and complete surgical remissions are candidates as well, owing to their high risk of relapse.

Many drugs have been studied in intraperitoneal regimens. Cisplatin, one of the most effective agents against ovarian cancer, is useful because of its dose-response relationship. Local side effects are minimal, but high doses will cause systemic effects. The concurrent use of sodium thiosulfate to negate systemic toxicities allow for greater dose delivery but has not demonstrated a response or survival advantage.[172] 5-Fluorouracil can produce local irritation but is effective, as are melphalan, hexamethylmelamine, doxorubicin, and mitoxantrone.

REFERENCES

1. Rowinsky EK, Onetto N, Canetta RM, et al. Taxol: the first of the taxanes, an important new class of antitumor agents. *Semin Oncol* 1992;19:646–662.

2. Runowicz CD, Wiernik PH, Einzig AI, et al. Taxol in ovarian cancer. *Cancer* 1993;71:159–166.

3. Arbuck SG, Christian MC, Fisherman JS, et al. *Clinical Development of Taxol.* Monographs of the National Cancer Institute 15. 1993, pp. 11–24.

4. Evans WE, Tsiatis A, Rivera G, et al. Anaphylactoid reactions to *E. coli* and *Erwinia asparaginase* in children with leukemia and lymphoma. *Cancer* 1982;49:1378–1383.

5. Vogelzang NJ. Adriamycin flare: a skin reaction resembling extravasation. *Cancer Treatment Reports* 1979;63:2067–2069.

6. Carter JJ, McLaughlin ML, Bern MM. Bleomycin-induced fatal hyperpyrexia. *Am J Med* 1983;74:523–525.

7. Quigley H, Brada M, Heron C, Horwich A. Severe lung toxicity with weekly low dose chemotherapy regimen in patients with non-Hodgkins lymphoma. *Hematol Oncol* 1988;6(4):319–324.

8. Von Hoff DD, Schilsky R, Reichert CM, et al. Toxic effects of cis-dichlorodiammineplatinum (II) in man. *Cancer Treatment Reports* 1979;63:1527–1531.

9. Bristow MR, Thompson PD, Martin RP, et al. Early anthracycline cardiotoxicity. *Am J Med* 1978;65:823–882.

10. Buzdar MR, Legha SS, Tashima CK et al. Adriamycin and mitomycin C: possible synergistic cardiotoxicity. *Cancer Treatment Reports* 1978;62:1005–1008.

11. Braverman AC, Antin JH, Plappert MT, et al. Cyclophosphamide cardiotoxicity in bone marrow transplantation: a prospective evaluation of new dosing regimens. *J Clin Oncol* 1993;9:1215–1223.

12. Beretta B, Villani F. Cardiomyopathy in adults after combination Adriamycin and DTIC. *Cancer Treatment Reports* 1980;64:353 (letter).

13. Praga C, Beretta G, Vigo PL, et al. Adriamycin cardiotoxicity: a survey of 1273 patients. *Cancer Treatment Reports* 1979;63:827–834.

14. Basser RL, Green MD. Strategies for prevention of anthracycline cardiotoxicity. *Cancer Treatment Reviews* 1993;19:57–77.

15. Carlson RW. Reducing the cardiotoxicity of the anthracyclines. *Oncology* 1992;6:95–100.

16. Allen A. The cardiotoxicity of chemotherapeutic drugs. *Semin Oncol* 1992;19:529–542.

17. Riegger GA. Lessons from recent randomized controlled trials for the management of congestive heart failure. *Am J Cardiol* 1993;71:38E–40E.

18. Hershko C, Link G, Tzahor M, et al. The role of iron and iron chelators in anthracycline toxicity. *Leukemia and Lymphoma* 1993;11:207–214.

19. Booser DJ, Hortobagyi GN. Anthracycline antibiotics in cancer therapy: focus on drug resistance. *Drugs* 1994;47:223–258.

20. Von Hoff DD, Layard MW, Basa P, et al. Risk factors for doxorubicin induced congestive heart failure. *Ann Intern Med* 1979;91:710–717.

21. Ayash LJ, Wright JE, Tretyakov O. Cyclophosphamide pharmacokinetics: correlation with cardiac toxicity and tumor response. *J Clin Oncol* 1992;10:995–1000.

22. Jeremic B, Jevremovic S, Djuric L, et al. Cardiotoxicity during chemotherapy treatment with 5-FU and cisplatin. *J Chemother* 1990;2:264–267.

23. Rowinsky EK, McGuire WP, Guarnieri et al. Cardiac disturbances during the administration of taxol. *J Clin Oncol* 1991;9:1704–1712.

24. Sonnenblick M, Rosin A. Cardiotoxicity of interferon. A review of 44 cases. *Chest* 1991;99:557–561.

25. Keefe DL, Roistacher N, Pierri MK. Clinical cardiotoxicity of 5-fluorouracil. *J Clin Pharmacol* 1993;33:1060–1070.

26. Allen A. The cardiotoxicity of chemotherapeutic drugs. In *The Chemotherapy Source Book*. Baltimore: Williams and Wilkins, 1992, pp. 583–597.

27. Bristow MR, Mason JW, Billingham ME, et al. Doxorubicin cardiomyopathy: evaluation by phonocardiography, endomyocardial biopsy, and cardiac catheterization. *Ann Intern Med* 1978;88:168–175.

28. Faulds D, Balfour JA, Chrisp P, et al. Mitoxantrone: a review of its pharmacodynamic and pharmacokinetic properties in the chemotherapy of cancer. *Drugs* 1991;41:400–449.

29. Corder MP, Flannery EF. Possible radiation pericarditis caused by actinomycin D. *Oncology* 1974;30:81–84.

30. Laughlin RA, Landeen JM, Habal MB. The management of inadvertent subcutaneous adriamycin infiltration. *Am J Surg* 1979;137:408–412.

31. Lebredo L, Barrie R, Weltering EA. DMSO protects against adriamycin-induced tissue necrosis. *J Surg Res* 1992;53:62–65.

32. Dorr RT. Antidotes to vesicant chemotherapy extravasations. *Blood Rev* 1990;4:41–60.

33. Bertelli G, Dini D, Forno GB, et al. Hyaluronidase as an antidote to the extravasation of vinca alkaloids: clinical results. *J Cancer Res Clin Oncol* 1994;120:505–506.

34. Mitchell EP, Schein PS. Gastrointestinal toxicity of chemotherapeutic agents. In *The Chemotherapy Source Book*, Baltimore: Williams and Wilkins, 1992, pp. 620–634.

35. Grunberg SM, Hesketh PJ. Drug therapy: control of chemotherapy-induced emesis. *New Engl J Med* 1993;329:1790–1796.

36. Sonis S, Clark J. Prevention and management of oral mucositis induced by antineoplastic therapy. *Oncology* 1991;5:11–18.

37. Cascinu S, Fedeli A, Fedeli SL, et al. Octreotide vs loperamide in the treatment of fluorouracil-induced diarrhea. *J Clin Oncol* 1993;11:148–155.

38. Rosenthal S, Kaufman S. Vincristine neurotoxicity. *Ann Intern Med* 1993;80:733–737.

39. Ehrlich AN, Stalder G, Gellew W, et al. The gastrointestinal manifestations of malignant lymphoma. *Gastroenterology* 1968;54:1115–1121.

40. Phillips TL, Wharam MD, Margolis LW. Modification of radiation injury to normal tissues by chemotherapeutic agents. *Cancer* 1975;35:1678–1684.

41. Henriksson R, Lomberg R, Israelsson G, et al. The effect of ondansetron on radiation-induced emesis and diarrhea. *Acta Oncologica* 1992;31:767–769.

42a. Vadell C, Segui MA, Gimenez-Arnau JM, et al. Anticachectic efficacy at megestrol acetate at different doses and versus placebo in patients with neoplastic cachexia. *Am J Clin Oncol* 1998;21:347–351.

42b. Beal JA. Appetite effect at dronabinol. *J Clin Oncol* 1994;12:1524–5.

43. DeVita VT, Carbone PP, Owens AH Jr, et al. Clinical trials with 1,3-bis (2-chloroethyl)-1-nitrosourea. *J Cancer Res* 1965;25:1876–1881.

44. Kremer WB. Cytarabine. *Ann Intern Med* 1975;82:684–688.

45. Berkowitz RS, Goldstein DP, Bernstein MR. Ten years' experience with methotrexate and folinic acid as primary therapy for gestational trophoblastic disease. *Gynecol Oncol* 1986;23:111–118.

46. Weinstein GD. Methotrexate. *Ann Intern Med* 1977;86:199–204.

47. Tran A, Housset C, Boboe B, et al. Etoposide (VP 16-213)-induced hepatitis. Report of three cases following standard dose treatments. *J Hepatol* 1991;2:36–39.

48. Raine J, Bowman A, Wallendszus K, et al. Hepatopathy-thrombocytopenia syndrome—a complication of dactinomycin therapy for Wilms' tumor. *J Clin Oncol* 1991;9:268–273.

49. Saghir NS, Hawkins KA. Hepatotoxicity following vincristine therapy. *Cancer* 1984;54:2006–2008.

50. Cersosimo RJ. Hepatotoxicity associated with cisplatin chemotherapy. *Ann Pharmacother* 1993;27:438–441.

51. Sutherland CM, Krementz ET. Hepatic toxicity of DTIC. *Cancer Treatment Rept* 1981;65:321–322.

52. Perry MC. Chemotherapeutic agents and hepatotoxicity. *Semin Oncol* 1992;19:551–565.

53. Shulman HM, Hinterberger W. Hepatic veno-occlusive disease—liver toxicity syndrome after bone marrow transplantation. *Bone Marrow Transplantation* 1992;10:197–214.

54. Rollins BJ. Hepatic veno-occlusive disease. *Am J Med* 1986;81:297–306.

55. Calabresi P, Parks R Jr. Antiproliferative agents and drugs used for immunosuppression. In Gilman AG, Goodman LS (Eds), *The Pharmacological Basis of Therapeutics.* New York: Macmillan Publishing Co., Inc., pp. 1256–1313.

56. Gastineau DA, Hoagland HC. Hematologic effects of chemotherapy. *Semin Oncol* 1992;19:543–550.

57. Henry DH, Abels RI. Recombinant human erythropoietin in the treatment of cancer and chemotherapy-induced anemia: results of double-blind and open-label follow-up studies. *Semin Oncol* 1994;21:21–28.

58. Wasserman TH, Slavik M, Carter SK. Clinical comparison of the nitrosureas. *Cancer* 1975;36:1258–1268.

59. Rosen PJ. Bleeding problems in the cancer patient. *Hematol Oncol Clin N Am* 1992;6:1315–1328.

60. Christie DJ, Howe RB, Lennon SS, et al. Treatment of refractoriness to platelet transfusion by protein A column therapy. *Transfusion* 1993;33:234–242.

61. Taylor KM. Perioperative approaches to coagulation defects. *Ann Thoracic Surg* 1993;56:S78–82.

62. Antman KS, Griffin JD, Elias A, et al. Effect of recombinant human granulocyte-macrophage colony-stimulating factor on chemotherapy-induced myelosuppression. *New Engl J Med* 1988;319:593–598.

63. Winston DJ. Prophylaxis and treatment of infection in the bone marrow transplant recipient. *Curr Clin Topics Infect Dis* 1993;13:293–321.

64. O'Reilly M, Silver GM, Greenhalgh DG, et al. Treatment of intra-abdominal infection with granulocyte colony-stimulating factor. *J Trauma* 1992;33:679–682.

65. Herrmann F, Schulz G, Lindemann A. Hematopoietic responses in patients with advanced malignancy treated with recombinant human granulocyte-macrophage colony-stimulating factor. *J Clin Oncol* 1989;7:159–167.

66. Rothschild N, Erickson B, Sisk B, et al. Cancer-associated hemolytic uremic syndrome: analysis of 85 cases from a National Registry. *J Clin Oncol* 1989;7:781–789.

67. Snyder HW Jr, Mittelman A, Oral A et al. Treatment of cancer chemotherapy-associated thrombotic thrombocytopenic purpura/hemolytic uremic syndrome by protein A immunoadsorption of plasma. *Cancer* 1993;71:1882–1892.

68. Haskell CM, Canellos GP, Leventhal BG, et al. L-asparaginase: therapeutic and toxic effects in patients with neoplastic disease. *New Engl J Med* 1969;281:1028–1034.

69. Whitecar JP Jr, Bodey GP, Harris JE, et al. L-asparaginase. *New Engl J Med* 1970;282:732–734.

70. Maraninchi D. The clinical consequences of hematological and non-hematological toxicity following bone marrow transplantation and the possible impact of hematopoietic growth factors. *Bone Marrow Transplantation* 1993;11:12–22.

71. Bodey GP, Rodriguez V, Chang H-Y, et al. Fever and infection in leukemic patients: a study of 494 consecutive patients. *Cancer* 1978;41:1610–1622.

72. Pizzo PA. Management of fever in patients with cancer and treatment-induced neutropenia. *New Engl Med* 1993;328:1323–1332.

73. Schimpff SC, Young VM, Greene WH, et al. Origin of infection in acute non-lymphocytic leukemia: significance of hospital acquisition of potential pathogens. *Ann Intern Med* 1972;77:707–714.

74. Pizzo PA, Ladisch S, Simon RM, et al. Increasing incidence of gram-positive sepsis in cancer patients. *J Med Pediatr Oncol* 1978;5:241–244.

75. Pizzo PA. Considerations for the prevention of infectious complications in patients with cancer. *Rev Infect Dis* 1989;11:81551–81563.

76. Bodey GP, Rodriguez V, Cabanillas F, et al. Protected environment-prophylactic antibiotic program for malignant lymphoma: randomized trial during chemotherapy to induce remission. *Am J Med* 1979;66:74–81.

77. Pizzo PA, Thaler M, Hathorn J, et al. New beta-lactam antibiotics in granulocytopenic patients: new options and new questions. *Am J Med* 1985;79:75–82.

78. Karp, JE, Dick JD, Angelopulos C, et al. Empiric use of vancomycin during prolonged treatment-induced granulocytopenia: randomized, double-blind, placebo-controlled clinical trial in patients with acute leukemia. *Am J Med* 1986;81:237–242.

79. Pizzo PA. After empiric therapy: what to do until the granulocyte comes back. *Rev Infect Dis* 1987;9:214–219.

80. Pizzo PA. Evaluation of fever in the patient with cancer. *Eur J Cancer Clin Oncol* 1989;25:S9–S16.

81. Schmitt HJ. New methods of delivery of amphotericin B. *J Clin Infect Dis* 1993;17:8501–8506.

82. Fraser IS, Denning DW. Empiric amphotericin B therapy: the need for a reappraisal. *Blood Rev* 1993;7:208–214.

83. Bonawitz SC, Hammell EJ, Kirkpatrick JR. Prevention of central venous catheter sepsis: a prospective randomized trial. *Am Surg* 1991;57:618–623.

84. Goodman JL, Winston DJ, Greenfield RA, et al. A controlled trial of fluconazole to prevent fungal infections in patients undergoing bone marrow transplantation. *New Engl J Med* 1992;326:845–851.

85. Lecciones JA, Lee JW, Navarro EE, et al. Vascular catheter-associated fungemia with cancer: analysis of 155 episodes. *J Clin Infect Dis* 1992;14:875–883.

86. Wadhwa NK, Cabralda T, Suh H, et al. Exit-site/tunnel infection and catheter outcome in peritoneal dialysis patients. *Adv Peritoneal Dialysis* 1992;8:325–327.

87. Mueller BU, Skelton J, Callender DP, et al. A prospective randomized trial comparing the infectious and noninfectious complications of externalized catheter versus a subcutaneously implanted device in cancer patients. *J Clin Oncol* 1992;10:1943–1948.

88. Groopman J, Molina J-M, Scadden D. Hematopoietic growth factors: biology and clinical applications. *New Engl J Med* 1989;321:1449–1459.

89. MacDonald DR. Neurologic complications of chemotherapy. *Neurol Clin N Am* 1991;9:955–967.

90. Postma TJ, Benard BA, Huijgens PC, et al. Long-term effects of vincristine on the peripheral nervous system. *J Neura-Oncol* 1993;15:23–27.

91. Jackson DV, Wells HB, Atkins JN, et al. Amelioration of vincristine neurotoxicity by glutamic acid. *Am J Med* 1988;84:1016.

92. Roelofs RI, Hrushesky W, Rogin J, et al. Peripheral sensory neuropathy and cisplatin chemotherapy. *Neurology* 1984;34:934–938.

93. MacDonald DR. Neurotoxicity of chemotherapeutic agents. In Peny MC (Ed), *The Chemotherapy Source Book*. Baltimore: Williams and Wilkins, pp. 666–679.

94. Allen JC, Rosen G. Transient cerebral dysfunction following chemotherapy for osteogenic sarcoma. *Ann Neurol* 1978;3:441–444.

95. Moore DH, Fowler WC, Crumpler LS. 5-Fluorouracil neurotoxicity. *Gynecol Oncol* 1990;36:152–154.

96. Phillips GL, Wolff SN, Pay JW, et al. Intensive 1, 3-bis (2-chloroethyl)-1-nitrosurea (BCNU) monochemotherapy and autologous marrow transplantation for malignant glioma. *J Clin Oncol* 1986;4:639–645.

97. Antman KH, Elias A, Ryan L. Ifosfamide and Mesna: Response and toxicity at standard and high-dose schedules. *Semin Oncol* 1990;17:68.

98. Miller LJ, Eaton VE. Ifosfamide-induced neurotoxicity: a case report and review of the literature. *Ann Pharmacother* 1992;26:183–187.

99. Manetta A, MacNeill C, Lyter JA, et al. Hexamethylmelamine as a second-line agent in ovarian cancer. *Gynecol Oncol* 1990;36:93.

100. Demicoff KD, Rubinow DR, Papa MZ, et al. The neuropsychiatric effects of interleukin-2/lymphokine activated killer cell treatment. *Ann Intern Med* 1987;107:293–300.

101. Herzig RH, Hines JD, Herzig GP, et al. Cerebellar toxicity with high-dose cytosine arabinoside. *J Clin Oncol* 1987;5:927–932.

102. Riehl JB, Brown WJ. Acute cerebellar syndrome secondary to 5-FU therapy. *Neurology* 1964;14:961–967.

103. Schweitzer VG. Ototoxicity of chemotherapeutic agents. *Otolaryngol Clin N Am* 1993;26:759–789.

104. Nakagawa H, Murasaw A, Kubo S, et al. Diagnosis and treatment of patients with meningeal carcinomatosis. *J Neuro-Oncol* 1992;13:81–89.

105. Allen JC, Rosen G, Mehta BM, et al. Leukoencephalopathy following high-dose IV methotrexate chemotherapy with leucovorin rescue. *Cancer Treatment Rept* 1980;64:1261–1273.

106. Resar, LM, Phillips PC, Kastan MB, et al. Acute neurotoxicity after intrathecal cytosine arabinoside in two adolescents with acute lymphoblastic leukemia of B-cell type. *Cancer* 1993;71:117–123.

107. Gutin PH, Levi JA, Wiernik PH, et al. Treatment of malignant meningeal disease with intrathecal thiotepa: a phase II study. *Cancer Treatment Rept* 1977;61:885–887.

108. Martin Algarra S, Henriquez I, Rebollo J, et al. Severe polyneuropathy and motor loss after intrathecal thiotepa combination chemotherapy: description of two cases. *Anti-Cancer Drugs* 1990;1:33–35.

109. Breuer AC, Pitman WS, Dawson NM, et al. Paraparesis following intrathecal cytosine arabinoside. *Cancer* 1977;40:2817–2822.

110. Wesseliue LJ. Pulmonary complications of cancer therapy. *Comprehensive Ther* 1992;18:17–20.

111. Kreisman H, Wolkove N. Pulmonary toxicity of antineoplastic therapy. In Perry MC (Ed), *The Chemotherapy Source Book*. Baltimore: Williams and Wilkins, 1992, pp. 598–619.

112. Cooper AD, White DA, Matthay RA. State of the art. Drug-induced pulmonary disease. *Am Rev Respir Dis* 1986;133:321–340.

113. Comis RL. Bleomycin pulmonary toxicity: current status and future direction. *Semin Oncol* 1992;19:64–70.

114. Phillips GL, Pay JW, Herzig GP, et al. Intensive 1,3-bis (2-chloroethyl)-1-nitrosourea (BCNU) and cryopreserved autologous bone marrow transplantation for refractory cancer. *Cancer* 1992;52:1792–1802.

115. Moormeier JA, Williams SF, Kaminer LS. High-dose tri-alkylator chemotherapy with autologous stem cell rescue in patients with refractory malignancies. *J Nat Cancer Inst* 1990;82:29–34.

116. Carr ME. Chlorambucil-induced pulmonary fibrosis: report of a case and review. *Virginia Med* 1986;113:677–680.

117. Miller H, Schwartz R, Rubio F, et al. Interstitial pulmonary fibrosis following busulfan therapy. *Am J Med* 1961;31:134–139.

118. Doll DC, Weiss RB, Issell B. Mitomycin: ten years after approval for marketing. *J Clin Oncol* 1985;3:276–286.

119. Comis RL. Detecting bleomycin pulmonary toxicity: a continued conundrum. *J Clin Oncol* 1990;8:765–767.

120. McKeage MJ, Evans BD, Atkinson C, et al. Carbon monoxide diffusing capacity is a poor predictor of clinically significant bleomycin lung. *J Clin Oncol* 1990;8:779–783.

121. Sorenson PG, Rossing N, Rorth M. Carbon monoxide diffusing capacity: a reliable indicator of bleomycin-induced pulmonary toxicity. *Eur J Respir Dis* 1985;66:333–340.

122. Santamauro JT, Stover DE, Jules-Elysee K, et al. Lung transplantation for chemotherapy-induced pulmonary fibrosis. *Chest* 1994;105:310–312.

123. Anderson BS, Cogan BM, Keating MJ, et al. Subacute pulmonary failure complicating therapy with high-dose ara-C in acute leukemia. *Cancer* 1985;56:2181–2184.

124. Jehn U, Goldel N, Rienmuller R, et al. Non-cardiogenic pulmonary edema complicating intermediate and high-dose ara-C treatment for relapsed acute leukemia. *Med Oncol Tumor Pharmacother* 1988;5:4147.

125. Jehn U, Goldel N, Rienmuller B, et al. Noncardiogenic pulmonary edema complicating intermediate and high-dose ara-C treatment for relapsed acute leukemia. *J Med Oncol Tumor Pharmacother* 1988;5:4147.

126. Maxwell I. Reversible pulmonary edema following cyclophosphamide treatment. *J Am Med Assoc* 1974;229:137–138.

127. Nesbit M, Krivit W, Heyn R, et al. Acute and chronic effects of methotrexate on hepatic, pulmonary, and skeletal systems. *Cancer* 1976;37:1048–1054.

128. Stern AC, Jones TC. The side-effect profile of GM-CSF. *Infection* 1992;20:5124–5127.

129. Gaynor ER, Vitek L, Sticklin L, et al. The hemodynamic effects of treatment with interleukin-2 and lymphocyte-activated killer cells. *Ann Intern Med* 1988;109:953–958.

130. Sostman HD, Matthay RA, Putman CE et al. Methotrexate-induced pneumonitis. *J Med* 1976;55:371–388.

131. Everts CS, Westcott JL, Bragg DG. Methotrexate therapy and pulmonary disease. *J Diagnos Radiol* 1973;107:539–543.

132. Clarysse AM, Cathey WJ, Cartwright GE, et al. Pulmonary disease complicating intermittent therapy with methotrexate. *J Am Med Assoc* 1969;209:1861–1864.

133. Jones SE, Moore M, Blank N, et al. Hypersensitivity to procarbazine manifested by fever and pleuropulmonary reaction. *Cancer* 1972;29:498–500.

134. Holoye PY, Luna MA, Mackay B, et al. Bleomycin hypersensitivity pneumonitis. *Ann Intern Med* 1978;88:47–49.

135. Cohen IJ, Loven D, Schoenfeld T, et al. Dactinomycin potentiation of radiation pneumonitis: a forgotten interaction. *Pediatr Hematol Oncol* 1991;8:187–192.

136. Bauer JH, Brooks CS, Burch RN. Clinical appraisal of creatinine clearance as a measure of glomerular filtration rate. *Am J Kidney Dis* 1982;2:337–346.

137. Patterson WP, Reams GP. Renal toxicities of chemotherapy. *Semin Oncol* 1992;19:521–528.

138. Calabresi P, Parks R Jr. Antiproliferative agents and drugs used for immunosuppression. In Gilman AG, Goodman LS (Eds), *The Pharmacological Basis of Therapeutics*, New York: Macmillan Publishing Co., Inc., 1980, pp. 1256–1313.

139. Pfeifle CE, Howell SB, Felthouse RD, et al. High-dose cisplatin with sodium thiosulfate protection. *J Clin Oncol* 1985;3:237–244.

140. Markman M, Clearly S, Howell SB. Nephrotoxicity of high-dose intracavitary cisplatin with thiosulfate protection. *Eur J Cancer Clin Oncol* 1985;21:1015–1018.

141. Cornelison TL, Reed E. Nephrotoxicity and hydration management for cisplatin, carboplatin, and ormaplatin. *Gynecol Oncol* 1993;50:147–158.

142. Shin AF, Rutkowski D, Wilner FN, et al. Dosage modification of cancer agents in renal failure. *Drug Intelligence and Clin Pharmacol* 1977;11:140–141.

143. Goren MP, Wright RK, Pratt CB, et al. Potentiation of ifosfamide neurotoxicity, hematotoxicity, and tubular nephrotoxicity by prior cisplatin therapy. *J Cancer Res* 1987;47:1457–1460.

144. Ries F, Klastersky J. Nephrotoxicity induced by cancer chemotherapy with special emphasis on cisplatin toxicity. *Am J Kidney Dis* 1986;8:368–379.

145. West WH, Tauer KW, Yannelli JR, et al. Constant infusion recombinant interleukin-2 in adoptive immunotherapy of advanced cancer. *New Engl J Med* 1987;316:898–905.

146. Patterson WP, Khojasteh A. Ifosfamide-induced renal tubular defects. *Cancer* 1989;63:649–651.

147. Calabresi P, Parks R Jr. Antiproliferative agents and drugs used for immunosuppression. In Gilman AG, Goodman LS (Eds), *The Pharmacological Basis of Therapeutics*, New York: Macmillan Publishing Co., Inc., 1980, pp. 1256–1313.

148. Schilsky RL, Anderson T. Hypomagnesemia and renal magnesium wasting in patients receiving cisplatin. *Ann Intern Med* 1979;90:929–931.

149. Perry MC, Hoagland HC, Wagoner RD. Uric acid nephropathy. *J Am Med Assoc* 1976;236:961–962.

150. Vogelzang NJ, Nelimark RA, Nath KA. Tumor lysis syndrome after induc-

tion chemotherapy of small cell bronchogenic carcinoma. *J Am Med Assoc* 1983;249:513–514.

151. Mohrmann M, Ansorge S, Schmich U, et al. Toxicity of ifosfamide, cyclophosphamide and their metabolites in renal tubular cells in culture. *Pediatr Nephrol* 1994;8:157–163.

152. Vose JM, Reed EC, Pippert GC, et al. Mesna compared with continuous bladder irrigation as uroprotection during high dose chemotherapy and transplantation: a randomized trial. *J Clin Oncol* 1993;11:1306–1310.

153. DeFronzo RA, Braine H, Colvin OM, et al. Water intoxication in man after cyclophosphamide therapy. *Ann Intern Med* 1973;178:861–869.

154. Slater LM, Wainer RA, Serpick AA. Vincristine neurotoxicity with hyponatremia. *Cancer* 1969;23:122–125.

155. Moore JL Jr, Martin JN Jr. Cancer and pregnancy. *Obstet Gynecol Clin N Am* 1992;19:815–827.

156. Doll DC, Ringenburg QS, Yarbro JW. Management of cancer during pregnancy. *Ann Intern Med* 1988;148:2058.

157. Jacob JH, Stringer CA. Diagnosis and management of cancer during pregnancy. *Semin Perinatol* 1990;14:79–87.

158. Wiebe VJ, Sipila PEH. Pharmacology of antineoplastic agents in pregnancy. *Crit Rev Oncol Hematol* 1994;16:75–112.

159. Hoover HC Jr. Breast cancer during pregnancy and lactation. *Surg Clin N Am* 1990;70:1151–1163.

160. Sahn SA. Malignant pleural effusions. *Semin Respir Med* 1987;9:43–53.

161. Sherman S, Grady KJ, Seidman JC. Clinical experiences with tetracycline pleurodesis of malignant pleural effusions. *Southern Med J* 1987;80:716–719.

162. Robinson LA, Fleming WH, Galbraith TA. Intrapleural doxycycline control of malignant pleural effusions. *Ann Thoracic Surg* 1993;55:1115–1121.

163. Albert DS, Chen HS, Mayersohn M, et al. Bleomycin pharmacokinetics in man. *Cancer Chemother Pharmacol* 1979;2:127–132.

164. Ruckdeschel JC, Moores D, Lee JY, et al. Intrapleural therapy for malignant pleural effusions: a randomized comparison of bleomycin and tetracycline. *Chest* 1991;100:1528–1535.

165. Walker-Renard PB, Vaughan LM, Sahn SA. Chemical pleurodesis for malignant pleural effusions. *Ann Intern Med* 1994;120:56–64.

166. Aelony Y, King R, Boutin C. Thoracoscopic talc poudrage pleurodesis for chronic recurrent pleural effusions. *Ann Intern Med* 1991;115:778–782.

167. Zimmer PW, Hill M, Casey K, Harvey E, Low DE. Prospective randomized trial of talc slurry vs. bleomycin in pleurodesis for symptomatic malignant pleural adhesion. *Chest* 1997;112:430–434.

168. Markman M, Cleary S, King ME, et al. Cisplatin and cytarabine administered intrapleurally as treatment of malignant pleural effusions. *Med Pediatr Oncol* 1985;13:191–193.

169. Suhrland LG, Weisberger AS. Intracavitary 5-fluorouracil in malignant effusions. *Archiv Intern Med* 1965;116:431–433.

170. Groth G, Gatzemeier U, Haussinger K, et al. Intrapleural palliative treatment of

malignant pleural effusion with mitoxantrone vs placebo (pleural tube alone). *Ann Oncol* 1991;2:213–215.

171. Markman M. Intraperitoneal chemotherapy. In Ferry MC (ed.), *The Chemotherapy Source Book*. Baltimore: Williams and Wilkins, 1992, pp. 226–231.

172. Howell SB, Pfeifle CL, Wung WE, et al. Intraperitoneal cisplatin with systemic thiosulfate protection. *Ann Intern Med* 1982;97:845–851.

PART V

SUPPORTIVE CARE

CHAPTER 19

PERIOPERATIVE PSYCHOSOCIAL CONSIDERATIONS

JUDITH McKAY, Ph.D.

Traditionally, healing has been associated with bringing a patient back into a sense of wholeness. Hippocrates's concept of health centered on an innate harmony within the individual. Restoring the harmony of the individual parts was the goal of medicine. The World Health Organization defines health as a "state of complete mental and social well-being."[1]

Surgery involves the cutting away of some part of the patient and, while it may be an unwanted or diseased part, it often represents a loss that must be adapted to. In no other type of surgery do these losses have as great an impact on the psychological, functional, and social existence of the patient as in gynecologic surgery.

Added to the generic fear that all surgery patients face regarding the physical trauma, general anesthetic, and the worry of what will be discovered, the residual effects of gynecologic surgery have been found to have ramifications far beyond the physical significance and effect of the operation.[2] High proportions of patients receiving radical gynecologic surgery report depression and anxiety postoperatively,[3–5] temporary or permanent loss of sexual function,[6–9] problems with body image,[10] in addition to gender identity problems associated with reproductive/menopausal issues, lowered libido, and decreased sexual confidence.[10–13] It is important to note that these psychological effects are not related only to radical gynecologic surgery. A simple hysterectomy can require a huge emotional adjustment on the part of the patient with regard to her femininity, her body image, even perhaps causing her to question her purpose in life. It is absolutely crucial that the surgeon recognize and administer to these other aspects of loss and healing that are concomitant to this type of surgery (Level II-2).

Perioperative and Supportive Care in Gynecologic Oncology: Evidence-Based Management,
Edited by Steven A. Vasilev.
ISBN 0-471-24788-X   Copyright © 2000 by Wiley-Liss, Inc.

The good news is that although patients are usually hesitant to initiate conversations around these concerns, they readily respond to and are able to discuss their problems when they are brought up by their physician, nurse-practitioner, or other member of the health care team.[14] The other hopeful aspect is that a trained sex therapist is not necessary to implement very supportive and beneficial strategies for this group of patients.

St. Bartholomew's Hospital in London provides a senior nurse with basic counseling training on an outpatient basis to see patients at their first routine postoperative checkup to screen for depression, anxiety, and sexual concerns. With regard to sexual dysfunction, the responsibility lies both with the physician, to initiate discussion about the possibility of these concerns and to provide relevant information, and with the couple, to address and be willing to work together to achieve a maximally satisfying sexual interaction.[15]

As early as 1980, Derogatis noted that with the expanded awareness and experience of sexuality at all ages, patients will demand not only that their disease process be treated but that "They will require and expect therapeutic interventions which will assist them in becoming psychosexually, as well as physically, rehabilitated."[16]

In designing the ideal treatment, therefore, the surgeon must be aware that "his object is not only to save life, but also to help make the life he saves worth living." This is especially true when considering treatment options for patients with cervical cancer. Although curing the disease is the primary objective, the surgeon needs to be mindful of the effect of surgery on other organs. The vagina is not essential to life, but the mutilation, shortening, or complete occlusion of the vagina may have such significance to the patient as to compromise post-surgical emotional and psychosocial adjustment.[11] In any gynecologic surgery, the surgeon needs to consider the broader impact of the treatment and what it will mean to the specific patient in question.

SEXUAL/EMOTIONAL PROBLEMS

Frequency of Sexual/Emotional Reactions

Cain found that the diagnosis and treatment of cervical, endometrial, ovarian, vaginal, or vulvar cancer significantly affected the mood level of patients.[12] He and his colleagues interviewed 60 women within a month of being diagnosed with carcinoma. As a group they reported significantly more depressed feelings than a large sample randomly selected from the community.

Since it was felt that psychosocial disabilities might correlate with the site, stage, and grade of cancer, as well as treatment, data were grouped by these variables. Women with ovarian cancer, women receiving triple-agent chemotherapy, and women with Grade 3 tumors of the uterus and ovary approached the level of depression typically obtained by patients entering outpatient psychiatric clinics as measured by the Hamilton Depression Scale, the Hamilton Anxiety Scale, and the Psychosocial Adjustment to Illness Scale. The women with gynecological cancer and treatment scored significantly higher on these measures than a large sample of women from the community without cancer. Many of these impairments such as ability to work, to perform domestic chores, or to function sexually resulted not from physical limitations but from the patients' psychosocial reaction to the cancer and its treatment.

Twenty-nine of the 60 women interviewed described a regular and satisfying sexual relationship before the diagnosis. After diagnosis, all 29 women ceased to have sexual intercourse. "Either they were told to abstain following surgery or they believed sexual intercourse would exacerbate vaginal bleeding or vaginal discharge."[12]

Abitol[17] suggests that sexual function is often not taken into consideration, especially with older women, since it is usually assumed that "intercourse is an unsuitable indulgence for any woman of or beyond middle age.[18] However, many early studies[19–21] have observed that women between 60 and 93 are sexually active and, if they are not, it is most usually not due to lack of interest but rather the absence of a partner or the partner's inability to have sex. Starr and Weiner surveyed 800 subjects from 60 to 91 years (65% were women) and found that the majority remained sexually active.[22] The older women in the study were interested in sex and wanted to feel and be perceived as sexual.

In comparing the posttreatment sexual functioning of 97 patients with invasive carcinoma of the cervix (Stages I and II of the International Classification), Abitol found that in 22 out of the 28 patients treated with radiotherapy there was significant disturbance of sexual function.[17] Only 2 of the 32 surgical patients experienced sexual interference. Of the 15 patients treated with both surgery and radiotherapy, 5 mentioned problems with sexual function. Abitol concludes, "Whenever the five-year cure rate is similar with different modes of therapy and the possibility of complication is limited, preference should be given to radical surgery over radiotherapy."

Although Abitol's point, that sexual functioning is an important aspect when choosing treatment options, is well taken, it should be noted that in Abitol's study, treatment groups were unmatched in terms of cancer staging. Also, the low evidence (6%) of sexual dysfunction among surgical subjects is markedly lower than that found in uncomplicated hysterectomy studies, which is surprising since with the compounding factors of malignancy and the more extensive procedure of a Wertheim hysterectomy, greater sexual dysfunction in this group would be predicted.[15]

Although in 90% of the patients in Abitol's study[17] there was some relationship between pelvic findings and sexual activity, this relationship was inverse in about 10%: Three women claimed a normal sexual life with a practically obliterated vagina, and five women complained of marked difficulty in spite of a normal vagina. Twolmby points out that sexual function may depend primarily on the motivation of the patient to succeed as well as her conception of gratifying sexual activity.[23]

In another study of 96 women (between 41 and 50 years of age) treated surgically for cervical cancer, 34% abstained completely from sexual activity because of "dyspareunia or psychic factors." This was at a 1- to 2-year follow-up.[24]

Weijmar Schultz[15] reviewed 44 posttreatment studies summarizing the psychosocial functioning of gynecological cancer patients. In all of the studies in which the patient compared her preoperative and postoperative states retrospectively, sexual functioning was considered to have deteriorated after treatment.

In spite of major physical limitations and significant emotional strain, the patients attempted to maintain a sexual life.[24] Weijmar Schultz discovered several prognostic variables with regard to postoperative sexual dysfunction: the magnitude of surgical intervention, the pretreatment libidinal level, age and presence of a stable relationship, and partnership-related factors such as availability, attitude, and health. In the Weijmar Schultz review it was found that with the cervical cancer patients there was a difference between treatment groups in the degree of posttreatment sexual disruption, with the major negative factor being inclusion of radiation therapy in the treatment.

After radical vulvectomy,[5,13,25,29] as many as 50% to 80% of the women in these studies had stopped all sexual activity. However, in a cohort of 10 women treated for vulvar cancer by radical vulvectomy, 8 of the 10 couples accomplished complete or partial sexual rehabilitation.[26] One of the women in this group became pregnant and had an uncomplicated vaginal delivery after the radical vulvectomy. It was felt that this high level of sexual rehabilitation was due to the fact that adequate information was offered to the patients and a safe venue for discussion was provided, although even these factors were not enough to guarantee a successful resumption of sexual activities with the entire group (Level II-2).[1]

Andersen did a study in 1988 comparing 42 women treated for vulvar cancer (6 treated with laser or chemotherapy, 26 treated with wide local excision, 9 with total vulvectomy, and 1 with radical vulvectomy) and 42 healthy women.[25] The treatment group had disruption in the excitement and resolution phases of sexual function, but did not lose their desire for sexual activity. There was two to three times more sexual dysfunction in this group compared to the healthy group. Thirty percent of the treatment group was sexually inactive at follow-up ranging from 1 to 10 years after surgery. The severity of the surgical intervention correlated with the sexual outcome: The more extensive the treatment, the greater the disruption of the desire and resolution phases of the sexual response cycle.

In an interesting study of 308 women treated for breast cancer or genital cancer, Wenderlein et al. found that patients with gynecological cancer have a 50% higher incidence of sexual problems and anxiety about sexual activity than do mastectomy patients.[27] Feelings of guilt are common with cervical cancer patients, as many have heard from the media that this is a sexually transmitted disease.[28,29] Guilt can also be experienced when vulval irritation, vaginal discharge and bleeding are exacerbated by sexual contact. This could obviously be easily mitigated to some extent by the simple provision of information and the open discussion of some of the very painful conclusions that patients have adopted. Again, this discussion will have to be initiated by the physician or some member of the health care team, as the patient is usually too embarrassed to mention her concerns.[6]

In a comparative study of 16 women treated for breast cancer (Stage II, treated by surgery and chemotherapy), 16 women treated for gynecological cancer (treated by surgery or surgery and radiotherapy), and 16 healthy women, 82% of the gynecological cancer sample reported poorer body image in contrast to 31% of the breast cancer patients. Although frequency of sexual behavior and level of sexual arousal were lower for both patient groups compared to healthy outpatients, there were no differences on indicants of sexual desire or orgasm.[3]

In Great Britain 105 women were retrospectively questioned about their psychosexual functioning after treatment for cancer of the cervix and vulva by radical vulvectomy, Wertheim's hysterectomy, and pelvic exenteration.[6] Ninety percent of the women in relationships had been sexually active prior to surgery. Sixty-six percent of those sexually active women had sexual function problems more than 6 months after surgery and 15% never resumed intercourse (two women had colpectomies and were not included). Eighty-two percent of those under 50 who had radiotherapy suffered sexual dysfunction.

Lack of desire was the most prevalent problem. Fifty percent of the women felt that their sexual relationship had deteriorated, yet only 16% felt that their marriage had worsened. Forty-six percent felt moderately to severely distressed. The authors comment, "As well as organic causes there is a strong psychogenic element brought about by loss of fertility, disfigurement, depression and anxiety about one's desirability as a sexual partner."[6] Again, a stable relationship helped mitigate the severity of the problems, and young, single women were at highest risk.

Sewell, using a semistructured interview and psychometric measures with 15 patients treated for vulvar cancer, found that sexual functioning and body image are significant problems postoperatively even though intercourse is possible.[28] Women reported levels of sexual arousal in the eighth percentile and body image in the fourth percentile. Although they reported levels of sexual activity comparable to healthy women preoperatively, postoperatively their sexual activity was half that of the normative sample. This sample did, however, report higher frequency of sexual activity as compared to a sample of patients who had a pelvic exenteration.[13] The vulvectomy patients' psychological distress as measured by the Symptom Checklist was 1 to 1.5 standard deviations above the mean expected for normal, healthy individuals.[30] Scores on the Beck Depression Inventory indicated mild to moderate levels of depression in these patients.[31]

A survey questionnaire of 18 patients treated with wide local excision rather than vulvectomy for microinvasive disease was reported by DiSaia and colleagues.[32] All women maintained their sexual responsiveness, in contrast to two radical vulvectomy patients who reported loss of orgasmic ability and dyspareunia.

Lack of Postsurgical Education

As previously cited, many patients experience a myriad of psychosocial problems after gynecologic surgery, including sexual dysfunction, depression, anxiety, poor body image, and lack of confidence in their femininity. These factors have been shown to be significantly improved with education and open discussion (Levels I-2 and III). However, the paucity of information given to patients and the lack of any provision for discussion of sexual function and how it might be affected subsequent to surgical procedures is alarming.

Andersen found that in a cohort of 42 women treated surgically for vulvar cancer, 60% to 84% received no information regarding sexual outcome.[25] Jenkins interviewed 27 sexually active women following surgical and radiotherapy treatment for endometrial and cervical cancer who experienced significant negative changes on four indicators of sexual function: frequency of intercourse, orgasm, and feelings of desire and enjoyment.[10] Fifty-nine percent of this group received no information at all about sexual or psychological sequelae to surgery. Eighty-eight percent of these women wanted sexual discussion to be initiated by their physician or nurse.

When interviewing 50 patients treated for cervical cancer, Vincent reported that 70% of the women had received no information on the sexual implications of their disease either before or after treatment.[33] Fifty-six percent wanted more information on sexual functioning than they received, and 79% of these said they would not ask their physician about these concerns. In another study by Kreuger et al., almost half of the 108 patients wanted nurses to initiate discussion about the effect of hysterectomy on sexuality.[34]

Many studies have reported that women are inadequately prepared for the sexual outcome of their treatment, and that they find it difficult or impossible to ask health care workers about this aspect of treatment. Patients report that they feel they should be grateful just to be alive and that they are being presumptuous to ask for more in terms of quality of life.

In addition, if a woman is uninformed about her body and does not have the appropriate vocabulary with which to describe her experience, she will be more reticent to discuss these matters. In the past, if a patient has not voiced concerns, health care givers have assumed that there were none.[5,29] It is imperative that the physician and his or her staff understand the danger of this assumption.

Cultural factors can also have a significant impact on the patient's feelings that she is entitled to have pleasurable sex and that it is her responsibility and right to address the problem if she is not. Corney et al. found in their interview of 105 women treated for gynecological cancer that over a quarter of the patients felt they would have benefited from more information, and 50% felt that more information should have been given to their husbands.[6] Corney notes, "Other difficulties such as loss of libido, anorgasmia and anxiety about one's sexual desirability are unlikely to be discussed spontaneously by the woman. Nevertheless, we were impressed that women will talk about very intimate aspects of sexuality if they feel that there is a willingness to discuss the subject." Women in this study were accepting of the necessity of making the adjustments necessary to adapt to disfigurement and sexual limitations (only five of the women reported postsurgically that they wished they had not had surgery), but they expressed a real need for, and lack of, adequate explanation and discussion of alternative means of sexual expression, if appropriate.

In a study of 27 women treated for endometrial and cervical cancer with surgery and radiation therapy, Jenkins found that 95% had not received any information on sexual functioning in spite of the fact that as a group they showed significant decrease in the actual frequency of intercourse, orgasm, and in their feelings of desire and enjoyment subsequent to treatment.[10] Seventy-six percent reported dyspareunia, 60% vaginal dryness, and 53% narrowed or shortened vagina. Eighty-eight percent of the sample indicated that they would have liked a health care professional to initiate discussion regarding sexual functioning and the possible effects of surgery.

Treatment

Capone compared two groups of patients diagnosed with cancer of the genital organs.[35] Both groups were interviewed using a semistructured interview followed by the administration of three psychometric measures assessing psychologic distress, affective state, and self-concept.

Return to employment and frequency of intercourse were two additional behavioral measures. One group ($N = 56$) received counseling a minimum of four times during their hospital stay that was aimed at developing realistic expectations and adaptive behavioral coping techniques. Patients were given an arena and permission to express feelings of anger, concern, and fears related to treatment or death. They were given information regarding their disease and possible treatment sequelae. Self-esteem, femininity, and interpersonal relationships were also covered during the counseling sessions.

For sexually active patients, a sexual rehabilitation component was added. Discussions of sexuality and sexual concerns were initiated early and continued throughout treatment. Counseling dealt with sexual misconceptions and fears and methods of working with anxieties associated with resumption of sexual activity. For women whose medical treatment precluded a return to prior sexual activities, options and alternatives were discussed and realistic expectations were set.

A control group ($N = 41$) was interviewed and assessed using the same procedures as were used for the experimental group. Patients in the control group were not counseled. It was found that the intervention had a significant effect in reducing sexual dysfunction and in enhancing the rate of return to pretreatment frequency of intercourse. Counseled patients who had been employed before treatment returned to work at a 2 : 1 ratio over the noncounseled group. There were no significant differences between the groups on the emotional measures. The subjects in the control group repeatedly emphasized the lack of opportunity for discussion of sexual adjustment, which replicates the findings of

the surgery and recovery process with previous exenteration patients preoperatively.

This discussion is extremely helpful to the patient and the team in clarifying the importance of the patient's decision and in establishing realistic expectations concerning the recovery process. It also gives the message to the patient and her partner that the quality of her life, especially her sexual life, is important to the team, and gives her permission and familiarity with discussing these often sensitive arenas of her functioning with various health care givers.

The enterostomal therapist also meets the patient preoperatively to discuss the care and placement of the ostomy. Postoperative meetings in hospital are also available as is counseling on an outpatient basis. Postoperative counseling is provided, encouraging the patient to be active and involved in the specific strategies of her recovery process, including dilation of the neovagina and the need for sexual activity to hasten recovery.

Counseling is afforded the patient to discuss any further problems relative to her surgery, ostomy care, or sexual rehabilitation. Visits vary from every 2 to 4 weeks in the first 6 months to every 3 to 6 months after that. If the patient and her partner are identifying problems, the surgeon and the sex therapist are available to supervise self-examination in the office with either the patient alone or with her partner if needed.

Although radical pelvic surgery means loss of sexually responsive tissue, women who lose their vagina and clitoris can often learn to have complete sexual response with stimulation of other erogenous areas—that is, the anus, urethra, ostomy of the ileo-conduit or colostomy, or even stimulation of the scar tissue in the area of the vulva. With counseling, the patient can learn that there is a wide range of sexually stimulating behaviors that she and her partner need to explore in order to maintain satisfying sexual function. Lack of sexual response and happiness in the woman who has been presurgically well adjusted sexually may have to do more with her feelings of being unattractive or the absence of information or support to deal with postoperative psychological reactions than her actual physical limitations.[9]

The Lamont report involved a group of 12 patients, and because the number was so small, few conclusions could be drawn. In this group, three neovaginas were constructed from peritoneum, five from sigmoid colon, and two from ileum. One patient did not need a neovagina because half of her vagina was preserved at the time of surgery. Eight of the women in this study were judged to have good adjustment preoperatively, and of these, seven resumed sexual activity and enjoyed good postoperative adjustment. Six of the seven patients were orgasmic within six months of their surgery. One patient was too newly discharged to be able to make an adequate assessment of her sexual functioning. One patient's postoperative adjustment was limited because of her emphasis on coital interaction, little opportunity to communicate with her partner about other sexual behaviors, and difficulty in accepting the care of her neovagina. The other three were not sexually active preoperatively. Two of these three remained inactive, and one was not assessed prior to Lamont's report.[38]

Patients need to be encouraged to not only engage in continued coital activity but to explore various aspects of foreplay (with an emphasis on "play"), allowing the couple to develop a range of stimulating experiences that will promote the same feelings and responses they enjoyed prior to surgery.[39] Lamont and his group feel that the most important factor in sexual rehabilitation is an educated partner who is accepting of the patient's surgery and who is willing to support her feelings of loss and will reinforce her feelings of her own femininity and self-esteem. Too often, if there is any sexual assessment, counseling, or education, the partner is left out.

ISSUES OF DEATH AND DYING

Patient Mortality

Often a physician is hesitant to bring up issues of mortality, fearing that the suggestion might frighten a patient or cause the patient to lose confidence in the surgeon or the proposed intervention. If there is the chance of cancer involvement or cancer is diagnosed preoperatively, the patient's fears may realistically be heightened. Interestingly, in the 1950s, patients were usually not told of their diagnosis of cancer, which put the surgeon in a difficult position when obtaining the informed consent for surgery. The diagnosis was kept from the patient, as it was deemed too painful for the patient to handle.[40]

Since then, psychological responses of patients to life-threatening diagnoses and procedures have been examined more closely. Strain and Grossman identified concerns of patients preoperatively as occurring within the broad categories of fears around turning one's life over to strangers, separation from the familiar environment of home and family, loss of control or death under anesthesia, being partially awake during surgery, and damage to body parts.[41] In addition to these specific fears, a patient may have more generalized reactions of feeling hopeless, helpless, and angry.

More extreme emotional reactions are exhibited with patients who have a history of anxiety, a high need for control, or specific negative associations around surgery. The relationship established with the surgeon preoperatively in laying the foundation for the patient to expect direct, understandable information on her condition, and the sense that her emotional reactions and concerns are important, is crucial. Dr. S. J. Stehlin notes, "If the doctor–patient relationship is one in which each feels free to communicate with the other, ... once the essentials of truth are explained in the proper manner, the way becomes clear for the next phase ... hope. A patient can tolerate knowing he is incurable; he cannot tolerate hopelessness" (Level III).[42]

Discussing candidly with a patient that there is always a possibility of death or complications that would render her incompetent to make decisions for herself at some later date allows the patient to establish what her choices are from a position of power. It is important to discuss the advantages of the patient's recording her wishes in writing, via advance directives, a durable power of attorney, and the provisions of a will, when she is healthy and competent, as opposed to having her family or hospital administration guess at what she would want in a time of crisis.

If dealt with compassionately and gently, this can be an empowering process for the patient at a time when she may feel that most of the control in her life is being eroded away. It can also be an important precedent for establishing trust between patient and surgeon by way of direct, honest communication while discussing matters of the greatest import. The patient learns through this interaction that her wishes are being asked for and listened to.[42]

The preoperative consultation visit with the surgeon is the appropriate venue to assess the patient's emotional stability and concerns, and to establish what the patient's wishes are in case of complications. As a part of securing the informed consent, it is important for the surgeon to explain clearly and in layperson's terms all aspects of the proposed treatment and to allow the patient adequate time for questions, the expression of her fears about death, and doubts and concerns about treatment. If the surgeon feels that the patient is significantly apprehensive or unable to face or discuss her mortality or the possibility of complications, a referral to a social worker or psychologist may be appropriate to provide support and increase the patient's feelings of safety. Personal confrontation of mortality is never easy, but the earlier and the more fully these issues are discussed, the easier the entire process will be for the surgeon, the patient, and her family.

In instances when the patient has not had a chance to complete advance directives, or "do not resuscitate" (DNR) orders, and family members are left to make decisions about treatment without the guidance of having written instructions on the patient's wishes, many states have adopted health care surrogate acts that delineate, in a specified order, those individuals who may make decisions on behalf of a patient. In states without such statutes, frequently a member of the family or a close friend may serve as surrogate decision maker.

Obviously, the patient's current condition and the expected outcome of resuscitation will be the primary variables to consider in making DNR decisions. However, when recovery is doubtful, it should be the responsibility of the attending physician to convey that information and to guide the patient's surrogate in attempting to ensure that the course of treatment is consistent with the known views of the patient, as reflected in oral statements, lifestyle commitments, and values. If the family member or friend is having difficulty with the decision, a referral to either a psychologist or social worker may be indicated to allow the surrogate decision maker to come to as clear a choice as possible with a minimum amount of guilt. Ferreting out the probable choices of the patient, were she competent, may take more time than the surgeon has available, but a timely referral can honor the needs of the family member in making these potentially guilt-producing decisions.

When in the course of surgery physical evidence of advanced disease and poor prognosis is discovered, the earlier foundation of honest communication about issues of death and dying will be of utmost benefit. In this case, the postoperative period not only involves recovery from the procedures but also confrontation with, and adaptation to, loss and possible death.

This process resembles anticipatory grieving and often involves the five stages of grief identified in the 1960s by Elizabeth Kubler-Ross: denial, anger, bargaining, depression, and acceptance.[43] Sometimes suicidal thinking will emerge in the patient's attempt to take control of a process she may believe is hopeless.

In order to interact honestly and humanely, it is important for the physician to examine his or her own attitudes toward death. Implicit throughout the medical student's training is the theme that "every death corresponds to a failure, either of the individual physician or, more commonly, of medicine as a whole."[44]

In a pilot study, Feifel found that compared to a control group of patients and other nonprofessionals, physicians thought less about death, but were more afraid of death.[45] Seeing death as the "enemy," which would be natural in this philosophical formulation, will jeopardize the surgeon's ability to discuss in an empathic, supportive way the possibility of a patient's death. It is imperative, therefore, for each physician to examine his or her own relationship and feelings about death so as to better model an acceptance of death as an integral part of life, as opposed to seeing death as a failure or an indignity that can be avoided if one is an "exceptional patient."

Fetal Death

Sometimes in the process of gynecologic treatment, elective fetal termination will be required. Death of a child is one of the greatest human tragedies. Often, physicians do not regard the interruption of fetal development as a significant loss compared to the death of an infant or child. Mothers are often plagued with guilt and suffer as much, if not more, adjustment to the loss of a fetus if that loss is a result of their own health requirements. Usually, only the physician can provide the kind of information necessary to allay that guilt.[46]

In a retrospective study of 26 families who had experienced perinatal death (7 stillborn infants: >20 weeks' gestation and 19 live-born infants, none of whom went home from hospital), Rowe found that only 7 of the mothers interviewed were satisfied with the information they had received from their physician.[47] Six mothers had a prolonged grief reaction of 12 to 20 months. There was a direct correlation between the degree of dissatisfaction and the mother's lack of understanding and/or her morbid grief response. A mother's level of dissatisfaction was not significantly related to age, economic class, marital status, the duration of survival of the infant, the cause of death, or the presence of a healthy child in the family. Mothers were more likely to feel dissatisfied if they had received no follow-up contact by a physician, either in person or by phone.

Rowe suggests it is not enough for a physician to simply inform the parents of the death of their child, whether a fetus or live-born. The physician has the "equal responsibility to present the information in a meaningful and empathetic

TABLE 19.1 Optimum Communication of Miscarriage, Still Birth, or Death of Neonate

The news should be given to both parents and they should be the first to know.
The information should be conveyed in a private place where the parents will feel comfortable expressing any emotions they feel.
The news should be factual, understandable and delivered by the surgeon directly.
Cliches of avoidance and denial such as "Forget about this" or "You can always have another child" are to be avoided.

Source: Adapted from Koop CE. The seriously ill or dying child: supporting the patient and family. In Schnaper N, et al. (Eds), *Management of the Dying Patient and His Family.* New York: MSS Information Corp., 1974.

context, in a personal interview if at all possible."[47] Rowe also recommends having a social worker assume responsibility for maintaining continuing communication with a family after they have had a perinatal loss.

Cullberg found that one-third of mothers experiencing a perinatal death suffer a morbid grief reaction.[48] In his survey, 19 out of 56 mothers studied 1 to 2 years after the deaths of their neonates had developed severe psychiatric disorders. The period of mental symptomatology was longer in those women whose feelings of grief were initially suppressed or denied. Koop has suggested some guidelines for the physician when discussing with parents the loss of a fetus or infant (Table 19.1).[49] When parents were asked what their most desperate need was after either a miscarriage, stillbirth, or death of a neonate, the most common response was the need to talk about it.[46]

In our culture death is not talked about. Giles observed that physicians dealt with perinatal death by treating the mother's physical symptoms and prescribing sedatives liberally.[50] They avoided, in about half of the cases, discussing the baby's death. When grieving parents feel they cannot share their feelings with friends and family, the physician may be the one avenue for the expression of their grief. Therapeutic listening, giving the patient permission to express her feelings, and providing ongoing resources for support are an important part of the physician's role as counselor/consoler. Giving the patient permission to seek grief counseling through individual or group work may be appropriate. There are many bereavement groups available, some of which have been formed for the specific purpose of dealing with infant death. Providing the patient with a referral to a social worker or psychologist who can help the patient find a support group during this difficult adjustment period is often beneficial.

Herzog has suggested that there are three stages of grief work (Table 19.2).[51] Although the surgeon's role cannot obviously encompass all of these stages, the initial interaction and support that is conveyed by the physician may permit the patient and her family to express their grieving in healthy ways and seek additional avenues of expression as needed for completing the grieving process.

TABLE 19.2. Three Stages of Grief Work

Resuscitation	Working through the initial shock during the first 24 hours
Rehabilitation	Consultation and discussion with family members for the first 6 months
Renewal	Healthy tapering of the mourning process from 6 months on

Source: Adapted from Herzog AA. A clinical study of parental response to adolescent death by suicide with recommendations for approaching the survivors. In Farberow NL (Ed), *Proceedings of the Fourth International Conference for Suicide Prevention.* Los Angeles: Delmar Publications, 1968.

PSYCHOLOGICAL COMPLICATIONS IN THE ICU

Postoperative stress in the intensive care unit (ICU) can have a significant impact on the mental and emotional status of the gynecologic surgery patient, which in turn can affect her physical state. In fact, Hackett mentions that psychological reactions to surgery postoperatively "frequently trouble the surgeon, harass the nursing staff, impede the course of recovery, and may be fully as dangerous as the infections or embolic complications of surgery."[52] The source of these complications can be classified as extrinsic or intrinsic.

Extrinsic Factors

Extrinsic factors have to do with the environment, the external milieu in which the surgical patient finds herself. The ICU may evoke fear and anxiety in the patient if the technology and equipment are perceived as intimidating or even harmful and overtax the already diminished resources of the patient. Extensive intravenous lines, arterial lines, monitoring wires, oxygen masks, and ventilator assistance equipment can create a feeling in the patient of being "tied down" or "trapped" and can increase feelings of helplessness.[53]

Twenty-four-hour management plans, employment of multiple invasive procedures, the use of omnipresent monitors, chronic high noise level, lack of privacy, continual activity, and light combine to create the paradoxical combination of sensory monotony and sensory overload, as well as sleep deprivation, in the patient. The combination of these myriad stressors on the critically ill patient can contribute to the development of postoperative depression, anxiety, or delirium, sometimes referred to as ICU delirium, ICU syndrome, or ICU psychosis.[54]

Intrinsic Factors

Factors intrinsic to the patient that increase the likelihood of psychological complications postsurgically are those which inhibit the patient's ability to adapt to stress. Increased age correlates with higher risk. Patients over 50 have a higher probability of developing delirium postoperatively.[55] Senile patients may show a deterioration of postoperative psychological functioning without a lucid interval.[56]

Prior psychiatric history is also associated with higher probabilities of psychological complications. Patients with depression, psychosomatic disease, sleep disturbance, anxiety disorder, phobias, or panic attacks have more limited resources to deal with the many stressors associated with gynecologic surgery and the subsequent physical, emotional, and sexual adaptations required.

Many of the drugs used after surgery may be potentiating factors for the development of depression, anxiety, delirium, or psychosis in a predisposed patient. Anticholinergic drugs, antitussives, tricyclic antidepressants, antihistamines, and anti-Parkinson agents are capable of promoting major psychological disturbance.[57]

Patients who have been addicted to drugs or alcohol, who have had cerebral damage, previous episodes of delirium, or chronic cardiovascular, metabolic, respiratory, or renal illness, are at higher risk for developing delirium. Metabolic and hemodynamic instability as a result of gastrointestinal hemorrhage, anoxia, liver failure, septic shock, respiratory failure, myocardial infarction, severe burns, drug overdoses, acid-base imbalances, electrolyte imbalances, infections, and pulmonary embolus have been correlated with instances of delirium. Sex does not appear to be a predisposing factor in the development of ICU delirium; the incidence is similar among men and women.[58] It is thus important for the physician to assess all of the predisposing factors that might be contributing to the patient's psychological imbalance, including environmental, pharmacologic, and medically related factors, as well as inherent psychological variabilities and coping abilities, before designing a treament plan (Levels II-3 and III; Table 19.3).

Delirium

The reversible, confusional state known as ICU psychosis or ICU syndrome is characterized by disorientation with regard to time, place, and person, difficulty in logical thinking, anxiety, apathy, sleep disturbance, incoherence, fear, excitement, illusions, hallucinations, and delusions. In more extreme cases, agitation, paranoia, and belligerence may cause the patient to be at risk to herself or others. Delirium differs from psychosis in that there is no consistent structure to the ideas as is found in psychotic states and there is no steady regressiveness. Instead, there is a fluctuation of consciousness with some intervals of lucidity.

Timely psychopharmacologic intervention may be of great benefit. However, the differential diagnosis is very extensive. Thus, the specific etiology must be identified prior to administering such agents. It is beyond the intent of this chapter to specifically address drugs and dosages in detail. An excellent review is provided within a recent Sociey of Critical Care Medicine *New Horizons* monograph.[56]

Postoperative delirium usually manifests as early as the second or third postoperative day and generally resolves within 48 hours after discharge from the

TABLE 19.3. Psychological Risk Factors in ICU

Extrinsic

Extensive and invasive equipment
Noise pollution
Lack of privacy
Continual activity
Anonymity
24-hour lighting
Sleep deprivation

Intrinsic

Increased age
Depression
Anxiety, panic attacks
Prior patterns of sleep disturbance
Significant psychopathology
Phobias
Multiple psychotropic drugs
Addictive patterns, drugs/alcohol

unit.[54,59] A lucid period of 2 to 3 days usually precedes the onset. The incidence in conscious patients admitted to critical care settings is estimated by Belitz at 12.5% to 38%.[60] However, in a random sampling of 200 general surgical patients, Titchener found that delirium was found in 78% of the patients.[61]

It has also been noted that some procedures "characteristically eventuate an affectual disturbance; hysterectomy particularly is indicated."[62] Thus, because of the very emotionally laden nature of gynecologic surgery, a higher incidence of delirium might be predicted postoperatively.

Treatment and Prevention of ICU Delirium

Preoperative assessment of a patient's predisposition to develop delirium can be ascertained by the physician or nurse. If any of the predisposing psychological or behavioral issues are evident, extra effort can be made to reassure and educate the patient as to the feelings and impaired perception that might develop, and to emphasize the importance for the patient to inform nursing staff if she notices any of the associated experiences.

Early intervention (either pharmacological or behavioral) has been shown to be effective and can obviate the development of more extreme symptoms.[56,63] If drug use is an issue preoperatively, detoxification may have to be completed before surgery can be undertaken.[58]

Personalizing nursing care has been found to greatly reduce the risk of the development of delirium. Arranging for continuity of care so that some type of

TABLE 19.4. Counseling for Gynecologic Surgery Patients

Goals

To initiate discussion, predict possible treatment sequelae, and provide support, information, and normalization of the myriad physical and emotional changes concomitant to gynecologic surgery. When patients are forewarned that they may have feelings of depression and loss, they feel more in control.

To inform the patient that her psychosocial functioning is an important aspect of healing.

Intervention

1. Evaluation
   - Assess degree of psychological distress
   - Ascertain prior psychiatric history
2. Provide appropriate consultations
   - Psychology—train in coping techniques for anxiety, provide supportive therapy for depression, grief work
   - Psychiatry—psychotropic medications for significant anxiety, depression
   - Nursing staff—discuss in detail predicted body and hormonal changes and adjustments required
   - Enterostomal therapist—discuss care and placement of ostomy
   - Sex therapy consultation—discuss in detail with patient and her partner about effects of surgery on sex life

1 Month Postsurgery
   - Sexual counseling with patient and partner
   - Supportive follow-up regarding emotional reactions of patient

6 Months Postsurgery
   - Ascertain overall psychosocial adjustment to surgery
   - Provide consults as necessary

---

rapport can be established between the patient and her nursing staff is crucial to reassure the patient. Depersonalization is often cited as a contributor to the development of delirium. "The more technological the environment—and the more technological the intervention—the greater is the need for human contact, for human responses to fundamentally human needs.[64] The use of names to continually reorient the patient as to who they are and who is taking care of them can be a simple reassurance available to the nursing staff. Giving permission to the family to touch their loved one, and making the patient more accessible to gentle contact, is often necessary in the intimidating environment of the ICU. Numerous researchers have cited the benefit of personal interactions between the patient and health care workers in helping to prevent delirium.[58,62,65]

Parker found that patients experiencing delirium, who were moved to a side room or transferred to a general medical floor and were allowed to interact with family members for extended periods of time, did better than those who were simply treated with pharmacologic sedation and soft cloth restraints.[54] Delirium is twice as frequent in windowless ICUs.[66,67] If possible, natural lighting should be relied upon as much as possible. Continuous lighting disturbs the structure by which the patient organizes the passage of time, inhibits the natural sleep cycle, and contributes to a sense of monotony that can be extremely disorienting. Large calendars and clocks with digital readouts in clear view will help the patient orient herself in time.[56]

It has been pointed out that if health care workers react to the patient's delirium with calm acceptance, promoted by discussion of the factors contributing to the delirium, the use of restraints can usually be avoided. Often the use of restraints compounds the patient's feelings of depersonalization and helplessness, thus exacerbating the symptoms.

Phenothiazines are an effective remedy for post operative delirium.[68,69] Hale suggests low dosages of perphenazine and haloperidol.[70] These medications lessen agitation, induce sleep, and help in managing the more belligerent patients. Minor tranquilizers such as the benzodiazapenes are only found to be transiently effective and often require dosages that cause sedation.

Anxiety

Heightened vigilance, insomnia, agitation, and tremulousness are frequently manifested symptoms of anxiety. Hackett feels that anxiety is consistently underdiagnosed in the ICU.[71] He attributes this to the hesitancy on the part of the patient to report feelings of anxiety because of associations with being "weak," especially in lower socioeconomic groups. Another factor in undermedicating anxiety is the failure of the physician to observe anxiety in patients who are reluctant to reveal it. The doctor usually relies on the patient's complaints of anxiety, objective and obvious signs of anxiety such as sweating or agitation, or the report of a nurse or family member.

Data suggest that it is most unusual to have an ICU patient complain of anxiety or request additional sedation.[72] Many physicians hesitate to ascertain the level of their patient's anxiety by direct questioning, as the questioning might be felt to be suggestive that the physician feels the patient should be frightened or anxious. This being the case, Hackett suggests that it is safest to assume that *all* patients are anxious to some degree, and treat them accordingly.

Treatment and Prevention of Anxiety

If there are any opportunities to increase the patient's sense of personal control, Easton suggests that this eases the patient's feelings of being immersed in a situation that is dangerous, depersonalized, and unpredictable.[58] Simple choices, such as the scheduling of a shower or the time of day they engage in physical therapy, can be surprisingly empowering to a patient.

Hale found that therapy involving a discussion of the frightening aspects of the patient's treatment and concerns about the future can also serve to enhance the patient's flagging ability to cope and to ease anxiety.[70] Reassuring a patient that anxiety, and sometimes delusional thinking, is a transient occurrence suffered by many patients postoperatively can allay fears that the patient might jump to regarding the loss of her sanity or the permanent impairment of memory or cognition.

The training of patients in meditation or self-hypnosis was found to reduce intraoperative and postoperative anxiety in ambulatory surgery patients.[73] When patients were trained using progressive relaxation techniques, length of stay was reduced and fewer analgesics were utilized by abdominal surgery patients.[74]

Consultations involving the judicious use of major tranquilizers and psychotherapy can also alleviate the patient's symptoms. Early referral for psychological or psychiatric intervention is recommended.

Depression

Depression, characterized by marked withdrawal, insomnia, lassitude, a sense of hopelessness, and sometimes suicidal ideation, can also surface as a reaction to the stresses of surgery. Depression subsequent to surgery for a benign condition with no complications usually diminishes by the third postoperative day.[75] The magnitude of the depressive reaction is often correlated with the significance of the disease process uncovered during surgery, and also the amount of postoperative pain experienced by the patient.[76]

The prospects of a lengthy, debilitating illness can often prompt a patient to worry about being a "burden" on the family and can promote a sense of hopelessness in the patient.[77] Suicidal ideation is common with this type of reaction when the patient is feeling that there is no point in continuing, or that a painful death is all that she has left. Again, early detection of these feelings is crucial in order to more adequately provide treatment.

Treatment of Postsurgical Depression

Often, supportive therapy, encouraging the patient to focus on the joyful aspects of her life that she has to be grateful for in spite of her losses, can be sufficient to allow her to rally her usual ego defenses and cope with the situation at hand. A therapeutic consultation in which a patient is given permission to cry and openly express her despair can be extremely beneficial. Normalizing her reactions and giving her a safe, neutral venue to express her feelings of fear and concerns for the future can allow the patient a cathartic experience as well as give the health care giver valuable information as to the level of her depression.

It is sometimes necessary to provide ongoing psychological support for a patient after she is discharged if her depressive symptoms continue. Families need help in planning care at home, especially if the patient is expressing suicidal thoughts or a sense of despair and hopelessness.

In addition to supportive therapeutic interventions in hospital, the use of antidepressants is often very helpful. If a patient has a preoperative history of taking an antidepressant, some psychiatrists and anesthesiologists suggest the conservative approach of suspending the use of all psychotropic drugs 2 weeks before surgery.[78] Jacobsen and Holland, instead, suggest that the anesthesiologist and the psychiatrist confer prior to surgery to generate a plan based on the particular patient's needs and the drug involved.[79]

The earlier the psychopharmaceutical or therapeutic intervention is initiated, the more effective is its impact. In two meta-analyses of psychological interventions facilitating adjustment to surgical procedures, the authors concluded that brief psychological interventions were superior to standard hospital care in reducing postoperative pain and in increasing satisfaction with care and psychological well-being.[80,81] Patients who received psychological preparation were discharged an average of 2 days sooner than patients who received standard care. The surgeon should continuously be mindful of the emotional well-being of the patient in order to make the appropriate referrals in a timely fashion, and if possible, provide psychological preparation for the stressful event preoperatively to avoid more significant emotional reactions including depression.

Effective physicians will be aware that a successful surgical procedure depends on more than the skillful manipulation of body parts. A surgeon may be a brilliant technician, but a great physician needs to address the broader spectrum of healing. Recognizing the patient in her wholeness will allow the physician to administer to all of a patient's needs.

REFERENCES

1. World Health Organization. *WHO Chron* 1943;1:29.

2. Clark J. Psychosocial responses of the patient. In Groenwald S, Frogge MH, Goodman M (Eds), *Cancer Nursing Principles and Practice*, 3rd ed. Boston: Jones & Bartlett, 1993.

3. Andersen BL, Jochimsen PR. Sexual functioning among breast cancer, gynecologic cancer and healthy women. *J Consult Clin Psychol* 1985;53:25–32.

4. Dempsey GM, Buchsbaum HJ, Morrison J. Psychosocial adjustment to pelvic exenteration. *Gynecol Oncol* 1975;3:325–334.

5. Moth I, Andreasson B, Jensen SB, Bock JE. Sexual function and somatopsychic reactions after vulvectomy. *Danish Med Bull* 1983;30:27–30.

6. Corney RH, Crowther ME, Everett H, Howells A, Shepherd JH. Psychosexual dysfunction in women with gynecological cancer following radical pelvic surgery. *Br Obstet Gynecol* 1993;100:73–78.

7. Andersen BL, Anderson B, Deprosse C. Controlled prospective longitudinal study of women with cancer: II. Psychological outcomes. *J Consult Clin Psychol* 1989;57:692–697.

8. Weijmar Schultz WCM, Van de Wiel HBM, Bouma J, Janssens J, Littlewood J. Psychosexual functioning after the treatment of cancer of the vulva: a longitudinal study. *Cancer* 1990;66:402–407.

9. Van de Weil HBM, Weijmar Schultz WCM, Hallensleben A, Thurkow FG, Bouma J, Verhoeven AC. Sexual functioning of women treated for cancer of the vulva. *Sex Marital Ther* 1990;5:73–82.

10. Jenkins B. Patient's reported sexual changes after treatment for gynecological cancer. *Oncol Nurs Forum* 1988;15:349–354.

11. Vasicka A, Popovich NR, Brausch CC. *Obstet Gynecol* 1958;11:403.

12. Cain EN, Kohorn EI, Quinlan DM, Schwartz PE, Latimer K, Rogers L. Psychosocial reactions to the diagnosis of gynecologic cancer. *Obstet Gynecol* 1983;62:635–641.

13. Andersen BL, Hacker NF. Psychosexual adjustment after vulvar surgery. *Obstet Gynecol* 1983;62:462–475.

14. Wilson-Barnett J. Providing relevant information for patients and families. In Corney R (Eds), *Developing Communication and Counselling Skills in Medicine*. London: Routledge, 1991.

15. Weijmar Schultz WCM, Bransfield DD, Van de Wiel HBM, Bouma J. Sexual outcome following female genital cancer treatment: a critical review of methods of investigation and results. *Sex Marital Ther* 1992;7:29–64.

16. Derogatis LR. Breast and gynecologic cancers: their unique impact on body image and sexual identity in women. In Vaeth JM (Ed), *Frontiers of Radiation Therapy and Oncology*, vol. 14. Basel: Karger S., 1980, pp. 1–11.

17. Abitol MM, Davenport JH. Sexual dysfunction after therapy for cervical carcinoma. *Am J Obstet Gynecol* 1974;119:181–189.

18. Masters WH, Johnson VE. *Human Sexual Response*. Boston: Little Brown & Company, 1966.

19. Kinsey AC, Pomeroy WB, Martin CE, Gebhard PH. *Sexual Behavior in the Human Female*. Philadelphia: WB Saunders Company, 1953.

20. Pfeiffer E, Verwoerdt A, Wang HS. Sexual behavior in aged men and women. *Arch Gen Psychiatry* 1968;19:753–758.

21. Newman G, Nichols CR. Sexual activity in postmenopausal women. *JAMA* 1960;173:33.

22. Starr BD, Weiner MB. *The Starr-Weiner Report on Sex and Sexuality in the Mature Years*. New York: McGraw-Hill, 1981.

23. Twombly GH. Sexual activity following pelvic reconstruction. *J Sex Res* 1968;4:275.

24. Kos L. As reported in Weijmar Schultz WCM, Bransfield DD, Van de Wiel HBM, Bouma J. Sexual outcome following female genital cancer treatment: a critical review of methods of investigation and results (1978). *Sex Marital Ther* 1992;7:29–64.

25. Andersen BL, Turnquist D, Lapolla J, Turner D. Sexual functioning after treatment of in situ vulvar cancer, preliminary report. *Obstet Gynecol* 1988;71:15–19.

26. Weijmar Schultz WCM, Wifma K, Vande Wiel HBM, Bouma J, Janssens J. Sexual rehabilitation of radical vulvectomy patients, a pilot study. *J Psychosom Obstet Gynecol* 1986;5:119–126.

27. Wenderlein JM. As reported in Weijmar Schultz WCM, Bransfield DD, Van de Wiel HBM, Bouma J. Sexual outcome following female genital cancer treatment: a critical review of methods of investigation and results (1979). *Sex Marital Ther* 1992;7:29–64.

28. Sewell HH, Edwards DW. Pelvic genital cancer: body image and sexuality. *Frontiers Radiat Ther Oncol* 1980;14:35–41.

29. Stellman RE, Goodwin JM, Robinson J, Dansah D, Hilgers RD. Psychological effects of vulvectomy. *Psychosomatics* 1984;25:779–783.

30. Derogatis LR. *The SCL-90R Administration, Scoring and Procedures Manual—*II. Maryland: Clinical Psychometric Research, 1983.

31. Beck AT, Ward CH, Mendelson M, Mock J, Erbaugh J. An inventory for measuring depression. *Archiv Gen Psychiatry* 1961;4:561–571.

32. DiSaia PJ, Creasman WT, Rich WM. An alternate approach to early cancer of the vulva. *Am J Obstet Gynecol* 1979;133:825.

33. Vincent CE, Vincent B, Greiss FC, Linton EB. Some marital-sexual concomitants of carcinoma of the cervix. *Southern Med J* 1975;68:552–558.

34. Krueger JC, Hassell J, Goggins DB. Relationship between nurse counselling and sexual adjustment after hysterectomy. *Nurs Res* 1979;28(3):145–150.

35. Capone MA, Good RW, Westie KS, Jacogson AF. Psychosocial rehabilitation of gynecologic oncology patients. *Arch Phys Med Rehabil* 1980;61:128–132.

36. Sadoughi W, Leshner M, Fine HL. Sexual adjustment in chronically ill and physically disabled population. *Arch Phys Med Rehabil* 1971;52:311–317.

37. Corney R, Everett H, Howells A, Crowther M. The care of patients undergoing surgery for gynecological cancer: the need for information, emotional support and counselling. *J Advanced Nursing* 1992;17:667–671.

38. Lamont JA, De Petrillo AD, Sargeant EJ. Psychosexual rehabilitation and exenterative surgery. *Gynecol Oncol* 1978;6:236–242.

39. Grinder RR. Sex and cancer. *Med Aspects Human Sex* 1976;10:130.

40. Jacobsen P, Holland JC. Psychological reactions to cancer surgery. In Holland JC, Rowland JH (eds), *Handbook of Psychooncology.* New York: Oxford University Press, 1989.

41. Strain JJ, Grossman S. Psychological care of the medically ill. New York: Appleton-Century-Crofts, 1975.

42. Stehlin SJ, Peach KH. Psychological aspects of cancer therapy. *JAMA* 1966;197:140–144.

43. Kubler-Ross E. *On Death and Dying.* New York: Macmillan Publishing, 1969.

44. Bohrod MG. Uses of the autopsy. *JAMA* 1974;193:810–812.

45. Feifel, H. The functions of attitudes toward death. In *Death and Dying: Attitudes of Patient and Doctor.* New York: Group for the Advancement of Psychiatry, 1965.

46. Knapp RJ, Peppers LG. Doctor-patient relationships in fetal/infant death encounters. *J Med Ed* 1979;54:775–780.

47. Rowe J, Clyman R, Green C, Mikkelsen C, Haight Ataide L. *Pediatrics* 1978;62(2):166–170.

48. Cullberg J. Mental reactions of women to perinatal death. In Morris N (Ed), *Proceedings of the Third International Congress of Psychosomatic Medicine in Obstetrics and Gynecology.* New York: S Karger, 1972.

49. Koop CE. The seriously ill or dying child: supporting the patient and family. *Pediatr Clin North Am* 1969;16(3):555–564.

50. Giles PFH. Reactions of women to perinatal death. *Aust NZ J Obstet Gynaecol* 1970;10:207.

51. Herzog AA. A clinical study of parental response to adolescent death by suicide with recommendations for approaching the survivors. In Farberow NL (Ed), *Proceedings of the Fourth International Conference for Suicide Prevention.* Los Angeles: Delmar Publications, 1968.

52. Hackett TP, Weisman AD. Psychiatric management of operative syndromes: II. Psychodynamic factors in formulation and management. *Psychosom Med* 1960;22:256–372.

53. Halm MA, Alpen MA. The impact of technology on patients and families. *Adv Clin Nurs Res* 1993;28:443–457.

54. Parker DL, Hodge JR. Delirium in a coronary care unit. *JAMA* 1967;201(9):132–133.

55. Heller SS, Frank KA, Maim JR. Psychiatric complications of open heart surgery. *N Engl J Med* 1970;283:1015–1019.

56. Fricchione G, Kohane DS, Daly R, Todred D. Psychopharmacology in the intensive care unit. *New Horizons* 1998;6:353–362.

57. Altschule MD. Postoperative psychosis: a biochemical disorder. *Med Counterpoint* 1969;(1):23–27.

58. Easton C, MacKenzie F. Sensory-perceptual alternations: delirium in the intensive care unit. *Heart Lung* 1988;17:229–237.

59. Ballard KS. Identification of environmental stressors for patients in a surgical intensive care unit. *Issues Ment Health Nurs* 1981;3:89–108.

60. Belitz J. Minimizing the psychological complications of patients who require mechanical ventilation. *Crit Care Nurs* 1983;3(3):42–46.

61. Titchener JL, Zwerling I, Gottschalk L, et al. Psychosis in surgical patients. *Surg Gynecol Obstet* 1956;102:59–65.

62. Lazarus HR, Hagens JH. Prevention of psychosis following open heart surgery. *Am J Psychiatry* 1968;124:76–81.

63. Layne OL jr, Yudofsky SC. Postoperative psychosis in cardiotomy patients: the role of organic psychiatric factors. *N Engl J Med* 1971;284:518–520.

64. Curtin L. Nursing: high-touch in a high-tech world. *Nurs Manage* 1984;15:7–8.

65. Kornfield DS, Heller SS, Frank KA, Moskowitz R. Personality and psychological factors in postcardiotomy delirium. *Arch Gen Psychiatry* 1974;31:249–253.

66. Keep P, James J, Inman M. Windows in the intensive therapy unit. *Anesthesia* 1980;35:257–261.

67. Wilsom LM. Intensive care delirium. *Arch Intern Med* 1971;130:225–226.

68. McKegney FP. The intensive care syndrome: the definition, treatment and prevention of a new "disease of medical progress." *Conn Med* 1966;30:633–636.

69. Blachly PH, Starr A. Postcardiotomy delirium. *Am J Psychiatry* 1965;121:371–375.

70. Hale M, Koss N, Kerstein M, Camp K, Barash P. Psychiatric complications in a surgical ICU. *Crit Care Med* 1977;5(4):199–203.

71. Hackett TP, Cassem NH, Wishnie H. Detection and treatment of anxiety in the coronary care unit. *Am Heart J* 1969;78(6):727–730.

72. Sgroi S, Holland J, Marwit SJ. Psychological reactions to catastrophic illness: com-

parison of patients treated in intensive care unit and medical ward. Presented at Twenty-fifth Annual Meeting, American Psychosomatic Society, March 29, 1968.

73. Domar AD, Noe JM, Benson H. The pre-operative use of the relaxation response with ambulatory surgery patients. *J Human Stress* 1987;13:101–107.

74. Wilson JF. Behavioral preparation for surgery: benefit or harm. *J Behav Med* 1981;4:79–102.

75. Chapman CR, Cox GB. Anxiety, pain and depression surrounding elective surgery: a multivariate comparison of abdominal surgery patients with kidney donors and recipients. *J Psychosom Res* 1977;21:1–15.

76. Massie MJ, Holland JC. The cancer patient with pain: psychiatric complications and their management. *Med Clin N Am* 1987;71:243–258.

77. Schmale AH. Giving up as a final common pathway to changes in health. *Adv Psychosom Med* 1972;8:20.

78. DiGiacomo JN. Preoperative considerations concerning psychotropic drugs. *Med Psychiatry* 1985;2:4–6.

79. Jacobsen P, Holland JC. Psychological reactions to cancer surgery. In Holland JC, Rowland, JH (Eds), *Handbook of Psychooncology.* New York: Oxford University Press, 1980.

80. Mumford E, Schlesinger HJ, Glass GV. The effects of psychological intervention on recovery from surgery and heart attacks: an analysis of the literature. *Am J Public Health* 1982;72:141–151.

81. Devine EC, Cook TD. Clinical and cost-saving effects of psychoeducational interventions with surgical patients: a meta-analysis. *Res Nurs Health* 1986;9:89–105.

CHAPTER 20

PAIN MANAGEMENT IN GYNECOLOGIC ONCOLOGY

LASZLO Z. GALFFY, M.D. and CLAYTON A. VARGA, M.D., M.H.S.M.

Pain is one of the most feared consequences perceived by patients suffering from cancer.[25,42,58] It is estimated that 50% to 60% of patients with incurable disease and as many as 90% of patients with advanced disease experience moderate to severe pain.[44,49,63,64,74] Patients with gynecological tumors most frequently complain of pelvic or abdominal pain but may also experience pain at a variety of locations. There is strong evidence that undertreatment of pain in patients with gynecological tumors is still quite common.[46,59,62] In the perioperative period, cancer pain, surgically related pain, or both may need to be addressed.

Unrelieved pain causes avoidable suffering, diminishes activity and appetite, and impairs sleep. It will further compromise an already debilitated patient. It may also lead to depression and loss of hope, and may signify inexorable progress of a fearsome and fatal disease. Suffering and a feeling of hopelessness can lead patients to reject potentially beneficial active treatment programs and increases the risk for suicide.[25,26,42] Even in the stable patient with ostensibly cured disease, untreated pain impairs productivity, impairs performance of family and social roles, and decreases quality of life.[21,24,33,35]

Current treatment paradigms allow for the vast majority of cancer patients to achieve comfort with relatively simple pharmacological measures, the cornerstone of which is the use of opiate analgesics. Almost all patients can be rendered comfortable using a comprehensive approach to pain management. This would include the use of opiate analgesics, coanalgesics, and surgical and rehabilitative interventions.[23,41,56,60,66,68,73]

The cancer patient may experience acute as well as chronic pain. Pain may be directly tumor related (about 65%), secondary to treatment (about 25%) such as

Perioperative and Supportive Care in Gynecologic Oncology: Evidence-Based Management,
Edited by Steven A. Vasilev.
ISBN 0-471-24788-X   Copyright © 2000 by Wiley-Liss, Inc.

surgery or chemotherapy, or completely unrelated to the cancer (about 10%) as in the case of acute or chronic back pain.[37,48,65] Overlap may be very significant when cancer patients receive surgical care.

Optimal treatment of pain necessitates that a detailed assessment of the patients and their pain complaints be carried out, in order to fully understand the etiology of the pain. Pain should be categorized by its physiologic mechanism as nociceptive (somatic or visceral), neuropathic, or mixed. This differentiation then allows the tailoring of treatment in a more specific fashion.[3,51] Consideration should be given not just to alleviating the patient's pain but to doing so in a manner that produces the fewest side effects and leaves the patient with the highest functional status and best possible quality of life.

CLINICAL ASSESSMENT

Identification of the types of presentation in the patient with gynecologic cancer will direct the overall management strategy. Proper diagnosis of the type(s) of pain a given patient has will determine the use of optimal pharmacological and nonpharmacological pain-control measures. Frequent reassessment of both the patient's pain and the overall condition is necessary, given the dynamic nature of the course of the disease and its associated pain syndromes.[9,10,51]

At the time of initial diagnosis of gynecological cancers, metastases are present in 70% of cases.[67,70] There is a paucity of well-conducted studies on the incidence of pain as the initial or presenting symptom. Pain can be caused by the primary mass or by metastases. The three most common gynecologic cancers—epithelial ovarian, cervical, and endometrial—may be associated with organ parenchymal metastases (liver, lungs, pleura, and less frequently the brain), skeletal and lymph node metastases.[70]

Epithelial ovarian carcinoma is diagnosed in 75% to 85% of patients at the time of peritoneal spread (Stage III), with the most common presenting symptom being vague abdominal pain or discomfort. Cervical cancer usually presents with vaginal bleeding or discharge. However, pain in the lumbosacral and gluteal area due to parametrial spread or lymph node involvement can be the initial presenting symptom in some advanced-stage patients. Endometrial cancer usually presents early with abnormal bleeding, but may be associated with pelvic pain when extrauterine spread is evident. At this point, pelvic and para-aortic node involvement may be associated with lumbosacral and gluteal pain. Breast cancer may be associated with treatment- or metastasis-related pain, including that due to pelvic masses. The principal types of pain presentation are listed in seven categories (Table 20.1).[48,64]

1. Tumor-related pain Pain in this case is caused by infiltration of soft tissue, bony or neurological structures. Pain may be the main symptom. It has a special significance as a marker of the disease. Recurring pain often signifies recurring disease and effective treatment of cancer "cures" the pain. It can be

TABLE 20.1. Types of Patients with Cancer Pain

1. Patients with tumor-related pain
2. Patients with therapy-related pain
3. Nonmalignant pain in the patient with cancer
4. Pregnant patients with cancer pain
5. Substance abusers with cancer pain
6. Psychiatric conditions associated with cancer pain
7. The dying patient with cancer pain

acute, chronic, chronically maintained acute, or incident pain. It may be maintained or amplified by the associated immunologic and neuroendocrine changes characteristic of some types of tumors (Table 20.2).

2. Therapy-related pain   Pain may be caused by surgery, radiation, chemotherapy, or various adjuvant therapies such as antibiotic therapy, hormonal therapy, or steroid withdrawal. It is present in approximately 25% of patients suffering from cancer. Chronic tumor and cancer therapy–related pain becomes an aspect of global suffering, along with immobility, sleep disturbance, and depression (Table 20.3).

3. Nonmalignancy-related pain in the patient with cancer   With or without cancer pain, there may be concomitant nonmalignancy-related pain occurring in 10% of patients.[37] For successful treatment it is important to establish the correct etiology and to avoid confusion with cancer-related pain. Preexisting chronic pain in a patient who subsequently develops cancer poses difficult diagnostic and therapeutic problems. This group is at high risk for developing escalating pain syndromes, therapy and procedure-related complications, and further functional incapacity. A subgroup in this category is that of AIDS-related pain syndromes (Table 20.4).

4. Cancer pain in the pregnant patient   This pain may be related to gynecological malignancies or tumors of other organs and systems. Personal decisions regarding abortion and efforts to minimize effects on the fetus will direct the use of available therapeutic options.

5. Drug abuse/addiction preceding cancer pain   In this group, pain is frequently undertreated and the diagnosis of cancer delayed. Appropriate opioid therapy should not be withheld. Cure of the cancer and control of cancer-related symptoms should be temporally coordinated with treatment of the addiction and psychological and social rehabilitation.[58]

6. Cancer pain in patients with psychiatric conditions   This group also present diagnostic and therapeutic challenges, since these patients may have increased difficulty in accurately reporting or describing their pain. Their complaints can change in a manner or degree disproportionate to changes in the course of the disease. They may either under- or overreport the intensity of their pain. Mental status changes, more frequent in the elderly population, may impair diagnostic accuracy and limit therapeutic choices.[24,45]

TABLE 20.2. Tumor-Related Pain Syndromes

1. Visceral nociceptive
   1.1. Abdominal pain (poorly localized), due to:
       - infiltration of the peritoneum
       - bowel obstruction
       - biliary/pancreatic duct obstruction
       - ureteral obstruction
       - stretch, compression of, or torsion of organ capsules or organ capsules or suspensive structures (e.g., right upper quadrant pain from distention of hepatic capsules)
2. Somatic nociceptive
   2.1. Involving soft tissues
       - invasion of muscle and connective tissue structures
       - invasion of mucous membrane
       - invasion of the skin and subcutaneous tissue
   2.2. Involving bone and joints
       2.2.1. Pathological fractures of
           - long bones
           - vertebra
             - atlanto-axial syndrome
             - C7-T1 syndrome
             - T12-L1 syndrome
             - sacral syndrome
       2.2.2. Incident pain related to mobilization of involved bone
           - from bone itself
           - due to reflex muscle spasm
           - from connective tissue
       2.2.3. Invasion of the skull
           - orbital syndrome
           - parasellar syndrome
           - sphenoid sinus syndrome
           - middle cranial fossa syndrome
           - clivus syndrome
           - jugular foramen syndrome
           - occipital condyle syndrome
       2.2.4. Generalized bone pain
           - multiple metastases
           - bone marrow replacement by tumor

Source: author.

7. Dying patient with cancer pain   The main therapeutic goal is maintaining the patient's comfort and addressing all the available modalities of easing the patient's and the family's suffering. Adequate pain control is of foremost importance and all available techniques in an optimal time frame should be attempted.[36,72,74]

TABLE 20.3. Therapy-Related Pain Syndromes

1. Postoperative pain syndromes
    1.1. Acute postoperative pain
    1.2. Postmastectomy syndrome
    1.3. Postthoracotomy syndrome
    1.4. Postradical neck dissection syndrome
    1.5. Postnephrectomy syndrome
    1.6. Phantom limb and stump pain syndrome
2. Postchemotherapy pain syndromes
    2.1. Mucositis
    2.2. Polymyalgias and polyarthralgias
    2.3. Pain secondary to tumor embolization
    2.4. Peripheral neuropathy
    2.5. Steroid pseudorheumatism
    2.6. Aseptic bone necrosis
3. Postradiation pain syndromes
    3.1. Enteritis or proctitis
    3.2. Radiation fibrosis of the lumbosacral plexus
    3.3. Radiation fibrosis of the brachial plexus
    3.4. Radiation myelopathy
    3.5. Radiation-induced peripheral nerve tumors

Source: author

TABLE 20.4. Pain Indirectly Related or Unrelated to Cancer

1. Pain associated with degenerative joint disease of the cervical and lumbar spine.
2. Myofascial pain
3. Postherpetic neuralgia
4. Chronic headache syndromes
5. Diabetic neuropathy
6. Pain associated with other therapies (i.e., Synercid)

Source: author

PAIN ASSESSMENT

The International Association for the Study of Pain has defined pain as "an unpleasant sensory and emotional experience associated with actual or potential tissue damage or described in terms of such damage." The activity produced in the different nervous system by a stimulus originating in damaged tissues or damaged nerves is described as nociception.[1]

Intense and sustained nociceptive input will result in reflex responses at several levels. Segmental and suprasegmental reflex responses produce increased general sympathetic tone. This will result in vasoconstriction in the cutaneous and splanchnic vessels, increased stroke volume and heart rate, increased blood pressure, increased metabolic rate and oxygen consumption. Decrease in gastrointestinal and urinary tract tone may progress to delayed gastric emptying, ileus, and urinary retention. It also causes increased skeletal muscle tone, which may progress to muscle spasms. Catabolic endocrine responses to nociceptive input are represented by increases in stress hormone levels and decreases in insulin and testosterone levels. Metabolic responses include changes in protein, carbohydrate, and fat metabolism, water retention, decreased functional extracellular fluid, and fluid shifts to the vascular and cellular compartments. Stimulation of the respiratory center results in hyperventilation, a response that may be overcome by splinting.

The patient's perception of pain and interpretation of its meaning is a complex phenomenon. It involves, along with physiologic processes (such as pain perception, pain transmission, and modulation), psychological, emotional, and behavioral changes. Pain intensity is influenced by multiple factors and may not be directly proportional to the extent of the injury. Pain perception consists of a complicated interplay between sensory impulses in the central nervous system ascending pathways and activation of descending inhibitory systems. The diencephalic and cortical responses lead to anxiety, causing a further increase in general sympathetic tone, increased blood viscosity, clotting time, fibrinolysis, and platelet aggregation, thus increasing the risk of thromboembolism and other coagulation disorders.

Given this complicated framework, it should be emphasized that there is no single effective approach to pain management. Diagnosis and management of pain should be strictly individualized, taking into account the stage of the disease, the presence of concomitant pathophysiologic states, the type of pain, and the psychological and sociocultural characteristics of the patient. Cancer pain assessment should be ongoing and active, necessitating frequent reassessment of pain quality, pain intensity, and treatment effectiveness.

CHARACTERISTICS OF PAIN

Pain assessment should include information about the temporal, physiologic, topographic, and etiologic characteristics. Based on temporal characteristics, two types of pain are described.

Acute pain has a well-defined onset in time, usually an obvious cause, limited duration, and is responsive to the available analgesic treatments. It has a protective function and it is regarded as being a symptom. It is usually focal, experienced at the site of the injury, self-limited, and with mild or no associated psychological disturbance. It is associated with obvious pain-related behavior, such as immobility, grimacing, and moaning. Severe acute pain is associated with all the physiological changes described above. Its prognosis is generally excellent.

Chronic pain is defined as pain lasting for more than 3 months, usually without a well-defined onset and a fluctuating course. Chronic pain may no longer serve any useful purpose as a warning sign of continued tissue damage and in this regard may be considered a disease process unto itself. Pain behavior may or may not be obvious and sympathetic hyperactivity may not be present. Patients may present with anger or depression, along with sleep disturbance, and may complain of symptoms involving uninjured tissue sites. Chronic pain may lead to physical disability such as muscular atrophy, contractures, and trophic changes. Treatment often requires multidisciplinary management efforts including intense physical therapy, vocational rehabilitation, and early psychological assessment and intervention.[53]

Pain can be discriminated on a *physiologic* basis into nociceptive and neuropathic pain. *Somatic nociceptive pain* is the result of nociceptor activation in the skin and subcutaneous tissues. The pain is associated with a lesion that can be identified and is commensurate with its extent. It is often described as an aching or pressure-like sensation; however, it can be throbbing or stabbing. It is described as well localized and sharp with stimulation of the affected tissue. Examples are postsurgical pain and pain caused by skeletal metastasis.

Visceral nociceptive pain has a cramping, poorly localized character resulting from distention, stretching, compression, or infiltration of the abdominal and thoracic organs. It is often referred to areas that are localized far from the site of the lesion, such as a shoulder pain caused by irritation of the diaphragm. Pain due to obstruction of a hollow viscus is described as crampy or gnawing. Involvement of organ capsules or peritoneal appendages may cause aching, throbbing, or sharp pain. Nociceptive pain responds well to opiate analgesics and to interventions directed to the resolution of the initiating lesion. Nerve blocks or other procedures that interrupt nociception may also be effective.

Neuropathic pain is the result of abnormal somatosensory processing in the periphery or the central nervous system. It results from direct injury to the nerves as a consequence of tumor invasion or from therapy-induced neural injury. It is often associated with loss of motor and sensory function along with sympathetic dysfunction. The pain occurs in the absence of detectable tissue-damaging processes. It may present as an abnormal, unpleasant sensation (i.e., dysesthesia), frequently with a burning quality, and a brief shooting-stabbing component. Its onset is delayed relative to the precipitating injury. Mild stimulation of the skin can be painful (i.e., allodynia). Repeated stimulation with an identical stimulus causes progressive buildup of pain intensity (i.e., hyperpathia), and the pain persists after the eliciting stimulus is withdrawn (i.e., afterreaction). Its hallmark is a dysesthetic and unfamiliar sensation perceived in an area of motor or sensory deficit.

There is disagreement in the literature about the response of neuropathic pain to opiate analgesics. It was initially felt that neuropathic pain was relatively nonresponsive to treatment with opiates. More recent studies, however, have called this finding into question.[53] Neuropathic pain is sometimes responsive to treatment with adjuvants, such as anticonvulsants, antidepressants, or antiarrhythmics. Preemptive analgesia may be useful in preventing the development of neuropathic pain syndromes.[53]

Topographically pain can be *localized*, *multifocal*, or *generalized*. This distinction is important in determining the usefulness of specific therapies, such as nerve block or neurosurgical interventions. *Localized pain* should be differentiated from *referred pain*, which could be:

- Pain referred along the course of an injured peripheral nerve
- Pain referred along the course of the fibers of a damaged nerve root (radicular pain)
- Pain referred to nondermatomal parts of the body from lesions involving the spinal cord or central pathways (funicular pain)
- Pain referred in a nondermatomal fashion from a visceral source (e.g., jaw from myocardium; shoulder from diaphragmatic irritation)

Etiologic characterization refers to the cause-effect relationships that are usually obvious in acute pain. In chronic pain, however, it may be difficult to link the pain to a specific injury. It is important that the etiology of the pain is considered in evaluation of cancer patients, due to the fact that this approach can lead to identification of an underlying recurrence and can also guide therapy. Previously unsuspected new lesions can be identified by analysis of changing pain patterns in over 60% of cancer patients.[51]

COMMON CANCER PAIN SYNDROMES

Common cancer pain syndromes are displayed in Table 20.2. Visceral pain syndromes that the gynecological cancer patient may experience are familiar to most clinicians. The distinction between visceral and some somatic or neuropathic pain syndromes is not always clear. Involvement of the celiac plexus causes a boring, dull epigastric pain. This pain radiates to the back in the upper lumbar or lower thoracic area and is by convention considered visceral rather than neuropathic.[63] Tumor infiltration of the bladder and deep pelvic masses may cause suprapubic and perineal pain. Pain in the deep pelvis may also result from sacral plexus involvement. Tumor invasion of the pelvis may cause pain referred to the inguinal region and anterior thigh. Metastases in the epidural space can cause focal back pain, which may present as the initial symptom. This pain is often confused in older patients with nonmalignancy-associated back pain. Tumor invasion of paravertebral or retroperitoneal chest-wall regions can cause mononeuropathies. Infiltration of the brachial plexus may manifest as rapidly increasing pain in the shoulder and upper extremity, associated with motor and sensory dysfunction.

Primary or metastatic invasion of bone causes several specific pain syndromes. Pain due to metastasis to the skull base can manifest as the first complaint, preceding neurological signs and symptoms. Jugular foramen syndrome consists of occipital headaches, exacerbated by head movement, referred to the vertex and the shoulder and arm on the same side.[50] Pain associated with hoarseness, dysarthria, and cranial nerve–related symptoms from the 6th to the 12th nerves is typical for clivus metastases. Breast cancer can cause a constant, dull pain radiating to both shoulders, originating at the spinous processes of C7–T1. Involvement of the first lumbar vertebra may cause referred pain to the sacroiliac region or superior iliac crest, along with midback ache exacerbated by sitting or laying and relieved by standing up.

Treatment-induced pain can be acute or chronic (Table 20.3). Acute therapy-related pain includes postsurgical pain, along with the mucositis of chemotherapy and the pain of radiation esophagitis. Chronic cancer therapy–related pain poses a diagnostic challenge. The distinction between recurring disease-related symptoms and complications from therapy is often impossible to make. For example, postmastectomy pain manifests as a burning sensation in the axilla, upper arm, or anterior chest wall, exacerbated by movement. It is a result of surgical or postsurgical damage to the intercostobrachial nerve. In some cases, the severity of pain with movement may lead to such limited use of the arm that a frozen shoulder develops.

Chemotherapy can cause a polyneuropathy, manifested by pain in the hands and feet, which is burning in character. Lymphedema, numbness, and pain are characteristic for radiation fibrosis of the brachial plexus. Radiation fibrosis of the lumbosacral plexus may cause pain in the anterior thigh and perineum. One of the radiation-related injuries most difficult to treat is radiation myelopathy, characterized by a localized or referred area of dysesthesia, below the level of cord damage.

Pain unrelated to cancer or cancer therapy most often manifests as back pain or neck pain related to degenerative joint disease of the cervical or lumbar spine (Table 20.4). Postherpetic neuralgia may cause severe neuropathic pain, which often precedes the presence of skin lesions. Early diagnosis and aggressive treatment with acyclovir, along with treatment of the pain, are recommended and may prevent the development of postherpetic neuralgia. Severe generalized pain syndromes can be present in patients treated for surgical or other therapy-related complications. As an example, therapy of VRE (vancomycin-resistant *Enterococcus faecium*) infections with Synercid may cause elevation of the liver enzymes, along with severe arthralgias and myalgias. This pain responds well to treatment with opiates.

MEASUREMENT OF PAIN

Pain measurement is inherently subjective and is based on the patient's self report. The simplest techniques of pain measurement rely on a single dimension, such as pain intensity. Pain intensity is measured by using numerical or linear analog scales (Fig. 20.1). These are usually clinically satisfactory. Verbal descriptors of pain intensity, such as mild, moderate, severe, and excruciating, or representations of facial expressions, are less sensitive. The restricted number of possible responses causes clustering to the middle of the scale.[3,14] Follow-up and a self-care pain management log can be used (Fig. 20.1).

More complex assessments of pain involve multiple-dimension reporting via pain questionnaires (such as the McGill pain questionnaire) coupled with a pain intensity score and a patient pain map. In patients with chronic pain, psychometric testing is indicated as part of the initial work-up. Commonly used techniques are the Minnesota Multiphasic Personality Inventory, Beck Depression Inventory, and Wisconsin Brief Pain Inventory. A measure of functional status such as the SPF 36 may also be indicated. Table 20.5 lists the components of a comprehensive initial pain assessment protocol.

MANAGEMENT OF PAIN

Common barriers to adequate cancer pain management are listed in Table 20.6. In the management of gynecologic cancer pain, a variety of options are available, including surgery, radiotherapy, chemotherapy, peripheral and neuraxial blockade, and pharmacological interventions. The suggested management interventions for cancer pain are presented in Figures 20.2, 20.3, and 20.4.

Pharmacological Management

Drug therapy is the cornerstone of cancer pain management, due to its effectiveness, comparatively lower risk, and economic advantages. The three major classes of drugs used alone or in combination are the nonsteroidal anti-inflammatory drugs (NSAIDs) and acetaminophen, the opiate analgesics, and the adjuvant analgesics.

Several principles outline the best approach to using medication in cancer pain management. The medication regimen must be individualized to the needs of the patient. The simplest dosage schedules and the least invasive route of administration should be used first. According to the World Health Organization three-step analgesic ladder developed in the early 1980s, acetaminophen or an NSAID should be the first step in managing mild to moderate pain.[76] U.S. formularies are largely limited to oral administration of the NSAIDs, the only parenteral nonsteroidal analgesic available being ketoralac. The second step on the ladder consists of adding an opiate and adjusting the dose according to the severity of the pain. The third step consists of the use of strong opiate agonists, with or without nonopioid or adjuvant therapy. The coanalgesics, which may be used in any step, include anticonvulsants, antidepressants, anxiolytics, steroids, dextroamphetamine, phenothiazines, antiarrhythmics, alpha-1 antagonists, and alpha-2 agonists.[16,19,38]

The preferred route of analgesic administration is oral. Rectal and transdermal routes should be considered when the patient cannot take medications orally, before considering systemic parenteral administration. There is strong evidence against the appropriateness of intramuscular administration of anal-

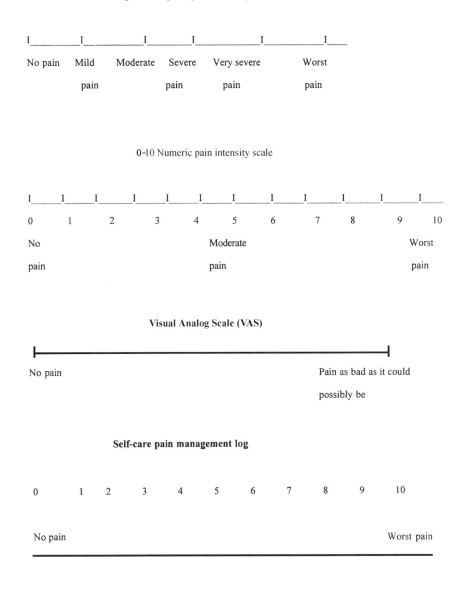

FIGURE 20.1. Pain intensity scales.

TABLE 20.5. Initial Pain Assessment

A. Assessment of Pain Intensity and Character

1. Onset and temporal pattern: When did your pain start? How often does it occur? Has its intensity changed?
2. Location: Where is your pain? Is there more than one site?
3. Description: What does your pain feel like? What words would you use to describe your pain?
4. Intensity: On a scale of 0 to 10, with 0 being no pain and 10 being the worst pain you can imagine, how much does it hurt right now? How much does it hurt at its worst? How much does it hurt at its best?
5. Aggravating and relieving factors: What makes your pain better? What makes your pain worse?
6. Previous treatment: What types of treatments have you tried to relieve your pain? Were they and are they effective?
7. Effect: How does the pain affect physical and social function?

B. Psychosocial Assessment

Psychosocial assessment should include the following:
1. Effect and understanding of the cancer diagnosis and cancer treatment on the patient and the caregiver
2. The meaning of the pain to the patient and the family
3. Significant past instances of pain and their effect on the patient
4. The patient's typical coping responses to stress or pain
5. The patient's knowledge of, curiosity about, preferences for, and expectations about pain management methods
6. The patient's concerns about using controlled substances such as opioids, anxiolytics, or stimulants
7. The economic effect of the pain and its treatment
8. Changes in mood that have occurred as a result of the pain (e.g., depression, anxiety)

C. Physical and Neurological Examination

1. Examine site of pain and evaluate common referral patterns
2. Perform pertinent neurologic evaluation
   - Head and neck pain–cranial nerve and fundoscopic evaluation
   Back and neck pain–motor and sensory function in limbs; rectal and urinary sphincter function

D. Diagnostic Evaluation

1. Evaluate recurrence or progression of disease or tissue injury related to cancer treatment
   - Tumor markers and other blood tests
   - Radiologic studies
   - Neurophysiologic (e.g., electromyography) testing
2. Perform appropriate radiologic studies and correlate normal and abnormal findings with physical and neurologic examination

TABLE 20.5. (*Continued*)

D. *Diagnostic Evaluation* (Continued)

3. Recognize limitations of diagnostic studies
   - Bone scan—false negatives in myeloma, lymphoma, previous radiotherapy sites
   - CT scan—good definition of bone and soft tissue but difficult to image entire spine
   - MRI scan—bone definition not as good as CT; better images of spine and brain

---

Source: Jacox A, Carr DB, Payne R, et al. *Management of Cancer Pain. Clinical Practice Guideline*. AHCPR Pub. No. 94-0592. Rockville, MD: Agency for Health Care Policy and Research, U.S. Department of Health and Human Services, 1994.

TABLE 20.6. Barriers to Cancer Pain Management

Problems Related to Health Care Professionals

Inadequate knowledge of pain management
Poor assessment of pain
Concern about regulation of controlled substances
Fear of patient addiction
Concern about side effects of analgesics
Concern about patients becoming tolerant to analgesics

Problems Related to Patients

Reluctant to report pain
Concern about distracting physicians from treatment of underlying disease
Concern about not being a "good" patient
Reluctance to take pain medications
Fear of addiction or of being thought of as an addict
Worries about unmanageable side effects
Concern about becoming tolerant to pain medications

Problems Related to the Health Care System

Low priority given to cancer pain treatment
Inadequate reimbursement
The most appropriate treatment may not be reimbursed or may be to costly for patients and their families
Restrictive regulation of controlled substances
Problems of availability of treatment or access to it

Source: Jacox A, Carr DB, Payne R, et al. *Management of Cancer Pain. Clinical Practice Guideline*. AHCPR Pub. No. 94-0592. Rockville, MD: Agency for Health Care Policy and Research, U.S. Department of Health and Human Services, 1994.

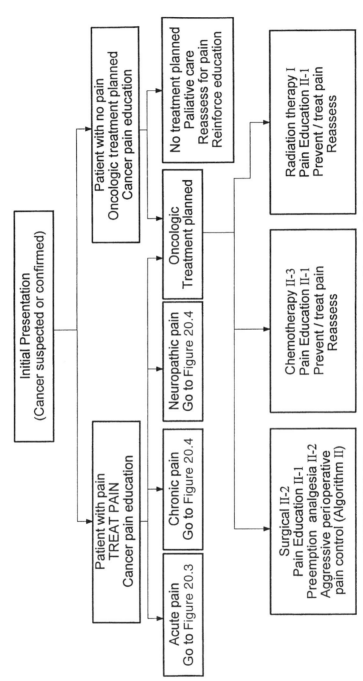

FIGURE 20.2. Management of pain in the patient with gynecologic can-

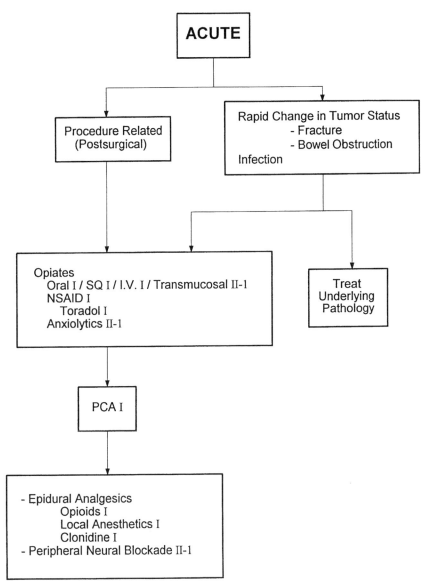

FIGURE 20.3. Management of acute procedure–related and tumor complication–in-duced pain.

gesics, given the unpredictable absorption rate, the duration of action, and the unpleasant and potentially harmful side effects caused by the injection.[46] Consideration of epidural or intrathecal analgesic systems should follow failure of maximal systemic doses of opiates to relieve pain, despite proper management of opiate-induced side effects.

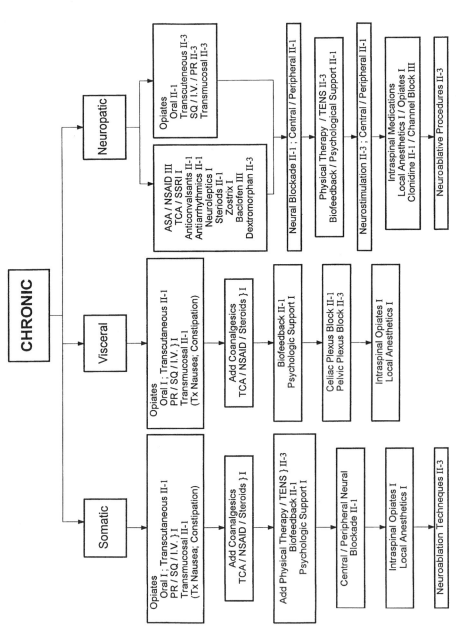

FIGURE 20.4. Mangement of chronic pain due to somatic, visceral, or neuropathic stimuli.

Nonopiate analgesics constitute a group of compounds that differ in chemical structure and pharmacological properties. Dosing data for these agents is summarized in Table 20.7. Initially, the group consisted of acetaminophen and the NSAIDs. Recently, other types of nonopiate analgesics are being added, such as tramadol, which has a combination of weak μ-1 agonist and serotonergic activity. Newer drugs, not yet released, target tumor necrosis factor alpha and interleukin-mediated mechanisms of nociception.

Acetaminophen is an oral analgesic with the potency of aspirin. It has antipyretic activity, but its anti-inflammatory potency as well as its antiplatelet activity are minimal. It causes minimal gastric irritation, but it may cause severe hepatotoxicity. Acetaminophen is used in combination with opiates in several commercially available combination analgesics. It is the first line of treatment for mild to moderate pain. It can be administered orally or rectally and the total daily dose for adults should be limited to 4,000 mg.

Nonsteroidal anti-inflammatory drugs are a group of structurally diverse compounds that have a common mechanism of action, consisting of central and peripheral cyclo-oxygenase activity inhibition that blocks prostanoid synthesis.[47] Cyclo-oxygenase has two main isoenzymes that are inhibited to varying degrees by the available nonsteroidal anti-inflammatory drugs. Inhibition of COX-1 is linked to gastrointestinal ulcerations, while inhibition of COX-2 is not. Recent development of selective COX-2 inhibitors may lead to important progress in analgesic therapy. The available NSAIDs vary from being COX-1 selective (flurbiprofen, ketoprofen), to nonselective (ibuprofen, naproxen), or COX-2 selective (mefenamic acid, diclofenac). Mefenamic acid is unique in its ability to inhibit production of both prostaglandins and leukotrienes. Enhanced production of leukotrienes is responsible for anaphylactoid reactions to NSAIDs.[43,56]

The main side effects of NSAIDs include gastritis, exacerbation of bronchospasm, platelet inhibition, nephrotoxicity, and water retention. Phenylbutazone may cause bone marrow toxicity. Naproxen may result in pulmonary infiltrates, while use of ibuprofen, sulindac, and tolmentin may result in aseptic meningitis. Misoprostol, 200 mg bid, effectively prevents NSAID-induced gastric ulcerations and is available in combination preparations. Extreme care should be taken to monitor renal function in patients on NSAIDs, due to the risk of severe renal failure secondary to renal prostaglandin synthesis inhibition.

Tramadol is useful in controlling mild to moderate cancer pain. A 50 mg dose has the analgesic potency of 60 mg of codeine. It can be combined with acetaminophen in patients in whom the NSAIDs are contraindicated, and in patients who wish not to use opioids.

Opiate analgesics are used in steps 2 and 3 of the WHO analgesic ladder. Dosing data for these agents is summarized in Table 20.8. Codeine, dihydrocodeine, hydrocodone, oxycodone, and propoxyphene, in combination with acetaminophen, are used in the treatment of moderate pain. The usefulness of fixed combinations is often limited by the excessive amount of acetaminophen they contain. Codeine has to be converted to morphine to pro-

TABLE 20.7. Dosing Data for Acetaminophen (APAP) and NSAIDs

Drug	Usual Dose for Adults and Children >50 kg body weight	Usual Dose for Children and Adults <50 kg body weight
Acetaminophen and Over-the-Counter NSAIDs		
Acetaminophen III	650 mg q 4 h	10–15 mg/kg q 4 h
	975 mg q 6 h	15–20 mg/kg q 4 h (rectal)
Aspirin IV	650 mg q 4 h	10–15 mg/kg q 4 h
	975 mg q 4 h	15–20 mg/kg q 4 h (rectal)
Ibuprofen (Motrin, others)	400–600 mg q 6 h	10 mg/kg q 6–8 h 5
Prescription NSAIDs		
Carprofen (Rimadyl)	100 mg tid	
Choline magnesium trisalicylate VI (Trilisate)	1,000–1,500 mg tid	25 mg/kg tid
Choline salicylate (Arthropan) VI	870 mg q 3–4 h	
Diflunisal (Dolobid) VII	500 mg q 12 h	
Etodolac (Lodine)	200–400 mg q 6–8 h	
Fenoprofen calcium (Nalfon)	300–600 mg q 6 h	
Ketoprofen (Orudis)	25–60 mg q 6–8 h	
Ketorolac tromethamine VIII (Toradol)	10 mg q 4–6 h to a maximum of 40 mg/day	
Magnesium salicylate (Doan's, Magan, Mobidin, others)	650 mg q 4 h	
Meclofenamate sodium (Meclomen) VIII	50–100 mg q 6 h	
Mefenamic acid (Ponstel)	250 mg q 6 h	
Naproxen (Naprosyn)	250–275 mg q 6–8 h	5 mg/kg q 8 h
Naproxen sodium (Anaprox)	275 mg q 6–8 h	

TABLE 20.8. Dose Equivalents for Opioid Analgesics in Opioid-Naive Adults and Children ≥50 kg Body Weight

Drug	Approximate Equianalgesic Dose		Usual Starting Dose for Moderate to Severe Pain	
	Oral	Parenteral	Oral	Parenteral
Morphine III	30 mg q 3–4 h (repeat around-the-clock dosing) 60 mg q 3–4 h (single dose or intermittent dosing)	10 mg q 3–4 h	30 mg q 3–4 h	10 mg q 3–4 h
Morphine, controlled-release III, IV (MS Contin, Oramorph)	90–120 mg q 12 h	N/A	90–120 mg q 12 h	N/A
Hydromorphone III (Dilaudid)	7.5 mg q 3–4 h	1.5 mg q 3–4 h	6 mg q 3–4 h	1.5 mg q 3–4 h
Levorphanol Levo-Duromoran)	4 mg q 6–8 h	2 mg q 6–8 h	4 mg q 6–8 h	2 mg q 6–8 h
Meperidine (Demerol)	300 mg q 2–3 h	100 mg q 3 h	N/R	100 mg q 3 h
Methadone (Dolophine, other)	20 mg q 6–8 h	10 mg q 6–8 h	20 mg q 6–8 h	10 mg q 6–8 h
Oxymorphone III (Numorphan)	N/A	1 mg q 3–4 h	N/A	1 mg q 3–4 h
Combination opioid/NSAID preparations [5]				
Codine [6] (with aspirin or acetaminophen)	180-200 mg q 3–4 h	130 mg q 3–4 h	60 mg q 3–4 h	60 mg q 2 h (IM/SC)
Hydrocodine (in Lorcet, Lortab, Vicodin, others)	30 mg q 3–4 h	N/A	10 mg q 3–4 h	N/A

vide analgesia. Thus, inhibitors of facilitating enzyme systems, such as quinidine, cimetidine, or fluoxidine, counteract its analgesic efficacy.

Persistent or severe pain should be medicated around the clock, with supplemental doses "as needed." Early aggressive treatment of side effects will permit upward titration to pain control and will prevent patient refusal of the drug. Opiates with no ceiling effect should be used for severe pain, and mixed agonists-antagonists should not be given at the same time with direct agonists, in order to avoid opiate withdrawal syndrome. Administration of naloxone for opiate side-effect reversal should be performed with small, titrated doses, to avoid reversal of analgesia. Opiates with potentially toxic active metabolites (such as propoxyphene and meperidine) should not be used if sustained opiate use is anticipated.[40]

Intravenous administration of opiates can provide rapid pain relief and, when used as patient-controlled analgesia (PCA), enhances the patient's sense of control. Along with the use of epidural opiates or opiate and local analgesic combinations, PCA is the preferred analgesic method for control of postoperative pain. Limitations in the intensive care unit may include the unconscious, heavily sedated, or confused patient. Physical limitations include patients with severe arthritis or other conditions that interfere with use of the PCA apparatus.

Potential complications include infiltration of the lines, infection, and the risk of excessive sedation if high doses of a continuous infusion are used. Additionally, total analgesic requirements show a large interpatient variability that is partly age related. Morphine is the most commonly used agent, although meperidine hydrochloride (Demerol), fentanyl citrate (Sublimaze), sufentanil, hydromorphone, and others can also be used.[75]

Initially, a loading dose may be appropriate if the patient has not been receiving other narcotics. Typically, 1–2 mg of morphine sulfate (or equi-analgesic) is administered every 15–30 minutes until pain relief is obtained. The PCA should then be adjusted to deliver the minimum effective analgesic concentration required to provide optimal analgesia with minimal side effects.[18,57] This can be easily achieved by appropriately setting the demand dose, lockout interval, and total hourly limit administered. Sample orders are shown in Table 20.9 and general guidelines for initial dosing are presented in Table 20.10. Otherwise, the amount of drug available for the patient should only be limited by the associated side effects. The PCA is intended to deliver a relatively constant analgesic dose range to patients in order to minimize wide fluctuations between underdosed pain and overdosed sedation and respiratory depression.

Infusion of the ultra-short-acting opiate remifentanil is useful in the ICU setting to wean patients from long-acting opiates. This drug is easily titrated and termination of the effect occurs minutes after cessation of use. PCA can also be administered via subcutaneous infusion of hydromorphone and morphine, providing rapid pain relief in the absence of IV access.[30]

Epidural opiates used in combination with local anesthetics tend to produce the best compromise between the quality of analgesia and the intensity of side effects in the control of postoperative pain.[20,28] Lipid-soluble drugs (opiates and

TABLE 20.9. Patient-Controlled Analgesia (PCA) Basic Sample Orders

1. Disregard previous analgesic and sedative orders.
2. Intravenous fluids as ordered previously or start IV D5/0.45 NS to keep open until PCA discontinued. If IV infiltrates and cannot be restarted, call MD.
3. PCA orders:
   A. Agent used _____
   B. Concentration _____ mg/ml
   C. PCA dose _____ mg
   D. Lockout interval _____ minutes
   E. Continuous-rate background _____ mg/hr
   F. 4-hour limit _____ mg
4. Keep 0.4 mg naloxone (Narcan) taped to PCA pump.
5. Side-effect medications:
   A. Droperidol 0.5 mg IV push q 4 hr prn nausea
   B. Benadryl 25 mg IV or PO q 4 hr prn pruritis
   C. If respiratory rate <8 or patient not arousable:
      1. Stop PCA STAT
      2. Administer Narcan 0.4 mg IVP STAT
      3. Notify MD STAT

local anesthetics) placed in the center of the segmental area targeted for the pain control will produce excellent analgesia and minimal side effects. Properly trained nursing personnel and good communication between the surgical and pain management team are essential to assure maximal benefits and minimal complications of this method. The most popular combinations are fentanyl 1–5 mcg/ml with bupivacaine 0.125–0.25%. Sufentanyl 0.2–0.5 mcg/ml and ropivacaine 0.1–0.2% are reasonable alternatives.

For patients with poor pain control or for those experiencing intractable side effects, intrathecal and intracerebral administration may prove advantageous. Local anesthetics added to epidural or spinal opiates may dramatically improve the quality of analgesia. The use of transdermal fentanyl provides an alternative delivery route for patients unable to tolerate oral drug delivery. The onset to peak plasma levels after placement of the initial patch or after increasing the

TABLE 20.10. Initial Morphine Sulfate PCA Dosing Guidelines[a]

	Age <50 Years	Age 51–60 Years	Age 61–70 Years	Age >70 Years
Bolus dose (mg)	2	1.5	1	0.5
Background dose (mg)	1–2	1–2	1	1
Lockout (minutes)	10	12	15	20
Total dose limit (mg/4 hours)	30	20	15	10

[a]The guidelines are intended to be very general in nature and should be adjusted to each patient's individual requirements and medical condition.

dose is about 12 hours. The rectal route is a useful alternative when the oral or parenteral administration is not available. The onset of action is slow and this route is not widely accepted by patients.

Tolerance and physical dependence are expected with long-term opiate use and should not be regarded as addiction. Abrupt discontinuation of opiates or administration of antagonists or agonists-antagonists will result in withdrawal, manifested by viral flu-like symptoms in mild cases. Severe pain, anxiety, chills, lacrimation, diaphoresis, nausea, and adbominal cramps and diarrhea may be seen in the more severe cases. The onset of withdrawal occurs from 6 to over 24 hours after treatment discontinuation, depending on the agent's half-life. If discontinuation of opiates is required, a tapering schedule that reduces the amount of drug by about 10% per day minimizes withdrawal symptoms. Clonidine 0.1–0.2 mg/day transdermally will reduce the autonomic hyperactivity and anxiety associated with opioid withdrawal.

Prevention and treatment of opiate side effects is an often disregarded, important aspect of management. Nausea may be treated by a centrally acting antiemetic. Early administration of a bowel stimulant and a stool softener will usually ensure one soft bowel movement every 1 to 2 days. Sedation typically resolves with time. It can be reduced with the use of methylphenidate, dextramphetamine, and caffeine. Myoclonic spasms can be treated with a long-acting benzodiazepine such as clonazepam. Changing to a different opiate may be necessary in some patients. Delirium may appear secondary to large doses of opiates or from other causes in the critically ill patient. If this occurs, decreasing the dose or changing to another potent opiate may be necessary.

The role of adjuvant therapy is to supplement opiate analgesia, treat specific types of pain, and control associated symptoms. Skeletal metastases, neuropathic pain syndromes, and visceral pain syndromes may respond well to coanalgesics. Commonly used drugs are antidepressants, anticonvulsants, corticosteroids, antiarrhythmics, alpha-1 antagonists and alpha-2 agonists. Other types of drugs that can be used for special therapeutic reasons are the skeletal muscle relaxants, antihistamines, and antipsychotics. Substance P inhibitors and local anesthetics are used externally for treatment of localized pain syndromes.[16,29,38] Dosing data for these agents is presented in Table 20.11.

The antidepressants are useful for the treatment of neuropathic pain. They also improve sleep as well as depression. However, anticholinergic, antihistaminic, antidopaminergic, and alpha-1 antagonist activity–related side effects may limit their therapeutic use. Also, pain relief may not be achieved for several weeks following initiation of therapy. Nortriptyline and desipramine are better tolerated than other tricyclic antidepressants. The initial dose should be low, followed by slow upward titration, limited by side effects.

Anticonvulsants are useful in the treatment of shooting, lancinating, or shock-like pain and enhance control of neuropathic pain when added to an antidepressant. A safer new agent in this class is gabapentin. Monitoring is required to avoid specific toxicities when other anticonvulsants are used. Antiarrhythmics are also effective in the treatment of neuropathic pain.

TABLE 20.11. Adjuvant Analgesic Drugs for Cancer Pain

Drug	Approximate Adult Daily Dose Range	Route of Administration	Type of Pain
Corticosteroids			
Dexamethasone II	16–96 mg	PO, IV	Pain associated with brain metastases and
Prednisone	40–100 mg	PO	epidural spinal cord compression
Anticonvulsants			
Carbamazepine III	200–1,600 mg	PO	Neuropathic pain
Phenytoin IV	300–500 mg	PO	
Antidepressants			
Amitriptyline V	25–150 mg	PO	Neuropathic pain
Doxepin VI	25–150 mg	PO	
Imipramine VII	20–150 mg	PO	
Trazodone VIII	75–225 mg	PO	
Neuroleptics			
Methotrimeprazine VIII	40–80 mg	IM	Analgesia; sedation; antiemetic
Antihistamines			
Hydroxyzine VV	300–450 mg	IM	Adjuvant to opioids in postoperative and other types of pain; relief of complicating symptoms including anxiety, insomnia, nausea
Local anesthetics/ antiarrythmics			
Lidocaine VVI	5 mg/kg	IV/SC	Neuropathic pain
Mexiletine VVII	450–600 mg	PO	
Tocainide VVIII	20 mg/kg	PO	

Corticosteroids are effective in pain associated with inflammation and may decrease pain due to CNS and spinal cord tumors. Alpha-1 antagonists and alpha-2 agonists are used in the treatment of sympathetically mediated pain. Blockade of alpha-receptors located on the peripheral nerve terminals by the alpha-1 antagonists and inhibition of norepinephrine release from the postganglionic sympathetic terminals are considered to be their mechanisms of action.

Several drugs are used to secure comfort of patients undergoing palliative care. Subcutaneous midazolam infusion, titrated intravenous barbiturates and propofol, and oral, parenteral, and intrathecal ketamine have been used along with opiates with often dramatic improvement of patient comfort.[23,30,36,52,60,71,72,74] Optimal use of coanalgesics often requires a pain specialist experienced in treatment of the targeted conditions.

Nonpharmacological Measures

Nonpharmacological measures are important for maximizing both patient comfort and functional status. The use of physical therapy interventions such as heat, cold, electrical stimulation, massage, hands-on mobilization, and stretching techniques as well as appropriate exercise programs may be very helpful in relieving pain such as mechanical low back pain or pain secondary to muscle spasm. Biofeedback and relaxation training, guided imagery conditioning, and cognitive restructuring may be helpful in decreasing pain and anxiety and in improving the patient's sense of self-control. Acupuncture has been used in the management of cancer pain, although outcome studies are inconclusive about its efficacy.

When pharmacological and other noninvasive means have proven insufficient in the management of a patient's pain, invasive management strategies may be appropriate. Palliative radiation therapy may be useful for the treatment of painful metastatic lesions. Neural blockade with local anesthetics and steroids can provide what is often temporary but significant relief of pain in localized areas.[22] Implanted epidural and intrathecal drug delivery systems may produce profound analgesia with minimal side effects in patients who experience insufficient pain relief or intolerable side effects from analgesics via other routes of administration. Neurolytic blockade and neurosurgical ablative procedures are usually steps of last choice.[5,12,22] These techniques bring with them the possibility of significant long-term side effects such as loss of motor or sensory function in the targeted area, and achieving the desired effect of pain relief is uncertain at best.

Monitoring of Pain Management Quality

The application of quality assessment and improvement methodologies is considered the most successful way to facilitate progress in the field of cancer pain relief. An interdisciplinary team effort is necessary to provide the required expertise and outcome analysis. Educational efforts should address the patients, their families, and their caregivers. Active assessment of pain at all levels of care and efforts to assure continuity of care at all levels is imperative. Availability of pain specialists and allocation of funds for treatment, education, and research are highly desirable.[1,2,9,10,32,51]

REFERENCES

1. Management of Cancer Pain Guideline Panel. *Management of Cancer Pain. Clinical Practice Guideline.* AHCPR Pub. No. 94-0592. Rockville, MD: Agency for Health Care Policy and Research, Public Health Service, U.S. Department of Health and Human Services, 1994.

2. Acute Pain Management Guideline Panel. *Acute Pain Management: Operative or*

Medical Procedures and Trauma. Clinical Practice Guideline. AHCPR Pub. No. 92-0032. Rockville, MD: Agency for Health Care Policy and Research, Public Health Service, U.S. Department of Health and Human Services, 1992.

3. Ad Hoc Committee on Cancer Pain of the American Society of Clinical Oncology. Cancer pain assessment and treatment curriculum guidelines. *J Clin Oncol* 1992;10(12):1975–1982.

4. Adams F, Fernandez F, Andersson BS. Emergency pharmaco-therapy of delirium in the critically ill cancer patient. *Psychosomatics* 1986;27(suppl 1):33–38.

5. Amano K, Kawamura H, Tanikawa T, Iseki H, Iwata Y, Taira T. Bilateral versus unilateral percutaneous high cervical cordotomy as a surgical method of pain relief. *Acta Neurochir (Wien)* 1991;52(suppl):143–145.

6. American Cancer Society. *Cancer and the Poor: A Report to the Nation.* American Cancer Society, 1989.

7. American Cancer Society. *Questions and Answers About Pain Control: A Guide for People with Cancer and Their Families.* American Cancer Society and the National Cancer Institute, 1992, p. 76.

8. American Cancer Society. *Cancer Facts and Figures—1994.* Atlanta: American Cancer Society Inc., 1994, p. 1.

9. American Pain Society, Committee on Quality Assurance Standards. Standards for monitoring quality of analgesic treatment of acute pain and cancer pain. *Oncol Nurs Forum* 1990;17:952–954.

10. American Pain Society. Committee of quality assurance standards. American Pain Society quality assurance standards for relief of acute pain and cancer pain. In Bond MR, Charlton JE, Woolf CJ (Eds), *Proceedings of the Sixth World Congress of Pain.* New York: Elsevier Science Publications, 1991, pp. 185–190.

11. American Pain Society. *Principles of Analgesic Use in the Treatment of Acute Pain and Chronic Cancer Pain: A Concise Guide to Medical Practice.* Skokie, IL: American Pain Society, 1992.

12. Arbit E, Galicich JH, Burt M, Mallya K. Modified open thoracic rhizotomy for treatment of intractable chest wall pain of malignant etiology. *Ann Thoracic Surg* 1989;48(6):820–823.

13. Attard AR, et al. Safety of early pain relief for acute abdominal pain (13 references). *Br Med J* 1992;305:554.

14. Au E, et al. Regular use of a verbal pain scale improves the understanding of oncology inpatient pain intensity (12 references). *J Clin Oncol* 1994;12(12):2751.

15. Avellanosa AM, West CR. Experience with transcutaneous electrical nerve stimulation for relief of intractable pain in cancer patients. *J Med* 1982;2(3):203–213.

16. Bach FW, Jensen TS, Kastrup J, Stigsby B, Dejgard A. The effect of intravenous lidocaine on nociceptive processing in diabetic neuropathy. *Pain* 1990;40(1);29–34.

17. Barbour LA, McGuire DB, Kirchhoff KT. Nonanalgesic methods of pain control used by cancer outpatients. *Oncol Nurs Forum* 1986;13(6):56–60.

18. Baumann TJ, Batenhorst RL, Graves DA, Foster TS, Bennett RL. Patient-controlled analgesia in the terminally ill cancer patient. *Drug Intell Clin Pharm* 1986;20(4):297–301.

19. Beck SL. The therapeutic use of music for cancer-related pain. *Oncol Nurs Forum* 1991;18(8):1327–1337.

20. Behar M, Magora F, Olshwang D, Davidson JT. Epidural morphine in treatment of pain. *Lancet* 1979;1(8115):527–529.

21. Bolund C. Suicide and cancer: II. Medical and care factors in suicide by cancer patients in Sweden 1973–76. *J Psychosoc Oncol* 1985;3:17–30.

22. Bonica KK, Buckley FP, Moricca G, Murphy TM. Neurolytic blockade and hypophysectomy. In Bonica JJ (Ed), *The Management of Pain*, 2nd ed., vol. 1. Philadelphia: Lea and Febiger, 1990, pp. 1980–2039.

23. Bottomley DM, Hanks GW. Subcutaneous midazolam infusion in palliative care. *J Pain Symptom Manage* 1990;5:259–261.

24. Breitbart W, Holland JC. Psychiatric complications of cancer. In Brain MC, Carbone PP (Eds), *Current Therapy in Hematology-Oncoloy*—3. Philadelphia: BC Decker Inc., 1988, pp. 268–274.

25. Breitbart W. Cancer pain and suicide. In Foley K, Bonica JJ, Ventafridda V (Eds), *Advances in Pain Research and Therapy*, vol. 16. New York: Raven Press, 1990, pp. 399–412.

26. Breitbart W. Suicide in cancer patients. *Oncology* 1987;1:49–53.

27. Brennan SC, Redd WH, Jacobsen PB, et al. Anxiety and panic during magnetic resonance scans. *Lancet* 1988;2(8609):512.

28. Bromage PR, Camporresi EM, et al. Rostral spread of epidural morphine. *Anesthesiology* 1982;56:4341–4346.

29. Brose WG, Cousins MJ. Subcutaneous lidocaine for treatment of neuropathic cancer pain. *Pain* 1991;45(2):145–148.

30. Bruera E, Brenneis C, et al. Continuous Sc infusion of narcotics for the treatment of cancer pain: an update. *Cancer Treat Rept* 1987;71(10):953–958.

31. Bruera E., Schoeller T, Montejo G. Organic hallucinosis in patients receiving high doses of opiates for cancer pain. *Pain* 1992;48(3):397–399.

32. Brunier G., et al. What do nurses know and believe about patients with pain? Results of a hospital survey (36 references). *J Pain Symptom Man* 1995;10(6):436.

33. Burkberg J, Penman D, Holland JC. Depression in hospitalized cancer patients. *Psychosom Med* 1984;46(3):199–212.

34. Byrne TN. Spinal cord compression from epidural metastases. *N Engl J Med* 1992;327(9):639–645.

35. Cassel EJ. The nature of suffering and the goals of medicine. *N Engl J Med* 1982;306(11):639–645.

36. Charap AD. The knowledge, attitudes and experience of medical personnel treating pain in the terminally ill. *Mt Sinai J Med* 1978;45:561.

37. Cherny NI, Portenoy RK. Cancer pain: principles of assessment and syndromes. In Wall PD, Melzack R (Eds), *Textbook of Pain*, 3rd ed. Edinburgh: Churchill Livingstone, 1994, p. 787.

38. Chinery R, Beauchamp RD, et al. Antioxidants reduce cyclooxygenase-2 expression, prostaglandin production, and proliferation in colorectal cancer cells. *Cancer Res* 1998;58(11);2323–2327.

39. Christensen O, et al. Analgesic effect of intraarticular morphine: a con-

trolled randomized and double-blind study (16 references). *Acta Anaesth Scand* 1996;40(7):842.

40. Clark RF. Meperidine: therapeutic use and toxicity (62 references). *J Emerg Med* 1995;13(6):797.

41. Cleeland CS, Gonin R, Hatfield AK, et al. Pain and its treatment in outpatients with metastatic cancer. *New Engl J Med* 1994;330:592.

42. Cleeland CS. The impact of pain on patients with cancer. *Cancer* 1984;54:263–267.

43. Cryer B, Feldman M. Cyclooxygenase-1 and cyclooxygenase-2 selectivity of widely used nonsteroidal anti-inflammatory drugs. *Am J Med* 1998;104(5):413–421.

44. Daut RL, Cleeland CS. The prevalence and severity of pain in cancer. *Cancer* 1982;50:1913–1918.

45. Derogatis LR, Marrow GR, et al. The prevalence of psychiatric disorders among cancer patients. *JAMA* 1983;249:751–757.

46. Edwards WT. Optimizing opioid treatment of postoperative pain. *J Pain Symptom Manage* 1990;5:S24.

47. Eisenberg E, et al. Efficacy and safety of nonsteroidal antiinflammatory drugs for cancer pain: a meta-analysis (47 references). *J Clin Oncol* 1994;12(12);2756.

48. Foley KM. Pain syndromes in patients with cancer. In Bonica JJ, Wentafridda V (Eds), *Advances in Pain Research and Therapy*, vol. 2. New York: Raven Press, 1979, p. 59.

49. Foley KM. The treatment of cancer pain. *N Engl J Med* 1985;313:84–95.

50. Forsyth PA, et al. Headaches in patients with brain tumors: a study of 111 patients. *Neurology* 1993;43(9):1678.

51. Gonzales GR, Elliott KJ, et al. The impact of a comprehensive evaluation in the management of cancer pain. *Pain* 1991;47:141.

52. Greene WR, Davis WH. Titrated intravenous barbiturates in control of symptoms in patients with terminal cancer. *South Med J* 1991;84:332–337.

53. Gupta R, Raja N. Chronic pain: pathophysiology and its therapeutic implications. *Curr Rev Pain* 1996;1:1–9.

54. Hagen NA, et al. Cancer pain emergencies: a protocol for management (28 references). *J Pain Symptom Manage* 1997;14(1):45.

55. Hanks GW, Justins DM. Cancer pain: management. *Lancet* 1992;339:1031–1036.

56. Janusz JM, Young PA, et al. New cyclooxygenase-2/5 lipoxygenase inhibitors. 3. 7-tert-butyl-2, 3-dihydro-3, 3-dimethylbenzofuran derivatives as gastrointestinal safe antiinflammatory and analgesic agents: variations at the 5 position. *J Med Chem* 1989;41(18);3515–3529.

57. Lehman KA. Patient-controlled analgesia for postoperative pain. In Max MM, Portenoy RK, Laska E (Eds), *Design of Analgesic Clinical Trials*. New York: Raven Press, 1991, p. 481.

58. Levin D, Cleeland CS, Dar R. Public attitudes toward cancer pain. *Cancer* 1985;56:2337–2339.

59. Marks RM, Sachar EJ. Undertreatment of medical inpatients with narcotic analgesics. *Ann Intern Med* 1973;78:173.

60. Moyle J. The use of propofol in palliative medicine. *J Pain Symptom Manage* 1995;10:643–646.

61. Niv D, Devor M. Preemptive analgesia in the relief of postoperative pain. *Curr Rev Pain* 1996;1:79–92.

62. Portenoy RK, Hagen NA. Breakthrough pain: definition, prevalence and characteristics. *Pain* 1990;41:273.

63. Portenoy RK, Kornblith AB, Wong G, et al. Pain in ovarian cancer: prevalence, characteristics, and associated symptoms. *Cancer* 1994;74:907.

64. Portenoy RK. Cancer pain: epidemiology and syndromes. *Cancer* 1989;63:2298.

65. Portenoy RK. Cancer pain: pathophysiology and syndromes. *Lancet* 1992;339: 1026–1031.

66. Rosen SM. Procedural control of cancer pain. *Semin Oncol* 1994;21:740–747.

67. Schirrmacher V. Cancer metastasis: experimental approaches, theoretical concepts, and impacts for treatment strategies. *Adv Cancer Res* 1985;43:1.

68. Schug SA, Zech D, Dorr U. Cancer pain management according to WHO analgesic guidelines. *J Pain Symptom Manage* 1990;5:27–32.

69. Schwartz PE. Cancer in pregnancy. In Gusberg SB. *Female Genital Cancer.* New York: Churchill Livingstone, pp. 725–754.

70. Sugarbaker EV. Patterns of metastasis in human malignancies. *Cancer Biol Rev* 1981;2:235.

71. Tobias JD, et al. Oral ketamine premedication to alleviate the distress of invasive procedures in pediatric oncology patients (18 references). *Pediatrics* 1992;90(4):537.

72. Twycross RG, Fairfield S. Pain in far-advanced cancer. *Pain* 1982;14:303.

73. Ventafridda V, Caraceni A, Gamba A. Field-testing of the WHO guidelines for cancer pain relief: summary report of demonstration projects. In Foley KM, Bonica JJ, Ventafridda V (Eds), *Proceedings of the Second International Congress of Cancer Pain*, vol. 16 of Advances in Pain Research and Therapy. New York: Raven Press, 1990, pp. 451–464.

74. World Health Organization. *Cancer Pain Relief and Palliative Care.* Geneva: World Health Organization, 1990.

75. Veselis RA. Intravenous narcotics in the ICU. *Crit Care Clin* 1990;6(2);305–313.

76. Ventafridda V, Saita L, Ripamonti C, DeConno F. WHO guidelines for the use of analgesics in cancer pain. *Int J Tissue React* 1985;7(1):93–96.

INDEX